Essentials of Pain Management

LIBRARY

College of Physicians and Surgeons
of British Columbia

Essentials of Pain Management

Editors
Nalini Vadivelu, MD
Associate Professor of Anesthesiology
Department of Anesthesiology
Yale University School of Medicine
New Haven, CT, USA

Richard D. Urman, MD, MBA
Assistant Professor of Anesthesia
Harvard Medical School
Director, Hospital Procedural Sedation Management
Department of Anesthesiology
Brigham and Women's Hospital
Boston, MA, USA

Roberta L. Hines, MD
Nicholas M. Greene Professor of Anesthesiology
Department Chair and Chief, Anesthesiology
Yale University School of Medicine
New Haven, CT, USA

Case Scenarios Editor

Dr. Sreekumar Kunnumpurath
MBBS, MD, FCARCSI, FRCA, FFPMRCA
Consultant in Anesthesia and Pain Management
Royal Free Hospital
London, UK

🖄 Springer

Editors
Nalini Vadivelu, MD
Department of Anesthesiology
Yale University School of Medicine
333 Cedar Street
New Haven, CT 06520-8051, USA

Richard D. Urman, MD, MBA
Department of Anesthesiology
Harvard Medical School and Brigham and
  Women's Hospital
75 Francis St.
Boston, MA 02115, USA

Roberta L. Hines, MD
Department of Anesthesiology
Yale University School of Medicine
333 Cedar Street
New Haven, CT 06520-8051, USA

ISBN 978-0-387-87578-1   e-ISBN 978-0-387-87579-8
DOI 10.1007/978-0-387-87579-8
Springer New York Dordrecht Heidelberg London

Printed on acid-free paper

Springer is part of Springer Science+Business Media (www.springer.com)

To my parents; my husband, Thangamuthu Kodumudi; my sons, Gopal and Vijay; and all my wonderful colleagues.

- N.V.

I would like to thank my parents, my wife Zina Matlyuk-Urman, MD for their love and encouragement, and all my colleagues and mentors for their inspiration.

- R.D.U.

I would like to dedicate this book to all my teachers and students who have been so instrumental in my career.

- R.L.H.

Preface to the Case Scenarios

When presented with pain, we, as healthcare professionals, are asked to find appropriate solutions. The clinical presentation may be acute or chronic, and successful management involves an accurate diagnosis and implementation of a suitable therapy or therapies. For a beginner in pain management, this can pose a significant challenge. We have placed a clinical scenario at the end of nearly all of the chapters, for a total of 33 cases, in an attempt to present a collection of common pain-related clinical problems and possible ways to manage them effectively.

Treatment of pain begins with a detailed history taking, a thorough clinical examination, specific investigations, and the right intervention. The importance of history and clinical examination in pain management cannot be overstressed. The knowledge, attitude, and skills needed in managing pain are acquired over time, and the management involves multidisciplinary teams and multimodal approaches. This is exemplified in the clinical scenarios. It is also important to re-explore and re-assess when there is a change in the clinical picture.

The clinical scenarios are presented in a question-and-answer format. The reader is encouraged to go through the questions first and to come up with a solution before reading the given answer. There is always a potential for a different approach to the given clinical problem.

Many of these scenarios were taken from our day-to-day practice of pain medicine. While we have presented the scenarios in a positive note with regard to the effectiveness of pain management strategies, we have the humility to admit that we may sometimes be too optimistic in our outlook.

Dr. Sreekumar Kunnumpurath,
MBBS, MD, FCARCSI, FRCA, FFPMRCA

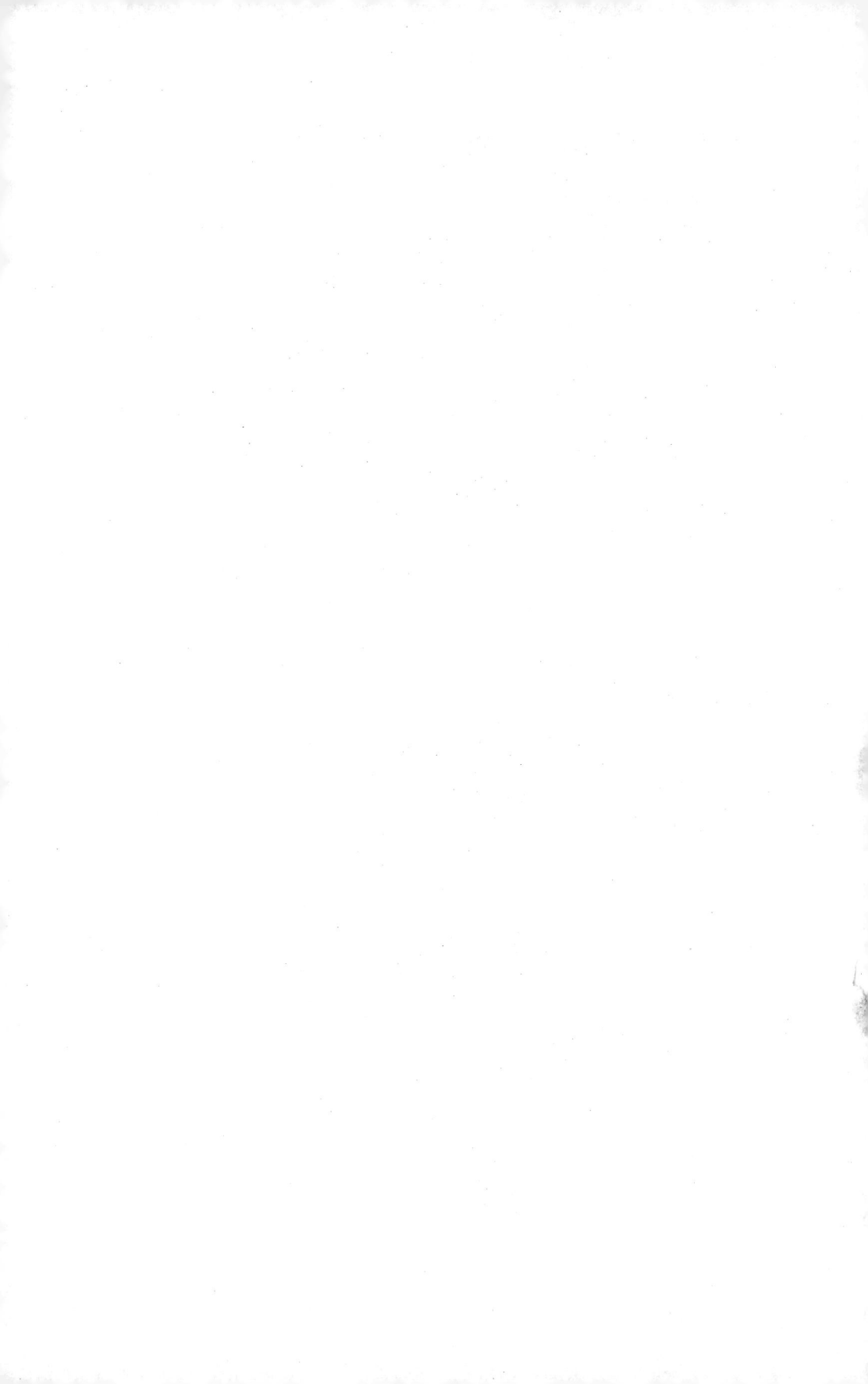

Preface

Essentials of Pain Management is a concise yet comprehensive evidence-based guide to what is now recognized as the "fifth vital sign." We wrote it to provide an in-depth review of clinical principles and procedures that stresses the multidisciplinary, practical approach to pain management. With contributions from a cross section of pain experts, the book is designed to help the pain management professional in any specialty and at any stage of training to provide the most up-do-date, evidence-based care.

We cover a wide variety of topics including pharmacology, palliative medicine, physical therapy, acupuncture, behavioral and interventional therapy, and pain management in pediatric and elderly populations. We also cover topics of importance to nurses and dentists. In addition, the book also contains the most up-do-date pain drug formulary for easy reference.

Another unique feature is a collection of multiple choice questions with detailed explanations, useful for chapter review and exam preparation. We also included practical case vignettes to follow each chapter. These vignettes illustrate specific pain management challenges and provide detailed sample solutions. The vignettes are a useful way to apply the knowledge obtained from reading the chapter to a real patient situation.

We would like the thank all of our contributors for their expertise, our colleagues and trainees for their inspiration, and our families for their patience and moral support. Whether you are a student or a practicing healthcare professional, we hope that you will find *Essentials of Pain Management* an indispensable guide to pain management.

Nalini Vadivelu, MD
Richard D. Urman, MD, MBA
Roberta L. Hines, MD

Foreword

"Just the facts, ma'am." Those who remember the early days of television recall this often used line by Sgt. Joe Friday in the long running series, *Dragnet*. Fast-forward 50 years and facts are as accessible as the swiftness of one's "thumb typing abilities." However, another time-honored adage, "caveat emptor" ("let the buyer beware") reminds us that fast facts obtained between cases or patient visits from Internet search sites can both produce a morass of too many "hits" and run the risk of obtaining misinformation from an unreliable source.

While the world continues to transition from libraries with stacks of periodicals to virtual libraries, the contemporary professional will still benefit from a handy, concise, and authoritative compendium of essential information written by expert faculty who have thoroughly researched and distilled the topics to their key points of information.

Drs. Vadivelu, Urman, and Hines have provided the interested practitioner with an informative and diverse text on practice topics pertinent to the multidisciplinary specialty of pain medicine. This book should especially appeal to health-related professions, trainees, and faculty as well as pain fellows and practicing physicians who need a source with a high probability of quickly providing the needed information. A novel feature included in the book assists the reader's understanding of the material within a clinical context by providing short case scenarios.

Essentials of Pain Management is logically divided into nine parts of pertinent pain topics and even includes a section on "Non-pharmacologic Management of Pain." The appendix contains multiple choice questions that will assist students and residents in preparing for examinations.

The editors should be congratulated for assembling an enthusiastic group of pain specialist authors to produce this handy reference manual useful to providers at all levels of the analgesic care continuum. In my program, every resident carries a smart phone, but it is more common for me to see them reading a text for their didactic instruction.

Buffalo, NY   Mark J. Lema, MD, PhD

Contents

Contributors

Shamsuddin Akhtar, MBBS
Associate Professor, Department of Anesthesiology, Yale University School of Medicine, New Haven, CT, USA

Muhammad Anwar, MD
Assistant Professor, Department of Anesthesiology, Yale University School of Medicine, New Haven, CT, USA

Joseph N. Atallah, MD
Chief, Pain Service, Department of Anesthesiology, University of Toledo Medical Center, Toledo, OH, USA

Amir Baluch, MD
Senior Resident, Department of Anesthesiology, University of Miami School of Medicine, Miami, FL, USA

Trevor Banack, MD
Resident, Department of Anesthesiology, Yale University School of Medicine, New Haven, CT, USA

Jack M. Berger, MS, MD, PhD
Professor of Clinical Anesthesiology, Keck School of Medicine, University of Southern California, Los Angeles, CA, USA

Erica Bial, MS, MD
Pain Physician, Department of Population Medicine, Havard Medical School, Boston, MA, USA

Ferne Braverman, MD
Professor, Department of Anesthesiology, Yale University School of Medicine, New Haven, CT, USA

Charles Brown, MD
Division of Pain Medicine, Department of Anesthesiology and Critical Care Medicine, The Johns Hopkins University School of Medicine, Baltimore, MD, USA

Doris K. Cope, MD
Professor, Department of Anesthesiology, University of Pittsburg School of Medicine, Pittsburg, PA, USA

May L. Chin, MD
Professor of Anesthesiology and Critical Care Medicine, George Washington University, University Medical Center, Washington, DC, USA

Paul J. Christo, MD, MBA
Division of Pain Medicine, Department of Anesthesiology and Critical Care Medicine, The Johns Hopkins University School of Medicine, Baltimore, MD, USA

Steven P. Cohen, MD
Associate Professor, Department of Anesthesiology & Critical Care Medicine, The Johns Hopkins University School of Medicine, Baltimore, MD, USA; Director of Pain Research, Walter Reed Army Medical Center (Colonel, U.S. Army), Washington, DC, USA

Darin J. Correll, MD
Assistant Professor of Anesthesia, Harvard Medical School, Boston, MA, USA; Director, Postoperative Pain Management Service, Brigham and Women's Hospital, Boston, MA, USA

Michael A. Cosgrove, MD
Pain Management Fellow, Department of Anesthesiology, Dartmouth Medical School, Dartmouth Hitchcock Medical Center, Lebanon, NH, USA

Susan Dabu-Bondoc, MD
Assistant Professor, Department of Anesthesiology, Yale University School of Medicine, New Haven, CT, USA

Michael H. Ebert, MD
Professor of Psychiatry and Associate Dean for Veterans Affairs, Yale University School of Medicine, New Haven, CT, USA; Chief of Staff, VA Connecticut Healthcare System, New Haven, CT, USA

Ryan P. Ellender, MD
Chief Resident, Department of Anesthesiology, Louisiana State University School of Medicine, New Orleans, LA, USA

Gilbert J. Fanciullo, MS, MD
Professor of Anesthesiology, Department of Anesthesiology, Dartmouth Medical School, Dartmouth Hitchcock Medical Center, Lebanon, NH, USA

Dr. Adam Fendius, BSC(Hons), MBBS, FRCA, DipIMC(RCSED), DipHEP
Specialist Registrar in Anaesthesia, Department of Anaesthesia, St. George's Hospital, London, UK

Debebe Fikremariam, MD
Resident, Department of Anesthesiology, West Virginia University School of Medicine, Morgantown, WV, USA

Charles J. Fox III, MD
Associate Professor of Anesthesiology, Tulane University School of Medicine, New Orleans, LA, USA

Elizabeth Freck, MD
Resident, Department of Anesthesiology, Yale University School of Medicine, New Haven, CT, USA

Dan Froicu, MD
Resident, Department of Anesthesiology, Yale University School of Medicine, New Haven, CT, USA

Xing Fu, MD
Resident, Department of Anesthesiology, Yale University School of Medicine, New Haven, CT, USA

M. Khurrum Ghori, MD
Assistant Clinical Professor of Anesthesiology, Department of Anesthesiology, VA Medical Center, Yale University School of Medicine, New Haven, CT, USA

Gerald W. Grass, MD, FAAMA
Assistant Professor of Anesthesiology, Yale University School of Medicine, New Haven, CT, USA; Chief, Pain Medicine VA Connecticut Healthcare System, New Haven, CT, USA

Amitabh Gulati, MD
Assistant Professor, Department of Anesthesiology, Memorial Sloan Kettering Cancer Center, Weill Cornell Medical College, New York, NY, USA

Thomas Halaszynski, DMD, MD, MBA
Associate Professor of Anesthesiology, Yale University School of Medicine, New Haven, CT, USA; Department of Anesthesiology, Yale-New Haven Hospital, New Haven, CT, USA

Anne M. Haskins, PhD, OTR/L
Assistant Professor, Department of Occupational Therapy, University of North Dakota School of Medicine and Health Sciences, Grand Forks, ND, USA

Henry A. Hawney, MD
Chief Resident, Department of Anesthesiology, Tulane University School of Medicine, New Orleans, LA, USA

Anita Hickey, MD
Director, Pain Research and Integrative Medicine, Department of Anesthesiology, Naval Medical Center, San Diego, CA, USA

Chris James, BA
Medical Student, Coney Island Hospital, Tampa, FL, USA

Janet S. Jedlicka, PhD, OTR/L
Associate Professor and Chair, Department of Occupational Therapy, University of North Dakota School of Medicine and Health Sciences, Grand Forks, ND, USA

Dr. Zacharia Jose, MBBS, MD, FRCA, FCARCSI
Consultant Anaesthetist, Department of Anaesthesia, East Surrey Hospital, Redhill, Surrey, UK

Alan D. Kaye, MD, PhD
Professor and Chairman, Department of Anesthesiology, Louisiana State University School of Medicine, New Orleans, LA, USA; Professor of Pharmacology, Louisiana State University School of Medicine, New Orleans, LA, USA; Director, Interventional Pain Services, Louisiana State University School of Medicine, New Orleans, LA, USA; Adjunct Professor, Department of Anesthesiology, Tulane University School of Medicine, New Orleans, LA,

USA; Adjunct Associate Professor, Department of Pharmacology, Tulane University School of Medicine, New Orleans, LA, USA

Dr. Ganesh Kumar, MBBS, DA, MRCA
Specialty Doctor, Department of Anaesthetics and Critical Care, East Surrey Hospital, Redhill, Surrey, UK

Rae Ann Kingsley, APRN
Section of Pediatric Anesthesia, Department of Anesthesiology, Yale-New Haven Children's Hospital, New Haven, CT, USA

Dr. Sreekumar Kunnumpurath, MBBS, MD, FCARCSI, FRCA, FFPMRCA
Consultant in Anesthesia and Pain Management, Royal Free Hospital, London, UK

Dr. Jones Kurian, MD, MRCP, FRCA, DIP Pain Med
Department of Pain Medicine, East Surrey Hospital NHS Trust, Redhill, Surrey, UK

Ian Laughlin, MD
Lieutenant Commander, Naval Medical Center, San Diego, CA, USA

Raphael J. Leo, MA, MD
Associate Professor, Department of Psychiatry, School of Medicine and Biomedical Sciences, State University of New York at Buffalo, Buffalo, NY, USA; Consultant, Center for Comprehensive Multidisciplinary Pain Management, Erie County Medical Center, Buffalo, NY, USA

Mark J. Lema, MD, PhD
Professor of Anesthesiology and Oncology, Chair of Anesthesiology, School of Medicine and Biomedical Sciences, State University of New York at Buffalo, Buffalo, NY, USA; Chairman of Anesthesiology, Perioperative Medicine, Pain Medicine, and Critical Care, Roswell Park Cancer Institute, Buffalo, NY, USA

Jeffrey Loh, MD
Resident, Department of Anesthesiology, Weill Cornell College of Medicine, New York, NY, USA

Timothy Malhotra, MD
Associate Professor, Department of Anesthesiology, Memorial Sloan Kettering Cancer Center, Weill Cornell College of Medicine, New York, NY, USA

Yogi Matharu, DPT, OCS
Director, University of Southern California Physical Therapy Associates, Los Angeles, CA, USA; HSC Director, Orthopedic Physical Therapy Residency, Los Angeles, CA, USA; Assistant Professor of Clinical Physical Therapy, Division of Biokinesiology and Physical Therapy, University of Southern California School of Dentistry, Los Angeles, CA, USA

Brenda C. McClain, MD
Section of Pediatric Anesthesia, Department of Anesthesiology, Yale University School of Medicine, Yale-New Haven Children's Hospital, New Haven, CT, USA

Dr. Suresh Menon, MBBS, DA, FRCA
Department of Anaesthetics, Royal London Hospital, Whitechapel, London, UK

Amit Mirchandani, MD
Resident, Department of Anesthesiology, Yale University School of Medicine, New Haven, CT, USA

Ali Nemat, MD
Assistant Professor of Clinical Anesthesiology & Medicine (Physiatry), Division of Pain Medicine, University of Southern California Keck School of Medicine, Los Angeles, CA, USA; Director, Pain Fellowship Program, Department of Anesthesiology, University of Southern California Keck School of Medicine, Los Angeles, CA, USA

Prasad Nidadavolu, MD
Department of Neurology, Jackson Memorial Hospital, University of Miami School of Medicine, Miami, FL, USA

Wendy J. Quinton, PhD
Adjunct Instructor, Department of Psychology, State University of New York at Buffalo, Buffalo, NY, USA

Dr. Suneil Ramessur, MBBS, BSc(Hons), FRCA, DipHEP
Department of Anaesthetics, St. Georges University Hospital, Tooting, London, UK

Roberto Rappa, MD
Resident, Department of Anesthesiology, Yale University School of Medicine, New Haven, CT, USA

Dr. Manoj Narayan Ravindran
Department of Anaesthetics, St. George's Hospital, Tooting, London, UK

Robby Romero, MD
Assistant Professor of Anesthesiology, Yale University School of Medicine, New Haven, CT, USA

Alecia L. Sabartinelli, MD
Resident, Department of Anesthesiology, University of Miami School of Medicine, Miami, FL, USA

Marianne Saleeb, MD
Resident, Department of Anesthesiology, Yale University School of Medicine, New Haven, CT, USA

Geremy L. Sanders, MD, MS
Assistant Professor of Anesthesiology, Louisiana State University School of Medicine, New Orleans, LA, USA

Mario Serafini, DO
Department of Anesthesiology, University of Vermont, Burlington, VT, USA

Raymond Sinatra, MD
Professor of Anesthesiology, Yale University School of Medicine, New Haven, CT, USA

Neil Sinha, MD
Resident, Department of Anesthesiology, Yale University School of Medicine, New Haven, CT, USA

Dr. Imrat Sohanpal, MbChB, FRCA, FFPM
Senior Registrar in Anaesthetics and Pain Medicine, Royal Free Hospital, London, UK

Dmitri Souzdalnitski, MD
Resident, Department of Anesthesiology, Yale University School of Medicine, New Haven, CT, USA

Michael P. Sprintz, DO
Clinical Staff, Department of Anesthesiology, Alton Ochsner Clinic and Hospital, New Orleans, LA, USA

Jan E. Stube, PhD, OTR/L
Associate Professor, Department of Occupational Therapy, University of North Dakota School of Medicine and Health Sciences, Grand Forks, ND, USA

Ellie Sutton, MBBS
GPVTS Specilaist Trainee, Department of Endocrinology and Renal Medicine, Whipps Cross University Hospital, London, UK

Arlyne K. Thung, MD
Assistant Professor, Department of Anesthesiology, Yale University School of Medicine, New Haven, CT, USA; Section of Pediatric Anesthesia, Yale-New Haven Children's Hospital, New Haven, CT, USA

David K. Towns, MD
Pain Management Fellow, Department of Anesthesiology, Dartmouth Medical School, Dartmouth Hitchcock Medical Center, Lebanon, NH, USA

Richard D. Urman, MD, MBA
Assistant Professor, Department of Anesthesia, Harvard Medical School/Brigham and Women's Hospital, Boston, MA, USA

Amarender Vadivelu, BDS, MDS
Professor, Faculty of Dental Sciences, Sri Ramachandra University, Chennai, India

Nalini Vadivelu, MD
Associate Professor, Department of Anesthesiology, Yale University School of Medicine, New Haven, CT, USA

Mani K.C. Vindhya, MD
Department of Anesthesiology, St. Joseph's Hospital, Tampa, FL, USA

Shu-Ming Wang, MSci, MD
Associate Professor, Department of Anesthesiology, Yale School of Medicine, New Haven, CT, USA

Richa Wardhan, MBBS
Resident, Department of Anesthesiology, Yale University School of Medicine, New Haven, CT, USA

Ena Williams, MBA, MSM, RN
Nursing Director, Yale-New Haven Hospital, New Haven, CT, USA

Shaaron Zaghi, MD
Fellow, Pain Medicine, Department of Anesthesiology, University of Southern California Keck School of Medicine, Los Angeles, CA, USA

Robert Zhang, MD
Resident, Department of Anesthesiology, Yale University School of Medicine, New Haven, CT, USA

Section I

Introduction

Chapter 1

Introduction to Pain Management, Historical Perspectives, and Careers in Pain Management

Erica Bial, MS, MD and Doris K. Cope, MD

Introduction: The Need for Historical Perspective on Pain

The importance of recognizing, assessing, understanding, and treating pain is central to the role of any caregiver. When a patient presents to the physician, he rarely comes labeled with a given diagnosis; rather, he more often has a chief "complaint" that he suffers in some manner. To the patient, the symptom, not the pathology or disease, is the affliction. As such, it is imperative that we respect and understand that pain and suffering are the often primary reasons that patients seek medical care for.

The necessary nature of pain treatment has long been categorized among other basic human rights, and in 1999 the Joint Commission on Accreditation of Healthcare Organizations formalized pain standards to ensure to all patients their right to appropriate assessment and management of their pain, describing pain as the "fifth vital sign (Lanser 2001)." Intrinsic to our capacity to treat pain is possession of perspective of the many cultural beliefs, philosophical ideologies, and scientific discoveries that have influenced and evolved into the modern Western conceptualization of pain.

Why would we stress the importance of the *history* of pain medicine? History helps us understand our own place in the universe as healers. We need to appreciate our past in order to gain a sense of connectivity and perspective that is inherent in establishing our identity as a professional. Hundreds of years hence, our theoretical constructs and clinical practices may be considered quaint and outmoded, but the essence of professionalism and the critical, scientific study of medicine will remain unchanged through the ages. Like the times before us, our current era is an exciting one for the study and treatment of pain. With rapidly evolving capacity to elucidate ever more microscopic scientific detail of the anatomy and physiology of pain, developing technologies yield a vast scientific understanding and lexicon of pain. As developments in laboratory and clinical science continue to increase our capacity to further reduce pain to its biological components, simultaneously we must possess the knowledge and vocabulary to discuss pain with our patients in this time of great renewed public interest in many of the "old" medical arts. With a majority of our patients now choosing to partake of complementary and alternative medicine approaches (Barnes 2002), there is a renewed and growing public interest in a more holistic medical model which requires us to recognize that

N. Vadivelu et al. (eds.), *Essentials of Pain Management*,
DOI 10.1007/978-0-387-87579-8_1, © Springer Science+Business Media, LLC 2011

"everything old is new again." Likewise, having an intercultural and historical appreciation and perspective on pain is an asset to any clinician.

Defining "pain" in a succinct manner is a great challenge. What is pain? It has been described as an emotional state, a physical experience, a spiritual sacrament, and a complex set of interconnected subcellular signals. This chapter will discuss this plurality of concepts. From the mind–body dilemma, through the larger context of how our intellectual constructs shape our understanding, we will consider some of the historical and evolving treatment approaches of this complex phenomenon we call pain. The chapter will close with a discussion of how the medical subspecialty of pain management is evolving within the broader context of medical specialization and thoughts for future development (Benedelow and Williams 1995).

Evolving Concepts of Pain

Over time and across cultures, the understanding and expression of pain reflects the contemporary spirit of the age. Universally, the human experience begins through the painful process of birth, and throughout our lifetimes, the experience of pains-physical, emotional, and spiritual-persists as a part of this common experience. The experience of suffering remains universal. However, the expression and meaning of pain have changed over recorded history with changing world views. There has been great debate and discussion as to the origin and nature of pain. It has been viewed as an imbalance of vital forces, a punishment or pathway to spiritual reward, an emotional or behavioral experience, and, relatively recently, as a biological phenomenon.

Among the earliest recorded systems of pain management, dating back over 4,000 years, is Chinese acupuncture. In this medical system, pain is felt to represent an imbalance between *yin* and *yang*, the two vital opposing attributes of life force, or *qi*. Later, the ancient Egyptians considered the experience of pain to be a god or disincarnate spirit afflicting the heart, which was conceptualized as the center of emotion. Aristotle and later Galen both described pain as an emotional experience or "a passion of the soul (Birk 2006)."

In different places and in different points over time, both Eastern and Western medical traditions have included a concept of imbalance as an important etiology of painful symptoms. Unsurprisingly, these ideas emerged alongside the thinking of agrarian societies, integrating the knowledge and experience emerging during that age. During the Han dynasty, approximately 2nd century BCE, the *Huang Di Nei Jing* described the body as a microcosmic representation of the forces of the universe and defined the physician's role as assisting in maintaining the harmonious balance of those forces, both internally as well as in relation to the larger external environment. As such, the concept of *Five Elements* evolved. External bodily invasions (by wind, heat, dampness, dryness, and cold), as well as internal susceptibility (to anger, excitement, worry, sadness, and fear), could affect the balance of energy and humors related to a traditional understanding of the functions of the internal organs. Descriptors from nature (wood, fire, earth, metal, and water) are still used today to codify these traits, symptoms, and imbalances, as summarized in Table 1.1 (Helms 1998).

Somewhat similarly, in the Western world, dating from antiquity and persisting until the 19th century, was the theory of the *Importance of the Four Humors*. This theory was first espoused by Greek philosophers in approximately 400 BC and later applied to medicine by Hippocrates, who described the humors as related to one of the four constitutions, each of which was also correlated with the changing seasons and representative natural elements, as

Table 1.1   Overview of the traditional Chinese *Five Elements*.

Element	Organ systems	Emotions	Taste	Basic function
Fire	Heart, small intestine	Excitement, joy	Bitter/roasted	Generation of warmth, energy, Circulation of blood, promotion of activity
Earth	Stomach, spleen	Sympathy, worry	Sweet	Digestion, metabolism, utilization of nutrients to build body
Metal	Lungs, colon	Grief, sadness	Pungent	Processing waste, protecting body from infection, regulating vital energy
Water	Kidneys, bladder	Fear, fatigue	Salty	Balance of water and minerals, storing and generating basic life force, strength and body integrity
Wood	Liver, gallbladder	Anger, irritability, emotional volatility	Sour	Builds and stores blood, regulates smooth flow of *qi*

Adapted from Rey (1955).

Table 1.2   Overview of the *Four Humors*.

Humor	Black bile	Blood	Phlegm	Yellow bile
Element	Earth	Air	Water	Fire
Constitution	Dry, cold	Hot, wet	Cold, wet	Hot, dry
Season	Autumn	Spring	Winter	Summer

Adapted from Rey (1955).

summarized in Table 1.2. Seasonal changes could evoke particular imbalances of the humors, yielding certain disorders. For example, headache was attributed to excessive cold humors thought to result in a mucus discharge requiring application of "hot effusions" to the head. Interestingly, a similar process of excess "liver fire" was one explanation of headache in the traditional system of Chinese medicine. Consistent with both ideologies was the custom of treating pain by applying "opposites," such as hot applications to the head to counterbalance and evacuate "cold" humors of headaches (King 1988) in the *Four Humors* system, while the imbalance of excess liver fire could be "dispersed" through needles inserted along the liver meridian and then cooled with alcohol. Used in both Eastern and Western tradition was the technique called *cupping*. Warm suction cups were applied to the skin that on cooling resulted in raised reddened welts thought to "draw out" any unbalanced humors (Rey 1955) or unblock stagnant *qi*. The practice of cupping continues today in traditional Chinese medicine, and the sight of healing cupping welts has been widely photographed on the backs of Hollywood's elite.

Another example of pain viewed as representative of energy imbalances in the body came as *vitalism*. Vitalism theory asserted that every part of a living thing was endowed with "sensibility" and the vital animating force of a living organism was capable of being either stimulated or consumed. In this model of disease, pain was necessary to produce a "crisis" in order to rid the patient of the original pain by stimulating his waning energy (Rey 1955). The work of German physician Franz Anton Mesmer, which developed into the well-known practice of mesmerism, was based on this belief. In 1766, he published his doctoral dissertation entitled "On the Influence of the Planets on the Human Body," wherein he described animal magnetism as a force to cure many ills (Académie nationale de médecine 1833). He used iron magnets to treat various diseases, making a spectacle of amplifying magnetic fields with room-sized Leyden jars, imbuing his actions with mystical rites by wearing colored robes in dimly lit ritualistic séances with soft music playing from a glass harmonium. Mesmerism was so well regarded that it represented an early rival to ether anesthesia as a way to relieve pain during surgical procedures (Zimmermann 2005). During his day, Robert Liston reportedly exclaimed after the successful administration of ether anesthesia, "This Yankee Dodge beats mesmerism hollow (Squire 1888)."

Religious explanations of pain have also been prevalent in various times and cultures. Pain has been explained as a possession of the body by an angry deity in many cultures. Much like the earlier Egyptians, coincident with the spread of Christianity during the Middle Ages in Europe, pain was explained in a spiritual, religious context. While little is known of if or how pain was actually treated during this period, the images of a suffering Christ, martyred saints, and the concept of physical pain in purgatory originated around the 12th century (Rey 1955, Bonica 1953). One clear example of pain as ennobling was St. Ignatius Loyola's habit of wearing ropes and chains cutting into the skin and encouraging other humiliations of the flesh to enhance his spiritual development (Birk 2006). The persistence of this practice in the current era was explored in the widely popular 2003 novel *The DaVinci Code* (Brown 2003).

Pain has also been viewed as an emotional or behavioral phenomenon. Beginning in the 17th century and persisting through the turn of the 19th century, huge numbers of female invalids filled convalescent homes, spas, and sanitariums, bearing the diagnosis of "hysteria." In 1681, Thomas Sydenham wrote, "Of all chronic diseases hysteria–unless I err–is the commonest (Epistolary Dissertation 1681)." The cardinal symptom of this outbreak was unexplained pain. The mysterious syndrome of hysteria afflicted only middle and upper class females and commonly was treated by social isolation, bed confinement, and a total prohibition on any form of intellectual activity, even the women's work of sewing or reading (Gilman 1935). However, as social and educational opportunities for women improved, this disorder almost totally disappeared—resolving hundreds of years of suffering on the order of magnitude of the eradication of influenza or yellow fever. Clearly, there are multitudes of modern day examples of painful disorders that can be linked to social and behavioral etiologies. A most prevalent example in the 21st century is fibromyalgia. While it is a commonly diagnosed disorder in Western countries, interestingly enough, it is either underreported or not significantly present in Asian and Third World populations. Additionally, this disorder is characterized by widespread, not-otherwise-explained pain, has a dramatic predilection for women, and a high degree of concomitance with depression and sleep disorders—not at all unlike the hysteria of eons past.

Further discussion of the mind–body pain connection would be incomplete without mention of the landmark development of Freudian theory in understanding the subconscious influences on pain perception and behavior. The link between the unconscious mind and physical sensation in hysterical conversion disorders was posited as an explanation for psychogenic pain and continues to be influential today. This conceptual paradigm was expanded in the 1970s by the psychiatrist George L. Engel, who demonstrated the link between chronic pain and psychiatric illness (Engel 1958). Depression, stress, and personality, in addition to physiological mechanisms, have proved to be critical grounds for investigation and therapy. In the 1980s, the cognitive behavioral school of pain therapy, which is widely employed today, expanded the role of the mind–body connection in pain medicine, emphasizing the development of coping mechanisms to deal with chronic pain. Cognitive behavioral therapy, with particular attention paid to coping mechanisms and avoidance of catastrophizing, is a basic component of interdisciplinary pain programs today.

The Anatomical Basis of Pain

The concept that the mind and the body are separable but interconnected, known as *dualism*, is commonly attributed to Rene Descartes. He described the *mind* as a nonphysical substance and distinguished the *mind* from the *brain*, which was physical (Descartes 1641). In his 1649 essay, "The Passions of the Soul," Descartes sought to delineate emotions from physiological processes and reductionistically compared the human body to a watch:

> ... the difference between the body of a living man and that of a dead man is just like the difference between, on the one hand, a watch or other automaton (that is, a self-moving machine) when it is wound up and contains in itself the corporeal principle of the movements for which it is designed ...; and, on the other hand, the same watch or machine when it is broken and the principle of its movement ceases to be active (Descartes 1664).

The philosophical mind-set of *mechanism*, suggesting that the human body functions as a simple machine, with pain being the result of its malfunction (Sawda 2007) was the outcome. This idea, the extension of which informs much of our current day scientific inquiry and clinical practice, had been evolving slowly over time and ultimately superseded more traditional philosophical and theological explanations of pain. Beginning with the early anatomical studies of Galen of Pergamum (130–201 AD) and Avicenna, the Persian polymath (980–1037 AD), evidence for a physical, visible basis of pain developed. During the Renaissance, the zeitgeist of the day encouraged questioning and cultural mores evolved to view science less as religious heresy. This change permitted scientific observation and inquiry, yielding advances in the anatomical, medical, and neurological knowledge. The study of the circulation of blood by William Harvey in 1628 (Harvey 1628), and the direct anatomical studies of Descartes in 1662 (Cranefield 1974) elucidating sensory physiology, became the theoretical basis for further exploration in the 18th and 19th centuries through today (Fig. 1.1).

In the years that followed those early anatomical observations, several important ideas added to our understanding of physiologic pain, including the specificity theory, pattern theory, summation theory, and gate theory.

Descartes described the concept of a pain pathway and theorized the transmission of pain signals, as illustrated in Fig. 1.2. Nearly 150 years later, Charles Bell in Scotland proffered the *specificity theory*. Specificity theory, the seminal concept that pain has a dissectible and demonstrable anatomical basis, and that individual sensory nerves exist and are specialized to perceive and transmit information from an individual stimulus type, cleared the initial path for considerable subsequent experimentation (Bell 1811). Bell discovered that ventral root stimulation caused motor contraction. In 1839, Johannes Muller advanced the idea of specialization of nerve fibers, considering the sensation of sound to be the "specific energy" of the acoustic nerve and the sensation of light the particular "energy" of the visual nerve (Muller 1839). In 1858, Moritz Schiff demonstrated a reproducible loss of tactile and painful sensation resulting from particular lesions of the spinal cord. In 1882, Francois Magendie demonstrated that sensory function occurred via stimulation of dorsal nerve roots (Bell 1811,

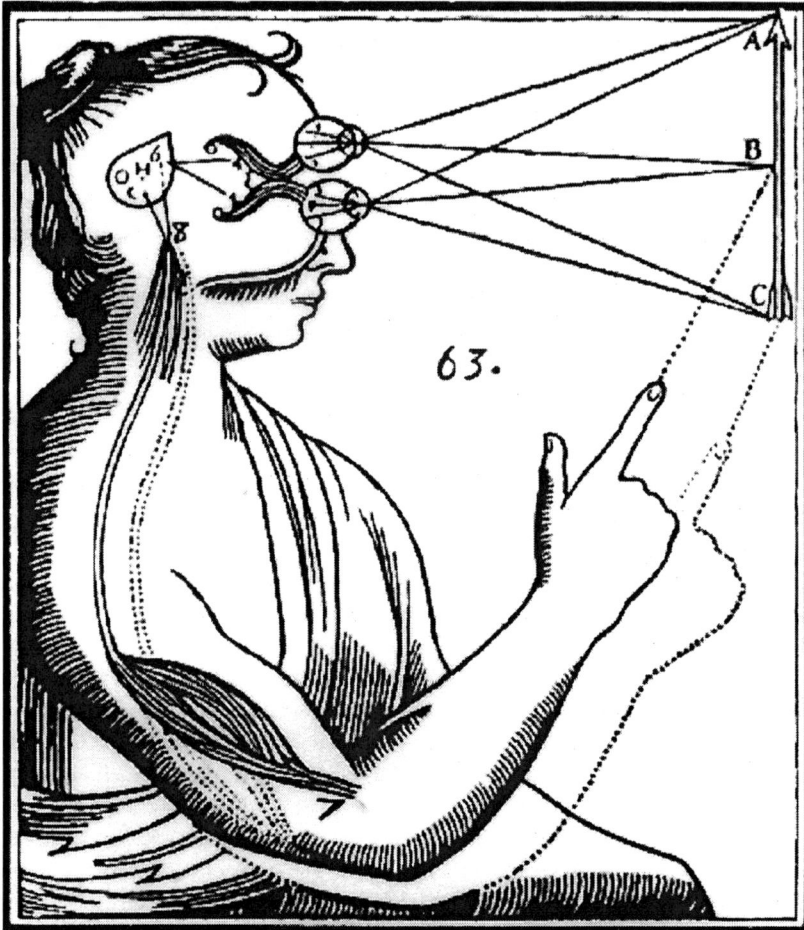

Figure 1.1 Rene Descartes (1596–1650) described the first systematic accounts of the mind/body relationship and mechanisms of action of sensory physiology. In this drawing, he depicts light entering the eye and forming images on the retina. Hollow nerves in the retina would then project to the ventricles, stimulating the pineal gland to release animal spirits into the motor nerves to initiate movement.

Magendie 1822). Ultimately, the sum of these and other discoveries was the specificity theory's advancing the idea of specific pathways and specific receptors for pain that continues to inform our thinking today.

The *pattern theory* was introduced by Alfred Goldscheider, a German army physician, in 1894. This theory proposed that particular, reproducible patterns of nerve activation were triggered by a summation of sensory input from the skin in the dorsal horn. Prior to this time, the skin was believed to be endowed with only one kind of sensation. However, Goldscheider demonstrated that skin contains several distinct perceptive organs. He described three distinct stimuli, pressure, warmth, and cold, and showed that localized points reacted only to a given stimulus and each point had a specific function (Goldscheider 1884). Nafe expanded the pattern theory to the concept that a perceived sensation is the result of spatially and temporally patterned nerve impulses rather than the simple conduction of an individual or specific

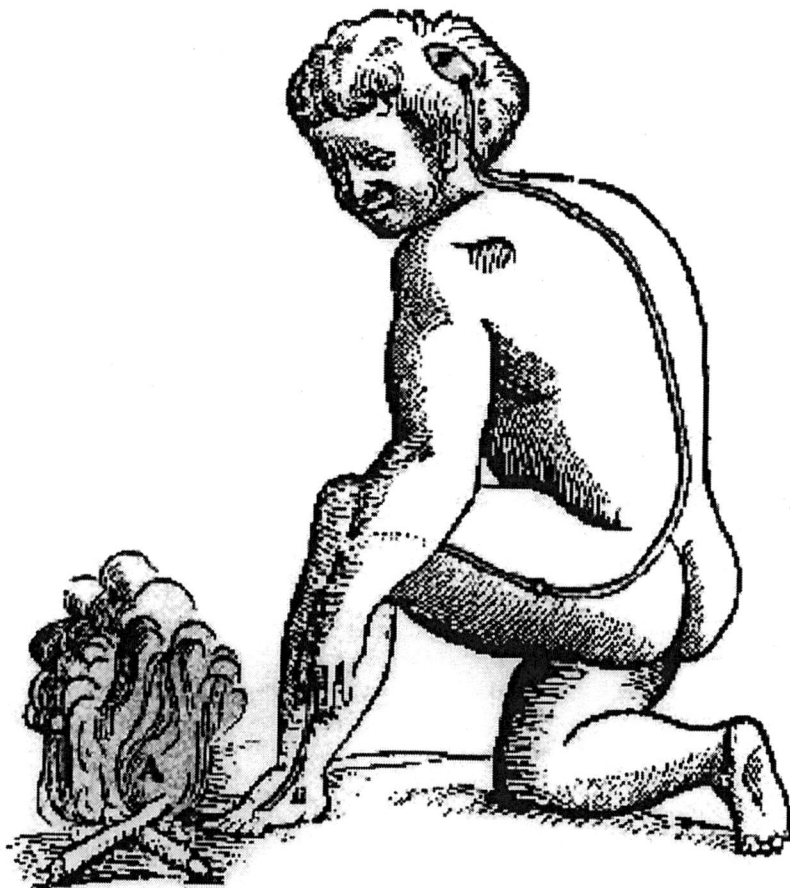

Figure 1.2 Descartes reduced reflex nerve function to hydraulic mechanisms, stating, "If the fire is close to the foot, the small parts of this fire, which...move very quickly, have the force to move the part of the skin of the foot that they touch, and by this means pull the small thread... opening the entrance of the pore, where this small thread ends...the entrance of the pore or small passage, being thus opened, the animal spirits in the concavity enter the thread and are carried by it to the muscles that are used to withdraw the foot from the fire."

receptors or pathway (Nafe 1929). Later, the pattern concept was further detailed by Sinclair and Weddell in 1955, who believed that all sensory fiber endings, except those innervating hair follicles, are similar, and it is the pattern of their activation that was felt to be necessary for sensory discrimination (Sinclair 1955, Weddell 1955).

The specificity theory or the pattern theory alone, or in combination could not fully explain many of the clinical observations that have been made about pain. Particularly confounding were the presence of discontinuous pain fields and the capacity for the development of hyperalgesia, the ability to increase pain sensitivity with repeated stimulation. It was also known that pressure sensation over time resulted in increased painful sensation and that pressure points could respond differently to stimulation than did adjacent areas (Perl

2007). Thus, the *summation theory* was proposed to explain these phenomena. Summation theory is based on the idea that there exist multiple interactions between and among neurons, not only within the sensory system, but also including overlap and contributions to pain sensation from internuncial neurons and the autonomic nervous system. The importance of these interactions was demonstrated by Livingstone, Hardy, and Wolff. In 1932, Dr. Charles S. Sherrington was awarded the Nobel Prize in Medicine for his development of the concept of the motor unit, comprised of a receptor, conductor, and effector; and he later identified polymodal receptors and selective excitability. These ideas are central to explaining the anatomy of the summation theory and began to examine the wide array of pain responses and great capacity for neuroplasticity that are well known in the clinical arena. These concepts, which Sherrington initially published in 1906, are still highly relevant today (Sherrington 1906).

In 1965, the ground-breaking *gate theory* was published by Canadian psychologist Ronald Melzack and British physiologist Patrick Wall (Melzack and Wall 1938) and remains a dominant theory in explaining many of the interrelationships seen in pain sensation and perception. Central to this theory is the concept of the presence of a "gate" that either permits or stops the conduction of a given pain signal based on intermodulation and summation of both painful and nonpainful nerve messages, by either turning on or off an inhibitory interneuron. The gate theory permitted the integration of the presence of specific pathways, patterns, and summation of stimuli and provided a paradigm through which to view the more complex interaction between the central and peripheral nervous systems. Despite the fact that many of the specific details of the theory were later refuted, gate control's central tenet of pain modulation through both central mechanisms and competing stimuli has allowed for a more complex understanding of pain and provides the basis for a considerable volume of current day research as well as pain therapy.

The Treatment of Pain

Clinically, pain can be described as a complex construct, integrating the physiologic, mechanical, and neurochemical responses with the social, behavioral, and psychological responses to noxious stimuli. It is therefore necessary to recognize myriad approaches to the treatment of pain and to assess and treat the patient within a larger biopsychosocial view. The choice of a given course of therapy for pain, therefore, is often more dependent on the beliefs of the caregiver and the prevalent world view of his/her place and time. Through history and continuing today, pain therapies have ranged from religious and spiritual practices, cognitive approaches, behavioral therapies, and pharmacotherapy, to highly anatomically specific treatment.

Physicians have long sought to categorize and form systematic means of understanding and addressing pain through the listing and classification of its causes. For example, during the time of the Roman emperor Trajan, who reigned from 98 CE until his death in 117 CE, 13 causes of pain were recorded. Avicenna, a noted Muslim healer and one of the early fathers of modern medicine, in the early 11th century described 15 separate causes of pain. Samuel Hahnemann, the founder of homeopathy, listed 75 (Fulop-Miller 1938). Despite these attempts at organization of pain etiologies, very few specific therapies for painful syndromes were utilized. Prior to the 18th century and the development of anatomical theories that could be clinically implemented in the treatment of pain, many nonspecific therapies were commonly used.

The view of the body as a representation of changes in the natural world, with energetic disproportions envisioned as the etiology of pain, required the development of treatments that would address these imbalances. Examples include the 4,000-year-old practice of acupuncture, which involves the insertion of needles at particular points or along particular meridians, which are then manipulated to either drive energies into or out of the affected system, thereby providing a direct revision of the imbalanced *qi*. Additionally, the application of humoral opposites (see Table 1.2), cupping, blood letting, purging, the use of topical and oral herbal compounds, and distraction by creating a competing, more severe pain, were all employed as means to return balance and alleviate pain.

The English word "pain" is derived from the Latin word *poena*, meaning punishment. It is then unsurprising that an early requirement for the relief of pain was through prayer (Parris 2004). This interpretation clearly reflects the idea of the painful stimulus as being harm inflicted by an omnipowerful presence in response to wrong doing. The iconography of tortured saints, with ecstatic faces, depicted pain as a spiritual discipline, primarily relieved by prayer, meditation, and righteousness.

The relationship between the psyche and the presence and importance of pain is not a new concept. Coping, learning, the role of anxiety, and concurrent psychiatric illness have all been identified as altering pain perception and success of pain therapies. In the 20th century, many new ideas in psychology emerged, which directly affected how pain is treated today. During World War II, Henry Beecher astutely noted that on the battlefield, seriously wounded soldiers reported less pain than civilian patients in the Massachusetts General Hospital recovery room. However, at a later time these same patients would complain vehemently about even minor physical insults. These observations caused Beecher to conclude that the experience of pain was derived from a complex interaction between physical sensation, cognition, and emotional reaction (Beecher 1946). In the 1950s, based on Freudian ideals, the link between psychiatric illness and pain was explored by Engel. By the mid-1960s, it was confirmed that chronic pain patients also often had coexisting psychiatric disease (Engel 1959) and behavior and cognitive therapies were emerging as rational alternatives to more traditional psychoanalytic thought.

The advent and advancement of pharmacological approaches to pain ultimately revolutionized the physician's capacity to provide a therapy that could yield direct relief. While pain-relieving drugs are alluded to in the writings of many ancient societies, the modern pharmacological treatment of pain has been mostly influenced by the cultivation of opioids. While it is not known precisely when in history the opium poppy was first cultivated, it is believed that the Sumerians isolated opium from its seed capsule by the end of the third millennium BCE and that its use spread along trade routes. Beginning in the 16th century, opioid abuse was identified in Turkey, Egypt, Germany, and England. Famously, Thomas Sydenham concocted the recipe for laudanum, consisting of opium, sherry, wine, and spices, in the mid-17th century, and it was quickly and widely employed to treat a broad range of ailments, from dysentery to hysteria and gout. In 1806, the active ingredient in opium was identified by Serturner, who dubbed it *morphine* after Morpheus, the god of dreams. Soon after, codeine was isolated (Brownstein 1993). Without the ability to inject medications, the routes of convenient administration of drugs were limited. This was revolutionized in the 1850s, following the development of the hypodermic needle by Rynd (1845) and the syringe by Wood (Mann 2006). In the years that followed, accompanying increased medicinal use of opiates, many attempts were made to synthesize a more potent, safer, less addicting alternative to morphine, yielding the development of heroin in 1898 and methadone in 1946 (Brownstein 1933).

Other classes of drugs still in use today take their roots in traditional medicines of antiquity. In South America, coca leaves were traditionally used as a remedy for altitude sickness, physical pain, and as a topical anesthetic. From the coca plant, the alkaloid anesthetic cocaine was isolated by Albert Niemann in the 1860s. Niemann touted the use of cocaine as a cure-all, including for treatment of alcohol and morphine addiction (Niemann 1860). Soon after, in 1884, Carl Koller demonstrated the local anesthetic effects of cocaine (Koller 1884). Additionally, nonsteroidal anti-inflammatory drugs are known to have been used in the form of myrtle leaf, a natural source of salicylates, by the ancient Egyptians. By 200 BCE willow bark, another natural source of salicylic acid, was in use by Greek physicians; however, the first scientific report of the power of willow derivatives was not published until 1763 by the Reverend Edmund Stone (Leake 1975). Salicylic acid was identified as the active ingredient in willow leaf extract by the French pharmacist Henri Leroux in 1829. A more palatable and well-tolerated version of the drug was prepared by Charles von Gerhardt in 1873 with the addition of an acetyl group, synthesizing what is commonly known today as aspirin (Fairley 1978). Quickly thereafter, in 1899, aspirin was registered and marketed by Bayer.

As the adage goes, "a chance to cut is a chance to cure," requiring that the medical caregiver believes that the nature of a pain lies in the body. Inspired by specificity theory and its derivatives, more and more refined specific anatomical treatments were developed for the treatment of pain, in both the peripheral and central nervous systems. Multitudes of surgical approaches to pain have been employed, predominantly based on the tenet of interruption of a specific path of sensory conduction, including neurotomies, dorsal root excision, thalamectomy, mesencephalic lesioning, psychosurgical lobotomies, and other procedures specifically designed to alter the anatomy and interrupt pain signal reception.

In addition to open surgical procedures, direct interventional approaches to the disruption of pain signals developed. As early as 1784, James Moore, a British surgeon, demonstrated that the compression of specific nerves could provide reversible surgical anesthesia, thereby piloting regional nerve blockade (Moore 1784). However, the use of injection of neurolytics to provide long-lasting interruption of nerve conduction was not performed until 1903 by Schloesser (1903). Later, in response to patients with sympathetic nerve injuries in World War I, René Leriche developed the technique of injecting the local anesthetic procaine and surgical sympathectomy, which later became a standard therapy (Leriche 1937). In the 1920s, nerve ablation procedures became a treatment of choice, even for chronic unexplained pain syndromes, cementing the role of nerve blocks, and in 1936, at Bellevue Hospital in New York City, the first nerve block clinic for pain management was established (Rovenstine 1941).

While electrical modalities for pain relief were used by the ancient Egyptians, Greeks, and Romans, typically by means of medical use of electric fish, the underlying explanation of how electricity caused pain relief was not explained until gate control theory became a part of the pain practitioner's lexicon (Sabatowski et al. 1992). Modern extrapolations of gate control theory now include implantable dorsal column stimulators, transcutaneous electric nerve stimulation (TENS) units, and deep brain stimulation.

The Specialty and Future of Pain Medicine

While ever finer and more targeted anatomical treatment for pain continues to become more prevalent, it is important to recognize that perhaps the greatest advance in modern thinking about pain medicine has come not in the form of choosing a single modality or approach or pain concept, but rather is the recognition that multiple pain theories, anatomical processes, and therapies must coexist. Although this joining of previously dichotomous thinking has been advocated for some time, as recently as a decade ago, French sociologist Isabelle Baszanger noted the presence of two disparate types of pain clinics in Paris: one based on "curing through techniques" and the second based on "healing through adaptation (Baszanger 1992)." Rather than our making a choice between the mind and the body, a holistic concept of patient-centered pain management has emerged. Initially this was devised by the mother of hospice medicine in Great Britain, Dame Cicely Saunders, through her idea of "total pain (Clark 1999)." After his experiences treating the pain of World War II veterans, the founder of interdisciplinary pain care, Dr. John Bonica, organized an early large-scale multidisciplinary conference of 300 clinicians and researchers, which ultimately gave rise to the International Association for the Study of Pain (IASP) (Liebeskind 1997). Now, more than 60 scientific disciplines are represented by the IASP. This multidisciplinary trend has continued with the establishment of formal subspecialty Board certifications in Pain Medicine through the American Board of Anesthesiology in 1991, followed by subspecialty certification from the American Board of Psychiatry and Neurology (ABPN) and the American Board of Physical Medicine and Rehabilitation (ABPMR) in 2000 (Fishman et al. 2004). Currently, in the United States, the expectation and preference of interdisciplinary pain care has impacted the training of physicians, and the Accreditation Council for Graduate Medical Education established new guidelines to provide for multidisciplinary pain education as a requirement for subspecialty pain fellows in 2007 (Official website of the ACGME 2008).

Pain is essentially so much a part of our common humanity and so central to the practice of medicine that without understanding of the assessment, diagnosis, and treatment of pain, our care of patients would be woefully inadequate. The dramatic breadth and depth of the field of pain medicine makes it a fertile ground for future innovation. In every aspect of pain care, from the subcellular to the community-wide level, advances are being made that not only influence theory but also practice. The rapid current acceleration in molecular biology, genetics, imaging modalities, and high technology provides constantly growing potential for discovery. At the same time, renewed interest in old world ideas and techniques encourages the development of the art of healing among caregivers. It is the goal of this chapter to provide a mental framework to understand the evolution of our current concepts and therapy for pain and to foster professionalism in this newly emerging and exciting focus of scientific and clinical study.

References

Académie nationale de médecine (France). Report of the experiments on animal magnetism made by a committee of the medical section of the French Royal Academy of Sciences, read at the meetings of the 21st and 28th of June 1831. Tr., and now for the first time published, with an historical and explanatory introduction, and an appendix, by J.C. Colquhoun. Edinburgh: R. Cadell; London: Whittaker, 1833.

Barnes PA, Powell-Griner E, McFann K, Nahin RL. Complementary and alternative medicine use among adults, United States, 2002. U.S. Department of Health and Human Services, DHHS Publication No. (PHS) 2004-1250, *Advance Data from Vital and Health Statistics* No. 343, May 27, 2004.

Baszanger I. Deciphering chronic pain. Soc Health Illn. 1992 Jun;14(2):181–215.

Beecher HK. Pain in men wounded in battle. Ann Surg. 1946;123:96–105.

Bell C. Idea of a new anatomy of the brain, submitted for the observations of his friends. London: Strahan & Preston; 1811.

Benedelow GA, Williams SJ. Transcending the dualisms toward a study of pain. Sociol Health Illn. 1995 Mar;17(2):139–65.

Birk RK. The history of pain management. Hist Anesth Soc Proc. 2006 Sept;36:37–45.

Bonica JJ. The management of pain. Philadelphia, PA: Lea & Febiger; 1953, p. 23.

Brown D. The DaVinci code. New York: Anchor Books; 2003.

Brownstein MJ. A brief history of opiates, opioid peptides, and opioid receptors. Proc Natl Acad Sci. 1993 Jun;90:5391–3.

Charlotte Perkins Gilman as quoted in Rey R. The history of pain. Gilman CP. The living of Charlotte Perkins Gilman: an autobiography. New York, NY: D. Appleton-Century Co.; 1935. p. 96.

Clark D. Total pain: disciplinary power and the power in the work of Cicely Saunders, 1958–1967. Soc Sci Med. 1999;49:727–36.

Cranefield PF. The way in and the way out: François Magendie, Charles Bell and the roots of the spinal nerves. Mount Kisco, NY: Futura Publishing Company; 1974.

Descartes R. L'Homme. Paris: e. Angot; 1664.

Descartes R. (1641) Meditations on first philosophy. In: The philosophical writings of René Descartes (trans: Cottingham J, Stoothoff R, Murdoch D). Cambridge: Cambridge University Press; 1984. vol. 2, pp. 1–62.

Engel GL. Psychogenic pain. Med Clin North Am. 1958 Nov;42(6):1481–96.

Engel GL. Psychogenic pain. Med Clin N Am. 1959;42:1481–96.

Epistolary Dissertation (1681). The works of Thomas Sydenham, M.D. (trans: Latham RG). London: Sydenham Society; 1848–1850. vol. 2, p. 85.

Fairley P. The conquest of pain. London: Michael Joseph; 1978.

Fishman S, Gallagher, RM, Carr DB, Sullivan LW. The case for pain medicine. Pain Med. 2004;5(3):281–6.

Fulop-Miller R. Triumph over pain. (trans: Eden P, Cedar P). New York, NY: Literary Guild of America; 1938. p. 396.

Goldscheider A. Die spezifische Energie der Gefühlsnerven der Haut. Mh Prakt Derm. 1884;3:283.

Harvey W. Exercitatio anatomica de motu cordis et sanguinis in anima. Animalibus Anno: 1628, Florence:R Live; 1928.

Helms JM. An overview of medical acupuncture. Altern Ther. 1998 May;4(3):32–45.

Kiersey D. Please understand me II: temperament, character, intelligence. Del Mar, CA: Prometheus Nemesis Book; 1998.

King H. The early anodynes: pain in the ancient world. In: Mann RD, editor. The history of the management of pain. Lancaster, UK: Parthenon Publishing Group Ltd.; 1988. pp. 51–60.

Koller C. On the use of cocaine for producing anaesthesia on the eye. Lancet. 1884;2:990.

Lanser P, Gesell, S. Pain management: the fifth vital sign. Healthc Benchmarks. 2001 Jun;8(6):62, 68–70.

Leake CD. An historical account of pharmacology to the twentieth century. Springfield, IL: CC Thomas; 1975. p. 160.

Leriche R. La Chirurgie de la Douleur. Paris: Masson; 1937.

Liebeskind JC, Meldrum ML, John JB. World champion of pain. In: Jensen TS, Turner JA, Wisenfeld-Hallin Z, editors. Proceedings of the eighth world congress on pain: progress in pain research and management. Seattle, WA: International Association for the Study of Pain Press; 1997. Vol. 8, pp. 19–32.

Magendie F. Experiments on the spinal nerves. J Exp Physiol Pathol. 1822;2:276–9.

Mann RD. The history of the non-steroidal anti-inflammatory drugs. Quoted in Birk RK. The history of pain management. Hist Anesth Soc Proc. 2006 Sept:37–45.

Melzack R, Wall PD. Pain mechanisms: a new theory. Science 1965;150:971–9.

Moore J. A method of preventing or diminishing pain in several operations of surgery. London: T. Cadell; 1784.

Muller J. Handbuch der physiologie des menschen. Vol. 2. (trans: Baly W). London: Taylor and Walton; 1839; Vol. 234, pp. 253–55.

Nafe JP. A quantitative theory of feeling. J Gen Psychol. 1929;2:199–211.

Niemann A. Über einer organische Base in der Coca. Ann Chem. 1860;114:213.

Official website of the ACGME. http://www.acgme.org/acWebsite/downloads/RRC_progReq/sh_multiPainPR707.pdf. Accessed Nov 2008.

Parris W. The history of pain medicine. In: Raj PP, editor. Practical management of pain. 3rd ed. St. Louis, MO: Mosby; 2000. p. 4.

Perl ER. Ideas about pain, a historical review. Nat Rev Neurosci. 2007 Jan;8:72.

Rey R. Christianity and pain in the Middle Ages. In: Rey R, editor. The history of pain. Cambridge: Harvard University Press; 1955. pp. 48–9.

Rovenstine EA, Wertheim HM. Therapeutic nerve block. JAMA. 1941;117:1599–603.

Rynd F. Neuralgia – introduction of fluid to the nerve. Dublin Med Press. 1845;13:167.

Sabatowski R, Schafer D, Kasper SM, Brunsch H, Radbruch L. Pain treatment: A historical overview. Curr Pharm Des. 2004 Mar;10(7):701–16.

Sawda J. Engines of the imagination: Renaissance culture and the rise of the machine. London, NY: Routledge; 2007. chapter 6.

Schloesser H. Heilung periphärer Reizzustände sensibler und motorischer Nerven. Klin Monatsbl Augenheilkd. 1903;41:244.

Sherrington CS. The integrative action of the nervous system. Cambridge: Cambridge University Press; 1906.

Sinclair DC. Cutaneous sensation and the doctrine of specific energy. Brain 1955;78:584–614.

Squire WW. On the introduction of ether inhalation as an anesthetic in London. Lancet 1888 December 22:1220–21.

Weddell G. Somesthesis and the chemical senses. Ann Rev Psychol. 1955;6:119–136.

Zimmermann M. The history of pain concepts and treatment before IASP. In: Merskey H, Loeser JD, Dubner R, editors. The paths of pain 1975–2005. Seattle, WA: IASP Press; 2005. p. 9.

Chapter 2

Multidisciplinary Approach to Pain Management

Debebe Fikremariam, MD and Mario Serafini, DO

In 1996 the International Association for the Study of Pain defined pain as "an unpleasant sensory and emotional experience associated with actual and potential tissue damage or described in terms of such damage." An estimated 50 million Americans live with chronic pain caused by disease, disorder, or accident. An additional 25 million are treated for acute pain related to surgery or accidental injury (National Pain Survey 1999). Approximately two-thirds of these patients have been living with pain in excess of 5 years. The loss of productivity and the quality of life due to pain is substantial (Chronic Pain America 1999). Million and even billions of dollars are lost from habitual health care utilization and disability compensation. In a study done in 2000 (Merck 2000), it was reported that 36 million Americans missed work in the previous year due to pain and 83 million indicated that the pain affected their participation in various activities.

In 1986, Koch estimated that 70 million office visits to physicians were motivated by pain complaints (Koch 1986). A 1994 estimate indicated that approximately one-fifth of adult population experience chronic pain and in 1999, Market Data Enterprise estimated that 4.9 million individuals saw a physician for chronic pain treatment (Joranson and Lietman 1994, Market Data Enterprise 1999). These statistics indicate that pain and its under treatment represents a major problem confronting society.

Acute pain is elicited by the injury of body tissues and activation of nociceptive transducers at the site of local tissue damage. The goals of acute pain management are to eliminate pain and to restore the patient's ability to function as rapidly as possible. Chronic pain is also elicited by an injury but may be perpetuated by factors that are both pathogenically and physically remote from the originating cause. Chronic pain is characterized by low levels of underlying pathology that does not correspond to the presence or extent of the pain experienced by the patient. Chronic pain prompts patients frequently to seek health care and it is rarely effectively treated in a primary care setting. Of the patients with chronic pain one-half to two-thirds are partially or totally disabled which all too often may become permanent. After the pain has become chronic its total eradication may be unrealistic.

Traditional biomedical methods of treating chronic pain have proven unsatisfactory both from the patients' and providers' prospective and this fomented a demand for effective therapy (Loeser). John Bonica first appreciated the need for a multidisciplinary approach to chronic pain during World War II after several months of experience in treating military personnel with the variety of pain problems (Loeser). Bonica put the concept of the multidisciplinary approach for the diagnosis and therapy of complex chronic pain problems during

N. Vadivelu et al. (eds.), *Essentials of Pain Management*,
DOI 10.1007/978-0-387-87579-8_2, © Springer Science+Business Media, LLC 2011

his practice at Tacoma General Hospital. This became the world's first multidisciplinary clinic. The group consisted of specialists who had developed interest and expertise in pain management and included an anesthesiologist, a neurosurgeon, an orthopedist, a psychiatrist, an internist, and a radiation therapist.

The importance of the multidisciplinary approach to the management of chronic pain has been emphasized by two important task groups, one in the United States and one in Canada. The Quebec Task Force suggested that if management by the treating physician specialist was not successful and the patient still had pain after 3–6 months, the patient should be referred to a multidisciplinary team, which should focus primarily on psychosocial and psychological elements on the premise that these factors are primarily responsible for the persistence of the pain.

Most multidisciplinary pain programs focus on patients who manifest chronic pain behavior and disability long after healing process should have been completed and have no treatable structural pathology. These principles of multidisciplinary diagnosis and treatment should be applied to patients with obvious chronic pathology not amenable to surgical or medical therapy, such as arthritis, cancer, deafferentation pain, and other chronic pain syndromes. Chronic pain that is not adequately treated causes the patient to develop psychological, psychosocial, and behavioral problems as well as progressive physical deterioration with marked interruption of activities of daily living.

Treating physicians who have been unsuccessful with the first or at most the second attempt in using surgery or medical therapies in managing complex pain problems are encouraged to refer such patient to a multidisciplinary pain center that can carry out a coordinated effort to establish a diagnosis and develop an effective treatment strategy.

Multidisciplinary Pain Assessment

The objectives of multidisciplinary pain assessment are to (1) identify those patients who could benefit from a physical and psychological rehabilitation program based on cognitive behavioral principles of effecting behavioral change and pain reduction, (2) to rule out those patients who have a medical or psychological contraindication to such a program, and (3) to identify other, perhaps more effective methods of treatment and to help establish appropriate therapeutic goals.

Pain center referrals from primary care physicians are usually made by either a letter or a telephone call from another physician or on occasion from another type of health care provider. The pain center physician may accept the patient for multidisciplinary evaluation, for emergency treatment, and for a consult, ask additional information, reject the patient, or the patient may have unresolved medical problem that should be addressed before referral to a pain center. Once referral is established to a multidisciplinary program the initial screening evaluation consists of medical and psychological evaluation, review of patients' diaries, referral letter, medical records, and spouse interview.

Description of Multidisciplinary Pain Process:

Concepts of treatment at multidisciplinary pain clinics include

- reconceptualization of the patient pain and associated problems from uncontrollable to manageable;
- overt to covert efforts are made to foster optimism and combat demoralization;

- flexibility is the norm with attempts to individualize some aspects of treatment to patient's needs and unique physical and psychological characteristics;
- emphasize active patient participation and responsibility;
- provide education and training in the use of specific skills such as exercise, relaxation, and problem solving;
- encourage feelings of success, self-control, and self-efficacy;
- encourage patients to attribute success to their own role.

Programs usually emphasize physical conditioning, medication management, acquisition of coping and vocational skills, and gaining knowledge about pain and how the body functions. Individual and group counseling addresses patient needs. In contrast to traditional Western health care, the emphasis is on what the patient accomplishes, not on what providers accomplish. The providers can be teachers, coaches, and sources of information and support.

Multidisciplinary pain management requires the collaborative efforts of many health care providers including but not limited to physicians, psychologists, physical therapists, occupational therapists, vocational counselors, social workers, ergonomists, and support staff.

Facilities

The facilities for a multidisciplinary pain treatment program can exist within a large hospital or medical center or they can be free standing. They can be associated with academic centers or private practice scenarios.

Patient Treatment Strategies

Each patient will present with different mixtures of functional limitations, pain behaviors, affective disturbance, physical disability, and vocational dysfunction. The original multidisciplinary pain management programs were all inpatient based. It is now apparent that outpatient programs can be equally successful if they have adequate intensity and duration (Turk et al. 1993).

There are no controlled studies to determine the optimal duration of treatment and hours per day, nor does the literature reveal which aspects of the various components are most important for a treatment program. It is clear that the effects of multidisciplinary pain treatment program are greater than the sum of its parts. Common features of all programs include physical therapy, medication management, education about how the body functions, psychological treatment (e.g., coping skills learning, problem solving, communication skill training), vocational assessment, and therapies aimed at improving function and the likelihood of returning to work. The overall length of a program depends in part on unique patient requirements. Typical programs operate 8 h a day, 5 days a week and last 3–4 weeks, although some programs meet less frequently and last for longer periods.

Role of the Physicians

The physicians are responsible for the initial history, physical examination, review of outside records, determination of the need for any future diagnostic tests. Other responsibilities of the physicians include:

- detailed assessment of the patient's medication history;
- implementation of medication management;

- reviewing the medical issues and the findings in diagnostic tests and imaging studies with the patient;
- education of the patient and legitimizing all of the other components of the program.

Role of The Psychologists

Roles of the psychologists are as follows:

- conducts the initial psychological evaluation;
- monitors and implements the cognitive and behavioral treatment strategies;
- teaches the patient coping skills;
- educates patients about the relationships among thoughts, feelings, behavior, and physiology;
- leads both individual and group educational and counseling sessions for the patients.

Role of the Nurse

The nurse is a key part of the treatment program and plays a major role in patient education regarding topics such as medication, diet, sleep, hygiene, and sexual activity. Another nursing function is assisting patients in the practice of newly learned skills, assessing medication response, and acting as a focal point of communication to coordinate patient care. The role of the nurse varies with their skills and the interaction with other providers. Since the nurses tend to be with patients throughout their active treatment course, they are a focal point for continuity in the treatment program.

Role of the Physical and Occupational Therapists

Physical and occupational therapists provide assessment and active physical therapy for patients to improve their strength, endurance, and flexibility. They do not provide passive modalities for treatment. Therapists assist the patient in developing proper body mechanics and strategies for coping with the physical demands of a job and everyday life. They function mainly as teachers and coaches.

The occupational therapists review the patient's work history, disabilities, and factors that may play a role in determining the ability of the patient to return to the work force. They help in the establishment of "work-hardening" and training activities.

Some programs heavily emphasize ergonomic issues and use high technology in physical therapies; however, the need for this type of treatment is unclear.

Role of the Vocational Counselor

The vocational counselor plays a critical role in the treatment of patients for whom return to work is a treatment goal. Initial assessment occurs as part of the screening process, but in-depth evaluation of interest, education, aptitude, physical capacities, learning capabilities, work experience, transferable skills, and vocational goals occurs on entry into the treatment program.

The goals are to identify vocational opportunities and barriers to effective employment. In addition to occupational counseling, the vocational counselor provides job-seeking skills training, placement counseling, job hardening, and information about educational options and liaisons services.

Treatment Principles

General Goals of the Multidisciplinary Pain Center (MPC)

- Identification and treatment of unresolved medical problems
- Elimination of inappropriate medications
- Symptomatic improvement
- Restoration of physical functioning
- Restoration of social and occupational functioning, social integration, and return to productive employment
- Reduction in use of the health care system
- Improvement in coping skills, foster independence

Principles of MPC Program

The single most important ingredient is the existence of health care providers who are willing to work as a team. The health care providers must care about chronic illness and not be totally locked into acute diseases as is fostered by the biomedical model. The commitment of the provider to the patient is essential. Patients must want to change their lives and must be willing to give the program a try. They must recognize that in this type of program the patients do the therapeutic work. The treatment is the start of a journey to reclaim one's life; long-term support is required to keep the patient on the road to recovery. The attempt to treat the untreatable leads to demoralization of the treatment team. Patients must be properly selected.

Physical Therapy

Physical therapy uses behavioral medicine principles and engages few, if any passive modalities (Turk et al. 2000). Biofeedback can be a useful adjunct because it teaches the patient that he or she can gain control over various bodily functions. The emphasis is on improving strength, endurance, and flexibility through the patient's physical activities. The therapist provides instruction, guidance, safety, and encouragement.

Medications

Medication is given on a time-contingent basis to uncouple the reinforcement of pain behavior medication. In general, patients in an MPC program do not derive adequate pain relief from analgesic medication, and thus they are usually tapered. This technique is simply a method of converting all opioids to an equivalent dose of sustained acting opioids or methadone. The dose is then tapered over the period of treatment, always with the full knowledge of the patient. Most medications may be discontinued; the common exceptions are antidepressants, which often help chronic pain patients. Pain clinics may also discourage long-term use of other medications both because of their potential side effects and because their use undermines the philosophical concept that the patient must learn to control his or her pain and not depend on health care providers or their prescriptions.

Psychological Strategies

Generally, the aim is to alter behavior rather than change the patient's personality. Patients learn coping skills because this is frequently a deficiency that has led to the patients many difficulties.

Another important aspect of multidisciplinary pain management is education. This is an activity shared by physicians, psychologists, and nurses. Topics cover a wide array of the problems facing those who suffer from chronic pain. Subject selection and content can be tailored to the needs of each group of patients, but a core set of issues to be discussed includes:

- Stress treatment
- Relaxation training
- Coping skills
- Anger treatment
- Pain behavior
- Sleep disorder
- Physiology of stress
- Assertion training
- Cognitive strategy
- Communication skills
- Dealing with depression
- Crisis management
- Cost/meaning of pain

Outcomes

Several epidemiologic studies have examined the characteristics of patients treated at MPC as compared to patients with chronic pain not treated at MPC facilities (Crook et al. 1986, Crook et al. 1989). The patients treated at MPCs had reports of constant pain, high levels of emotional distress, work-related injuries, significantly lower levels of education, high levels of health care utilization, high levels of opioid use, high levels of functional impairment, and negative attitudes about the future.

Criteria for Treatment Success

The evaluation of treatment success must include several considerations listed below:

1. *Pain reduction*: The most common criterion measure of outcome in various treatment approaches for pain problem. Dvorak and colleagues studied 575 patients who were operated on lumbar disk herniation and concluded that 70% continued to complain of back pain 4–17 years after surgery (Dvorak et al. 1988). Pain reduction following treatment at MPCs ranged from 20 to 40% (Flor et al. 1992). Studies investigating the long-term maintenance of pain reduction observed at discharge tend to be maintained at follow up of up to 2 years. In a direct comparison, Gallon showed that only 17% of the surgical patients viewed themselves as improved as compared to 38% of non-surgical-treated patients.
2. *Iatrogenic complications*: Surgical procedures themselves sometimes may cause additional problem that may require repeat surgery. In a series of 78 surgical patients, Long et al.

observed that 11.6% developed serious complications from the procedure. In contrast to surgery, MPCs rarely report any significant iatrogenic problems following treatment.

3. *Elimination or reduction of opioid medication*: Flor et al. found that over 50% of patients treated at MPCs were taking opioid medication on admission (Flor et al. 1992). Because of potentially detrimental effects of opioids and attempts to encourage self-initiated pain treatment elimination or reduction of opioids intake is an important part of most multidisciplinary treatment programs.

   In general, MPCs appear to be effective in eliminating or greatly reducing opioid intake in chronic pain patients. Studies report that up to 100% of patients decrease opioid use by the time of treatment terminations at MPCs. Over 65% of treated patients remain opioid-free at 1-year follow up.

4. *Utilization of health care system*: MPCs effectively reduce utilization of the health care system following treatment. About 60–90% of patients did not seek any additional treatment for their pain during a 3–12-month post-treatment period. Compared to conventionally treated patients (i.e., medication and/or surgery), MPCs consistently show superior rate of reduced health care utilization (Fig. 2.1).

5. *Increase in activity*: According to quantitative review of outcome studies (Flor et al. 1992), substantially greater increase in activity level occurred in patients treated at MPCs (65%) compared to conventionally treated patients (35%).

6. *Return to work*: Although return to work is an important outcome as it has significant socioeconomic implications, several factors impede patient's return to work aside from their pain. Return to gainful employment for chronic pain patients depends on factors such as local economy, job availability, and the aggressiveness of care managers. The average time off from work is 7 years. Skills that were useful prior to the pain onset may be outdated making patients less marketable. The results of 11 studies with 259

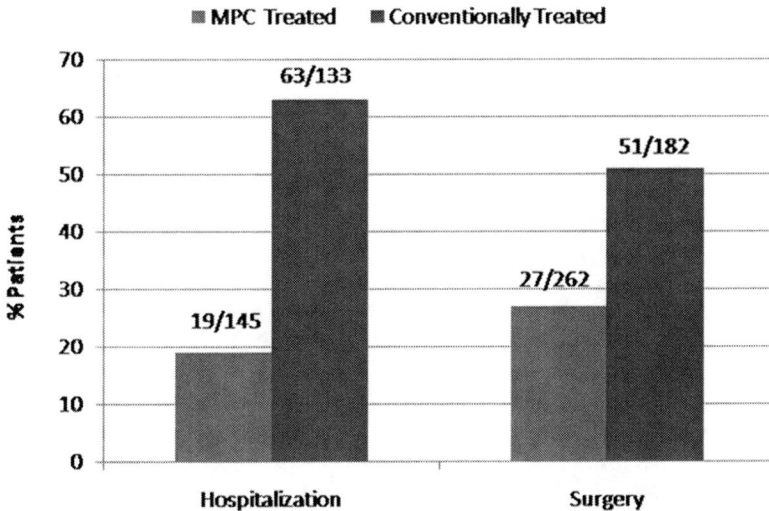

Figure 2.1   Frequency of patients receiving additional surgery and hospitalization following treatment: comparisons between multidisciplinary pain center (MPC) and conventional treatments. Modified from Loeser and Turk (2001, p. 2075).

conventionally treated and 435 MPC-treated patients indicate the rate of returning to work among treated patients is substantially higher (67%) when compared to the rate among the untreated patients (24%).

7. *Closure of disability claims*: Chronic pain is costly for society due to loss of productivity and disability payments to patients. Painter et al. followed patients for a longer period and reported that the proportion of patients receiving compensation declined from 70 at admission to 45% at 2-year follow up.

Cost-Effectiveness of MPCs

Treatment at MPCs results in impressive reduction on health care utilization. Simon and colleagues reported a 62% reduction of medical costs as a result of treatment at MPCs. Using the figure of 176,000 patients treated at MPCs annually, the estimated medical cost saving during the first year following treatment at MPCs well over 1.87 billion dollars. The average age of patients treated at MPCs is 45 years and assuming a mean life expectancy of 75, the estimated saving in 30 years would be 45 billion dollars (Flor et al. 1992). As a result of treatment at MPCs there is a significant decline in the proportion of patients receiving disability compensation which translates to savings of billions of dollars.

Systematic comparison of cost-effectiveness across different modalities needs a common index. The index of cost-effectiveness can be defined as:

$$\text{Cost - effectiveness} = \frac{\text{improvement} \times 100}{\text{cost of treatment}}$$

Using the return to work rate as the improvement score, the cost-effectiveness index score for each treatment modality is shown in Fig. 2.2.

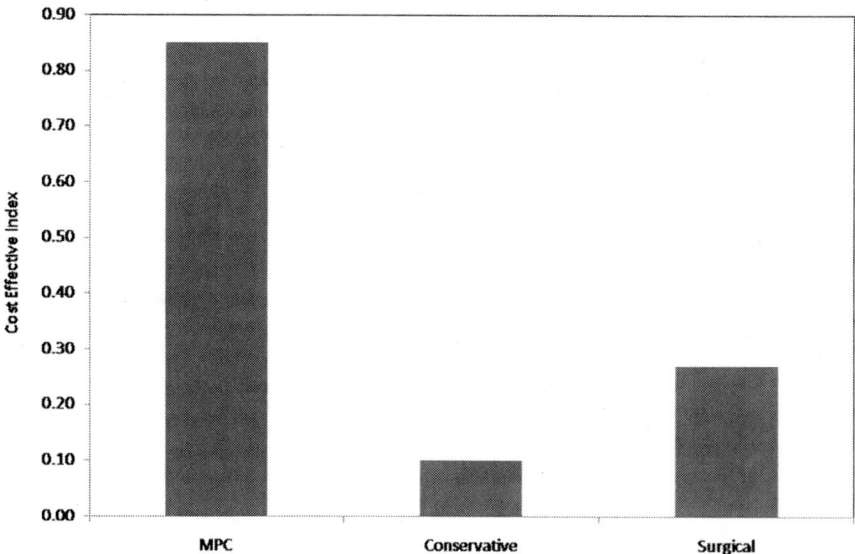

Figure 2.2 Cost-effective index by treatment modalities; MPC = multidisciplinary pain center. Modified from Turk and Okifuji (1998).

The cost-effectiveness index score of MPCs treatment far exceeds medical and surgical treatment. In fact, based on the index scores, multidisciplinary treatment can be considered nine times as cost-effective as conservative treatment and three to six times as cost-effective as surgical treatment in helping patients return to work.

Flor et al. concluded that "overall MPCs are efficacious. Even at long-term period, patients who are treated in such a setting are functioning better than 75% of a sample that is either untreated or that has been treated by conventional unimodal treatment approach."

Conclusion

A substantial body of literature supports the assertion that multidisciplinary pain treatment is effective in reducing pain, the use of opioid medications and health care services. Multidisciplinary pain management also increases activity, improves activity of daily living, returns people to work, aids in the closing of disability claims. Eventhough treatment at MPC targets patients with the most recalcitrant problem, the benefits appear to exceed those for conventional treatments such as surgery. Moreover in contrast to surgery there are no known iatrogenic complications of treatment at MPCs. Not only do MPCs appear to be clinically effective, but they also appear to be cost-effective, with the potential to provide substantial savings in health care costs and disability payments.

The treatment principles developed in MPCs should be applied much earlier in the management of chronic pain patients. It is also important to remember that prevention is always better than remediation. Even for patients who have been disabled for prolonged periods, multidisciplinary pain management can offer restoration to normal life.

Case Scenario

Sreekumar Kunnumpurath, MBBS, MD, FCARCSI, FRCA, FFPMRCA

Vincent is a 54-year-old artist who has made significant contributions to the world of art in the recent past. About 9 months ago, he was involved in a fight at a local bar and an assailant stabbed him in the left shoulder. Although the injury was deep, he underwent immediate surgery and his shoulder injury was repaired without much problem. He had an uneventful recovery. However, after discharge from the hospital, he continued to suffer from pain in the left shoulder, which slowly started to involve his left arm. He was under the care of his primary care physician who prescribed him various analgesics, physiotherapy, TENS, and even suggested acupuncture. Unfortunately, he failed to respond to all these therapeutic measures. He was then referred to the pain physician who found that Vincent's initial injury had healed well, and noted a few trigger points over his left shoulder which he treated with injections. He yet again failed to respond. He was then started on gabapentin without any improvement; in fact, he became depressed. His misery was compounded by the fact that he used his left hand to hold the brush while he painted. Now he has opted to undergo the pain management program and is here to consult you as a pain specialist.

Do you think this referral is appropriate?

Vincent's pain is persisting long after the resolution of the primary injury, and there is nothing in the history suggesting any ongoing complications of the injury (which you

may have to rule out). The conventional treatment strategies have obviously failed. Hence, this referral is justified at this point.

Q. How will you assess the suitability of Vincent for the pain management program?
Initial screening evaluation consists of medical and psychological evaluation and review of patient's diaries, referral letter, and medical records.

Vincent's clinical examination reveals a long scar on his left shoulder (which looks well healed) and a small patch of skin with sensory loss over the shoulder. There are no signs of complex regional pain syndrome (CRPS). He tells you that the pain is a constant ache with sharp shooting episodes during the night which is "worrying him a lot" and "keeps him awake." The pain score varies from 5 to 8 out of a maximum of 10. He is worried about moving his neck for fear of worsening of the pain. His medications include acetaminophen, codeine, oral morphine, tramadol, and gabapentin. He mentions that he feels sleepy during the day ever since he has started taking gabapentin. His appetite has increased and he has "put on a several pounds." Vincent feels that the medications are harming his creativity.

The pain center psychologist further assesses Vincent. The interview reveals that Vincent is suffering from depression which was present even before the injury. He is upset that the pain is preventing him from going out and painting outdoors. At the end of the evaluation and in consultation with your team, you conclude that Vincent is a suitable candidate for the multidisciplinary pain management program.

Describe your multidisciplinary pain management process for Vincent?
The emphasis of the strategies would be on physical conditioning, medication management, acquisition of coping and vocational skills, and gaining knowledge about pain and how the body functions. Vincent needs counseling addressing his needs. The most important aim is to change Vincent's pain from uncontrollable to manageable.

It is advisable to have realistic expectations regarding the outcome from the program. Vincent tells you that he is really upset that he cannot use his left hand effectively to paint and he would be happy if he could do so for at least an hour a day.

As a physician, you are responsible for implementation of medication management. How are you going to achieve this?
Pain medications should be given on a contingent basis to uncouple the reinforcement of pain behavior and medication. Patients in the MPC program do not derive adequate pain relief from analgesics. An attempt to taper the pain medications by means of the pain cocktail technique should be made. Instead of multiple opioids, generally a single long-acting medication should be prescribed.

It is worth considering stopping gabapentin altogether. Gabapentin is not currently indicated and furthermore can cause side effects such as increased appetite and disturbed sleep patterns which can further aggravate his symptoms. He might benefit from an addition of an antidepressant to help with depression and pain symptoms.

Vincent undergoes the MPC program whole-heartedly and cooperates with the multidisciplinary team, which includes physical therapists, pain nurses, and vocational counselors. He learns more about his body and the basic mechanism of chronic pain, which helps him to get over the fear of losing his livelihood. He learns to paint with his right hand with the help of the occupational therapist, and at the end of the program he is able to go out into the open and paint landscapes. Though he still has pain, it no longer bothers him. The MPC program has been a great success for him.

References

Chronic Pain America; road blocks to relief, survey conducted for the American Pain Society, the American Academy of Pain Medicine and Jansen Pharmaceutical, 1999.

Crook J, Tunks E, Rideout E, et al. Epidemiologic comparison of pain sufferers in a specialty pain clinic and in the community. Arch Phys Med Rehab. 1986;67:451–5.

Crook J, Weir R, Tunks E. An epidemiologic follow-up survey of persistent pain sufferers in a group family practice and specialty pain clinic. Pain 1989;36:49–61.

Dvorak J, Gauchat M, Valach L. The outcome of surgery for lumbar disk herniation. A 4–17 yrs follow-up with emphasis on somatic aspects. Spine 1988;13:1418–22.

Flor H, Fydrich T, Turk DC. Efficacy of multidisciplinary pain treatment centers; a metaanalytic review. Pain 1992;49:221–230.

Loeser JD, Turk DC. Bonica's management of pain. 3rd ed. 2001. pp. 2067–79.

National Pain Survey, conducted for Ortho-McNeill Pharmaceutical, 1999.

Pain in America: a research report, survey conducted for Merck by the Gall up Organization, 2000.

Pain management programs: a market analysis. Tampa, FL: Market Data Enterprise; 1999.

Koch, HJ. The management of chronic pain in office-based ambulatory medical care survey. Advance data from vital and statistics no. 123, No PHS 86-1250, Hyattsville, MD; 1986.

Joranson D, Lietman R. The McNeill national pain study. New York, NY: Louis Harris Associates; 1994.

Turk DC, Okifuji A, Sherman J. Behavioral aspects of low back pain. In: Taylor J, Twomey L, editors. Physical therapy of the low back. 3rd ed. New York, NY: Churchill Livingstone; 2000. pp. 351–83.

Turk DC, Okifuji A. Treatment of chronic pain patients: clinical outcomes, cost-effectiveness and cost-benefits of multidisciplinary pain centers. Crit Rev Phys Made Rehab. 1998;10: 181–208.

Turk DC, Rudy T, Sorkin B. Neglected topics in chronic pain treatment outcome studies; determination of success. Pain 1993;53:3–16.

Section II

Anatomy and Physiology

Chapter 3

Anatomic and Physiologic Principles of Pain

Xing Fu, MD, Dan Froicu, MD, and Raymond Sinatra, MD

If you are distressed by anything external, the pain is not due to the thing itself, but to your estimate of it. This you have the power to revoke at any time.

–Marcus Aurelius

Introduction

Pain is the most frequent cause of suffering and disability and is the most common reason that people seek medical attention. It is a major symptom in many medical conditions, significantly interfering with a person's quality of life and general functioning. To understand the physiology and the mechanism of pain as well as optimal methods of control, one must appreciate the anatomical pathways that transmit nociceptive information to the brain. For a better comprehension of the anatomical pathways we divided it into four parts: the *peripheral system*, the *spinal and medullary dorsal horn system*, and the *ascending and supraspinal system*.

The pain pathway can be envisioned as a three-neuron pathway that transmits noxious stimuli from the periphery of the cerebral cortex.

The primary afferent neurons are located in the *dorsal root ganglia*, which lie in the vertebral foramina at each spinal cord level. Each primary afferent neuron has a single bifurcating axon, one end going to the peripheral tissue it innervates and the other going to the dorsal horn of the spinal cord, which receives sensory input.

In the *dorsal horn of the spinal cord*, the primary afferent neuron synapses with a *second-order neuron* whose axons cross the midline of the cord and ascend in the contralateral spinothalamic tract to reach the thalamus. Once in the dorsal horn, in addition to synapsing with second-order neurons, the axons of first-order neurons may synapse with interneurons, sympathetic neurons, and ventral horn motor neurons.

Second-order neurons synapse in *thalamic nuclei* with *third-order neurons*, which in turn send projections through the internal capsule and corona radiata to the postcentral gyrus of the cerebral cortex. At each point along the pathway there are several options for longer routes and for modification, and or integration of the information (Fig. 3.1) (Besson 1999).

The Peripheral Receptor System

The sensation of pain starts with a physical event such as a cut, burn, inflammation that excites sensory nerve fiber terminal endings including:

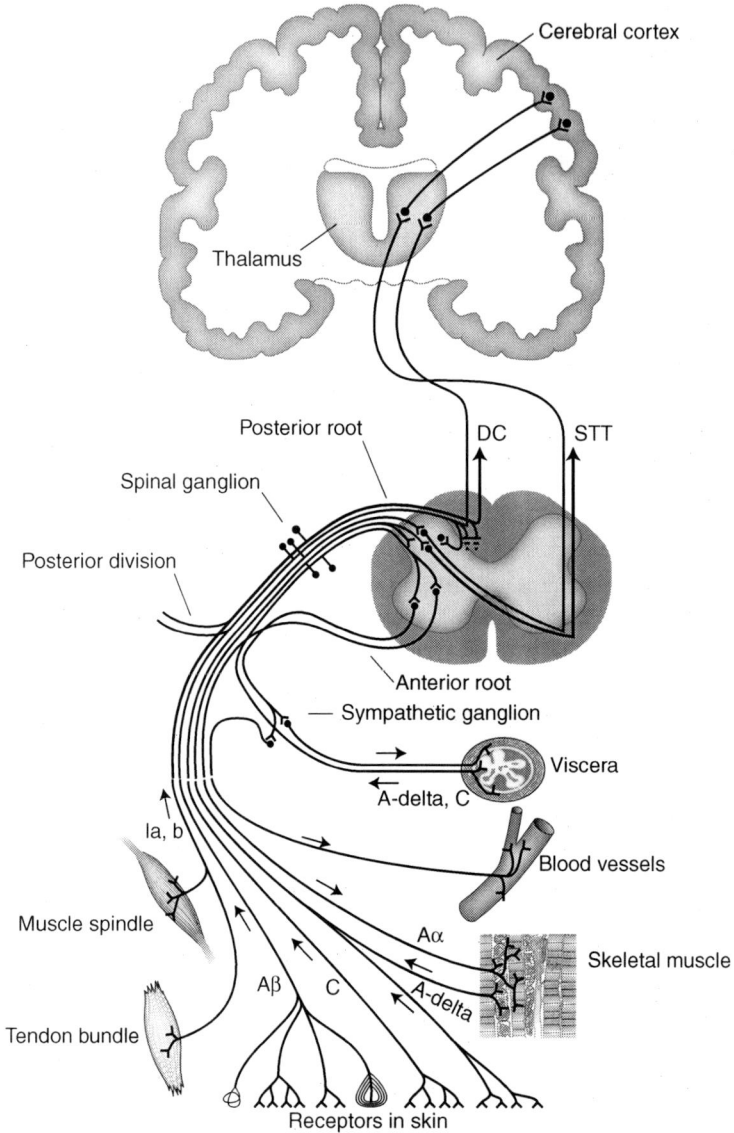

Figure 3.1   Pain pathways. Primary afferent neuron in spinal ganglion. Second-order neuron in dorsal horn. Third-order neuron in thalamic nuclei.

- *unmyelinated C and A-delta fibers* with bipolar cell bodies in the dorsal root ganglion (mentioned above) with proximal endings in the dorsal horn and distal endings in peripheral tissues
- *autonomic preganglionic neurones* with cell bodies located in the motor nuclei of the brainstem or in the anterolateral horn of the spinal cord

    These receptors and associated fibers are called *nociceptors*.

Nociceptors

The nociceptors are divided into several types, based on the stimuli they perceive. Nociceptor types include:

1. Mechanical (pressure, swelling, incision, tumor growth)
2. Chemical (excitatory neurotransmitter, toxic substance, ischemia, infection)
3. Thermal (burn)
4. Polymodal (i.e. the capability to respond to different stimuli: a combination of stimuli, respond to excessive pressure, extremes of temperature and halogens)

The nociceptors are distributed in the somatic structures and visceral structures.

Somatic Structures

Somatic structures (*skin and deep tissues*: muscles, tendons, bones, joints) respond to a variety of mechanical, chemical, and thermal stimuli leading to a well-perceived and well-localized sensation. Deep somatic nociceptors in tissue are less sensitive to noxious stimuli than cutaneous nociceptors, but are easily sensitized by inflammation. Specific nociceptors may exist in muscles and joint capsules; they respond to mechanical, thermal, and chemical stimuli, this would explain the presentation of most sports injuries. The cornea and tooth pulp are unique in that they are almost exclusively innervated by nociceptive A-delta and C fibers (cornea) and A-delta, A-beta, and C fibers (teeth).

Visceral Structures

Visceral structures (visceral organs such as liver, gastro-intestinal tract) respond to pain induced by ischemia, spasm, or inflammation of smooth muscle as well as mechanical stimulation such as distension of the mesentery. These fibers run in sympathetic and parasympathetic nerves, and the pain induced is poorly localized.

Visceral organs are generally insensitive and mostly contain silent nociceptors. Some organs appear to have specific nociceptors, such as the heart, lung, testis, and bile ducts. Most other organs, such as the intestines, are innervated by polymodal nociceptors that respond to smooth muscle spasm, ischemia, and inflammation. These receptors generally do not respond to the cutting, burning, or crushing that occurs during surgery. A few organs, such as the brain, lack nociceptors altogether; however, the brain's meningeal coverings do contain nociceptors. This phenomenon explains the need for adequate anesthesia and analgesia only during the beginning of neurosurgical procedures for the dissection and exposure of brain tissue.

Like somatic nociceptors, those in the viscera are the free nerve endings of primary afferent neurons whose cell bodies lie in the dorsal horn. These afferent nerve fibers, however, frequently travel with efferent sympathetic nerve fibers to reach the viscera. Afferent activity from these neurons enters the spinal cord between T1 and L2.

Nociceptive C fibers from the esophagus, larynx, and trachea travel with the vagus nerve to enter the nucleus solitarius in the brainstem. Afferent pain fibers from the bladder, prostate, rectum, cervix and urethra, and genitalia are transmitted into the spinal cord via parasympathetic nerves at the level of the S2–S4 nerve roots. Though relatively few compared to somatic pain fibers, fibers from primary visceral afferent neurons enter the cord and synapse more diffusely with single fibers, often synapsing with multiple dermatomal levels and often crossing to the contralateral dorsal horn. This nonspecific synapsing of visceral afferents explains the reason why somatic musculoskeletal pain is arranged in dermatomes but the visceral pain are usually nonspecific and variable in nature.

Somatic nociceptive pain has a dermatomal pattern (Fig. 3.2) and is sharp, crushing, or tearing in character. Somatic nociceptive pain is very well localized, whereas visceral nociceptive pain is nondermatomal and cramping or colicky and poorly is localized. Sometimes

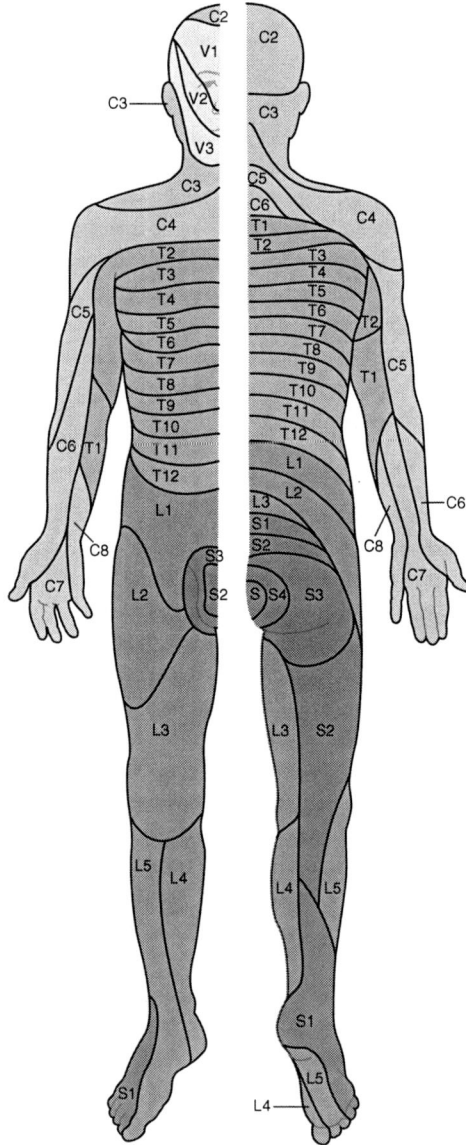

Figure 3.2   Dermatomes.

visceral pain is radiating has a somatic dermatomal pattern, and is known as *referred* pain. Referred pain represents a convergence of noxious input from visceral afferents activating second-order cells that are normally responsive to somatic sensation and leads to a well-delineated somatic discomfort at sites adjacent to or distant from internal sites of irritation or injury.

When there is prolonged noxious stimulation, the nociceptors can become sensitized. *Pain hypersensitivity* presents when either the thresholds are lowered so that stimuli that would normally not produce pain now begin to (allodynia), or the responsiveness is increased and the noxious stimuli produce an exaggerated and prolonged pain (hyperalgesia). Sensitization can be peripheral and central.

Peripheral Sensitization
Peripheral sensitization represents a reduction in threshold and an increase in responsiveness of the nociceptors from peripheral targets such as skin, muscle, joints, and the viscera in response to inflammatory chemicals or mediators such as adenosine triphosphate (ATP) or prostaglandin PGE_2.

Inflammation
Inflammatory factors released as a direct result of tissue injury or peptides released from collaterals of activated nociceptive nerve terminals (e.g., calcitonin gene-related peptide [CGRP] and substance P) induce increased vascular permeability and escape of plasma proteins into the tissue leading to edema at the injury site (Fig. 3.3). Primary afferent peptides, neurotransmitters, injury products like prostaglandins, as well as infiltrating immune cells and blood products like bradykinin escape from the vasculature, they combine to make important contributions to inflammation and to the pain resulting from the injury. Activation of receptors on peripheral terminals of "pain fibers" can initiate action potentials. Endogenous prostaglandins, bradykinin, and cytokines have strong peripheral actions and can sensitize as well as excite nociceptors.

Hyperalgesia
Hyperalgesia is an exacerbation of pain in response to sensations that normally would not be perceived as painful as a result of the damage of the nociceptors or of the peripheral nerves. *Primary hyperalgesia* occurs directly in the damaged tissues due to sensitization of peripheral nociceptors to thermal stimulation, whereas *secondary hyperalgesia* occurs in surrounding undamaged tissues due to sensitization within spinal cord and central nervous system (CNS) to mechanical stimulation (Fig. 3.4). Hyperalgesia is mediated by platelet-activating factor (PAF) that leads to an inflammatory response.

Allodynia
Allodynia is pain induced by a stimulus which does not normally provoke pain. Allodynia can be mechanical allodynia (pain in response to light touch/pressure) or thermal allodynia (pain from normally mild skin temperatures in the affected area). Allodynia is a result of neuronal sensitization both in the thalamus and in the dorsal horns. In the thalamus cysteine-cysteine chemokine ligand 21 (CCL21) induces production of prostaglandin E_2 (PGE_2) that can sensitize nociceptive neurons and lower their threshold to pain. In the dorsal horns of the spinal cord, tumor necrosis factor-alpha (TNF-alpha) increases the number of

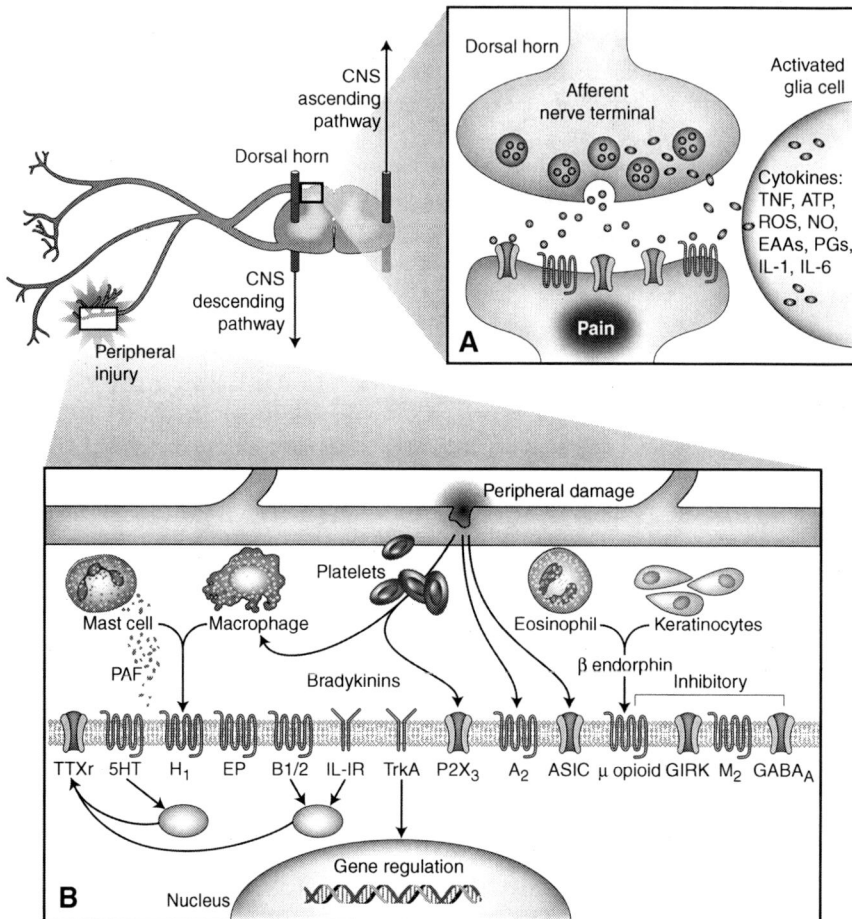

Figure 3.3 Inflammation leads to the release of numerous chemicals from mast cells, macrophages, and injured cells that act directly or indirectly to alter the sensitivity of receptors and ion channels on peripheral nerve terminals.

amino-3-hydroxyl-5-methyl-4-propionic acid (AMPA) receptors and decreases the number of gamma-aminobutyric acid (GABA) receptors on the membrane of nociceptors leading to easier activation of the nociceptors and increases PGE_2 production with a mechanism and effect similar to the ones in the thalamus.

Afferent Pain Fibers

The nociceptors have two types of axons either myelinated or unmyelinated and are divided into the C fibers and the A-delta fibers.

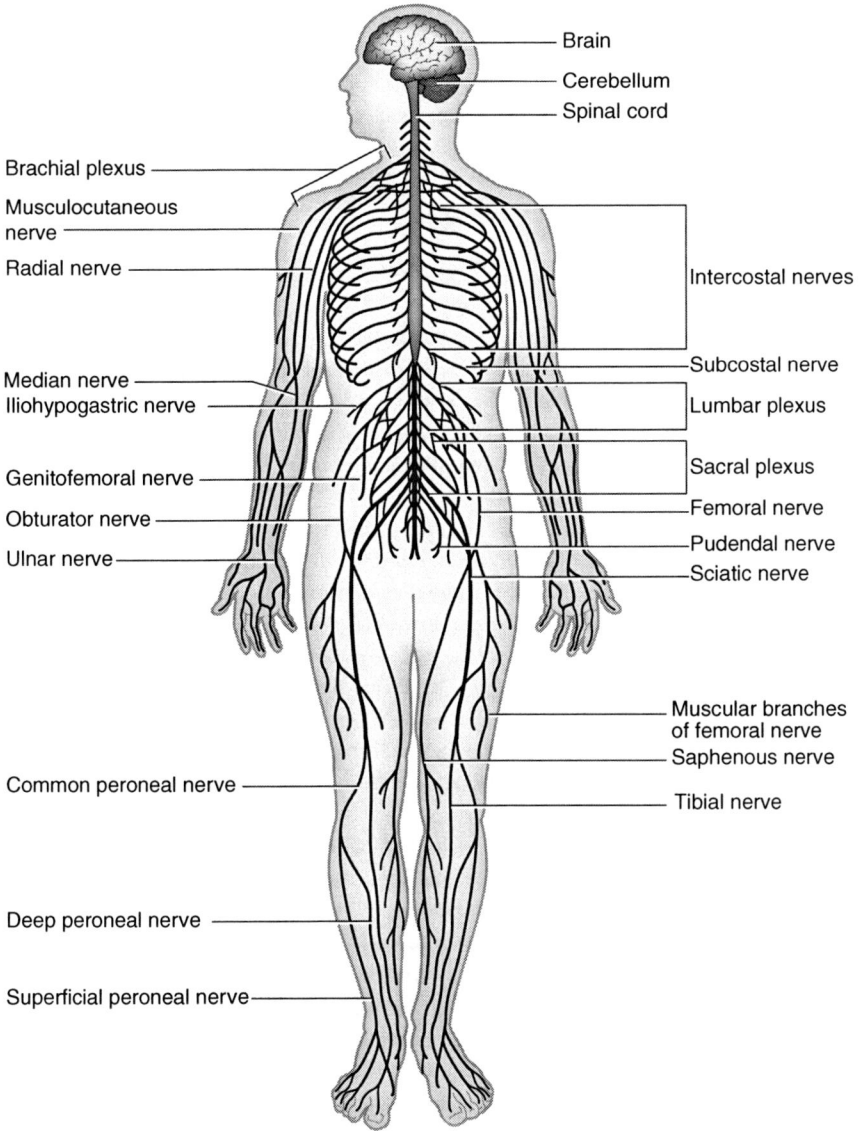

Figure 3.4   CNS in *red* and PNS in *blue.*

The C Fibers

These are primary afferent fibers, small in diameter, slow conducting (travel rate 2 m/s), and unmyelinated. They respond to a multitude of noxious stimuli such as chemical, thermal, and mechanical and are associated with aching, diffuse, dull, or burning quality of pain.

The A-Delta Fibers

These are primary afferent fibers, large in diameter, fast conducting (travel rate of 20 m/s), and myelinated. They respond only to mechanical stimuli over a specific intensity and are associated with a sharp, localized, and pricking quality of pain.

The Spinal and Medullary Dorsal Horn

The Dorsal Horn

The dorsal horn is the rostral projection of C and A-delta fiber afferents in *Lissauer's tract* (LT) which enter the spinal column, ascend or descend one or two spinal segments in this tract before penetrating the gray matter of the dorsal horn where they synapse on second-order neurons. The synapse is an important checkpoint in modulation of the nociceptive information and is affected by various biochemical excitatory or inhibitory substances (Zeilhofer 2005).

For A-delta fiber the neurotransmitter in the dorsal horn is glutamate acting on AMPA receptors. For C fiber, the neurotransmitter in the dorsal horn is glutamate along with certain peptides such as substance P and the receptors for glutamate are AMPA and *N*-methyl-D-aspartate (NMDA). NMDA receptors are stimulated by prolonged depolarization. Continual stimulation of C fibers cause excitation in the post synaptic neurons in the dorsal horn which is intensified by concurrent NMDA activity (Rygh et al. 2005).

Algesic or pain-producing substances include serotonin, histamine, prostaglandins, bradykinin, substance P, substance K, the amino acids glutamate and aspartate, calcitonin gene-related peptide, vasoactive intestinal peptide, cholecystokinin, adenosine triphosphate, and acetylcholine.

Analgesic or pain-inhibiting substances are inhibitory neuromediators and include the endogenous opioids (enkephalins, dynorphins, and beta-endorphins), somatostatin, serotonin, norepinephrine, gamma-aminobutyric acid, and neurotensin. Endogenous analgesics activate opioid, alpha-adrenergic, and other receptors that either inhibit release of Glu from primary nociceptive afferents or diminish postsynaptic responses of second-order neurons.

Histologically the gray matter of the spinal cord is divided into ten "laminae" (Fig. 3.5). The dorsal horn is divided into (I–V), components of which deal with most incoming pain fibres: *Lamina I*: posterior marginal nucleus, *Lamina II/III*: substantia gelatinosa, *Lamina III/IV/V*: nucleus proprius, *Lamina VI*: nucleus dorsalis. Lamina VII is in between these laminae and the more ventral Laminae VIII (motor interneurons) and IX (motor interneurons), and X refers to the gray matter around the central canal of the spinal cord.

Axons in LT once within the dorsal horn give off branches that contact neurons located in several of Rexed's laminae. The A-delta and the C fibers give branches to innervate neurons in Rexed's Laminae I and II. From Rexed's Lamina II the information is transmitted to second-order projection neurons in Laminae IV, V, and VI. The axons of these second-order neurons in Laminae IV–VI cross the midline and ascend into the brainstem and thalamus in the anterolateral quadrant of the contralateral half of the spinal cord. These fibers, together with axons from second-order Lamina I neurons, form the spinothalamic tract. This pathway is referred to as the *anterolateral system*.

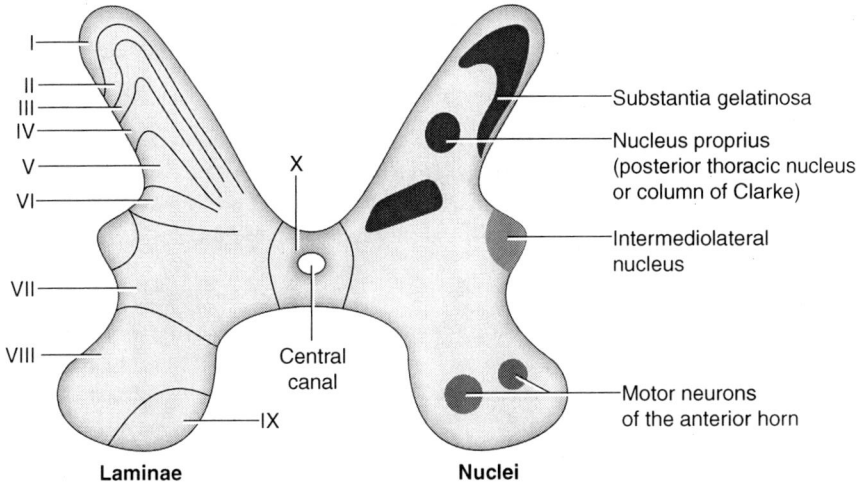

Figure 3.5 Histologically, the gray matter of the spinal cord is divided into ten "Laminae." The dorsal horn is divided into five Laminae (I–V), components of which deal with most incoming pain fibres: *Lamina I:* posterior marginal nucleus, *Lamina II/III:* substantia gelatinosa, *Lamina III/IV/V:* nucleus proprius, *Lamina VI:* nucleus dorsalis. *Laminae VII* is in between these laminae and the more ventral *Laminae VIII* (motor interneurons) and IX (motor interneurons), and X refers to the gray matter around the central canal of the spinal cord.

The Ascending System

The ascending system that transmits the nociceptive impulses from the dorsal horn to supraspinal targets is constituted from several systems, discussed in detail below:

1. The spinothalamic tract
2. The spinoreticular tract
3. The spinomesencephalic tract

Spinothalamic Tract

The spinothalamic tract (STT) is the major ascending pathway for information about pain, temperature, and "simple" touch and is localized in the anterolateral quadrant of the spinal cord. The STT mediates the discriminative components of these sensations into the "fast" (discriminative aspect) and "slow" (affective aspect) components of pain in different regions of the tract that are transmitted in parallel to the thalamus.

The STT is divided into the *lateral STT* (fast and slow pain and temperature) and the *anterior STT* (simple touch). The STT ascends the entire length of the cord and then enters the brainstem where the fast pain STT axons terminate in the ventroposterior nucleus. The slow pain STT axons terminate in the nonspecific intralaminar nuclei of the thalamus and the reticular formation in the brainstem, and these axons transmit information about the affective quality (unpleasantness and fear of further injury) of pain. The projections to the reticular formation are involved in the arousal effects of painful stimuli that activate noradrenergic neurons in the locus coeruleus and decrease the upward pain transmission by a negative feedback loop.

Spinoreticular Tract

The spinoreticular tract (SRT) ascends on both sides of the spinal cord and transmits sensory information from Laminae VII and VIII to neurons in reticular formation, which then project to intralaminar nuclei (part of paleospinothalamic tract). The SRT is involved in arousal and neural activity underlying the motivational and affective aspects of pain.

Spinomesencephalic Tract

The spinomesencephalic tract (SMT) arises from the Laminae I and V, courses through the medulla and pons with the STT and SRT and terminates in midbrain tectum and periaqueductal gray, where it integrates somatic sensation with visual and auditory information.

The Supraspinal System

The supraspinal system is involved in processing the nociceptive information and includes the reticular formation, thalamus, limbic system, cortex, and hypothalamus.

The neospinothalamic tract (nSTT), a component of the STT, is a direct relay to the ventrobasal group of the thalamus, whereas the paleospinothalamic tract (pSTT) has neurons with axons that form synaptic contact with medullary, pontine, midbrain and medial thalamic structures. The pSTT system produces a diffuse pain sensation that is difficult to localize, while the nSTT system permits perception of different types of pain and allows localization. Projections of the nSTT ascend directly and terminate within the ventroposterior lateral (VPL) and ventroposterior medial (VPM) regions of the neothalamus. The neothalamus is a highly somatotopically organized region. Axons from dorsal horn cells synapse with thalamic cells, which in turn transmit nociceptive impulses directly to the somatosensory cortex. This three-neuron pathway is responsible for rapid perception, localization, and prompt withdrawal from the noxious stimulus. Thalamo-cortical connections made other sites discriminative in terms of intensity and account for sensory qualities, such as throbbing or burning.

Distal projections of the pSTT contact neurons in medial thalamus. In contrast the VPL connections made in the medial thalamus are not somatotopically organized. Medial thalamic cells in turn project to the various regions in the limbic system including the amygdale, cingulate gyrus, and frontal cortex. Connections made within the limbic system are responsible for the suffering aspects of acute and persistent pain and the diffuse, unpleasant emotions that develop and persist long after an injury has occurred. Projections from the limbic cortex also activate motor cortex, hypothalamus, and pituitary gland. Connections to these areas mediate persistent supraspinal, hypothalamic, and pituitary effective responses that affect muscle tone, circulatory, respiratory, and endocrine functions.

Brain functional magnetic resonance imaging (fMRI) and positive emission tomography (PET) have helped clinicians better understand central sites of pain processing by revealing in real-time, discrete cortical and thalamic regions that are activated by noxious input. (Davis et al. 1997; Craig et al. 1996). Cortical pain processing may be divided into sensory-discriminative and affective-motivational components. The neocortical sensory-discriminative domain localizes the stimulus and determines its intensity. The limbic affective-motivational domain determines the unpleasantness and other qualities of pain. Connections made with cells in frontal cortex and amygdala also underlie emotional and behavioral responses such as fear, anxiety, helplessness, and learned avoidance.

Following standardized nociceptive stimulation and PET scan imaging, several well-connected regions in the CNS including the contralateral insula, secondary somatosensory cortex (SII), and the anterior cingulate cortex (ACC) were found to be consistently activated. Primary somatosensory cortex (SI), thalamus, brainstem, cerebellum, supplementary motor area, and the primary motor cortex are some of the other regions which become activated, but not as consistently as the insula and ACC.

In human studies of experimental electrical pain using fMRI, regional blood flow in the anterior cingulate gyrus, parieto-insular cortex, and somatosensory cortex was markedly increased. Increased blood flow in parieto-insular cortex corresponded to the physical sensation of pain and its intensity (pain thresholds). Activity in the cingulate cortex, specifically the dorsal anterior cingulate gyrus was related to the unpleasantness of pain and emotional affective responses to severe discomfort. The posterior aspect of the anterior cingulate gyrus is located in the medial frontal cortex and processes pain thresholds and affective components of pain such as its unpleasantness (Rainville et al. 1997). Sensory regions demonstrating opioid-induced metabolic suppression included the ipsilateral thalamus and amygdale, however, opioid binding and metabolic alterations were not observed in the primary sensory cortex.

Descending Pathways

Descending modulatory neural pathways function to reduce pain perception and efferent responses by inhibiting pain transmission in the dorsal horn, Periaqueductal gray (PAG), and brainstem rostral ventral medulla (RVM), and other regions of the CNS. The cerebral cortex, hypothalamus, thalamus, PAG, nucleus raphe magnus (NRM), and locus coeruleus (LC) all send descending axons that synapse with, and modulate pain transmission in, noxious cells located in the brainstem and spinal cord dorsal horn. Components of the descending system that play critical roles in modulating pain transmission include the previously mentioned endogenous opioid system, the descending noradrenergic system, and serotonergic neurons (Vanegas and Schaible 2004).

The PAG is an enkephalinergic brainstem nucleus responsible for both morphine-produced and stimulation-produced analgesias. Descending axons from the PAG project to nuclei in the reticular formation of the medulla, including NRM, and then descend to dorsal horn where they synapse with and inhibit wide dynamic range (WDR) and nervous system (NS) neurons. Axon terminals from NRM project to dorsal horn, where they release serotonin and norepinephrine (NE). Stimulation of the RVM activates the serotonergic system descending to the spinal dorsal horn resulting in analgesia. Although serotonin plays an important role in pain, the multiple subtypes of these receptors have confounded development of analgesics acting via these receptors. Axons descending from LC modulate nociceptive transmission in dorsal horn primarily via release of NE and activation of postsynaptic alpha 2-adrenergic receptors. The role of NE in this pathway explains the analgesic effects of tricyclic antidepressants and clonidine. GABAergic and enkephalinergic interneurons in the dorsal horn also provide local suppression of pain transmission. Descending inhibition is enhanced during periods of inflammation because of an overall increased descending inhibitory flow and increased sensitivity of neurons to descending noradrenergic and opioid-mediated inhibition. Unlike the other senses, pain has important subjective and emotional components. Outflow of descending inhibitory impulses from frontal cortex, cingulate gyrus, and hypothalamus contribute are influenced by the patient's psychological and emotional state. Anxiety, psychological stressors, and depression can reduce descending inhibition, thereby lowering the threshold for central sensitization and increasing pain intensity scores. Conversely, psychological support, including imagery, biofeedback, and music therapy can reduce pain intensity by either facilitating descending pathways or inhibiting cortical perception. This may explain the beneficial role of cognitive therapies, which marshal descending inhibitory mechanisms to reduce long-term synaptic strength in acute and persistent pain states.

Case Scenario

Sreekumar Kunnumpurath, MBBS, MD, FCARCSI, FRCA, FFPMRCA

Anita is a 28-year-old model with a very successful career. She has been living with her boyfriend, Leonardo, for the past 5 years. Through Leonardo, Anita has found the ultimate happiness in life and she is keen to keep this relationship forever. She decides to undergo laparoscopic-assisted tubal ligation. After careful evaluation and counseling, the surgeon decides to comply with Anita's wish and perform the procedure. You are the attending anesthesiologist involved with the case. The operation goes on without any glitch and completed in half an hour. You administer ketorolac and fentanyl as analgesics. At the end of the operation, the surgeon infiltrates abdominal incisions with bupivacaine at your request. You transfer Anita to the recovery room and hand her over to the recovery staff. Half an hour later you are called back to recovery: Anita is fully awake and in agony. When you see her in the PACU, she is thrashing about in her bed and screaming. She says that her pain is coming from her "tummy and chest."

What is your impression of Anita's pain?
She could be suffering from pain in three different anatomical locations due to three different physiological mechanisms. The pain might be coming from (1) visceral pain from the pelvics and from organs such as uterus, tubes, ovaries, or peritoneum; (2) somatic pain from the abdominal wound; (3) shoulder pain that is most likely a referred pain from the diaphragm due to distension from the collected CO_2 gas during laparoscopy.

Sometimes the diaphragmatic pain may be felt in the sub-phrenic region. It is also very important to make sure that the pain is not due to a serious complication of surgery such as injury to the internal organs or a major blood vessel.

How will you distinguish between these different types of pain?
Somatic pain is localized around the site of injury; visceral pain is poorly localized, cramp-like, or colicky in nature and could be associated with nausea and vomiting; diaphragmatic pain is characterized by its location and radiation to the shoulder.
A thorough clinical assessment could indicate the source of the pain. If you suspect visceral injury, you may have to order appropriate investigations such as a CT scan.

Somatic pain will respond to simple analgesics such as NSAIDS, and visceral pain responds well to appropriate dosing with opioids. Pain due to collections of gas under the diaphragm is common, and is best treated by implementing preventive measures such as completely suctioning out CO_2 at the end of the procedure, heating and humidifying the CO_2, or spraying local anesthetic aerosol inside the abdomen. Analgesia also can be provided by blocking nerve conduction using various local anesthetic agents alone or in combination with other pharmacological agents, and can be undertaken at various levels of the pain pathway. This involves a range of techniques from local infiltration to neuraxial blockade depending on the invasiveness of surgery performed. Pain is mediated by various physiologically active substances and pharmacological agents are available to counteract their effects, culminating in pain relief. The final perception of pain occurs at the cortical level and this is what ultimately matters in your final management of pain. It is essential to apply logic and knowledge in optimal proportions for successful, safe, and effective management of pain.

The pain from laparoscopic tubal ligation is usually of moderate intensity and Anita responds to further doses of opioid and ketorolac. She is discharged 2 days later. Three months after her surgery Anita is back to see you in the pain clinic. She has been referred to you by her primary care physician for the evaluation of a tender scar above the belly button. She tells you that the scar sometimes "burns". She mentions that ever since the laparoscopic her surgery, she has been suffering from severe and unbearable colicky pelvic pain radiating to her lower back. The pain comes during her mid-menstrual cycle. Anita is convinced that it is related to her ovulation. Her primary care physician has tried various analgesics and antidepressants without any benefit. Anita is concerned that her relationship with Leonardo is on the verge of breaking up. On examination you find that she has a very tender mass in the left iliac fossa.

What is your analgesic of choice for Anita? Since the pain is colicky in nature, would you prescribe an antispasmodic to treat the pain or would you inject her scar straight away? **You probably would not consider the last two options at this point. The clinical assessment is suggestive of a pelvic pathology. The presence of a possible organic intra-abdominal lesion may warrant an immediate surgical referral.** So you refer Anita to the surgeon who decides to do a diagnostic laparoscopy, which reveals a clip that had been applied onto the left ovary and which is now interfering with ovulation. There is also scarring and inflammation of this ovary. The surgeon removes the clip, releases the adhesions around the ovary, and performs the necessary repair. A few months later you inject the scar with local anesthetic and steroid with very good results. In about 6 months, Anita is pain-free.

References

Besson JM. Theneuro biology of pain. Lancet. 1999 May 8;353(9164):1610–5.

Craig AD, Reiman EM, Evans A, Bushnell MC. Functional imaging of an illusion of pain. Nature. 1996 Nov 21;384(6606):258–60.

Davis KD, Taylor SJ, Crawley AP, Wood ML, Mikulis DJ. Functional MRI of pain- and attention-related activations in the human cingulate cortex. J Neurophysiol. 1997 Jun;77(6):3370–80.

Rainville P, Duncan GH, Price DD, Carrier B, Bushnell MC. Pain affect encoded in human anterior cingulate but not somatosensory cortex. Science. 1997 Aug 15;277(5328):968–71.

Rygh LJ, Svendsen F, Fiska A, Haugan F, Hole K, Tjolsen A. Long-term potentiation in spinal nociceptive systems – how acute pain may become chronic. Psychoneuroendocrinology. 2005 Nov;30(10):959–64.

Vanegas H, Schaible HG. Descending control of persistent pain: inhibitory or facilitatory? Brain Res Rev. 2004 Nov;46(3):295–309.

Zeilhofer HU. Synaptic modulation in pain pathways. Rev Physiol Biochem Pharmacol. 2005;154:73–100.

Chapter 4

Acute and Chronic Mechanisms of Pain

Amit Mirchandani, MD, Marianne Saleeb, MD, and Raymond Sinatra, MD

Introduction

Pain is defined by the International Association for the Study of Pain as "an unpleasant sensory and emotional experience associated with actual or potential tissue damage." Caregivers involved in pain management suggest that pain and the intensity of discomfort are whatever the patient states and should be managed accordingly.

In addition to reducing discomfort and suffering, inadequate treatment of acute pain can increase morbidity, delay recovery, and increase medical costs of post-surgical patients, as well as lead to the development of chronic pain. In this chapter, we will outline the basic anatomy of the pain pathway, identifying key neurochemical mediators along the way. In addition, we will highlight important physiological processes which drive the transition from acute to chronic pain. In order to optimally administer analgesics and improve acute and chronic pain management, the caregiver must appreciate the anatomy and physiology of pain transmission and processing, in addition to the humanitarian responsibility.

Classification of Pain

Pain is a complicated physiological process that can be classified in terms of its duration, etiology, and physiology. Acute pain, which usually follows trauma to tissue, is limited in duration and is associated with temporal reductions in intensity. In contrast, chronic pain is of longer duration, often 3–6 months longer than expected. Chronic pain often has an unclear etiology and its prognosis is more unpredictable when compared to acute pain. Although acute pain and chronic pain have distinguishing characteristics, there is often overlap, making the diagnosis and management of pain challenging. Table 4.1 highlights some of these characteristics.

The etiologic classification of pain refers to the clinical context in which pain perception takes place. Thus, pain can be categorized as benign or adaptive, malignancy related, post-surgical, or degenerative. Identifying the etiology of pain is valuable in predicting prognosis and personalizing a patient's treatment strategy. For instance, a patient suffering from terminal pancreatic cancer may call for increasingly aggressive narcotic treatment with less concern for narcotic dependence and more concern for patient comfort.

N. Vadivelu et al. (eds.), *Essentials of Pain Management*,
DOI 10.1007/978-0-387-87579-8_4, © Springer Science+Business Media, LLC 2011

Table 4.1 Pain characteristics: Acute vs. Chronic

Acute pain	Chronic pain
1. Usually obvious tissue damage	1. Multiple causes (malignancy, benign)
2. Distinct onset	2. Gradual or distinct onset
3. Short, well-characterized duration	3. Persists after 3–6 months of healing
4. Resolves with healing	4. Can be a symptom or diagnosis
5. Serves a protective function	5. Serves no adaptive purpose
6. Effective therapy is available	6. May be refractory to treatment

Physiologic pain is defined as rapidly perceived non-traumatic discomfort of very short duration, alerting the individual of a dangerous stimulus. This is adaptive and initiates the withdrawal reflex that prevents and/or minimizes tissue injury.

Physiologic pain can be divided into neuropathic pain and nociceptive pain. Nociceptive pain can be further divided into somatic and visceral pain. Neuropathic pain results from irritation or damage to nerves. It is usually characterized as burning, electrical, and/or shooting in nature. However, a common characteristic of neuropathic pain is the paradoxical coexistence of sensory *deficits* in the setting of increased painful sensation.

Nociceptive pain is defined as noxious perception resulting from actual tissue damage following surgical, traumatic, or disease-related injuries. This pain is detected by specialized transducers called nociceptors, which are the peripheral endings of A-delta (Aδ) and C fibers. Nociceptive pain involves peripheral inflammation and the release of inflammatory mediators, which play a major role in its initiation and development.

Somatic nociceptive pain is well-localized sharp, crushing, or tearing pain that usually follows a dermatomal pattern and often occurs after mechanical trauma. In contrast, visceral nociceptive pain is poorly localized dull, cramping, or colicky pain generally associated with peritoneal irritation, dilation of smooth muscle, or tubular passages. Visceral pain radiating in a somatic dermatomal pattern is described as referred pain. Differences between the physiologic, neuropathic, and nociceptive pain are described in Table 4.2.

Table 4.2 Differences between the physiologic, nociceptive/inflammatory, neuropathic, and mixed pain.

Category	Cause	Symptoms	Examples
Physiologic	Brief exposure to a noxious stimulus	Rapid, yet brief pain perception	Touching a pin or hot object
Nociceptive/inflammatory	Somatic or visceral tissue injury with mediators impacting on intact nervous tissue	Moderate to severe pain, described as crushing or stabbing; usually worsens after the first 24 h	Surgical pain, traumatic pain, sickle cell crisis
Neuropathic	Damage or dysfunction of peripheral nerves or CNS	Severe lancinating, burning, or electrical shock-like pain	Neuropathy, chronic regional pain syndrome, post-herpetic, neuralgia
Mixed	Combined somatic and nervous tissue injury	Combinations of symptoms; soft tissue pain plus radicular pain	Low back pain, back surgery pain

Qualitative Aspects of Pain Perception

Appreciating the clinical features of the different types of pain not only helps to properly classify pain and its etiology, but also guide the often complex multimodal medical management that accompanies pain management. The health care provider must be detailed in attaining the qualitative factors and history associated with a patient's pain. Table 4.3 outlines the qualitative aspects of pain perception.

Table 4.3   Qualitative aspects of pain perception.

Temporal	Onset and duration
Variability	Constant, effort-dependent, waxing and waning, episodic "flare"
Intensity	Average pain, worst pain, least pain, pain with activity of living
Topography	Focal, dermatomal, diffuse, referred, superficial, deep
Character	Sharp, aching, cramping, stabbing, burning, shooting
Exacerbating/relieving	Worse at rest, with movement or no difference
Quality of life	Interfere with movement, ambulation, daily life tasks, work, etc.

The Pain Pathway—The Initial Insult

After having discussed the subjective qualities and different classification of pain, we will spend the core of this chapter discussing the pain pathway from the periphery to actual perception of pain which takes place at the level of the cerebral cortex.

The pain pathway begins with the activation of peripheral nociceptors. Nociceptors are located anywhere in the body and convey noxious sensation, either externally (i.e., skin, mucosa) or internally (i.e., joints, intestines). Nociceptors can be triggered by any painful stimuli, most of which can be categorized as either mechanical, chemical, or thermal in nature. Nociceptors are classified by the specific stimulus they respond to (i.e., "thermal nociceptor") and have a sensory specificity. Therefore, they will only be activated and an action potential when a certain threshold has been reached.

Transduction refers to the process in which noxious stimuli, chemical, thermal, or mechanical, are translated into electrical activity at the level of the nociceptors. The cell bodies of these nociceptors are found in the dorsal root ganglia (DRG) of the spinal cord. After the sensory threshold has been reached, nociceptor activation initiates a depolarizing Ca^{2+} current or generator potential, which depolarizes the distal axon and further initiates an inward Na^+ current which self-propagates action potential. In addition, following the initial insult, or tissue injury, several cellular mediators activate the terminal endings of the nociceptors such as potassium, hydrogen ions, prostaglandins, and bradykinin. Prostaglandin (PGE), which is synthesized by cyclooxygenase-2 (COX-2), is responsible for nociceptor sensitization and plays an important role in peripheral inflammation. Action potential through sensitized nociceptors also leads to the release of several peptides in and around the site of injury. These include substance P (sP), cholecytokinin (CCK), and calcitonin gene-related peptide (CGRP). Substance P is responsible for the further release of bradykinin and also fuels the release of histamine from mast cells and serotonin (5-HT) from platelets, which further increases vascular permeability and nociceptor irritability (Wang et al. 2005). The interactions of the mediators and peptides that are released during transduction exacerbate the inflammatory response, recruit adjacent nociceptors, and result in peripheral nociceptor sensitization (Treed et al. 1992).

Conduction

Pain stimuli are conducted from peripheral nociceptors to the dorsal horn via both unmyelinated and myelinated fibers. Nociceptive nerve fibers are classified according to their degree of myelination, diameter, and conduction velocity. Nociceptors have two different types of axons that transmit pain impulses to the dorsal root ganglion. The first are the Ad-fiber axons. These axons are myelinated and allow action potentials to travel at a very fast rate of approximately 20 m/s toward the central nervous system (CNS). The other type is the more slowly conducting non-myelinated C-fiber axons. These only conduct at speeds of about 2 m/s. Thus, in the classic example of touching a hot stove, the Aδ fibers transmit the "first pain," a rapid onset well-localized, sharp pain of short duration while the C fibers are responsible for the "second pain" or delayed pain. Second pain is associated with a delayed latency and is described as a diffuse burning, stabbing sensation that is often prolonged and may become progressively worse.

Transmission

Transmission refers to the transfer of noxious stimuli from primary nociceptors in the periphery to cell bodies in the spinal cord dorsal horn. As described above, Aδ and C fibers are the axons of unipolar neurons that have distal projections known as nociceptive endings. After the synapse in the dorsal root, the second-order neurons send their signals contralaterally and upward through the spinothalamic tract. The signals of the spinothalamic tract travel up the spinal cord through the medulla and synapse on neurons in the thalamus. Nerves from the thalamus then relay the signal to various areas of the somatosensory cortex, where pain perception takes place. Glutamate, the excitatory amino acid implicated in transmission from primary afferent nociceptors to dorsal horn neurons, has a number of receptors [amino-3-hydroxyl-5-methyl-4-propionic acid (AMPA), kainate, N-methyl-D-aspartate (NMDA), and metabotropic] it activates. The various combinations of these receptors exist on neurons in various laminae of the dorsal horn.

Modulation

Modulation describes inhibitory and facilitatory effects of spinal interneurons on noxious transmission. In other words, modulation can be described as manipulating a noxious stimulus so it is perceived as a pain-suppressive transmission. This occurs at higher levels of the brainstem and midbrain. It is accomplished by an electrical or pharmacological stimulation of certain regions of the midbrain producing relief of pain. Not all analgesics are exogenous. Since opioid receptors in the brain are unlikely to exist for the purpose of responding to the administration of opium and its derivatives, then it must be *endogenous* compounds for which these receptors had evolved. Endogenous analgesics, including enkephalin (ENK), norepinephrine (NE), and gamma-aminobutyric acid (GABA) activate opioid, alpha-adrenergic, and other receptors that either inhibit release of glutamate from primary nociceptors or diminish post-synaptic responses of second-order neurons.

Ascending and Descending Pathways

Several ascending tracts are responsible for transmitting nociceptive impulses from the dorsal horn to supraspinal targets. Of these, the spinothalamic tract is considered the primary perception pathway.

The descending pathways originate in the somatosensory cortex, which relays to the thalamus and the hypothalamus. Thalamic neurons descend to the midbrain. There, these neurons synapse on ascending pathways in the medulla and spinal cord and inhibit ascending nerve signals, producing an analgesic effect which comes from the stimulation of endogenous endorphins, dynorphins, and enkephalins. The extent of autonomic responses to pain (tachypnea, tachycardia, hypertension, diaphoresis, etc.) can be depressed in the cortex through descending pathways. Of interest, the influences of the descending pathways may also be responsible for psychogenic pain (pain perception that has no obvious physical cause).

Transition from Acute to Persistent Pain

Neural plasticity, "the capacity of neurons to change their function, chemical profile, or structure," is the basis for learning and memory and is also responsible for alterations in noxious perception. More so, neural plasticity underlies peripheral and central sensitization. The sensitization theory of pain perception suggests that brief high-intensity noxious stimulation in the absence of tissue injury activates the nociceptive endings of unmyelinated or thinly myelinated (high-threshold) fibers, resulting in physiologic pain perception of short duration. Other low-threshold sensory modalities (pressure, vibration, touch) are carried by larger-caliber (low-threshold) fibers. Large and small fibers make contact with second-order neurons in the dorsal horn (Woolf and Mannion 1999).

Following tissue injuries and release of noxious mediators, peripheral nociceptors become sensitized and fire repeatedly. Peripheral sensitization occurs in the presence of inflammatory mediators, which in turn increases the sensitivity of high-threshold nociceptors as well as the peripheral terminals of other sensory neurons. This increase in nociceptor sensitivity, lowering of the pain threshold, and exaggerated response to painful and non-painful stimuli is termed primary hyperalgesia.

The ongoing barrage of noxious impulses sensitizes second-order transmission neurons in the dorsal horn via a process termed windup. This creates several problems, including sprouting of Wide Dynamic Range (WDR) neurons and induction of glutamate-dependent N-methyl-D-aspartate (NMDA) receptors.

The NMDA receptor is an important four-subunit, voltage-gated, ligand-specific ion channel. Glutamate is the primary agonist of the NMDA receptor and therefore, the primary excitatory agonist for noxious transmission. Glutamate binding to NMDA receptors sustains an inward Ca^{2+} flux. Second messengers are then upregulated, which slowly prime and maintain excitability of these NMDA receptors. These changes increase neuronal excitability and underlie subsequent plasticity. The NMDA receptor appears to be responsible for not only amplifying pain, but also causing opioid tolerance.

As pain signals continue to enter the dorsal horn and synapse with the nerve cell bodies, WDR neurons can be found in areas of the dorsal horn, where they were not previously located. Specifically, they grow into the areas where pain-receiving nerve cell bodies are located. WDR neurons can experience a broad range of stimulating signals and pass these on to the brain or spinal cord. Once C-nociceptive fibers are activated and continue to over-whelm the nerve cells in the dorsal horn, Aβ touch sensitive fibers begin to fire and this affects nerve cell bodies in the DRG and the dorsal horn. Glutamate, an extremely fast neuro-transmitter, is released at the DRG presynaptic membrane and attaches to non-NMDA nerve cell receptors in the dorsal horn. After continued bombardment by C fibers and Aβ fibers the magnesium ion, which normally prevents NMDA post-synaptic receptors from receiving glutamate, is displaced and a process known as "windup" begins. Due to ongoing pain signals reaching and being amplified at the dorsal horn, the nerve cells begin to increase the num-ber of NMDA receptors at the post-synaptic membrane. This further increases windup and exhibits increased tolerance to opioids.

"Windup" is a term used to describe the process of increased central sensitization of the body's pain pathways in response to sustained input from nociceptive afferents. Central sensitization results in secondary hyperalgesia and the spread of the hyperalgesic area to nearby uninjured tissues. Inhibitory interneurons and descending inhibitory fibers modulate and suppress spinal sensitization, whereas analgesic under medication and poorly controlled pain favors sensitization. In certain settings, central sensitization may then lead to neuro-chemical/neuroanatomical changes (plasticity), prolonged neuronal discharge and sensitivity (windup), and the development of chronic pain. Activation of spinal and supraspinal NMDA receptors and increased Ca^{2+} ion influx are major requisites for the development of cen-tral sensitization. It is the sensitization of CNS neurons that underlies the transition from acute to persistent pain. Excitatory neurotransmitters are believed to cause spinal cord hyper-sensitivity to nociceptive inputs from the periphery. Excitotoxicity defines the pathological alterations observed in nerve cells stimulated by overactivation of NMDA.

There are certain mediators responsible for central sensitization and associated plastic-ity changes. Inflow of Ca^{2+} ions initiates the upregulation of COX-2, nitric oxide systems (NOS), and second messengers that initiate transcriptional and translational changes. Central sensitization can be divided into transcription-dependent and transcription-independent processes. Transcription-independent sensitization reflects neurochemical and electrical alterations that follow acute traumatic injury. It includes stimulus-dependent neuronal depolarization and stimulus-independent long-term potentiation. Windup is a form of transcription-independent central sensitization (Woolf 1983).

Transcription-dependent sensitization describes delayed-onset, long-lasting, noxious facilitation that follows genomic activation, transcription of messenger RNA (mRNA), and subsequent translational modifications. Following transcription of mRNA, inducible enzymes and reactive proteins are synthesized that mediate neuroanatomical and neu-ropathologic plasticity (Ji and Woolf 2001).

Opioid-induced hyperalgesia is a process that is associated with the long-term use of opioids for pain management. Opioid-induced hyperalgesia is a clinical picture which is characterized by increasing pain in patients who are receiving increasing doses of opioids. With time, individuals using opioids can develop an increasing sensitivity to noxious stimuli, sometimes even staging a painful response to non-noxious stimuli. Therefore, patients given opioids for acute pain may have a paradoxical increase in pain. Opioid-induced hyperalgesia is a result of glutamate-associated activation that occurs at the level of the NMDA recep-tor in the dorsal horn of the spinal cord. There is evidence that NMDA antagonists, such as ketamine, have a role in preventing opioid-induced hyperalgesia.

Conclusion

Understanding pain pathways and pain processing is the key to the optimal management of both acute and chronic pain. Our understanding of pain perception is evolving as we now recognize that humoral factors as well as neural transmission are responsible for the activation and sensitization of regions involved in pain perception, suffering, and avoidance behavior. Although acute pain initiates withdrawal reflexes that minimize further tissue injury, chronic pain serves no adaptive benefit and can lead to long-term disability. Chronic pain is persistent and reflects altered neural transmission as well as long-term plasticity changes in the peripheral and central nervous systems. Preventing these alterations by employing a balanced multimodal analgesic approach, using functional MRI (fMRI) to measure and correct alterations in CNS activity, and aggressive physical therapy and rehabilitation may reduce the transition from acute to chronic pain.

Case Scenario

Manoj Narayan Ravindran, MD

Andreas, a 35 year old marine, was leading a night patrol in the battlefield. He stepped over a land mine and sustained a blast injury to his right leg. The blast shattered the bones of his leg and feet and produced extensive damage to soft tissues. After the initial resuscitation at the frontline he was airlifted to the regional command hospital. He is now awaiting urgent surgery and having a lot of pain. As an anesthesiologist, you are requested to see him to provide effective pain relief. He is otherwise a healthy man with no significant past medical history.

What is the mechanism of acute pain in Andreas?
Andreas's pain has resulted from traumatic injury to foot and is thus an example of nociceptive pain. This pain results from the release of inflammatory mediators at the site of trauma and their stimulation of the peripheral pain receptors called nociceptors. The pain sensation is then carried to central nervous system by Aδ and C fibers. These fibers first synapse in the thalamus and then the sensory cortex.

How would you deal with his acute pain?
It is important to first determine the full medical history, drug history and find out any drug allergies that may be present. In this situation it is difficult to follow the WHO pain ladder. **Andreas needs strong opioid analgesics. Though we can supplement this with acetaminophen, using NSAIDS in hypovolemic patients with major trauma should be done with care as there is risk of renal toxicity and platelet dysfunction.** Adding weak opioids is another option. Neuraxial block can provide good quality analgesia, though this could prove risky in the presence of hypovolemia and coagulopathy.

How do these drugs relieve acute pain?
NSAIDs are used to overcome mild to moderate pain. **They act by preventing the production of prostaglandins and thromboxanes by inhibiting the enzyme cyclooxygenase.** This translates into reduction of inflammatory mediators such as prostaglandins.

The exact mechanism of action of acetaminophen is still not entirely understood. Its antipyretic action is thought to be due to **inhibition of prostaglandin synthesis in the central nervous system.**

Opioids are very effective analgesics because of their affinity for the opioid receptors. The opioid receptors are divided into mu-1 (μ1), mu-2, kappa (κ) and delta (δ) receptors. Mu-1 receptors are mainly involved in analgesia and euphoria, while mu-2 cause respiratory depression and inhibition of gut mobility. Kappa receptors are associated with spinal analgesia, meiosis and sedation, whereas delta receptors cause respiratory depression, physical dependence and analgesia. Opioid receptors activate G1 proteins and cause hyperpolarization of the cell membrane.

Could you suggest an intervention to block the transmission of nociceptive impulses in the above situation?
A combined femoral and sciatic nerve block using catheters could be used. This technique can provide adequate acute pain relief. It has the advantage of being useful in providing adequate surgical anesthesia even during a limb salvage operation which Andreas might be undergoing.

Andreas undergoes extensive limb salvage surgery and after evaluation of the clinical situation, you decide to err on the side of caution and administer morphine PCA along with acetaminophen for pain relief; you also prescribe tramadol as needed. Andrea's pain is now reasonably well-controlled. Unfortunately, over the following week the limb became unsalvageable due to infection. His surgeon decides that amputation is the best option and hence takes him to the operating room for a below-the-knee amputation. Andreas is worried about phantom limb pain, as he has heard dreadful stories about it.

What is phantom limb pain?
Phantom limb is **a type of chronic pain. It results in a sensation that an amputated limb is still attached to the body. More than half of amputees experience some phantom sensation in their amputated limb, with pain being the most common sensation.** It is most common if amputation is delayed after initial injury and it is more common in arm amputations. The perceived limb may be felt to be in an abnormal position.

Could you elaborate on the mechanism of phantom limb pain?
The exact mechanism is still unknown. Various theories that have been suggested to explain this, including abnormal re-growth of nerve endings in the stump of the amputated limb. These nerve endings then cause altered and painful discharges, leading to phantom limb pain. There is also possibility of altered nervous activity in the spinal cord and brain in these patients.

Is there any way of preventing this?
Effective control of pain before amputation can prevent dorsal root sensitization and help prevent or reduce severity of phantom limb pain. For this reason patients are

routinely prescribed opioids, anti-depressants, and anti-convulsants. Ketamine, which is an NMDA receptor antagonist, also has been tried for this purpose. Use of epidural analgesia before the actual amputation has been claimed to prevent the development of phantom limb pain.

List the various forms of treatments available for phantom limb pain?

Traditional treatment options include:

- Simple analgesics
- Anti-convulsants and anti-depressants, e.g. phenytoin, carbamazapine and gabapentin.
- TENS
- Dorsal column stimulation
- Injection around the stump neuroma with local anesthetic and depot steroid, if pain is thought to be due to neuroma in the stump.
- Prosthetic assessment: a correct fitting prosthesis may help phantom limb pain due to stump neuroma.
- Surgery to refashion the stump is advised if the pain is thought to be due to the presence of neuroma in the stump, close to weight-bearing area when a prosthesis is used.
- Acupuncture, hypnosis
- Biofeedback

Other options include:

- Mirror box: Ramchandran et al, found that stimulation of the motor cortex can help reduce phantom limb pain. In this study patients were asked to put their normal limb in a mirror box, so that they saw their normal limbs mirror-reversed to look like their amputated limb. When they moved their normal limb in the mirror box, their brains were fooled to believe that they were moving their amputated limb – this helped to reduce pain.
- Merely getting patients to imagine their paralyzed arms moving in relation to a moving arm on a screen in front of them can relieve phantom limb pain.
- Virtual reality: By attaching an interface to the patient's amputated limb, the amputee is able to see both of his limbs being moved in a computer generated simulation – this also has been shown to relieve phantom limb pain.

Cite the key differences between acute and chronic pain?
Acute pain occurs at the time of injury and disappears once the healing process is complete. It protects the body from further harm. The mechanism involved in acute pain is better understood. Whereas in the case of chronic pain, the onset is delayed and pain persists long after the healing process is completed; does not serve any perceived usefulness. It is different in character, mechanism and therapeutic options.

Andreas undergoes amputation under general anaesthesia and he continues on his PCA and other medication. Luckily, he does not experience the dreaded phantom limb pain which you attribute to your effective preoperative pain relief.

References

Ji RR, Woolf CJ. Neuronal plasticity and signal transduction in nociceptive neurons: implications or the initiation and maintenance of pathological pain. Neurobiol Dis. 2001;8(1):1–10.

Treed RD, Meyer RA, Raja SN, Campbell JN. Peripheral and ventral mechanisms of cutaneous hyperalgesia. Prog Neurobiol. 1992;38(4):397–421.

Wang H, Kohno T, Amaya F, et al. Bradykinin produces pain hypersensitivity by potentiation spinal cord glutamatergic synaptic transmission. J Neurosci. 2005;25(35):7986–92.

Woolf CJ. Evidence for a central component of post-injury pain hypersensitivity. Nature. 1983;306(5944):686–88.

Woolf CJ, Mannion RJ. Neuropathic pain: etiology, symptoms, mechanisms, and management. Lancet. 1999;353(9168):1959–64.

Section III

Clinical Principles

Chapter 5

Assessment of Pain: Complete Patient Evaluation

Amitabh Gulati, MD and Jeffrey Loh, MD

Introduction

Throughout history, physicians believed that the perception of pain could be explained by a single, simplified physiologic pathway (Loeser et al. 2001a). Their theories described pain as its own sensory apparatus, independent of touch and other senses, or as a result of excessive stimulation from the touch sensation. While the exact mechanisms were unknown, most physicians agreed that pain required a triggering stimulus and that removal of the stimulus should relieve pain. More recently, practitioners focus on pain that occurs during the absence of tissue damage or other organic pathology. While most pain experienced may have an initial inciting event, continuation of pain after removal of the stimulus indicates that many factors and biological pathways interact to cause the sensation of pain. Hence, the initial assessment of an individual's pain is important in determining the underlying cause and the possible treatments available for that individual (Loeser et al. 2001b, c; Garratt et al. 1993).

History of Present Illness
The Basics of History Taking

To accurately determine the cause of an individual's pain, physicians need an initial assessment including a thorough history and physical (Harden and Bruehl 2006). Physicians can differentiate pain into acute and chronic, malignant and non-malignant, somatic and neuropathic, but because management strategies may differ, accurate assessment of an individual's pain complaint is essential for formulating treatment plan.

While many lab tests and diagnostic studies help aid in the diagnosis of an individual's pain, initial history often plays the most important role in the evaluation of that individual. Most experienced clinicians rely on a detailed history obtained from a patient in order to successfully arrive at a diagnosis that can explain the individual's pain.

While taking a patient's history, the physician should avoid a hasty interaction. This legitimizes the patient's concerns and ultimately strengthens the patient–physician relationship. While the natural tendency for interviewing a patient is to follow a stereotyped form or a list of questions, each patient brings a unique history. As such, each patient should tell his/her own story, while the physician obtains a complete, logical, and well-organized history.

N. Vadivelu et al. (eds.), *Essentials of Pain Management*,
DOI 10.1007/978-0-387-87579-8_5, © Springer Science+Business Media, LLC 2011

Detailed information about the onset of a patient's pain is essential to help determine the underlying cause. Information regarding the precise start of the pain, circumstances surrounding the cause, the location, distribution, quality, intensity or severity, and duration should all be ascertained. The patient should also be questioned about any sensory, motor, or autonomic disturbances around the initial time of the injury as disorders such as complex regional pain syndrome is often associated with these types of disturbances. After describing the patient's initial onset of pain, information should then be gathered about the patient's subsequent pain state. Has the pain or location changed over time are important questions.

Because a patient may visit multiple doctors prior to seeing a pain specialist that individual may have tried many medication regimens. Physicians must be aware of therapies which were effective and alternatives not used. Accordingly, interventional and surgical procedures should be discussed before deciding on a pain treatment plan. If a certain medication or procedure relieved aspects of a patient's initial pain that information may lead to future therapies for the patient.

Focusing on both alleviating and aggravating factors of a patient's pain complaint often proves beneficial. Factors that could potentially affect one's pain, such as emotional disturbances, exercise, pressure, temperature, sneezing, and straining, should be investigated and recorded. Questions about the effect of one's pain on his/her daily life should also be asked, including the effect of pain on a patient's ability to perform activities and to sleep. All these discussions help a physician tailor an appropriate pain treatment regimen.

Pain History

When determining the characteristic of one's pain, descriptive questions should be asked of the patient's pain. Specifically, the physician should explore the quality, duration, location, exacerbating factors, and mechanism of injury in regard to a patient's pain.

Quality

Determining the quality of pain helps to deduce whether one's pain is superficial or deep. Questions should be asked about the specific characteristics of the pain, whether it is sharp, dull, or burning in nature. Superficial lesions will likely be sharp, burning, and well localized, whereas pain caused by deep somatic or visceral disease may be dull, diffuse, and poorly localizable. To better understand the severity behind a patient's pain, descriptive scales are effective.

Various patterns also help distinguish different pain states. For example, tic douloureux will often present as a brief flash, while inflammatory pain or migraines will demonstrate a rhythmic nature. Unfortunately, the quality of many patients' pain description varies, blurring the boundaries between whether the pain is due to a somatic, visceral, or neuropathic process.

Duration and Periodicity

To determine the duration and temporal characteristics regarding one's pain, the patient should be asked whether the pain is continuous, intermittent, pulsatile, or characterized by a wavelike rise and fall in intensity. Some physicians advocate the use of time–intensity curves to characterize how the pain starts, the rapidity with which it increases, the duration, and the manner by which the pain declines (Fig. 5.1). Additionally, the relationship of the pain

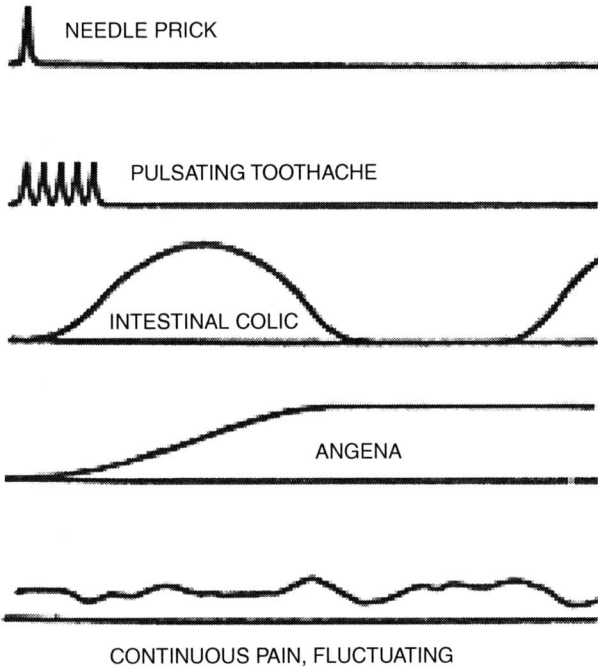

Figure 5.1   Time–intensity curve.

to a time-point (day, week, and season) or to a stressor (emotional or environmental) also provides vital information to the cause of an individual's pain.

Location and Distribution

While pain arising from a peripheral source is highly localizable, pain that arises from a deep somatic or visceral structure may be elusive to locate. Visceral pain can often be referred. For example, kidney pathology may cause pain in the inguinal or testicular area. Thus, depending on location and involvement of neural signaling of the injury, a patient's pain may range from a precise location to whole body pain.

When determining the location and distribution of an individual's pain, the classification of the pain as localized, projected, referred, of sympathetic distribution, or psychogenic nature proves helpful. Localized pain, as described by its name, remains confined to its site of origin. This type of pain does not tend to radiate to any other locations, and presentations of this pain can range from cutaneous hyperalgesia to deep tenderness. Examples of localized pain include arthritis, tendinitis, and incisional scar pain.

Projected pain, otherwise known as transmitted or transferred pain, is perceived by the patient as traveling along the course of a nerve or a peripheral distribution. An example of projected pain with a segmental distribution is radicular pain, which can be caused by either infectious etiologies like herpes zoster, or other processes involving the nerve root or nerve trunk, like a herniated disk. Examples of projected pain with peripheral distribution include trigeminal neuralgia, brachial plexus neuralgia, and meralgia paresthetica.

Referred pain is the result of pain originating from a deep somatic or visceral structure correlating with pain in a distant region due to nervous innervations from the same segment. Descriptions of this pain can include hyperalgesia, hyperesthesia, deep tenderness, muscle spasm, and autonomic disturbances. However, no changes should be seen with reflexes or muscle strength. Examples of referred pain include diaphragmatic pain presenting as shoulder pain or appendiceal pain initially presenting as epigastric pain.

Unlike the previously described locations of pain, reflex sympathetic pain does not conform to any segmental or peripheral nerve distribution or to any other recognizable pattern. Reflex sympathetic pain tends to be associated with hyperalgesia, hyperesthesia, and vasomotor and trophic changes. This pain has now been labeled as complex regional pain syndromes (CRPS) types I and II and may incorporate sympathetically mediated (vs. independent) pain.

Furthermore, psychological and psychiatric disorders may cause pain states that are difficult to localize with history taking (Schaffer et al. 1980). Examples of psychological or psychiatric pain include pain involving the entire body or pain scattered all over the body. To properly use the diagnostic term of psychogenic or psychiatric pain, the physician must have positive findings suggesting that mental processes are the sole cause of the patient's complaints (Bair et al. 2003). It is important to realize that psychological causes of pain are not a diagnosis of exclusion but supported with the history and physical examination (Magni et al. 1985).

Exacerbating and Relieving Symptoms

Exacerbating and alleviating mechanical factors, such as different positions or postures, sitting, standing, walking, bending, and lifting, all help to further delineate pain states. In addition, psychological questions about depression, stress, or emotional issues should be investigated. Furthermore, questions regarding the effects of biochemical changes (e.g., electrolyte abnormalities, hormonal imbalances) and environmental triggers (e.g., dietary influences, weather changes) also provide important diagnostic clues, and as previously discussed, medications and procedures all help determine what may effectively treat the patient's pain.

Past Medical/Surgical History

The past medical history helps provide insight into the general health of the patient before the onset of his/her current pain as well as determine if the patient has suffered from previous pain issues. The past medical/surgical history includes periods of disability, operations, injuries, and accidents sustained, with their duration, nature, and sequelae recorded. The past medical history provides an opportunity to ensure that pertinent information is not overlooked.

By having a good understanding of an individual's medical history, the physician is able to understand the patient's expectations during the treatment phase. Compared to patients with multiple medical issues, patients with few medical complaints are more likely to improve with effective therapy. In addition, by having a good knowledge of a patient's co-morbidities, a physician can develop a therapeutic strategy which will not jeopardize a patient's health.

Medications

A list of all medications, pain related or not, should be documented. Usually overlooked, holistic treatments and herbal medications must also be discussed. While going over a patient's medication history, the physician should determine which treatments the patient is willing to use, whether westernized or alternative. The practitioner should also analyze the negative or positive interactions of different medications as well as monitor any potential adverse reactions.

Allergies
Allergies, both to medications and non-medications, should be noted as part of the initial evaluation. Based on the patient's allergy profile, certain medications for the treatment of patient's pain will be indicated or contradicted.

Family History
Information about the health of parents and siblings offers important clues about the patient's genetic profile. Evidence of unusual disorder or disabilities in parents or siblings helps elucidate possible causes of a patient's pain. The family history also provides insight into any history of chronic pain or substance abuse, which should alert the physician to medication or prescription abuse.

Social History
The social history provides valuable insight into the patient's social structure, coping mechanisms, and support systems (Jamison and Virts 1990). A history of substance abuse, employment issues, or family difficulties affects an individual's ability to cope with his/her pain. Studies show that patients who are married or have children have a more positive outlook and are better capable of managing their pain. In addition, job satisfaction and one's general attitude toward life play a significant role in a patient's ability to cope with difficulties. The history of drug use or alcohol abuse is another important factor in alerting the physician about potential medication abuse.

Psychiatric History
The evaluation should go beyond simply questioning the patient about his/her mood and investigate whether the patient has displayed increased irritability, insomnia, weight changes, suicidal ideation, and depression. Within the elderly population, atypical depression often presents as non-specific pain symptoms. Without concurrently treating a patient's underlying psychiatric issues, the medical treatment of one's pain is often incomplete.

Review of Systems
The review of systems provides an opportunity to evaluate whether other physiologic systems, not discussed during history of present illness, are involved with the patient's presenting symptoms. The review also highlights physiologic systems which might affect the prescribed medications and treatment plan.

Physical Examination
Because pain may have widespread causes, an appraisal of the general physical, neurologic, musculoskeletal, and psychiatric status of the patient should be performed.

General Physical Examination
The first step in the evaluation is to record the patient's height, weight, and vital signs (e.g., body temperature, heart rate, blood pressure, respiratory rate). Observation should include the individual's general appearance, with an assessment of the patient's grooming and nutrition. The patient's facial expressions, signs of flushing or paleness, sweating, tears, tremors,

muscular tension, or psychiatric manifestations, such as anxiety, fear, or depression, should be noted.

The physician should also be attentive to the patient's posture and evaluate lordosis, kyphosis, and pelvic posturing. The examination room should then be scanned for the presence of any assistive devices used by the patient.

Starting with the head, the patient should be examined for any signs of trauma. Careful attention should be paid to the patient's sclera and pupils. An examination of the patient's oral cavity may uncover dental issues or other oral processes. The practitioner should next inspect the patient's head and neck for lymphadenopathy. While examining the patient's neck, the patient's thyroid should be noted for signs of abnormal enlargement, goiter, or nodules.

During examination of the chest, back, and abdomen, careful auscultation of the lungs can help uncover pulmonary co-morbidities [e.g., pneumonia, chronic obstructive pulmonary disease (COPD), or heart failure]. While examining the patient's lungs, the patient's back should be observed for structural abnormalities like scoliosis. Auscultation of the heart should include signs of irregular rhythms, tachycardia, and murmurs. Systolic murmurs suggest the possibility of aortic stenosis which restricts the types of treatment possible for a patient. Any irregular cardiac rhythms, like atrial fibrillation, should raise the suspicion of anticoagulation in the patient. Finally the abdomen should be methodically inspected, with the practitioner first visually inspecting the patient's belly. Auscultation of the abdomen should then be performed before any attempts at palpation or percussion. Abnormalities in bowel sounds or sensitivity to palpation and percussion may indicate underlying intra-abdominal issues.

The patient's skin should then be evaluated for color, temperature, and signs of rashes or edema. The practitioner should also be attentive to a patient's hair and nails, as patients with complex regional pain syndrome may present with hair loss over the affected extremity and the nails may show abnormalities in texture and smoothness. The skin's color and temperature allow the physician to assess the vascular status of a patient, as poorly perfused regions may appear cyanotic and cool to the touch. Often times, patients with vascular abnormalities will suffer from concurrent neuropathic pain.

Examination of the Painful Region

After performing the general inspection of the patient, the specific region causing pain should be examined. Similar to the initial general assessment, examination of the painful region consists of inspection, palpation, and percussion, with occasional auscultation of the region.

Inspection

When initially inspecting the region of pain, the appearance and color of the skin overlying the painful area should be closely observed with documentation of any abnormalities, trophic changes, cyanosis, flushing, or hypertrichosis. The presence of cutis anserina can indicate autonomic dysfunction due to nerve root damage, while cyanosis may indicate poor perfusion and ischemic nerve damage.

Palpation

Deep tenderness is best elicited by palpation using the finger to exert firm deep pressure on the painful site. The anatomical area and involved neural segments of tenderness should be determined. While palpating the affected area, the practitioner should be attentive to signs of subjective (e.g., grimacing, groaning, verbal and non-verbal expressions) and objective (e.g., sweating, flushing, tachycardia, muscle spasm) manifestations of pain and determine if any discrepancies exist.

Because the underlying sensitivity of a patient affects his/her expressiveness to painful stimulation, palpation of the patient's opposite symmetric non-painful side should be performed. As a result, the practitioner gains a better understanding of the sensitivity of the patient to noxious and non-noxious stimuli, as well as information about the sensitivity of the painful region.

Tests such as the brush test, pinch test, pinprick test, and scratch test help distinguish whether pain provoked by palpation results from overlying skin or deeper structures. The brush test consists of lightly stroking the skin with a cotton wisp. If the patient reports pain indicative of allodynia, the underlying cause of pain is suggestive of spinal cord dysfunction. The pinch test consists of squeezing skin between the thumb and index finger, first over an adjacent non-painful area, continuing over to the painful location, and then farther past to an asymptomatic region. The pinprick and scratch tests, which are performed as described, provide a means by which to examine a patient's sensation to superficial pain. For a baseline comparison of the effects of all these tests, the practitioner should perform the same tests on the opposite non-painful area as a control.

Examination of the Musculoskeletal System

Following the initial examination of the painful area, a full musculoskeletal exam should be performed. The musculoskeletal examination starts with inspection of the patient, including front, side, and back. Attention is directed to the posture, any deviations with limb alignment, or other abnormalities, such as flattened foot arches. Symmetry within the body, especially the arms, pelvis, and legs, is important as asymmetry can lead to poor posture or strained extremities, contributing to development of painful symptoms.

After the gross inspection, an assessment of the patient's gait should be performed. The practitioner should note the patient's arm swing, stride length, push off and heel strike, and abnormal side-to-side movements while walking. Next, the patient should walk on his/her toes to test the motor function of the S1 nerve root, followed by walking on his/her heels to test L5 nerve root.

The patient's soft tissues, bony structures, and stationary or moving joints should be palpated for signs of temperature differences, edema, fluid collections, crepitus, gaps, clicks, or tenderness. A functional comparison of the left and right sides may identify possible mechanisms and locations of underlying pathologic processes.

Examination of the range of motion should be done with both active and passive participation by the patient. Active movement of the joint allows the practitioner to determine the range, muscle strength, and willingness of the patient to co-operate. In contrast, passive movements test for pain and range. The physician should also assess for the presence of hypermobility and hypomobility of the joint.

The range of motion of the neck should be measured in full flexion and extension, lateral flexion, and rotational movement. With normal function, the chin touches the chest in full flexion and the examiners pointer and middle fingers are trapped between the occiput and the C-7 spinous process in full extension. With rotation of the head, the patient should be able to turn more than 70 degrees from the sagittal plane. Lateral flexion should be equal bilaterally and at least 45 degrees from neutral.

To evaluate muscle function of the upper extremity, the patient is tested for hand grip, raising of the shoulder, abduction of the arms, flexion, extension, supination, and pronation of the forearm, flexion, and extension of the wrist, abduction and adduction of the fingers, and touching the fifth finger with the thumb. By asking the patient to fully abduct his/her arms and place his/her palms together above his/her head, the functional range of the shoulder, acromioclavicular, rotator cuff, sternoclavicular joints, and lateral rotation of the humerus can be evaluated.

When assessing the passive range of motion, the examiner instructs the patient to flex and extend his/her arm, thereby eliciting signs of discomfort or decreased range of motion. Abduction to 90 degrees, adduction, and internal and external rotation of the shoulder assess range of motion and muscular involvement of shoulder pain. While stabilizing the scapula with one hand, the shoulder should then be externally and internally rotated to evaluate glenohumeral motion.

To evaluate range of motion of the lower extremity, first have the patient step up, raise his/her leg, rise from a squatting position, flex, and extend the leg, foot, and toes. By studying the manner in which the patient sits and stands, the physician can obtain an overall impression of the patient's muscle function. The hip can be externally and internally rotated, abducted, and adducted. Both the knee and ankle have extension and flexion of the joint, while the ankle can be internally and externally everted.

To assess spinal flexibility, the examiner should have the patient flex, extend, rotate as well as laterally flex his/her spine. Immobility secondary to pain may result from disease of the zygapophyseal joint or discogenic, muscular, or ligamentous pathology.

Finally, assessment of the sacroiliac joint is performed by pushing the ilia outward and downward in the supine position. The ilia should then be compressed midline to test the posterior sacroiliac ligaments. To evaluate ligamentous strain (i.e., Patrick's test), the patient's femur is flexed, abducted, and externally rotated while the contralateral side is held flush to the examination bed.

Neurologic Examination
A neurologic examination should be performed on every new patient regardless of the region or type of pain. The neurologic exam should focus on an examination of the cranial nerves, motor strength, sensory system, and deep tendon reflexes. Except for strength, the right and left sides of the body should be identical on testing. Neurologic deficits should follow the distribution of peripheral nerves, dermatomes, or hemibody and should not end abruptly at the midline as nerves partially overlap from either side (Shea et al. 1973).

Cranial Nerve Examination
Testing the patient's papillary response to light, visual acuity, and visual field evaluation is essential to evaluate cranial nerve II. Conjugate gaze should be observed superiorly, inferiorly, laterally, and medially, with the presence or absence of nystagmus noted, to test cranial nerves III, IV, and VI. The trigeminal nerve is evaluated by bilateral light touch and pinprick sensation over the forehead (cranial V1), the maxillary process (cranial V2), and the

mandibular process (cranial V3). Checking the patient's corneal reflexes provides an assessment not only of cranial nerve V, but also of cranial nerve VII. Evaluation of cranial nerve VII includes observing facial tone and symmetry with eye closure, raising eyebrows, and smiling. Cranial nerve VIII can be assessed with the Rinne and Weber tests using a tuning fork. To assess cranial nerves IX and X, an applicator stick is lightly placed in each tonsillar region to stimulate the patient's gag reflex. Examination of the strength in the trapezius and sternocleidomastoideus muscles, by having the patient shrug his/her shoulders and by turning his/her head against resistance, provides an assessment of cranial nerve XI. Finally, tongue protrusion and lateral movements complete the screening examination by assessing cranial nerve XII.

Motor Strength Examination

The evaluation of a patient's motor strength is graded on a scale of 0 to 5, with 3 being movement against gravity. Examination should test the patient's strength in the flexors and extensors of the shoulders, elbows, wrists, and fingers, as well as the flexors and extensors of the hips, knees, and ankles. Table 5.1 highlights the grading scale for motor strength.

Table 5.1   Motor strength scales.

Score	Description
0	Absent voluntary contraction
1	Feeble contractions that are unable to move a joint
2	Movement with gravity eliminated
3	Movement against gravity
4	Movement against partial resistance
5	Full strength

Sensory Examination

To assess the function of a patient's sensory system, a tuning fork should first be applied to each hand and foot to assess vibratory sensation. A cotton wisp brushed over each extremity, chest and abdomen, ascertains the patient's sensation to light touch. With the sharp end of a broken tongue depressor, the patient's pinprick sensation over each extremity, chest and abdomen, should be determined. Finally, using a fresh alcohol swab, the patient's sensation to temperature should be tested.

Deep Tendon Reflex Examination

Using a reflex hammer, the patient's reflexes at the triceps, biceps, quadriceps, and gastrocnemius should be tested. Reflexes are graded on a 0 to 4+ scale, with 2+ reflexes being normal. The presence or absence of a Babinski's response should also be noted, as this response can help in determining upper versus lower motor neuron damage. In general, absent reflexes or clonus is never normal.

Psychiatric Examination

Often times, psychiatric illnesses are associated with health behaviors and pyschophysiologic changes that promote medical illness. Attributing a patient's pain to solely a psychiatric cause is not a diagnosis of exclusion. More importantly, undertreated psychiatric disease may exacerbate pain states (Hudson et al. 1985). Thus, to assess the psychiatric status of the chronic pain patient, a physician should perform a Mini-Mental status exam and discuss any existing depression or anxiety symptoms (Wittink et al. 2004).

Mini-Mental Examination

The Mini-Mental examination is an initial tool for evaluating a patient's psychological status. The examination tests five areas of mental status; orientation, registration, attention and calculation, recall, and language, with a maximum score of 30 and any score less than 23 considered abnormal. While the Mini-Mental exam allows the physician to assess an individual's cognition, this test does not provide any information about the potential source of a patient's mental deficit. Furthermore, highly educated individuals are capable of performing well on this test, even with mild to moderate levels of dementia, and poorly educated individuals may perform poorly on this test without any underlying mental deficits.

Depression

Because depression is a treatable disorder, the practitioner should assess all chronic pain patients for this illness. While some patients may admit feelings of sadness, many patients deny or minimize the likelihood of being depressed. Thus, the practitioner should also screen the patient for symptoms characteristically found in depression, including anhedonia, fatigue, insomnia, appetite changes, and suicidal ideation. If a patient does admit to suicidal thoughts and impulses, the practitioner should contact psychiatric services and consider hospitalization to protect the patient.

Anxiety

Since most chronic pain patients display some symptoms of anxiety, a practitioner must be attuned to the possibility of a patient developing a true anxiety disorder. As an example, studies have shown that 30% of patients with fibromyalgia suffer from symptoms of anxiety. Commonly, pain patients with anxiety will present with other mood disorders, such as depression or dysthymia. In these circumstances, treatment of the mood disorder may correct the patient's underlying anxiety.

When evaluating a patient for an anxiety disorder, the physician should discover underlying disorders that can cause symptoms of anxiety. These include hyperthyroidism, adrenal dysfunction, seizure disorder, and drug intoxication or withdrawal. To accurately screen for issues of anxiety, the practitioner should question the patient regarding the presence of heart palpitations, sweating, trembling, feeling short of breath or choking, chest pain, nausea, dizziness, fear of dying or of losing control, temperature changes, and paresthesias.

Differential Diagnosis

Pain can be pathophysiologically categorized as nociceptive, neuropathic, sympathetically mediated, neuralgia, radicular, central, psychogenic, and referred. However, most clinicians specifically focus on somatic, visceral, psychogenic, neuropathic, and referred pain when determining the diagnosis of patient's underlying pain.

Somatic and visceral pains are categorized as nociceptive pain, with the degree of pain experienced proportional to activation of afferent pain fibers. Superficial somatic pain is caused by injury to the skin or superficial tissues and produces a sharp, well-defined, localized pain of short duration. Deep somatic pain originates from ligaments, tendons, bones, blood vessels, fascia, or muscles and produces a dull, aching, poorly localized pain of longer duration than cutaneous pain. Visceral pain originates from bodys viscera, or organs, with pain usually more aching and cramping and may have longer duration than somatic pain. Visceral pain is often extremely difficult to localize and may exhibit referred pain, where the sensation is localized to an unrelated site. Common manifestations of referred pain include cutaneous and deep hyperalgesia, autonomic hyperactivity, tenderness, and muscular contractions.

In contrast, neuropathic pain results from injury or disease to the peripheral or central nervous system and is characterized by pain out of proportion to tissue injury, dysesthesia, and signs of nerve injury detected during neurologic examination. As mentioned previously, psychogenic pain is characterized by pain existing with no apparent organic pathology despite extensive evaluation and commonly presents with pain inconsistent with the likely anatomic distribution.

Many disease processes present with pain, thus associated pain syndromes should be part of the physician's differential diagnosis (Overcash et al. 2001). Diabetic neuropathy (Tesfaye et al. 1994) is a frequently encountered pain, characterized by burning, muscle cramps, lancinating pain, metatarsalgia, hyperalgesia, allodynia, loss of proprioception, tingling, and numbness in lower extremities. Human immunodeficiency virus (HIV) patients present with pain including neuropathic, somatic, visceral, and headache symptoms. Patients suffering from autoimmune disease will often present with joint pain associated with inflammation, achiness, and stiffness. Post-surgical pain is commonly encountered and is usually somatic or visceral in nature. Infectious processes involving intra-abdominal organs are more likely to present with visceral pain while infectious processes involving the skin (e.g., herpes zoster) will present with somatic or neuropathic pain.

Indicated Studies

To help determine the underlying cause of a patient's pain, practitioners can utilize imaging, laboratory work, or questionnaires.

Imaging

The history and physical exam may help physicians decide which imaging modalities are indicated. Radiography can be used to evaluate bony abnormalities (fractures, osteophytes), ligamentous changes (ossification), and degenerative joints (Waldman 2006a). Pain physicians oftentimes work with radiologists to decide which views are necessary to adequately evaluate structures. While radiography provides a decent initial workup of bony structural abnormalities, this study modality (unless modified) is unable to provide an assessment of underlying soft tissue or vascular abnormalities.

Computerized tomography (CT) (Waldman 2006b) scan utilizes X-rays to provide a more comprehensive radiographic image. Unlike radiography, CTs provide highly detailed, sequential images of the scanned area. These images can be viewed in a number of different dimensions: axial, sagittal, and frontal, with three-dimensional reconstructions available. CT scans provide an assessment of bony and joint abnormalities, readily detecting fractures, subluxations, cystic bone lesions, and assessing bone mineral density. Additionally, CT scans produce images of soft tissue pathology.

Magnetic resonance imaging (MRI) (Waldman et al. 2006c) captures absorption and emission energies of molecules in the body to reproduce images of the scanned area. MRI provides excellent soft tissue contrast resolution. Spinous abnormalities like degenerative disk disease, joint disease, fractures, and neoplasms are readily discernable using MRI images. While tendons and ligaments prove hard to evaluate on CT, MRI is able to evaluate these soft tissue structures for sprains, tears, and inflammation. Gadolinium contrast further enhances MRI by enabling the detection of vascular abnormalities and epidural scarring.

When CT and MRI images prove insufficient or when MRI is contraindicated (pacemakers, ferromagnetic aneurysm clips), CT myelography may be a useful alternative. Myelography consists of instilling dye into the subarachnoid space while radiographic images are taken in the anteroposterior, lateral, and oblique planes. Based on defects within the dye column, one can determine areas of neural compression. With CT imaging in conjunction with myelography, a physician can see interactions of bony structures and neural elements. However, unlike CT and MRI, CT myelography poses the additional risks associated with invasively injecting dye into the subarachnoid space.

Ultrasonography avoids effects associated with ionizing radiation and also provides real-time assessment of soft tissue structures. Nerves and blood vessels within soft tissue structures, muscles, tendons, and many internal organs can be assessed with ultrasound techniques. Ultrasound, however, does not provide the resolution capacity with CT or MRI for imaging soft tissue structure, nor does ultrasound penetrate through bone well or provide a good assessment of anatomically deep structures like the spinal cord.

Laboratory Testing

Because there are numerous laboratory tests available, the physician must use the patient's history and physical to accurately determine which laboratory tests to perform. Commonly used tests include a complete blood count (CBC), acute-phase proteins [erythrocyte sedimentation rate (ESR), c-reactive protein (CRP)], blood chemistry, rheumatologic, and infectious disease studies.

The CBC helps provide an estimate of a person's general health. Based on the hematocrit level, an indication of that person's medical and nutritional health can be inferred. The shape of red blood cells allows for the determination of pain-inducing diseases such as sickle cell anemia. White blood cells when elevated can point to infections or underlying hematologic malignancies. Similar to white blood cells, platelet levels help elucidate underlying myeloproliferative disorders. Platelet levels also influence whether the patient is a candidate for invasive therapeutic procedures.

Acute-phase proteins such as the ESR and CRP provide a general indication of inflammatory issues within the patient. Abnormal values of these two tests are often seen with infection, trauma, surgery, burns, cancer, inflammatory conditions, and psychological stress and also help corroborate findings of thrombocytosis, leukocytosis, and anemia.

Coagulation parameters are a useful laboratory test as they determine the potential application of invasive therapeutic pain treatments as well as provide an assessment of the patient's liver function. Deficiencies in the clotting studies should make the practitioner wary of unrecognized bleeding into limited spaces (retroperitoneal, joints) as a possible cause for a patient's pain.

Blood chemistry values include sodium, urea, creatinine, and glucose. While hyponatremia itself may cause generalized symptoms of pain, the physician should determine whether a patient's hyponatremia is indicative of an abnormal hormonal process such as syndrome of inappropriate antidiuretic hormone (SIADH), which occurs with certain types of cancers. Monitoring glucose and hemoglobin A1c levels may uncover diabetes, a common cause of painful neuropathies. Abnormalities in the urea and creatinine levels can indicate issues of renal insufficiency, which may alter the pharmacologic and invasive treatment options. For example, worsening renal function may worsen side effects from morphine because of decreased excretion of morphine metabolites.

Diseases such as systemic lupus erythematosus and rheumatoid arthritis are associated with diffuse body pain and are characterized by inflammation of the joints, muscle, or skin. Screening for rheumatologic disorders includes testing for autoantibodies, antinuclear antibodies (ANA), rheumatoid factor, antineutrophil cytoplasmic antibody, anti-Ro, anti-Sm, and anticentromere. Diffuse pain and joint pain warrant consideration of a rheumatologic evaluation.

Because certain infectious diseases produce generalized pain symptoms, screening for diseases like HIV, syphilis, and lyme disease should be performed when indicated. HIV commonly causes abdominal pain, neuropathies, oral cavity pain, headaches, and reactive arthritis. Spirochetal diseases like syphilis and lyme disease can range in severity of symptoms including headaches, irritability, neck stiffness, or gummata. The Venereal Disease Research Laboratory (VDRL) and rapid plasma regain (RPR) tests are the initial tests used to screen for syphilis. Lyme disease, like syphilis, can range in pain symptoms from cranial neuritis, radicular pain, and weakness, to symptoms of Bell's palsy. Screening for lyme disease typically requires an enzyme-linked immunosorbent assay (ELISA) test.

Electromyography

Electromyography (EMG), in the most simplistic of descriptions, is a test of muscle function. However, EMG tests often include nerve conduction studies for an assessment of nerve, nerve root, and anterior horn cell function. Based on the EMG and nerve conduction studies, one can localize neuromuscular disease sites as well as determine the nature of the disease process (demyelinating, axonal, primary muscle disease, or radiculopathy).

Clinical Assessment Tools

Because pain is highly subjective between individuals, clinical assessment tools have been developed to aid physicians in understanding and characterizing pain symptoms. Simple scales measuring the severity of a patient's pain include the visual analog scale (VAS), the numerical rating scale (NRS), and the Wong–Baker FACES scale.

Single-Dimension Surveys

The VAS consists of a straight 100-mm line with the words "no pain" at the left-most end and "worst pain imaginable" at the right-most end (Fig. 5.2). Patients are instructed to mark on the line the amount of pain they feel at the current time. By measuring the distance from the left-most end of the line to the patient's mark, a numeric representation of the patient's pain

No Pain   Worst Pain Imaginable

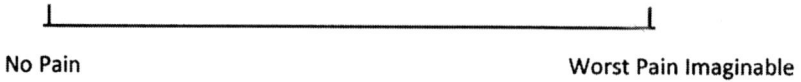

Figure 5.2   Visual analog scale.

can be determined. This simple survey method makes the VAS highly effective because of its ease of use as well as its understandability.

The NRS lists the numbers 0–10, with "no pain" at the left-most end and "worst pain imaginable" at the right-most end (Fig. 5.3). With the NRS, patients are instructed to circle the number that best represents the amount of pain they are currently experiencing. However, the disadvantage of both the NRS and VAS scales lies in their attempt to assign a numerical value to a complex, multifactorial process. Both tests have a ceiling for the worst pain experienced, which limits a patient's ability to convey a worsening of his/her pain if that patient marks his/her pain as being the worst pain imaginable on initial evaluation.

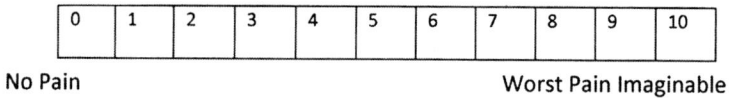

0	1	2	3	4	5	6	7	8	9	10

No Pain   Worst Pain Imaginable

Figure 5.3   Numerical rating scale.

Because children have more difficulty in quantifying their level of pain, assessment tools like the Wong–Baker FACES scale (Fig. 5.4) and the Faces Pain Scale provide a reliable and easily understood survey for children. The main disadvantage posed by these surveys is their inability to be used in children under the age of 3.

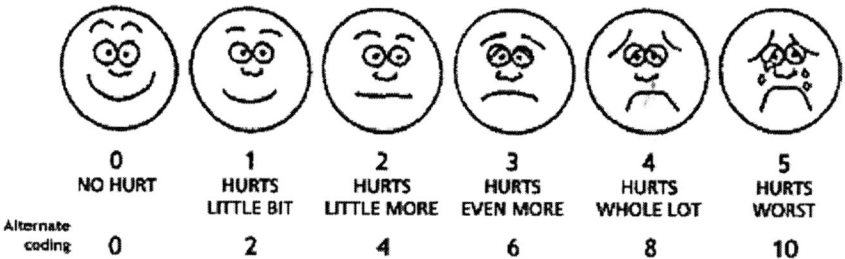

0	1	2	3	4	5
NO HURT	HURTS LITTLE BIT	HURTS LITTLE MORE	HURTS EVEN MORE	HURTS WHOLE LOT	HURTS WORST

Alternate coding

0	2	4	6	8	10

Figure 5.4   Wong–Baker FACES scale.

Multiple-Dimension Surveys

In comparison to the simplistic, quick, and easy NRS and VAS surveys, multidimensional surveys like the McGill Pain Questionnaire and the Brief Pain Inventory Questionnaire provide more complete information about a patient's underlying pain. These questionnaires are more useful in the chronic pain population than in patients with pain of acute onset.

The McGill Pain Questionnaire utilizes three different components to assess a patient's pain. The first part consists of a drawing of both the front and back of a human body, which the patient marks to indicate where they are experiencing pain. The second part is a six-word verbal descriptive scale that patients use to record their current pain intensity. The final part consists of 20 sets of adjectives that the patient selects to describe the sensory, affective, and evaluative qualities of his/her pain. Though the questionnaire has the disadvantage of being time-consuming, the McGill Pain Questionnaire is highly reliable and consistent, allowing for the differentiation of pain syndromes and the discrimination of the therapies effect on a patient's pain.

The Brief Pain Inventory (BPI) questionnaire asks patients to mark the location of their pain on a drawing of the front and back of a human body. Patients also fill out 11 different NRS surveys that assess their pain intensity and activities of daily living. Like the McGill Pain Questionnaire, the BPI provides an excellent tool to monitor the effect of pain or the treatment of pain over time, but has the disadvantage of being time-consuming to complete.

Quality of Life and Disability Questionnaires

To further determine the effects of a patient's pain on his/her quality of life, questionnaires such as the Oswestry Disability Index (ODI), the Short Form 36 (SF-36), and the Fact G may prove useful. The ODI consists of ten questions that investigate the patient's pain intensity, personal care, lifting, walking, sitting, standing, sleeping, sex and social life, and traveling; the higher the patient's score, the greater that individual's disability. Studies have shown that the ODI is an easy, comprehensive pain assessment tool that provides a means to monitor an individual's pain.

In contrast to the ODI, the SF-36 assesses eight different health domains: physical and social functioning, role limitations to physical and emotional problems, bodily pain, vitality, general health perception, and mental health. Each item is scored on a scale from 0 to 100 with higher scores indicating better health. The ability to quickly complete the SF-36 and accurately monitor a change in a patient's pain has made this questionnaire one of the most widely used health status instruments worldwide.

The Fact G questionnaire gained acceptance as an assessment for the cancer population, with studies showing the Fact G to be as efficacious as the SF-36 in the evaluation of an individual's quality of life. The domains explored in the Fact G consist of physical well-being, social/family well-being, emotional well-being, functional well-being, and relationship with the physician, with higher scores often correlating with better outcomes and quality of life for the patient. Similar to both the ODI and SF-36, the Fact-G is a valid, reliable, user-friendly questionnaire that has the added benefit of being sensitive enough to differentiate between different stages of cancer.

Case Scenario
Zacharia Jose, MBBS, MD, FRCA, FCARCSI

Kate is an 18-year-old woman who is studying business management. You are a primary care physician and Kate has come to see you with the following problem: she is under stress of her examination and has been suffering from a headache at least once every 2–3 days for the last few months. Red wine and menstruation precipitate the headache. She describes it as "pain behind the eye radiating to the face and the back of the head."

The pain is predominantly right-sided and rarely occurs on the left. It is also associated with visual aura with blurred peripheral vision. These headaches last for 1–3 days and are associated with nausea, photophobia, and phonophobia. Kate has tried acetaminophen and aspirin without much relief. She is desperate and anxious that the headache might affect her performance in the coming school exam. She believes that she is suffering from migraine and requesting you to prescribe "migraine spray."

How would you deal with Kate's request?

It is very tempting to jump to a conclusion that Kate is suffering from classical migraine. The cause of the headache could be inflammatory, vascular, tumor, psychological, or drugs. It could be due to a combination of these. Hence, you need to take a detailed history, a brief psychological assessment, a thorough physical examination, and undertake appropriate investigations which could include a CT or MRI scan of the head.

During your interview, Kate reveals that she gets the symptoms following alcohol intake, on which she indulges during most weekends. She also consumes alcohol when she is having her periods to ward off the premenstrual tension. Sometimes she gets the headache when she is stressed. She admits to occasionally smoking "weed" with her friends. The clinical examination is normal. The routine laboratory investigations are normal as well.

Do you agree with Kate's self-diagnosis of migraine?

Your diagnosis of migraine is justified if it satisfies the set criteria (see text). The migraine headache could be the result of alcohol and cannabis. Alternatively, she could be indeed suffering from migraine which is triggered by wine and stress. In order to have a proper diagnosis she needs to come off all these drugs. She needs the help of a psychologist/psychiatrist for detailed assessment and management of drug-related issues.

You explain your reasoning to Kate and she consults a psychologist. You advise Kate to take acetaminophen and ibuprofen for her headaches as an interim measure.

Kate returns after a month for a follow up. She is now off alcohol and cannabis. She tells you that she is still getting migraines, although now less frequently. Her symptoms likely point to a common migraine. She thinks that acetaminophen and ibuprofen are helping her to some extent.

How would you treat migraine?

You should recommend that Kate continue to avoid the precipitating agents. She should try to avoid stress (easily said than done!). This might keep the frequency of the migraine down. She is advised to take acetaminophen or ibuprofen during an acute attack, as well as the sumatriptan nasal spray. It is also worth considering propranolol 80 mg daily, a sustained release preparation as a preventive measure. It has the added advantage of having an anti-anxiety effect. Other preventive measures that could be used are amitriptyline or sodium valproate. Alternative medicine options include relaxation techniques and acupuncture.

Kate responds very well to your treatment and she completes high school successfully. Several years later, she returns to see you. She tells you that the migraine has returned and she frequently experiences right-sided headaches. She is requesting an urgent repeat prescription of the same medications that she had before, and she in a hurry to leave to attend an important meeting.

What would you like to tell Kate?
Recurrence of a migraine is, of course, a possibility. However, it could be an entirely different disease process. Therefore, further investigation is necessary. Your management must always include history, examination, and diagnostic testing. You tell Kate that she needs to be properly assessed before she can have any medications.

Kate agrees and you explore the history and note that she has been suffering from the headache for the last 12 months. Her headaches occur in clusters with symptom-free periods of a few months. The pain is intense and non-throbbing. Most of the time it occurs during nighttime without any warning. The pain is confined to over her right eye and is associated with lacrimation and rhinorrhea. On physical examination, you notice conjunctival injection and ptosis. Her blood pressure is normal and there is no neurological deficit. You order an MRI scan of head, which comes back normal.

What is your management plan?
On this occasion, Kate is suffering from what appears to be a cluster headache. Since it is in its early stage, oxygen therapy could be prescribed. Other options include sumatriptan, intra-nasal lidocaine, capsaicin or ergometrin for the prevention of the attack (see text).

References

Bair MJ, Robinson RL, Katon W, Kroenke K. Depression and pain comorbidity: a literature review. Arch Intern Med. 2003;163(20):2433–45.

Garratt AM, Ruta DA, Abdalla MI, et al. The SF36 health survey questionnaire: an outcome measure suitable for routine use within the NHS? BMJ. 1993;306(6890):1440–4.

Harden R, Bruehl S. Diagnosis of complex regional pain syndrome: signs, symptoms, and new empirically derived diagnostic criteria. Clin J Pain. 2006;22(5):415–9.

Hudson JI, Hudson MS, Pliner LF, et al. Fibromyalgia and major affective disorder: a controlled phenomenology and family history study. Am J Psychiatry. 1985;142(4):441–6.

Jamison RN, Virts KL. The influence of family support on chronic pain. Behav Res Ther. 1990;28(4):118–20.

Loeser J, Butler S, et al. History of pain concepts and therapies. Bonica's management of pain. 3rd ed. Philadelphia, PA: Lippincott Williams & Wilkins; 2001a. pp. 7–11.

Loeser J, Butler S, et al. Medical evaluation of the patient with pain. Bonica's management of pain. 3rd ed. Philadelphia, PA: Lippincott Williams & Wilkins; 2001b, pp. 276–78.

Loeser J, Butler S, et al. Medical evaluation of the patient with pain. Bonica's management of pain. 3rd ed. Philadelphia, PA: Lippincott Williams & Wilkins; 2001c, p. 270.

Magni G, Schifano F, De Leo D. Pain as a symptom in elderly depressed patients: relationship to diagnostic subgroups. Eur Arch Psychiatr Neurol Sci. 1985;235(3):143–5.

Overcash J, Extermann M, Parr J, et al. Validity and reliability of the FACT-G scale for use in the older person with cancer. Am J Clin Oncol (CCT). 2001;24(6):591–6.

Schaffer CB, Donlon PT, Bittle RM. Chronic pain and depression: a clinical and family history survey. Am J Psychiatry. 1980;137(1):118–20.

Shea JK, Gioffre R, Carrion H, Small MP. Autonomic hyperreflexia in spinal cord injury. South Med J. 1973;66(8):869–72.

Tesfaye S, Malik R, Ward JD. Vascular factors in diabetic neuropathy. Diabetologia 1994;37(9):847–54.

Waldman S. Radiography. Pain Management. 2nd ed. Philadelphia: WB Saunders, 2006a: 74 84.

Waldman S. Computed Tomography. Pain Management. 2nd ed. Philadelphia: WB Saunders, 2006b:93–106.

Waldman S. Magnetic Resonance Imaging. Pain Management. 2nd ed. Philadelphia: WB Saunders, 2006c:106–117.

Wittink H, Turk DC, Carr DB, et al. Comparison of the redundancy, reliability, and responsiveness to change among SF-36, Oswestry disability index, and multidimensional pain inventory. Clin J Pain. 2004;20(3):133–42.

Chapter 6

Diagnostic Imaging in Pain Management

Timothy Malhotra, MD

Introduction

When diagnoses in pain management are uncertain and information scant, radiologic imaging can be used to make the unseen seen. Differentials may be narrowed, decisions made more certain, and therapy commenced with greater effect. As powerful as it may be, imaging is no substitute for clinical examination and diagnoses; therapeutics should not be based solely on a radiologic result but in conjunction with the clinical findings. Much can be found if one looks, but if it does not hurt, is it of significance, and does it need to be treated?

All radiologic techniques rely on two qualities for their efficacy: contrast and dimension. Whether through the use of radiation or magnetism, by applying an exogenous stimulus and detecting the response, different tissues are transformed into shades of gray. The shades of gray and the *contrast* they provide give information as to the shape, quality, and boundaries of both normalcy and pathology. Images may exist in two-dimensions or constructed into three-dimensions using many images providing a multitude of views be they coronal, sagittal, axial, or more.

X-Ray

X-rays or plain radiographs rely on an external beam of X-radiation to pass through tissue and be detected and transformed into four fundamental shades of gray reflective of four different tissues: air (black), fat (dark gray), soft tissue (light gray), and bone (white) (Mettler 2005). Air allows the greatest transmission of X-rays to the detector and thus appears black; likewise, bone provides the greatest hindrance and appears white (Fig. 6.1). Detectors may include simple plain photographic film or digital plates that display the results on a computer screen.

Plain radiographs provide the greatest contrast at the extreme shades, white (bone) and black (air). They are therefore of great use in providing detail on the relative positions, densities, and shapes of bones and joints (Bogduk 2003) as may occur in fractures, dislocations, osteomyelitis, osteoporosis, and lytic lesions from cancer. Also, because they demonstrate the contrast between air (black) and other tissues well, X-rays have been a mainstay in chest radiographs.

When tissues themselves are not inherently "contrasty," radioopaque contrast agents may be given orally, rectally, or intravenously to contrast "enhance" hollow visci and vessels. When using intravenous contrast agents, there is a risk of a contrast reaction. Reactions are

N. Vadivelu et al. (eds.), *Essentials of Pain Management*,
DOI 10.1007/978-0-387-87579-8_6, © Springer Science+Business Media, LLC 2011

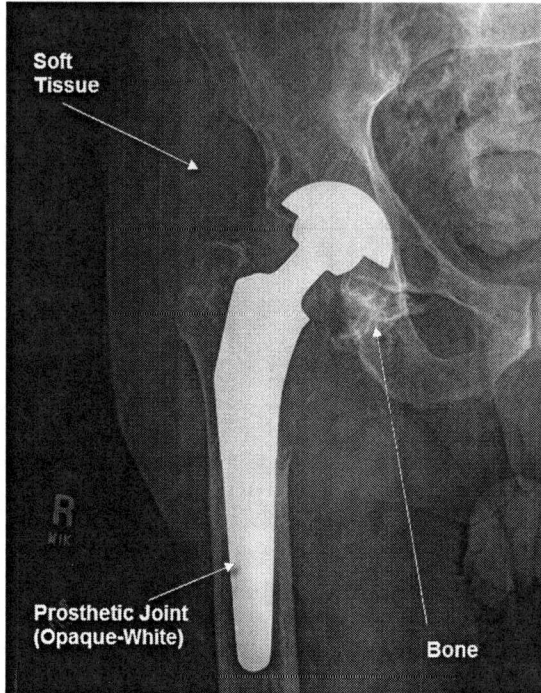

Figure 6.1 X-rays or plain radiographs rely on an external beam of X-radiation to pass through tissue and be detected and transformed into four fundamental shades of *gray* reflective of four different tissues: air (*black*), fat (*dark gray*), soft tissue (*light gray*), and bone (*white*) [1]. Air allows the greatest transmission of X-rays to the detector and thus appears *black*. Likewise, bone provides the greatest hindrance and appears *white*.

most common with iodinated contrast agents and may be classified as idiosyncratic (dose-independent) and non-idiosyncratic. Idiosyncratic reactions are true anaphylactic reactions occurring 20 min after injection and may include the following symptoms: urticaria, pruritus, nausea, vomiting dizziness progressing to bronchospasm, palpitations, bradycardia, hypertension, headache, further progressing to severe bronchospasm, pulmonary edema, hypotension, severe arrhythmias, seizures, and death (Siddiqi 2008).

Non-idiosyncratic reactions may include sensations of warmth, metallic taste, bradycardia, vasovagal reactions, and other autonomic reactions. The similarity to idiosyncratic reaction makes distinction difficult. Of great concern is contrast-induced nephropathy which may occur 1–3 days following injection, peaking at 3–7 days and "is manifested by elevation of the serum creatinine by a level greater than 0.5 mg/dL or more than 50% of the baseline level (Siddiqi 2008)." Although its incidence is low at 2–7%, its effect can be sustained in those who succumb.

Radiographs are two-dimensional and a single view provides little information as to the depth of an object. Dense objects can easily be *on* a patient or *in* a patient. A lateral view, in addition to a frontal view, may be required to elucidate greater information and increase the "dimensional" view.

Table 6.1 Conditions for which plain radiograph may be used as initial test.

Plain radiograph may be sufficient
- ☐ Arthritis (non-septic)
- ☐ Arthritis (septic)
- ☐ Fracture

Plain radiograph initially, then bone scan if needed
- ☐ Metastases
- ☐ Prosthetic joint, infection, or joint loosening

Plain radiograph initially, then triple-phase bone scan if needed
- ☐ Reflex sympathetic dystrophy
- ☐ Osteomyelitis

Plain radiograph initially, then MRI if needed
- ☐ Joint pain, monoarticular
- ☐ Osteomyelitis

Plain radiograph initially, then CT if needed
- ☐ Facial fracture

Adapted from Mettler (2005).

Although more sophisticated imaging techniques such as computer tomography (CT) or magnetic resonance imaging (MRI) may provide a more dimensional view, radiographs are sometimes sufficient for many situations. Table 6.1 lists conditions for which plain radiographs are indicated as an initial diagnostic test.

CT Scan

CT scanning utilizes the information from multiple radiographs rotated around a patient at a given "slice" to create three-dimensional "slices" through a patient. By processing the data from the multiple radiographs, every point within that slice may be "triangulated" and reconstructed to form a CT scan "allowing one to see the shape and position of the egg yolk without breaking the egg." What is demonstrated is only the "location, shape and density" of the yolk and not its internal architecture (Bogduk 2003). This slicing is repeated at various levels along a patient to form several such images, much like cutting ham slices. Because CT scan fundamentally uses radiographs, the same basic four gray shades of density are used to define the contrast that is obtained (bone, fat, soft tissue, and air); however, because multiple images are used in reconstruction, averaging of shades permits subtleties in shading with the potential for visualizing small details (Fig. 6.2).

CT scans, like ham, come in a variety of styles including helical (spiral) and single slice. Helical CT uses data from multiple slices by traveling in a spiral fashion around the patient. As a result it provides better resolution of high-contrast structures such as bone and air and thus is useful in identifying bony fractures (as in facial fractures) and pulmonary emboli. Single slice CT scanning is advantageous over helical CT in providing detail.

There are two fundamental uses for CT scans in pain management: identification of intra-cavitary tumors (such as within the thorax, abdomen, and pelvis) and imaging of the spine (Table 6.2). With respect to tumors, CT scan can provide data on progression and recurrence of primary and secondary tumors pointing to potential causes of pain. Back pain without neurologic findings is initially managed conservatively without initial imaging. MRI of the

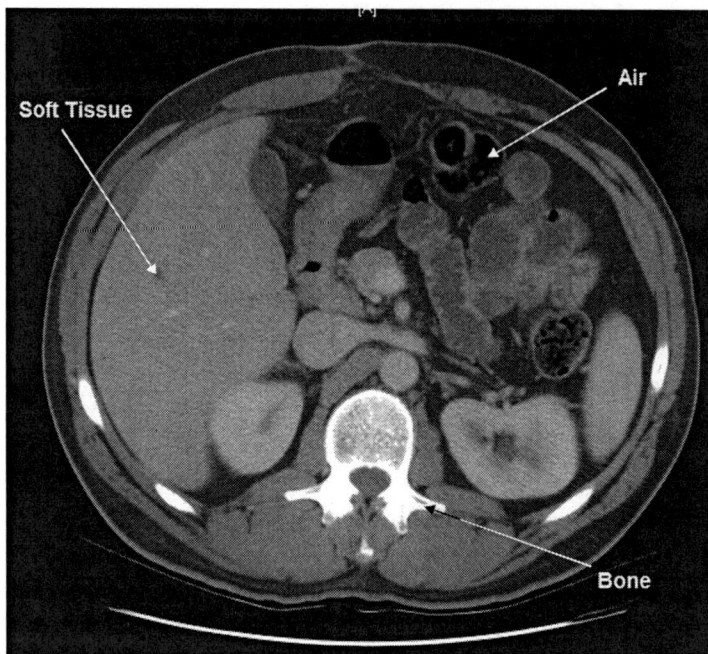

Figure 6.2   CT scan fundamentally uses radiographs, the same basic four *gray* shades of density are used to define the contrast that is obtained (bone, fat, soft tissue, and air). However, because multiple images are used in reconstruction, averaging of shades permits subtleties in shading with the potential for visualizing small details.

Table 6.2 Conditions for which computed tomography (CT) scan may be used as initial or follow-up test.

CT scan as primary modality
  ☐ Abscess
  ☐ Suspected pulmonary embolism
  ☐ Cancer
  ☐ Low back pain with radiculopathy [if magnetic resonance imaging (MRI) not possible]
CT scan after initial plain radiograph
  ☐ Facial fracture

Adapted from Mettler (2005).

spine is indicated when back pain occurs with a neurologic finding, such as radiculopathy. When MRI is contraindicated and spinal imaging is needed, CT myelography remains an option and results may be equivalent in detecting lesions (Modic 1986). CT may also be more useful when spinal hardware is present because of MRI artifacts.

Much as in plain radiography, contrast agents may be used to enhance detail and such is the principle behind CT myelography. A needle is inserted into the spinal fluid and contrast agent given. A plain radiograph or CT scan of the spine is performed and the outline of the contrast observed. Any extradural indentations of the thecal sac (such as from herniated disks, bone spurs, spinal stenosis, or tumors) suggest that a lesion is present, although the detail of that lesion may not be discernible (Kleefield 2004). Lesions that are present but do not impinge upon the thecal sac may be missed. Minor risks of this procedure include headache from the spinal injection. One of the more dreaded complications includes arachnoiditis, in which the nerves of the cauda equina become matted down from scarring and inflammation of the arachnoid as a reaction to the contrast agent (Eldevik 1978). The symptoms of this complication may be far worse than the condition for which this study was ordered.

While the typical CT scan provides images along an axial plane, it is possible through reconstruction of the computerized data to provide coronal and sagittal views as well. CT scans, however, are inferior to MRI in providing detail of soft tissues and thus fail to provide information about intrinsic problems within the spinal cord itself.

MRI

In MRI, a strong external magnetic field is applied to tissues to align the atoms in those tissues with the magnetic field. The field is then released and the atoms lose their alignment. Different tissues lose their alignment at different rates and this loss results in the production of radio waves. Because each type of tissue produces a different frequency of radio waves, different tissues can be distinguished by the different frequencies they produce. Two fundamental types of decay, T1 and T2, produce distinct frequencies when the magnetic field within tissues relaxes. Also, consequently, each of these produces different contrasts within tissue which is reconstructed to define the boundaries and innards of these tissues (Table 6.3).

Table 6.3 Relative weighting under T1 and T2 imaging of magnetic resonance imaging (MRI).

Tissue	T1 Image	T2 Image
Fat	White	Black
Water (or CSF)	Black	White
Brain and muscle	Gray	Gray

CSF = cerebrospinal fluid.

Compared to both plain radiography and CT, MRI is most useful for depicting the structure of soft tissues (Fig. 6.3). It is not as useful for depicting bone; any visualization of bone (i.e., white on T1-weighted images) really represents the marrow fat within bone and not the calcium itself (Mettler 2005). For bone structures, plain radiographs and CT scan remain the preferred modality. Furthermore, because MRI does not use ionizing radiation, it is potentially safer in some individuals (e.g., pregnant women beyond the first trimester (Wilkinson and Paley 2008)). Unfortunately, any ferromagnetic materials within or on a person may be pulled violently into the field and this remains a major contraindication to the use of MRI. In very high fields, people have reported seeing spherical visual hallucinations and have even had vertigo (Wilkinson and Paley 2008).

Specifically, the following remain major contraindications to the use of MRI:

- Cardiac pacemaker;
- Implanted cardiac defibrillator;
- Aneurysm clips;

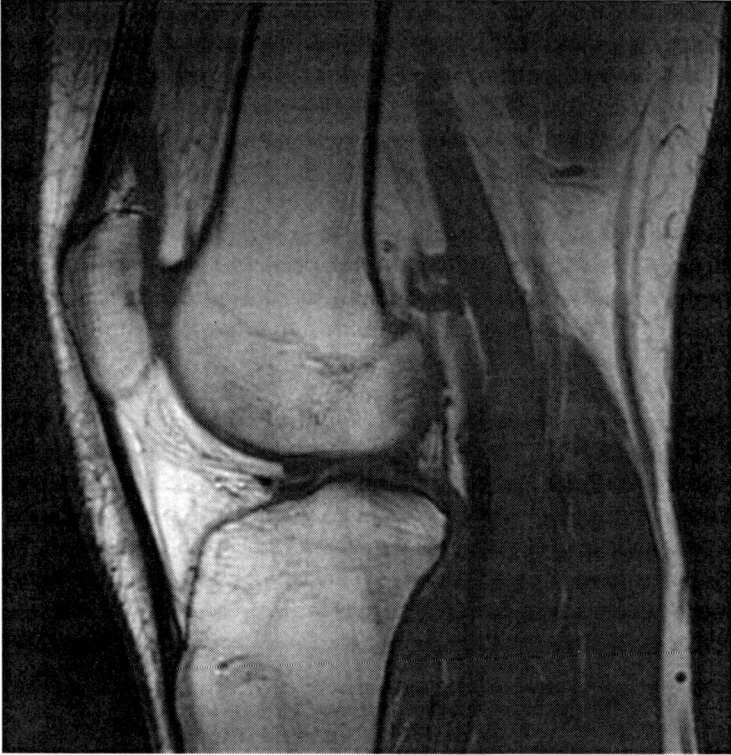

Figure 6.3   Compared to both plain radiography and CT, MRI is most useful for depicting the structure of soft tissues.

- Carotid artery vascular clamp;
- Neurostimulator;
- Insulin or infusion pump;
- Implanted drug infusion device;
- Bone growth/fusion stimulator;
- Cochlear, otologic, or ear implant (DCMR-Contraindications to MRI 2009).

Interestingly, presence of an implanted intrathecal pumps used for pain, such as a Medtronic Synchromed® pump (Medtronic Corporation, Minneapolis, MN, USA), do not comprise an absolute contraindication to MRI. The pump itself will stop functioning during the MRI exposure but will resume thereafter. It is recommended that the pump programming be checked immediately after the MRI to verify that it has not been altered (Important Safety Information for Drug Delivery Systems 2009).

Because of its superiority in demonstrating the intrinsic detail of soft tissue and because of its sensitivity to movement, MRI is most useful in imaging static soft tissue structures such as the spine, brain, and joints (Table 6.4). As such, it is the preferred means of evaluating back pain with radiculopathy. Furthermore, it is useful for detecting abnormalities within single joints and osteomyelitis as it provides soft tissue contrast in relation to the surrounding bone.

Table 6.4 Conditions for which magnetic resonance imaging (MRI) may be used as initial or follow-up test.

MRI as primary modality
  ☐ Low back pain with radiculopathy
  ☐ Occult hip fracture
  ☐ Occult knee fracture
MRI following plain radiograph
  ☐ Joint pain, monoarticular
  ☐ Osteomyelitis

Adapted from Mettler (2005).

When plain radiographs fail to demonstrate a hip or knee fracture, MRI is also useful for delineating an occult fracture.

Many patients complain of claustrophobia with MRI. To help alleviate this problem, open MRI systems have been developed. The strength of an MRI magnet is measured in Tesla (T) (Wilkinson and Paley 2008); most MRI scanners are in the range of 0.2–3.0 T, with the majority being 1.5 T. To generate a field above 1 T, a superconducting magnet must be cooled with liquid helium. Such a system requires a closed MRI system, i.e., a non-open MRI system (Wilkinson and Paley 2008). The open systems use weaker magnets and consequently provide lower resolution and less contrast, both of which affect diagnostic ability.

Much as in CT scanning, contrast agents enhance images. Gadolinium is the most commonly used contrast agent in MRI scanning. It is a toxic metal that is rendered safe by combining it with a chelating agent (Wilkinson and Paley 2008). This contrast agent accumulates where the blood–brain barrier has been compromised as in the case of tumors, abscesses, and demyelination (Wilkinson and Paley 2008). Their greatest value is in the distinguishing of tumor from edema.

Although the complications associated with gadolinium are far less than those with the contrast agents used in CT scanning, some still do exist (Prince et al. 1996). The most common reactions are simple allergic-like reactions that include pruritus, rash, hives, and facial swelling. Patients with pre-existing renal insufficiency or failure are at risk for developing the fibrosing condition known as nephrogenic systemic fibrosis caused by deposition of gadolinium in the tissues (Information for Healthcare Professionals Gadolinium-Based Contrast Agents for Magnetic Resonance Imaging 2009). It is characterized by a scleroderma-like syndrome involving the following organ symptoms: "burning or itching, reddened or darkened patches, and/or skin swelling, hardening and/or tightening [of the skin], yellow raised spots on the whites of the eyes, joint stiffness, limited range of motion in the arms, hands, legs, or feet; pain deep in the hip bone or ribs; and/or muscle weakness (Information for Healthcare Professionals Gadolinium-Based Contrast Agents for Magnetic Resonance Imaging 2009)." No known treatment exists.

Ultrasound

Ultrasound uses high-intensity sound waves in the range of 2–20 MHz to generate images of internal structures (Cosgrove et al. 2008). It is attractive in that it is portable and images can be achieved in real time. Further, this modality does not employ ionizing radiation or contrast agents, thus minimizing side effects and damage.

Sound waves are generated at the ultrasound transducer and are propagated through the tissue particles from one particle to the next much like marbles hitting one another. Some of the sound is absorbed and some is reflected, particularly at tissue boundaries (Cosgrove et al. 2008). By fixing the frequency of the transducer, the time required for sound waves to reflect back to the transducer can be related to depth; this is how ultrasound determines dimension. Wave reflection occurs at tissue boundaries, with the degree of reflection being related to the change in density of those two tissues. Thus ultrasound is very poor at imaging that for which radiographs are good: bone and air boundaries (Mettler 2005). Attempting to image the brain is near impossible as the sound waves do not traverse well past bone. Similarly, imaging lung is also difficult as the air boundary does not reflect sound and attenuates transmission. Contrast is achieved by the amount of reflection and absorption that returns to the transducer.

The utility of ultrasound in diagnosing pain conditions is quite limited. Because ultrasound is good for identifying tendons, it has a potential role in diagnosing tendonitis. However, the diagnosis of this condition is primarily clinical and does not require imaging to confirm or refute the diagnosis (Bogduk 2003). Ultrasound is of greater benefit therapeutically as it aids in the positioning of needles for nerve blocks. Such blocks may include aspiration and injection of joints or intercostals nerve blocks.

Bone Scans

The previous imaging techniques discussed create contrast by differential reaction of tissues to the stimulus of the modality being used, whether it is radiation, sound waves, or magnetic spin. Bone scans act in a similar fashion: Technetium 99-m-labeled diphosphonates (a radiotracer "contrast agent") are injected and differentially taken up by the tissues (Love et al. 2003). This compound initially disperses throughout all tissue and is ultimately taken up by bone, particularly in areas of rapid bone formation and good blood flow (Love et al. 2003). Patients are initially injected and then told to drink fluids and come back in 2–6 h for detection. By waiting and by encouraging fluid intake, the labeled diphosphonates are washed out of non-bony tissue and allowed to concentrate in bone resulting in greater distinction of uptake of the radiolabeled compounds and a more detailed picture. This picture is obtained by asking patients to lie in front of a gamma camera for about an hour (Love et al. 2003). Front and back images are typically obtained as well as any specific locations required. Thus dimension is limited to flat views much like in plain radiographs except that the entire body (front and back) may be imaged at once. The images do not carry the resolution detail that an MRI may have; they are actually somewhat "fuzzy" by comparison (see Fig. 6.4) but do offer good sensitivity (Love et al. 2003). Specificity is obtained by examining the pattern and distribution of the radiotracer uptake. For example, radiotracer accumulation in both the vertebral body and pedicles is suggestive of metastatic disease while sparing of the pedicles suggests benign disease. Patterns are not always constant and thus specificity is not superb, but the good sensitivity of this test and its ability to image the entire body make it a good screening test, particularly in its principle use: identification of distant metastases in cancer. It is more sensitive than plain radiograph and more efficient when imaging of the entire body is needed (Love et al. 2003).

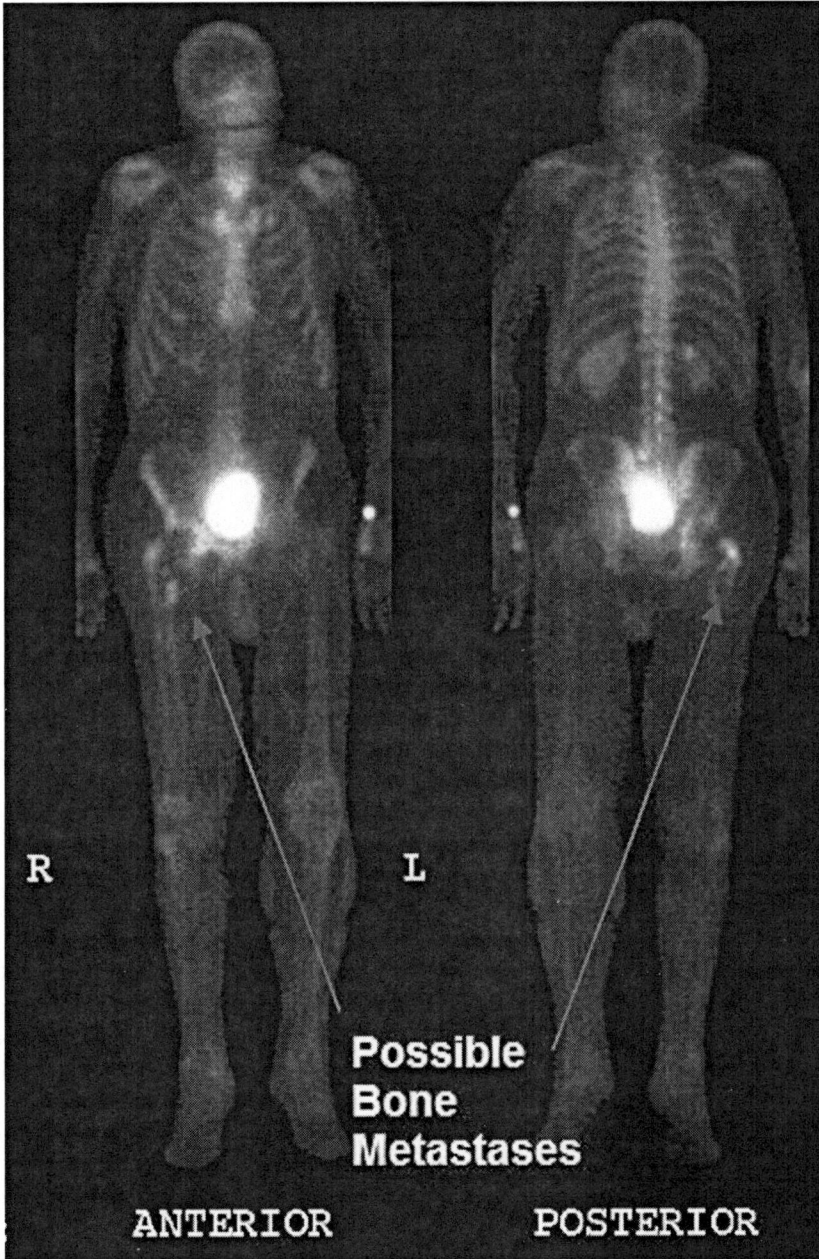

Figure 6.4 Bone scan images do not carry the resolution detail that an MRI may have; they are actually somewhat "fuzzy" by comparison but do offer good sensitivity.

In identification of metastases, the radiotracer concentrates in areas of bone formation and thus osteoblastic metastases may preferentially be identified compared to osteoclastic metastases. Furthermore, following hormone therapy or other chemotherapies, bone lesions may "flare" as part of the treatment response for about 3 months and worsening of the bone scan may simply reflect this "flare" and not worsening disease. However, a worsening bone scan beyond 6 months should raise concern for metastases (Love et al. 2003).

Bone scans are also useful for diagnosing acute stress fractures. This is only natural because fracture repair involves both bone formation and increased blood flow factors which concentrate the radiolabeled diphosphonates (Love et al. 2003). Furthermore, when plain radiographs fail to identify occult fractures (such as in the hip), a bone scan may be useful because of its greater sensitivity in determining areas of bone formation (Mettler 2005).

Shin splints, "or medial tibial stress syndrome, can be described as a clinical entity characterized by diffuse tenderness over the posteromedial aspect of the distal third of the tibia" caused by inflammation of the tibialis and soleus muscle insertions at the tibia (Love et al. 2003, Wilder and Sethi 2004). In a similar fashion, excessive walking or standing can cause inflammation of the plantar fascia on the bottom of the foot, referred to as plantar fasciitis. Sometimes referred to as a heel spur, it is aggravated by excessive use but is also worse in the morning as the plantar fascia may contract overnight and increase pain. Bone scan is useful in these diagnoses as radiotracers localize at the site of tendinous insertion of the muscles and fascia onto the bone.

Triple-phase bone scan is an imaging modality classically used to identify pain from complex regional pain syndrome but is more useful for osteomyelitis (Love et al. 2003). A triple-phase bone scan, as its name applies, has three phases: a dynamic phase (performed immediately after radiotracer injection), a blood pool phase (performed 3–5 min after injection), and a delayed bone phase (performed 2–6 h after injection) (Nagoya et al. 2008). In this scan, both blood flow and bone turnover are also evaluated as opposed to evaluation of only bone turnover in a plain bone scan. In the dynamic phase, the general amount of blood flow to an area is determined; in the blood pool phase, the amount of extravasation of tracer into the surrounding tissue is detected; while in the delayed phase, bone uptake is measured (Love et al. 2003). Because infections lead to increased blood flow in the area of infection as well as leaky tissue (osteomyel-"*itis*"), the two initial phases of at three-phase bone scan are useful in their diagnosis. The final phase, the delayed bone scan phase, localizes this infection to the bone ("*osteo*"-myelitis) by demonstrating increased bone turnover. Both fractures and metastases, as well as infections, may cause hyperperfusion and hyperemia resulting in positive three-phase bone scans. When diagnostic doubt exists and greater specificity is needed, a subsequent scan using indium-111 tagged leukocytes will be positive for infection but not the other conditions. In this scan, leukocytes are withdrawn from a patient, labeled with indium-111 and re-injected. Detection is performed 24 h later with the belief that these labeled leukocytes will concentrate at an area of infection.

Some have advocated use of bone scans to assess problems with prosthetic joints such as loosening and infection. Radiographs can provide some initial information on loosening but cannot elucidate presence or absence of infection (Nagoya et al. 2008). While CT scan and MRI can provide image on infection with the use of contrast, the presence of joint hardware can obscure the images by creating artifacts. Studies have indeed demonstrated good sensitivity and specificity for both prosthetic joint infection and loosening when all three phases

Table 6.5 Conditions for which bone scan may be used as initial or follow-up test.

Bone scan as primary modality
☐ Metastases
☐ Stress fracture
☐ Tendonitis and fasciitis
Bone scan following plain radiograph
☐ Occult hip fracture
☐ Prosthetic joint, infection, or loosening

of a bone scan are conducted, but follow-up tissue diagnosis is recommended (Nagoya et al. 2008). What may be of greatest benefit is a negative triple-phase bone scan as that strongly argues against any pathology and obviates the need for tissue specimens (Love et al. 2003) (Table 6.5).

Quantitative Sensory Testing

Sensory examinations are inherently subjective, both in the manner in which they are performed by an examiner and in the responses the examinee may report. While more of a diagnostic technique than an imaging technique, Quantitative Sensory Testing (QST) can aid in the diagnosis of pain syndromes by standardizing techniques of examination and evaluation. It is defined in its name: a means to perform sensory testing in a quantitative manner, rather than a subjective and qualitative manner. It is loosely analogous to the hearing exam performed in elementary school where fixed stimuli are given and response noted. Unfortunately, QST tests the entire sensory axis rather than localizing the pathology (Gruener and Dyck 1994). Viewing the results in the context of other available signs and symptoms helps pinpoint pathology.

The goal of QST is to standardize the stimuli and create a consistent algorithm for gauging the response in a manner that is reproducible between exams and patients (Gruener and Dyck 1994). QST devices test either vibration or thermal stimuli (Shy et al. 2003). There are two ways to apply such stimuli: (1) by gradually increasing the strength of stimulus in a continuous fashion until a response is detected or (2) applying fixed strength of stimulus for a specific time and noting absence or response (analogous to a hearing exam). Both methods of assessment have strengths and weaknesses; but that no single method is ideal points to the inherent subjectivity of human responses and this method of testing. As a result, concerns have been raised that subject response variability makes this test not entirely reproducible or appropriate for medico-legal disputes to assess malingering (Shy et al. 2003).

Case Scenario

Timothy Malhotra, MD

Omar is a 63-year-old retired teacher with a previous history of prostate cancer (now with no evidence of disease). He has been complaining of right knee swelling for the last few weeks. As his primary care physician, you prescribe acetaminophen, ibuprofen, and tramadol for 2 weeks. He returns to see you at the end of 2 weeks. He is still suffering from pain and you note that his knee is swollen and tender. There are no other signs of inflammation. You suspect an effusion of the knee joint.

How would you confirm your diagnosis?
An X-ray of the knee joint could confirm the effusion around the knee joint. Ultrasound scan is another imaging option. Nevertheless, to identify the nature of the effusion requires aspiration of the joint.

You order an immediate X-ray of the knee joint, which shows a collection of fluid inside the joint. You refer Omar to an orthopedic surgeon who aspirates the joint under ultrasound guidance. The aspirate is straw colored, and it is sent to the laboratory for analysis.

Two days following knee aspiration, Omar complains of increased pain, redness, warmth, and swelling around the aspirated area. In addition, he has fever and an elevated white blood count. A diagnosis of joint infection is made secondary to the procedure performed. To confirm the diagnosis and to rule out osteomyelitis, another X-ray is ordered. However, this x-ray is equivocal and fails to demonstrate a firm diagnosis of osteomyelitis.

What would be your investigation of choice in this situation?
An MRI scan of the knee joint with contrast can confirm the presence of osteomyelitis.

An immediate MRI scan is arranged and it shows not only the presence of osteomyelitis, but also demonstrates bony metastases to the knee. Further demonstrated on the MRI is an occult knee fracture not seen on plain radiograph. Omar mentions that he does have generalized bone pain in addition to the knee pain.

How would you rule out the presence of widespread bony metastasis in this case?
Because there is a concern for additional bony metastases, a bone scan should be performed. As suspected, the scan demonstrates widespread bony metastatic disease as well as the occult knee fracture. Meanwhile, you receive the result of examination of the aspirate from the laboratory and it reveals the presence of cancer cells. Omar undergoes chemotherapy which results in remission of the disease.

However, a few months later Omar is back in your clinic with sudden onset low lumbar back pain. You undertake a detailed clinical examination but there are no radicular signs. You order an X-ray of lumbar spine to rule out any fractures. The X-ray is negative and you advise Omar to continue to take the analgesics that you had prescribed earlier.

Two days later, Omar begins to experience radicular symptoms. You order an MRI of the lumbar spine, but the radiologist has difficulty interpreting the results as Omar has bullet fragments lodged in his lumbar spine from a shooting incident that happened years ago. The lead bullet fragments had caused streak artifact on the MRI. Because imaging is needed urgently, the radiologist decides to perform a CT scan of the spine with myelography, instead of the MRI.

While in the CT scanner, Omar develops symptoms of urticaria, pruritus, nausea, vomiting, and dizziness. Moments later he complains of bronchospasm, palpitations, bradycardia, hypertension, and headache.

What is your diagnosis and how will you manage this?
This is an idiosyncratic reaction to the contrast agent and is considered a medical emergency. It should be managed swiftly and effectively as per the anaphylaxis protocol (The ABC's of *Airway, Breathing, Circulation*). Immediately stop injecting the contrast. Oxygen and epinephrine should be administered without any delay. Also, consider administration of an antihistamine and steroid. Fortunately, the reaction is treated successfully and Omar is admitted overnight for observation.

His CT scan in fact demonstrates that he has a wedge fracture of L4 and a herniated disk at the L4–L5 level with impingement on the thecal sac. Omar undergoes a course of radiotherapy to help control the pain from the wedge fracture. In a few weeks Omar responds favorably to the radiotherapy.

However, one month later, he complains of severe sacral low back pain radiating down both legs with burning and electric shock sensations. As imaging options were limited, an MRI (without contrast) of the sacrum is ordered as it is somewhat distant from the bullet fragments. This demonstrates arachnoiditis-likely a reaction to myelographic dye. He prefers conservative pain management with oral medications. Unfortunately, he fails to respond and opts for the placement of an intrathecal pump with very good results.

References

Bogduk N. Diagnostic procedures in chronic pain. In: Jensen TS, Wilson PR, Rice ASC, editors. Chronic pain. London: Arnold; 2003. pp. 125–44.

Cosgrove DO. Ultrasound: general principles. In: Adam A, Dixon AK, editors. Adam Grainger & Allison's diagnostic radiology. Philadelphia, PA: Elsevier; 2008.

Eldevik OP, Haughton VM. Risk factors in complications of aqueous myelography. Radiology 1978;128(2):415–6.

Gruener G, Dyck PJ. Quantitative sensory testing: methodology, applications, and future directions. J Clin Neurophysiol. 1994;11(6):568–83.

Kleefield J. Radiological evaluation of spinal disease. In: Warfield C, Bajwa ZJ, editors. Principles and practice of pain medicine. New York, NY: McGraw-Hill; 2004. pp. 83–111.

Love C. Radionuclide bone imaging: an illustrative review. Radiographics 2003;23(2):341–58.

Mettler F. Essentials of radiology. Philadelphia, PA: Elsevier Saunders; 2005.

Modic MT. Lumbar herniated disk disease and canal stenosis: prospective evaluation by surface coil MR, CT, and myelography. Am J Roentgenol. 1986;147(4):757–65.

Nagoya S. Diagnosis of peri-prosthetic infection at the hip using triple-phase bone scintigraphy. J Bone Joint Surg Br. 2008;90(2):140–4.

Prince MR, Arnoldus C, Frisoli JK. Nephrotoxicity of high-dose gadolinium compared with iodinated contrast. J Magn Reson Imaging. 1996;6(1):162–6.

Shy ME. Quantitative sensory testing: report of the Therapeutics and Technology Assessment Subcommittee of the American Academy of Neurology. Neurology 2003;60(6):898–904.

Siddiqi NH. Contrast medium reactions, recognition and treatment. Available from: http://emedicine.medscape.com/article/422855-overview. Accessed 11 Feb 2008.

Unknown. DCMRC-Contraindications to MRI. [Web Page] 2009. Available from: http://dcmrc.mc.duke.edu/resources_physicians/contraindications.html. Accessed 27 Feb 2009.

Unknown. Important safety information for drug delivery systems. [Web Page] 2009. Available from: http://www.medtronic.com/your-health/painful-neuropathy/important-safety-information/drug-pumps/index.htm. Accessed 26 Feb 2009.

Unknown. Information for healthcare professionals gadolinium-based contrast agents for magnetic resonance imaging (marketed as Magnevist, MultiHance, Omniscan, OptiMARK, ProHance) [Web Page 2009; FDA ALERT]. Available from: http://www.fda.gov/cder/drug/InfoSheets/HCP/gcca_200705.htm. Accessed 28 Feb 2009.

Wilder RP, Sethi S. Overuse injuries: tendinopathies, stress fractures, compartment syndrome, and shin splints. Clin Sports Med. 2004;23(1):55–81, vi.

Wilkinson ID, Paley MNJ. Magnetic resonance imaging: basic principles. In: Grainger & Allison's diagnostic radiology. Philadelphia, PA: Churchill Livingstone; 2008.

Section IV

Pharmacology

Chapter 7

Opioids: Pharmacokinetics and Pharmacodynamics

Charles J. Fox III, MD, Henry A. Hawney, MD, and Alan D. Kaye, MD, PhD

Opiate History

Opiates have been used for pain control for several thousands of years, dating back to the times of the ancient Sumerians. The Sumerians documented poppy in their pharmacopoeia and called it "HU GIL," the plant of joy (Benedetti 1987). In the third century BC, Theophrastus has the first documented reference to poppy juice (Macht 1915). The word opium is derived from the Greek name for juice obtained from the poppy, *Papaver,* and the Latin name for sleep inducing, *somniferum.* Arab traders brought opium to the Orient, where it was used to treat the symptoms of dysentery. Opium contains approximately 20 distinct naturally occurring alkaloids, called opiates, such as morphine or codeine. In 1805, a German pharmacist Sertüner isolated a pure substance in opium and called it morphine. Morphine is named after Morpheus, the Greek god of dreams. After this initial discovery, many more opium alkaloids were discovered. Robiquet isolated codeine in 1832, and Merck isolated papaverine in 1848. In 1898, Bayer Pharmaceuticals launched an alternative to opium and morphine, diacetylmorphine or heroin, from the German word for hero. By the middle of the nineteenth century, pure opium alkaloids, rather than basic opium preparations, spread throughout the medical community. Until the early twentieth century, opioid abuse in the United States increased because of unrestricted availability of opium along with a massive influx of opium-smoking immigrants from the Orient. In fact, Thomas Jefferson grew opium poppies at Monticello. In 1942, the Opium Poppy Control Act banned opium production in the United States (Booth 1999). It is important to differentiate "opioids," which are substances that act on the opiate receptor, and the term "narcotic," which is a substance that produces narcosis and can be abused, such as cocaine, cannabis, and barbiturates (Reisine 1996). Narcotics are derived from the Greek word for stupor. Narcotics were initially used for sleeping aid medications rather than for opiates. Narcotic is now a legal term for drugs that are abused. In 2007, 93% of the opiates on the world market originated in Afghanistan (United Nations Office on Drugs and Crime 2007). This amounts to an annual export value of about $64 billion.

N. Vadivelu et al. (eds.), *Essentials of Pain Management,*
DOI 10.1007/978-0-387-87579-8_7, © Springer Science+Business Media, LLC 2011

Endogenous Opioid Peptides

The existence of an endogenous opioid system had been described as early as 1969. When certain areas of the rat brain were electrically stimulated, analgesia was produced, then reversed rapidly by the opioid antagonist naloxone. In 1975, the first endogenous opioid peptide was identified and named enkephalin. Shortly after, two other opioid peptides, endorphin and dynorphin, were identified. The endogenous opioid peptides are derived from one of three precursor polypeptides and released during stressful times. These precursors undergo complex cleavages and modifications to yield multiple active peptides which act at discrete receptors throughout the body. All of these opioid peptides share a common amino-terminal sequence, called the "opioid motif." The opioid effects of these peptides are quickly terminated by endogenous peptidases.

β-Endorphins are derived from preproopiomelanocortin (Pre-POMC), found in the central nervous system, and act primarily as μ1 opioid receptor agonists. Additionally, Pre-POMC can be cleaved into other nonopioid peptides such as adrenocorticotropic hormone (ACTH), melanocyte-stimulating hormone (MSH), and β-lipoprotein (β-1-LPH), demonstrating that endogenous opioid peptides are linked to numerous hormones. Preproenkephalin serves as the precursor for met-enkephalin and leu-enkephalin. Dynorphin A, Dynorphin B, and α-neoendorphin and β neoendorphin arise after cleaving preprodynorphin. The enkephalins act as *delta* (δ)-opioid receptor agonists and are found in areas of the central nervous system, gastrointestinal tract and adrenal medulla. Dynorphins have a bodily distribution similar to enkephalin, but lack their analgesic strength. They act as agonists at *kappa* (κ)-opioid receptors. All endogenous peptides produce their pharmacologic effects through membrane-bound, G-protein-coupled receptors.

Opioid Receptors

Opioid receptors are glycoproteins found in cell membranes at multiple sites in the central nervous system and in the periphery. Opioid receptors have multiple subtypes; the most important are μ, κ, and δ, and the opioid receptor-like receptor (ORL) (Table 7.1). Morphine and morphine-like opioids bind primarily to the μ receptors. These receptors are located in the periaqueductal gray matter (brain) and the substantia gelatinosa (spinal cord) (Carr and Lipkowski 1993). μ receptors can be further subdivided into μ1 and μ2 receptors. μ1 activation produces analgesia, and μ2 activation produces euphoria, respiratory depression, nausea, vomiting, decreased gastrointestinal motility, urinary retention, tolerance, dependence, histamine release, miosis, and/or anorexia (Ferrante 1993). The structural and pharmacochemical differences between opioid agonists can affect the binding and affinity with the mu receptor leading to varied analgesic responses.

At present, pharmaceutical researchers are trying to develop a μ1 opioid-specific agonist to eliminate the many unwanted side effects caused by activation of μ2 receptors. These *mu* receptor subtypes can lead to a patient responding better to one opioid versus another for adequate pain control and also to the phenomenon of cross-tolerance. Cross-tolerance is related to different subtypes of receptors, such as the activity of *kappa* and *delta* opioids mediating analgesia in the presence of high doses of *mu* opioid agonists. κ receptor activation causes analgesia (visceral and spinal), sedation, dysphoria, hallucinations, and less respiratory depression compared to μ receptors (Mogil and Pasternal 2001). Peripheral κ

Table 7.1   Four major subtypes of opioid receptors.

Receptor	Subtypes	Location	Function
Delta (δ)	δ_1, δ_2	• *Brain* o Pontine nuclei o Amygdala o Olfactory bulbs o Deep cortex	• Analgesia • Antidepressant effects • Physical dependence
Kappa (κ)	$\kappa_1, \kappa_2, \kappa_3$	• *Brain* o Hypothalamus o Periaqueductal gray o Claustrum • *Spinal cord* o Substantia gelatinosa	• Spinal analgesia • Sedation • Miosis • Inhibition of ADH release
Mu (μ)	μ_1, μ_2, μ_3	• *Brain* o Cortex (laminae III and IV) o Thalamus o Striosomes o Periaqueductal gray • *Spinal cord* o Substantia gelatinosa • *Intestinal tract*	μ_1: • Supraspinal analgesia • Physical dependence μ_2: • Respiratory depression • Miosis • Euphoria • Reduced GI motility • Physical dependence μ_3: • ?
Nociceptin receptor	ORL$_1$	• *Brain* o Cortex o Amygdala o Hippocampus o Septal nuclei o Habenula • *Hypothalamus*	• Anxiety • Depression • Appetite • Development of tolerance to μ agonists

Modified from Janet C. Hsieh and Daniel B. Carr, Massachusetts General Hospital Handbook of Pain Management, Lippincott Williams and Wilkins, 2005.

receptors have been found in the gastrointestinal tract, muscle, skin, connective tissues, and kidneys, where their activation can result in oliguria and antidiuresis. The primary endogenous ligand for κ receptors is dynorphin A. The δ receptor facilitates μ receptor activity and enhances supraspinal and spinal analgesia. The primary endogenous ligand for δ receptors is enkephalin. The ORL receptor is similar in structure to the classical opioid receptors (μ, κ, and δ), but the classical ligands do not have a high affinity for it. A new neuropeptide, termed orphanin FQ (nociceptin), was found to have a high affinity for the ORL-1 receptor (Borsook 1994). Orphanin FQ has potent anti-analgesic actions supraspinally and analgesic actions spinally. Other orphanin FQ activities are less clear. The diversity of responses might reflect ORL-1 receptor heterogeneity, but more studies are needed on this novel substance. The N-methyl-D-aspartate (NMDA) receptor is associated with opioid tolerance and is involved with nociceptive transmission in the spinal dorsal horn (Borsook 1994), as shown for the μ receptor in Fig. 7.1. The NMDA receptor is an inotropic receptor for glutamate and is distinct in that it is both ligand-gated and voltage-dependent. Methadone, dextromethorphan, ketamine, and tramadol are all examples of NMDA receptor antagonists. NMDA receptor antagonists can reduce the incidence of tolerance to morphine or other opiate agents.

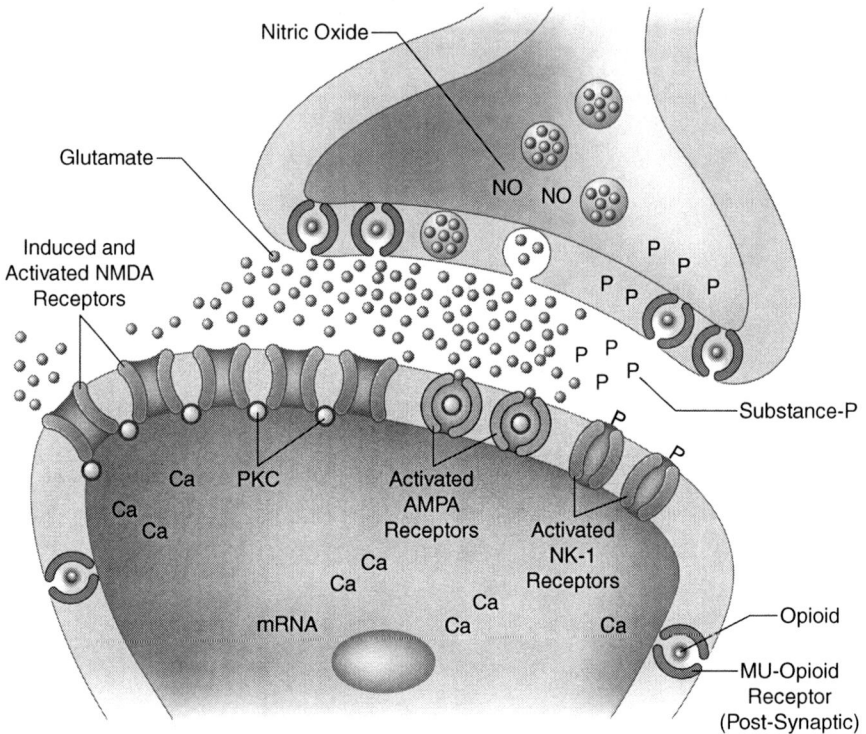

Figure 7.1 μ-**Receptor function.**

Classification of Opioids

There are multiple systems used to classify opioids. They may be categorized according to receptor affinity or by their intrinsic activity at that receptor site. According to the latter, they are classified as agonist, partial agonists, agonist/antagonist, or antagonist (Table 7.2). When classified according to receptor affinity, they may be classified as either weak or strong opioids. Based on derivation, opioids may be grouped as natural (morphine and codeine), semisynthetic, or synthetic (Table 7.3). Chemical classes of opioids include phenanthrenes, benzomorphans, phenylpiperidines, and diphenylheptanes.

Opium serves as the main source for production of the two naturally occurring alkaloid opioid chemical classes. One alkaloid group, consisting of morphine, codeine, and thebaine, contains the three-ringed phenanthrene nucleus. The other group consists of benzylisoquinoline alkaloids, papaverine, and noscapine, which lack analgesic activity. The semisynthetic opioids are produced by altering the alkaloid ring structure of naturally occurring opioids. Thebaine serves as precursor for the potent opioid oxycodone and the antagonist naloxone, while morphine serves as the building block for heroin. Synthetic opioids belong to one of the four chemical classes listed above. These chemical classes result after progressively reducing rings from the original five-ring structure of morphine. Phenanthrenes consist of a four-ring nucleus while phenylpiperidines contain only a two-ring nucleus (Gustein and Akil 2006).

Table 7.2 Classification of opioids: intrinsic receptor activity.

Class	Definition	Example
Agonist	A drug which causes maximal stimulation of the opioid receptor when bound	Morphine, fentanyl, sufentanil, remifentanil
Antagonists	A drug which fails to cause any stimulation of the receptor when bound	Naloxone
Partial agonists	A drug that, when bound to the receptor, stimulates the receptor below maximal intensity	Buprenorphine
Mixed agonists/ antagonists	A drug which acts simultaneously on several receptor subtypes. Drug acts as agonist on one or more subtypes and as antagonist at one or more subtypes	Nalbuphine, butorphanol

Modified from Wall (1994).

Table 7.3 Classification of opioids by derivation.

Naturally occurring	Semisynthetic	Synthetic
Phenanthrene	Morphine	Morphinans
Morphine	Diacetylmorphine	Levorphanol
Codeine	Dihydromorphinone	Nalbuphine
Thebaine	Dihydrohydroxymorphinone	
Benzylisoquinoline	Thebaine derivatives	Phenylheptylamines
Papaverine	Buprenorphine	Methadone
Noscapine	Oxycodone	l-Alpha-acetylmethadol (LAAM)
		Propoxyphene
		Phenylpiperidine
		Alfentanil
		Alphaprodine
		Fentanyl
		Ketobemidone
		Meperidine
		Remifentanil
		Sufentanil

Modified from Uppington (2005).

Mechanism of Action

Opioids bind to the G protein of the opioid receptors, which are widespread in the central nervous system, the peripheral nervous system, and other tissues. The sites in the central nervous system are associated with the processing of the affective and suffering aspects of pain perception. These include the cortex, central gray medial thalamus, amygdala, limbic cortex, midbrain, and spinal cord. It appears that opioids are not concentrated on the somatosensory cortex, which is important for pain localization. Sites in the peripheral nervous system include the mesenteric plexus of the gastrointestinal tract and the afferent neurons. Sites in other tissues include the lung and the joints. The presynaptic receptors are both excitatory and inhibitory, while the postsynaptic receptors are only inhibitory (Crain and Shen 1990). Opioids can bind to both the presynaptic and postsynaptic receptors. Presynaptic binding of the opioid receptors by opioids decreases adenylate cyclase activity, inhibits calcium channels that are voltage sensitive, and decreases the release of neurotransmitters such as glutamate, serotonin, norepinephrine, acetylcholine, and substance P (Herz 1993). The binding of the opioid receptors to the postsynaptic receptors leads to an increase in the outward conductance of potassium, hyperpolarization, and a corresponding decrease in neural transmission.

Pharmacokinetics of Opioids

Absorption

Absorption refers to the rate and extent at which a drug leaves the site of administration. Opioids must cross at least one membrane to arrive at the site of action. Although most opioids are well absorbed when administered orally, subcutaneously, or intravenously, opioid onset, duration, and potency depend on numerous factors.

Lipid solubility, protein binding, ionization state, molecular size, and membrane physiochemical properties significantly influence the absorption of opioids (Miyoshi and Leckband 2001).

Opioids are basic molecules which are highly ionized at physiologic pH. The pKa of a given opioid refers to the pH of a drug at which 50% of the drug exists in the ionized form and 50% in the nonionized form. The drugs with an increased nonionized component have an increased rate of absorption. Likewise, lipophilic opioids quickly traverse membranes compared to their hydrophilic counterparts. Smaller molecular size permits easier negotiation through membranes. The ideal opioid for absorption would be highly nonionized at physiologic pH, lipophilic, and of smaller molecular size.

Distribution

The volume of distribution is the concentration of the drug in the body divided by the plasma concentration. Distribution is to three compartments: the vascular compartment (5% of body weight), the intracellular compartment (30% of body weight), and the extracellular compartment (15% of body weight). Molecular size, lipid solubility, and protein binding influence the volume of distribution. Highly lipophilic drugs easily traverse membranes and are easily distributed to all three compartments, whereas lipid-insoluble drugs do not easily cross tissue membranes and experience only a small volume of distribution. Large molecular size or highly protein-bound drugs rarely leave the vascular compartment and result in a limited volume of distribution.

After a drug enters the systemic circulation, it is distributed throughout the body. Distribution is generally uneven because of differences in regional blood flow related to "directed" cardiac output. Because of this, there are two phases of distribution within the body. In the first phase, the drug is distributed to the highly perfused vital organs (kidney, brain, and liver). In the next phase, drug is delivered to the lesser perfused organs (skin, fat, and muscle).

Metabolism/Elimination

After the opioids are distributed throughout the body, there is termination of the drug's pharmacological activity and elimination of drug metabolites. To accomplish this, biotransformation of the opioid must take place. Biotransformation is a chemical process whereby drugs undergo structural change through a series of endogenous enzymatic reactions, which terminate their action and prepare the drug for elimination. For example, this mechanism transforms nonpolar molecules into more polar molecules, thus preventing reabsorption by the kidney in favor of excretion.

Biotransformation occurs primarily in the liver and consists of two phases. Phase I reactions may involve oxidation, hydrolysis, reduction, or hydration of the opioid to produce a more water-soluble and less active metabolite. The majority of metabolites produced during this phase are hydroxylated by the cytochrome P-450 enzyme system. Phase II involves a conjugation reaction which covalently attaches a small polar endogenous molecule, such as glucuronic acid, sulfate, or glycine, to a functional group on the opioid compound. This process yields a large molecular weight compound which is usually inactive and is more easily excreted.

While most opioid metabolites produced through Phase I and Phase II reactions are inactive and nontoxic, certain opioid metabolites are more toxic or potent than the parent compound. Meperidine is metabolized to normeperidine. This metabolite is potentially neurotoxic in patients placed on chronic therapy or who have poor renal function. Morphine is metabolized into two major metabolites: morphine-3-glucuronide (M3G) and morphine-6-glucuronide (M6G), which rely on renal elimination. M3G possesses antinociceptive effects and M6G has analgesic properties which appear more potent than morphine (Christup 1997).

Parent opioid drugs or their metabolites are eliminated through many routes (renal, liver, sweat, tears, breast milk, and saliva). The kidneys are the primary elimination route, with almost 90% eliminated in the urine. Some opioid metabolites experience biotransformation in the liver, and their metabolites are excreted by the gastrointestinal tract after gaining entrance through bile.

Routes of Administration

Opioids are the mainstay for pain management and are available in oral, neuraxial, rectal, transdermal, and intravenous forms for delivery. Oral administration is an easy, relatively inexpensive, and effective method for delivery of opioids. Despite significant first-pass effect with some oral opioids (e.g., oral morphine only has 25% of total dose available), the vast majority of patients are able to use oral dosing to provide for their analgesic needs. Concerns over incomplete bioavailability, peak levels, and analgesic onset are overcome with proper scheduling and dosing adjustments. Duration of action can be increased with sustained release preparations.

Intravenous opioid administration is practical for treatment of acute pain following surgery or trauma. Intravenous delivery provides a quicker onset of analgesic activity, but offers no difference in potency, despite popular belief. Intravenous patient-controlled analgesia is commonly used to treat acute pain postoperatively and allows the patient to self-administer analgesics. Hourly limits and lock-out intervals add to the safety profile of this device. Chronic pain patients, for various reasons, occasionally need intravenous administration of opioids. The major disadvantage of this route is the need of continuous intravenous access. Indwelling central or peripheral catheters incur significant cost with placement and maintenance. Additionally, they serve as an entry point for infection. Frequently, home health services are needed to administer the opioid intravenous infusion and maintenance care for the access catheter.

Intraoperatively, the primary intravenous agents used are morphine or a member of the phenylpiperidine family (fentanyl, sufentanil, or remifentanil). Sufentanil is the most powerful opioid mu-receptor agonist available for human clinical use and has been used for many years by cardiac anesthesiologists. Additionally, it has gained popularity in the intensive care unit. Critical care patients under mechanical ventilation require medications to enhance comfort and control noxious stimuli. Sufentanil provides fewer adverse respiratory effects than traditional opioids and enables quicker awakening than standard sedation medications for patients requiring frequent neurological evaluations (Giorgio et al. 2004, Conti et al. 2005).

Hydromorphone, morphine, and oxymorphone are available in rectal suppositories. Some of these preparations provide a more controlled release rate and higher bioavailability than oral preparations. Slow release morphine tablets have been given rectally when the oral route is not tolerable. Insertion of the suppository directly above the anal sphincter minimizes first-pass metabolism. The inferior and middle rectal veins do not drain into the portal circulation. However, higher placement of the suppository in the rectal vault can lead to drainage into the superior rectal vein and first-pass effect.

Another option for patients unable to take oral medications is the transdermal route. It is a noninvasive, avoids many of the gastrointestinal side effects, and, overall, is an effective manner for opioid delivery. Presently, fentanyl (Duragesic patch®, Janssen Pharmaceutica, Titusville, NJ) is the only medication available in this form. The delivery system includes a fentanyl reservoir, which contains a 3-day supply of fentanyl, and a controlling membrane. The medication is delivered through passive diffusion. The transdermal patches take up to 12 h to reach maximal blood levels and provide analgesia for 72 h (Giorgio et al. 2004). The major disadvantage of this route is the inability to rapidly increase or decrease blood levels. Transient and mild skin irritation can occur with transdermal patches. Rotation of skin sites has helped minimize this issue. Overall, this delivery system is well tolerated by chronic pain patients on chronic opioid doses.

Epidural and intrathecal administration of opioids is frequently used for management of postoperative pain. It is utilized by chronic pain physicians when other routes of administration are unable to provide adequate analgesia or when they are causing significant side effects. When placed neuraxially, small opioid doses provide profound analgesia. Fentanyl and morphine are the two most common opioids delivered by this route. The most worrisome side effect is delayed respiratory depression, which can occur up to 12 h after intrathecal administration. Because morphine is hydrophilic, it spreads rostrally and is a more common offender in causing delayed respiratory depression (Gupta et al. 1992).

Effects of Opioids

Central Nervous System

There are several effects of opioids on the central nervous system. One of the most common effects of opioids is the occurrence of nausea and vomiting because of the direct stimulation of the chemoreceptor trigger zone (CTRZ) on the floor of the fourth ventricle. Different classes of anti-emetics have been used to treat nausea and vomiting associated with opioid use. These include anticholinergics such as scopolamine, serotonin antagonists such as ondansetron, and the antidopaminergics such as droperidol and metoclopramide. Opioids can relieve the sensation of pain without affecting other sensations, such as temperature and pressure. They can, however, change the affective response and can produce dysphoria (activation of κ) and euphoria (activation of μ).

Confusion, delirium, and seizures can be seen with high doses of morphine in animal models. Seizures have been seen with meperidine in elderly patients and in patients with renal failure (in the latter group, the seizures are related to meperidine's metabolite, normeperidine). A common finding with opioid overuse is the presence of miosis by the stimulation of the parasympathetic Edinger–Westphal nucleus of the occulomotor nerve (Koyyalagunta 2006). Miosis can be seen with opioids having mu and kappa agonist effects. Muscle rigidity is another unwanted side effect seen with opioid administration. The mechanism is unknown, but studies hypothesize that it is located in the striatum, which has numerous opioid receptors (Monk 1998).

Respiratory Effects

Morphine acts directly on the respiratory centers of the brain stem and produces decreased minute ventilation by decreasing tidal volume. Respiratory depression is more likely with high doses of opioids. Respiratory depression is seen less with partial agonists/antagonists since they are mostly selective for kappa receptors. Morphine decreases the responsiveness to carbon dioxide, shifting the carbon dioxide response curve downward and to the right (Martin 1983). The cough center in the medulla can also be depressed with morphine (Grossman 1988). Naloxone is very effective in reversing respiratory depression quickly.

Neuroendocrine Effects

Opioids can decrease the body temperature by altering the equilibrium point of the hypothalamic heating mechanism (Koyyalagunta 2006). Opioids have neuroendocrine effects by suppressing the release of the hypothalamic releasing factors. There can be disruption of menstrual cycles with prolonged use of opioids (Koyyalagunta 2006). Opioids reduce the release of stress hormone and can also possibly suppress immune responses. Ongoing research has provided early evidence that opioids can enhance many types of infections and neoplastic conditions.

Gastrointestinal Effects

Opioids act on the gastrointestinal system to decrease gastric, duodenal, and large intestinal motility which can lead to delayed gastric emptying and induce an ileus (Murray 1984). The secretion of pancreatic, biliary, intestinal, and gastric secretions can be delayed, causing a stoppage in food digestion. With opioid administration, patients can develop a constriction of the sphincter of Oddi and an increased common bile duct pressure (Gustein and Akil 2001). Constipation is an extremely common problem with the use of opioids.

Bladder and Ureter

Opioids cause an increase in ureteral and external sphincter tone along with a decrease in the urinary voiding reflex (detrusor tone) (Thomass et al. 1992). These mechanisms can lead to urinary retention. Bladder volume is also seen to be increased in patients taking long-term opioids.

Skin

The release of histamine is probably the reason for the vasodilatation seen with morphine. Histamine may also be responsible for the local urticaria seen with local injection. Pruritus associated with opioid use could be due to a central mechanism and is more likely to do with neuraxial administration (Giorgio et al. 2004). Naloxone and antihistaminics are useful in relieving pruritus, but not the histamine effects (Conti et al. 2005).

In summary, opioid pharmacology is still in its infancy and each day brings about improved appreciation of its diverse pathways and functions. We should expect an ever-increasing understanding of the structure–activity relationship, agonist–receptor dynamics, and clinically relevant therapeutics in the very near future.

Case Scenario

Suresh Menon, MBBS, DA, FRCA and Sreekumar Kunnumpurath, MBBS, MD, FCARCSI, FRCA, FFPMRCA

As a fellow in pain medicine, you are approached by Emma, an intern on her nephrology rotation for advice regarding a patient, Michelle. Michelle is a 26-year-old female who is waiting for a renal transplant for end-stage renal failure. She is on dialysis and has been in and out of the operating room for various procedures such as fistula formation and insertion of peritoneal dialysis catheters. She has an infected peritoneal dialysis catheter, which was recently inserted as an interim measure. She is in excruciating pain. Antibiotics have been started and she is waiting a procedure to remove the catheter. Michelle is taking acetaminophen and codeine regularly for her pain. Unfortunately, her pain control is poor and she is complaining of constipation, nausea, and vomiting. Emma is worried and concerned about administering medication in the presence of renal failure. Her main concern is the administration of opioids, which so far have not given her any pain relief.

What is your interpretation of the observed discrepancy of lack of therapeutic effect and the evident side effect of codeine?
Both codeine and morphine are naturally occurring alkaloids found in poppy seeds. Morphine exerts its action by acting on various receptors in the brain and the spinal cord. There are mainly three receptors which morphine acts on: mu, kappa, and delta. Of these three receptors, pain relief is mainly mediated by mu receptors. Mu receptor has two subclasses, $\mu 1$ and $\mu 2$. Of these two, $\mu 1$ produces pain relief and $\mu 2$ mediates majority of the side effects of morphine. The side effects of opioids include euphoria, respiratory depression, nausea, vomiting, decreased gastrointestinal motility, urinary retention, tolerance, dependence, histamine release, miosis, and/or anorexia. This explains the constipation and nausea experienced by Michelle. Codeine, for its pain relieving effect, needs to be converted in the body into morphine by cytochrome P-450 enzyme system. There are large genetic variations in different population groups in their ability to do this. Different studies quote various figures, and it is estimated that about half of the population has decreased activity of this particular codeine-converting enzyme system. In fact, in a quarter of the world's population there is no

activity of this enzyme. As a result these population groups either get less analgesia from codeine or no pain relief at all.

What is the role of the route of administration on the effect of opioids?
There is a misconception among the public and even medical professionals that opioids need to be given intravenously or intramuscularly to produce good effects. In fact, the potency of opioids is not affected by the route; only the bioavailability is affected. For example, when morphine is given orally only about 30% is available. Again, various factors are responsible for this, such as absorption of the drug, first-pass metabolism, other drug interactions, and food intake. There are various preparations designed to circumvent these problems such as buccal and rectal preparations designed to avoid the first-pass metabolism.

Morphine is converted into water-soluble compounds by the liver and excreted by the kidney. Some of these metabolites are active forms and can produce toxicity if accumulated. About 90% of the drug is excreted by the kidney. Liver impairment and renal failure can adversely affect the metabolism and result in accumulation of the drug. However, this does not mean that opioids should be completely avoided in this group of patients. But caution should be exercised when prescribing opioids for these patients. The strategy should be to space the drug properly, avoid long-acting preparations and background infusions in case of patient-controlled analgesia, and monitor for the side effects carefully.

What are the analgesic options for Michelle?
Pain relief involves a multimodal approach. Patients like Michelle should be carefully evaluated before surgery and various analgesic options discussed. The components of her pain relief can be simple analgesics like acetaminophen, regional anesthesia if there are no contraindications, local anesthetic infiltration by the surgeon, and opioids such as hydromorphone, morphine. Another option would be fentanyl administered as needed or delivered by patient-controlled analgesia (PCA).

Hydromorphone, morphine, and fentanyl can be used as a patient-controlled analgesia if you expect the pain to be strong during the immediate postsurgical period. Fentanyl is a synthetic opioid which is about 100 times more potent than morphine but has a shorter duration of action. It may be safer to use fentanyl than morphine in patients with marked renal impairment. Again, whichever opioid is selected for the PCA (morphine, hydromorphone, fentanyl), the key to safety is careful monitoring for the side effects, particularly over sedation and respiratory depression.

References

Benedetti C. Intraspinal analgesia: an historical overview. Acta Anaesthesiol Scand. 1987;85:17.

Booth M: Opium: a history. New York, NY: St. Martin's Griffin; 1999.

Borsook D. Opioids and neurological effects. Curr Opin Anesthesiol. 1994;7:352–7.

Carr D, Lipkowski A. Mechanisms of opioid analgesic actions. In: Rodgers M, Tinker J, Covino B, et al., editors. Principles and practice of anesthesiology. St. Louis, MO: Mosby-Year Book; 1993:1105–30.

Christup L. Morphine metabolites. Acta Anaesthesiol Scand. 1997;41:116.

Conti G, Costa R, Pellegrini A, et al. Analgesia in PACU: intravenous opioids. Curr Drug Targets. 2005;6:767–71.

Crain B, Shen S. Opioids can evoke direct receptor mediated excitatory effects on sensory neurons. Trends Pharmacol Sci. 1990;11:77–81.

Ferrante M. Opioids. In: Ferrante M, VadeBoncouer T, eds. Postoperative pain management. New York, NY: Churchill Livingstone; 1993.

Giorgio A, Arcangeli C, Antonelli A, et al. Sedation with sufentanil in patients receiving pressure support ventilation has no effects on respiration: a pilot study. Can J Anesth. 2004;51:5:494–9.

Grossman A. Opioids and stress in man. J Endocrinol. 1988;119:377–81.

Gupta SK, Southam M, Gale R. System functionality and physiochemical model of fentanyl transdermal system. J Pain Symptom Manage. 1992;3(Suppl):17S.

Gustein H, Akil H. Opioid analgesics. In: Hardman J, Gilman A, et al, editors. Goodman and Gilman's the pharmacological basis of therapeutics, 10th ed. New York, NY: McGraw-Hill; 2001:569–619.

Gutstein HB, Akil H. Opioid analgesics. In: Brunton LL, Lazo JS, Parker KL, editors. Goodman & Gilman's the pharmacological basis of therapeutics, 11th ed. New York, NY: McGraw-Hill; 2006. pp. 547–90.

Herz A, ed. Handbook of experimental pharmacology. Opioids I. Berlin: Springer; Vol. 104/I, 1993.

Hughes J, Smith TW, Kosterlitz HW, et al. Identification of two related pentapeptides from the brain with potent opiate agonist activity. Nature 1975;258:577–80.

Koyyalagunta D. Opioid analgesics. In: Waldman S, editor. Pain management. New York, NY: Saunders-Elsevier; 2006:939–64.

Macht D. The history of opium and some of its preparations and alkaloids. JAMA 1915;46:477.

Martin W. Pharmacology of opioids. Pharmacol Rev. 1983;35:285–323.

Miyoshi HR, Leckband SG. Systemic opioid analgesics. In: Loeser JD, Butler SH, Chapman CR, Turk DC, editors. Bonica's management of pain, 3rd ed. Philadelphia, PA: Lippincott Williams & Wilkins; 2001. p. 1682.

Mogil, J, Pasternal G. The molecular and behavioral pharmacology of the orphanin FQ/nociceptin peptide and receptor family. Pharmacol Rev. 2001 Sept;53:381–415.

Monk J. Sufentanil: a review. Drugs 1998;36:249–381.

Murray K. Prevention of urinary retention associated phenoxybenzamine during epidural morphine. Br Med J. 1984;288:645.

Pasternak G, Goodman R, Snyder SH. An endogenous morphine like factor in mammalian brain. Life Sci. 1975;16:1765.

Reisine T, Pasternak G. Opioid analgesics and antagonists. In: Hardman J, Gilman A, et al, editors. Goodman and Gilman's the pharmacological basis of therapeutics, 9th ed. New York, NY: McGraw-Hill; 1996:521–555.

Reynold, RV. Surgery in the rat during electrical analgesia induced by focal brain stimulation. Science 1969;164:444.

Thomass D, Williams G, Iwata K, et al. Effects of central administration of opioids on facial scratching in monkeys. Anesth Analg. 1992;585:315.

United Nations Office on Drugs and Crime. Afghanistan opium survey 2007. http://www.unodc.org/pdf/research/AFG07_ExSum_web.pdf. 8-2007. Accessed 23 Oct 2009.

Uppington J. Opioids. Mass general handbook of pain management, 3rd ed. Philadelphia, PA: Lippincott Williams & Wilkins; October 2005.

Wall PD, Melzack R, eds. Textbook of pain, 3rd ed. Edinburgh, New York: Churchill-Livingstone; 1994.

Chapter 8

Opioids: Basic Concepts in Clinical Practice

Geremy L. Sanders, MD, MS, Michael P. Sprintz, DO, Ryan P. Ellender, MD,
Alecia L. Sabartinelli, MD, and Alan D. Kaye, MD, PhD

Opioid Uses

For centuries, opioids have been utilized to relieve pain and suffering. In current practice, opiates are employed to provide analgesia arising from both acute and chronic conditions. Acutely, opioids are most commonly used to treat pain following injury, surgery, or labor and delivery. They are also used to treat discomfort arising from exacerbations of medical disorders. In addition, opiates have been used in lower doses to treat cough; and they can also be effective in causing constipation or treating diarrhea. It is important to remember, however, that opiates merely treat these symptoms; the underlying disease remains.

Opioid Therapy

Opioid therapy involves the use of either weak or strong opiates, and often both are prescribed in conjunction to adequately control acute pain. Weak opiates typically come in oral preparations and are combined with varying formulations of acetaminophen, aspirin, or ibuprofen. All of these drugs have ceiling doses related to the non-opioid ingredient. For example, acetaminophen poisoning is one of the common causes of acute liver failure in the United States, and oftentimes these patients are on acetaminophen-containing opiates. Acetaminophen, also known as paracetamol or N-acetyl-p-aminophenol, causes centrilobular necrosis leading to nausea, vomiting, abdominal pain, renal failure and can progress to fulminant hepatic failure (Abram 2006).

Strong opiates are not mixed with other combination medications and are indicated for severe pain. These drugs do not have ceiling doses and toxicity relates directly to the dose-dependent effects of the opiate, for example, respiratory depression. Formulations include immediate release and sustained release preparations. Patients must be instructed not to crush sustained or extended release tablets as this can potentially lead to toxicity. Strong opiates often have additional routes beyond oral administration. Some of these include transdermal, parenteral, and neuraxial.

Prescribing Principles

Opiate prescribing principles in the acute setting are based on a variety of factors; however, it is imperative to understand that no standard therapy exists. Opioid doses should be

N. Vadivelu et al. (eds.), *Essentials of Pain Management*,
DOI 10.1007/978-0-387-87579-8_8, © Springer Science+Business Media, LLC 2011

titrated to a response. Some patients may require considerably more than the average dose of a drug to experience part or complete relief from pain; while others may require a dose at more frequent intervals. Treatment often depends on the patient population, is multifactorial, and can be heavily influenced by prior experience with opiates and other adjuvant agents.

Opioid Populations

Individuals who are naïve to opiates or substances of abuse often require minimal opiates due to a lack of tolerance and can be sensitive to overdose. On the other hand, patients who have had previous opiate treatment or have substance abuse problems often require stronger and more frequent therapy. Lastly, patients receiving opiates on an intermittent or chronic basis often require maximum recommended doses. Many communities have pain specialists available to help manage these more challenging patients.

In addition, some patients are poor metabolizers of opiates. For example, it is now understood that poor metabolizers of CYPD26, a key enzyme in codeine and dihydrocodeine metabolism, may not have success in attaining analgesia. Clinical signs, such as tachycardia and hypertension, may indicate that a patient is in acute pain. Likewise, a very long constellation of signs and symptoms, including tachycardia and hypertension, can be seen with opiate withdrawal and central nervous system hyperarousal states. An important clinical pearl is to not automatically assume abuse if a patient reports pain despite receiving medication. Lack of understanding of opioids and concern about governmental retaliation for prescribing opioids can result in many clinicians to utilize overly conservative dose adjustments that often lead to treatment failure (Tollison 2002).

Opioid Settings

If the patient is to be managed as an outpatient, weak opiates are often utilized. These medications are often prescribed on an as needed basis or in chronic states and are administered around the clock. Patients can be instructed to alternate acetaminophen-containing opiates with non-steroidal anti-inflammatory drugs in order to reduce acetaminophen-related potential injury to the liver. Currently, no more than 4 g of acetaminophen is recommended to be consumed in a 24-h period. In some countries outside of the United States, acetaminophen is deemed so toxic that it is not sold or used in clinical practice.

More options exist in managing patients with acute pain in the hospital setting. If a patient is able to tolerate oral intake, then weak opiates in elixir or tablet form are often prescribed as first-line therapy with mild and even moderate pain states. Patients taking opiates prior to their hospitalization should be maintained on their home regimen and also receive additional medications for acute pain. Home medications or first-line weak opiates can be given as scheduled around the clock doses as mentioned above, with strong opiates reserved for breakthrough pain on an as needed basis. Patients with severe pain and severe chronic pain states may need strong opiates on a 24-h/day regimen. Having scheduled doses available to treat patients can relieve anxiety, provide some level of control for the patient, and help to avoid unnecessary suffering. Delays in administration of doses often lead to subtherapeutic plasma concentrations of the drug and continued pain states. To avoid such complications, an increasing number of facilities employ patient-controlled analgesia (PCA) in both parenteral and neuraxial preparations. Another advantage of PCA is limiting the dose to ensure that too much is not given, which can result in toxicity, morbidity, and even mortality.

Opioid Duration

The duration of therapy has a huge impact on the approach to treating a patient's pain. When used in the acute pain setting, opioids can potentially obscure the progress of the disease or the location or intensity of pain. Goals of therapy are relief of sufferings without the development of adverse side effects such as decreased respiratory ventilation, reduced bowel motility, and urinary retention. Undertreatment can result in an increase in adrenocorticotropic hormone, cortisol, catecholamines, and interleukin (IL)-1 release along with sodium and water retention. Additionally, atelectasis, impaired ventilation, coronary vasoconstriction, decreased venous emptying, decreased intestinal motility, and urinary retention can be seen with inadequate pain management. Further, undertreatment of acute pain can lead to the development of certain chronic pain states (Tollison 2002).

In recent years, the chronic management of pain has emerged as a unique aspect of medicine. Medications with long half-lives are often used in the treatment of patients with chronic pain. Long-term treatment with opioids requires an opiate contract signed by the patient and the practitioner. Frequently, these patients suffer from pain associated with musculoskeletal conditions or malignancy. Patients with musculoskeletal pain often require treatment with analgesics for either intermittent pain exacerbations or constant disabling pain. Continued opioid treatment in these patients must be contingent on treatment compliance and achievement of functional improvement goals (Marcus 2005). Opiates are also used in the treatment of patients suffering chronically from pain arising from malignancy. Opioids are not indicated in all cases of terminal illness, but the analgesia, tranquility, and even the euphoria afforded by the use of opioids can potentially make the final days far less distressing for the patient and family (Ballantyne 2009). Achieving and sustaining an acceptable quality of life is a desired endpoint in the treatment of patients with chronic pain.

Opioid Limitations

Despite being the standard of analgesia therapy, opiates do have adverse clinical effects which can limit their use. Most of the side effects of opioids are dose-dependent and these effects are often magnified when used with other sedatives or substances of abuse. These side effects can cause patients to discontinue opiate therapy. Opioids cause a decrease in central nervous system function marked by sedation. Currently, however, there are no limitations on driving while taking opiates (Tollison et al. 2002). It should be noted that there is a great effort in the pharmaceutical industry to develop mu1 selective agonist agents with all of the positive features of opiates but without the many side effects.

Perhaps the most important effect of opiates is respiratory depression, which can ultimately lead to apnea. Care must be taken in the treatment of an obese patient with opiates as this group is more likely to experience respiratory complications. Special consideration must be given for the use of opiates during obstetrical analgesia, as the fetus is more susceptible to the respiratory-depressant effects of opiates than the mother (Hardman and Limbird 2009).

Opiates can cause nausea, vomiting, and as described earlier decreased gastric motility, potentially leading to constipation. Tolerance to the constipating effects of opioids does not develop. Opiates can also cause significant clinically relevant urinary retention. Recently data, including work by Dr. Johnathan Moss at the University of Chicago, suggest that opiates are associated with immunosuppression and can increase the rate of growth of infection as well as neoplastic cells, a feature *not* seen in patients who are without infection or cancer states. However, prolonged exposure to opioids appears much more likely to suppress immune function than do short-term exposure to these drugs (Ballantyne et al. 2009).

Opioid Overview

The important role opioids play in the treatment of pain, including non-malignant causes, is well supported (Savage 2003). However, an obstacle to effective use of opioids in pain treatment is the misunderstanding of the nature and risk of addiction when using opioids. The prevalence of drug abuse, dependence, or addiction in chronic pain patients has been stated to range from 3 to 19%. The concern of the medical community to not "fuel" this problem in chronic pain patients has led to less than optimal treatment of these patients. With these data, 81–97% of chronic pain patients were undertreated for fear of misuse or abuse of prescription medication.

Significant variation in the definitions and even diagnostic criteria of addiction is found within the medical, scientific, and political communities, as well as the general population. Such disparities result in misdiagnosis and undertreatment of addiction and pain syndromes. For the patient suffering from either one or even both conditions, could lead to a continued decrease in function, prolonged disability and pain, misuse of medications, and a decreased quality of life.

Historically, addiction-related terminology was confusing and ill-defined. This was most likely attributed to a poor understanding of the disease of addiction and its neurobiologic basis. Advances in addiction research have led to a greater understanding of the neurobiological basis of addiction, as well as the genetic and environmental influences that may effect its expression, and of course, the behavioral pathology that results in significant harm to the patient as well as any individuals affected by such behavior. With such a strong need for clarification of terminology, consensus definitions were established through collaboration of the American Academy of Pain Medicine, the American Pain Society, and the American Society of Addiction Medicine.

The defined addiction-related terminology is based on the following three points and is also summarized in Table 8.1:

1. Although some drugs produce pleasurable reward, critical determinants of addiction also rest with the user.
2. Addiction is a multidimensional disease with neurobiological and psychosocial dimensions.
3. Addiction is a phenomenon distinct from physical dependence and tolerance.

Historically, past definitions of addiction and dependence included references to tolerance and physical dependence as necessary elements of addiction. Although physical dependence and tolerance *may occur* in addiction, they *do not necessarily have to be present*. Moreover, physical dependence and/or tolerance may occur in the absence of addiction.

Table 8.1 Addiction-related terminology.

Tolerance	A state of adaptation in which exposure to a drug induces changes that result in a diminution of one or more of the drug's effects over time
Physical dependence	A state of adaptation that is manifested by a drug class-specific withdrawal syndrome that can be produced by abrupt cessation, rapid dose reduction, decreasing blood level of the drug, and/or administration of an antagonist
Addiction	A primary, chronic neurobiologic disease, with genetic, psychosocial, and environmental factors influencing its development or manifestations. It is characterized by behaviors that include one or more of the following: impaired control over drug use, compulsive use, continued use despite harm, and craving

The clinical relevance is that misunderstanding the definitions of physical dependence, tolerance, and addiction can lead to overdiagnosis of addiction with the therapeutic use of opioids and other drugs, as well as underrecognition of addiction to substances that do not result in demonstrable physical dependence.

For example, beta-blockers as well as clonidine, an α-2 agonist, used to control hypertension, can cause profound rebound hypertension upon abrupt cessation of the drugs, reflecting physical dependence, although no behavioral compulsions or psychological aberrations result from discontinuation of the drug. Intranasal phenylephrine (Afrin$^{®}$) can cause significant physical dependence, even after short-term use, as severe rebound nasal congestion can occur with continuous use of intranasal phenylephrine for as little as 3 consecutive days. Tolerance can also occur in the absence of addiction.

Cross-Tolerance

Cross-tolerance occurs when tolerance to the repeated use of a specific drug in given class of drugs is generalized to other drugs with the same or similar structural or mechanistic category (Ries et al. 2009). An individual with a high tolerance for alcohol will have a cross-tolerance for benzodiazepines, as both types of drugs work on the gamma-aminobutyric acid (GABA) receptor, albeit a different binding site on the receptor.

Opioid Rotation

Opioid rotation is the concept of transitioning from one opioid to another in a patient on chronic opioid therapy. The circumstances warranting rotation may include, but are not limited to, increasing tolerance with loss of analgesic efficacy, patient choice, significant side effects which persist, or a patient who must be nil per os.

The theory behind opioid rotation is based on the idea of incomplete cross-tolerance to the analgesic and non-analgesic effects of the opioids as well as the high degree of individual variation of patient response to opioids. The goal is to optimize the patient's relief, capitalizing on the benefits, while minimizing the risks.

Different mechanisms, including receptor activity, the asymmetry in cross-tolerance among different opioids, different opioid efficacies, and accumulation of toxic metabolites can explain the differences in analgesic or adverse effect responses among opioids in the clinical setting. Opioid rotation may be useful in opening the therapeutic window and establishing a more advantageous analgesia–toxicity relationship. By substituting opioids and using lower doses it is possible in most cases to reduce or relieve the symptoms of opioid toxicity and to manage highly tolerant patients with previous opioids while improving analgesia and, as a consequence, the opioid responsiveness.

Although studies evaluating the risks and benefits of opioid rotation are lacking, and there is no sufficient evidence to guide specific recommendations for opioid rotation, reports indicate that opioid rotation often results in improved analgesia in highly tolerant patients and may occur on a significantly lower equivalent dose of the new opioid. Tolerance or unacceptable side effects can develop to the new opioid, at which time switching to the original opioid or another alternative one might be considered.

When switching opioids in a chronic opioid patient, it is important to calculate equianalgesic doses of the opioids to avoid side effects and maintain adequate analgesia (Tables 8.2, 8.3, and 8.4). Many rotation protocols are available as well as tables to calculate equianalgesic doses, which often use parenteral morphine as the standard reference (Ries et al. 2009).

Table 8.2 **Principles of pain management/conversion rules.**

Principles of opioid conversion in pain management

1. Perform a comprehensive pain assessment, including history and physical, which includes onset, duration, location; intensity; quality; aggravating/alleviating factors; effect on function, quality of life; patients' goals; response to prior treatment
2. Avoid intramuscular (IM) route, if possible – unpredictable absorption
3. Treat persistent pain with scheduled, long-acting medications – minimize "clock-watching"
4. Ordinarily two drugs of the same class [e.g., non-steroidal anti-inflammatory drugs (NSAIDs)] should not be given concurrently; however, one long-acting and one short-acting opioid may be prescribed concomitantly
5. Short-acting strong opiates (morphine, hydromorphone, oxycodone) should be used to treat moderate to severe pain. Long-acting strong opiates (e.g., oxycontin, MS-contin, fentanyl patch) should be started once pain is controlled on short-acting preparations. Never start an opioid-naïve patient on long-acting medications
6. Titrate the opiate dose upward if pain is worsening or inadequately controlled: increase dose by 25–50% for mild/moderate pain; increase by 50–100% for moderate/severe pain. Continue to monitor for signs of addictive behavior versus pseudoaddiction
7. Manage breakthrough pain with short-acting opiates. Dose should be 10% of total daily dose. Breakthrough doses can be given as often as Q 60 min if PO; Q 30 min if SQ; Q 15 min if IV, assuming the patient has normal renal/hepatic function. Dose must be adjusted to compensate in the presence of renal or hepatic dysfunction
8. When converting patient from one opioid to another, decrease the dose of the second opioid by 25–50% to correct for incomplete cross-tolerance
9. Manage opioid side effects aggressively. Constipation should be treated prophylactically

Before converting

• Rule out disease progression and patient-related pharmacokinetic changes, such as absorption, metabolism, and drug–drug interactions
• Consider the possibility of unrealistic patient perceptions and expectations, non-compliance, or diversion
• Maximize the use of non-opioid analgesics where appropriate

Reminder: There is insufficient evidence to demonstrate any difference between opioids in their ability to relieve pain. Analgesia is more dependent on dose than drug. Therefore, unrelieved pain alone may not be sufficient reason to switch from one opioid to another

Adapted from University of Chicago, Department of Palliative Care, http://champ.bsd.uchicago.edu/PalliativeCare/documents/Pallpaincard2009update.pdf.

Table 8.3 Principles of opioid conversion and opioid switching in pain management.

Basic conversion equation

$$\frac{\text{Equianalgesic dose in route of } current}{\text{24 h dose and route of } current \text{ opioid}} = \frac{\text{Equianalgesic dose in } opioid \text{ route of } new \text{ opioid}}{\text{24h dose and route of } new \text{ opioid}}$$

Ex: Patient is taking 4 mg hydromorphone IV every 4 h and you want to switch to PO route. The equation would be

$$\frac{\text{4 mg IV hydromorphon}}{\text{24 mg IV hydromorphone}} = \frac{\text{1.5 mg PO dyromophone}}{\text{X mg PO hydromorphone}} \rightarrow \frac{\text{9 mg PO hydromorphone}}{\text{over 24 h}}$$

Converting to transdermal fentanyl
Calculate PO morphine equivalent and divide by two.
Ex: MS 100 mg PO = fentanyl 50 mcg patch. Patch duration of effect = 48–72 h
Takes 12–24 h before full analgesic effect of patch occurs after application.
**Must prescribe short-acting opioid for breakthrough pain.

Converting to methadone
Conversion varies with daily oral morphine dose, as the ratio of methadone to morphine changes with higher morphine doses. Additionally, methadone has a long and variable half-life (12–60 h), with a complicated dosing regimen. *Conversion to methadone should only be accomplished by a pain practitioner experienced with the use of methadone*

Adapted from University of Chicago, Department of Palliative Care, http://champ.bsd.uchicago.edu/PalliativeCare/documents/Pallpaincard2009update.pdf.

Table 8.4 Principles of opioid equianalgesics.

Conversion from one opioid to an equianalgesic dose of another
The following chart is to be used as a guide only. Individual patients may require adjustments in dosing, as well as frequency of administration.

Opioid equianalgesic dosing chart

Opioid	IV dose (mg)	Oral dose (mg)	Duration of effect
Morphine	5	15	3–4 h
Fentanyl	0.1	N/A	20–45 min
Hydrocodone	N/A	15	3–4 h
Hydromorphone	1.5	4	3–4 h
Levorphanol	1	2	6–8 h
Meperidine[a]	50	150	2–3 h
Codeine	60	100	3–4 h
Oxycodone	N/A	10	3–4 h

[a]Meperidine is not recommended for
1. *Patients with impaired renal function:*
   ■ The active metabolite, normeperidine, may accumulate, causing CNS toxicity manifesting as seizures
2. *Patients taking MAOI's:*
   ■ Due to risk of hypertensive crisis, hyperpyrexia, and cardiovascular system collapse

Adapted from University of Chicago Department of Palliative Care, http://champ.bsd.uchicago.edu/painControl/documents/Pallpaincard2009update.pdf.

Pseudoaddiction

Another situation can occur in which patients with unrelieved, real pain exhibit behaviors that suggest addiction. Termed *pseudoaddiction*, This behavior can mimic that of true addiction, including illicit drug use, lying, and manipulation in an attempt to relieve their pain (Savage 2003). Pseudoaddiction can be distinguished from true addiction by the cessation of drug-seeking behaviors when effective analgesia is achieved via opioid or non-opioid means. A patient with true addiction will continue drug-seeking behaviors despite appropriate increases in pain treatment modalities or may acquiesce for a short while, but soon commences drug-seeking behavior again, as the disease of addiction progresses.

Ultimately, it is close observation, vigilance, detailed documentation, and good clinical judgment that will enable the clinician to determine the presence of such behaviors.

Clinical Correlations of Opioid Agents and Practice Pearls

1. Meperidine is highly addictive, and overdose can cause generalized seizures. It is not reversible by naloxone. When taken with monoamine oxidase inhibitors (MAOIs), meperidine can cause serotonergic syndrome, characterized by hyperthermia, excitation, delusions, and seizures (Melzack and Wall 2003).
2. Codeine, dihydrocodeine, and diamorphine are prodrugs of morphine. They are converted to active forms by CYP2D6 enzymes in the liver (Thorn et al. 2009). Patients lacking this enzyme cannot metabolize medications containing codeine, resulting in treatment failure. Conversely, patients who are ultra-metabolizers can experience toxicity.
3. Morphine causes histamine release which can lead to pruritus. Furthermore, morphine is glucuronidated in the liver to an active metabolite, morphine-6-glucuronide, which is then excreted via the kidney (Warfield and Bajwa 2004). Therefore, morphine should not be used in renal failure patients.
4. Rapid infusion of large doses of fentanyl can cause increased muscle tone of the thorax leading to chest wall rigidity and the development of rigid chest syndrome (Ballantyne 2009). Also the Food and Drug Administration (FDA) has recently issued warnings due to deaths in patients using fentanyl patches and there is no one specific dose that causes this potentially lethal syndrome.
5. Methadone is very long acting, with a 23 h half-life. It has been associated with torsades de pointes, therefore a baseline electrocardiogram is now recommended prior to initiating treatment (Krantz et al. 2009).

Nomenclature for the Pain Practitioner and Summary

When assessing any type of pain, physicians must categorize the patient's symptoms based on severity, onset, duration, and chronicity as treatment will vary depending on its nature and etiology. Acute pain is initially treated with short-acting non-opioid pharmacologic agents or combination opioid drugs (e.g., Percodan®, Lortab®, Vicodin®, Tylenol® #3).

Acute versus chronic pain is important to clearly differentiate. Acute pain is rapid in onset, self-limiting, a symptom of the disease, and the patient often presents in acute distress. Examples of acute pain include postoperative pain, obstetrical labor pain, and trauma or injury-related pain (Table 8.5) and characteristically is described as sudden, sharp, and localized pain. It is usually self-limited and may be associated with physiologic changes such as diaphoresis and increases in heart rate and blood pressure.

Table 8.5 Common diverse acute pain syndromes.

Postoperative pain
Traumatic injury-related pain
Burn pain
Acute herpes zoster
Acute pain in obstetrics
Sickle cell pain
Cancer-related pain

Headache
-Muscle tension
-Vascular, migraine, aneursym
-Complex: compound headache

Chest pain
-Angina/ischemia
-Esophagitis/reflux
-Pleuritic pain: effusion, pneumonia, inflammation

Abdominal pain
-Acute pancreatitis
-Acute abdomen: perforation, obstruction, ischemic
-Renal colic

Musculoskeletal pain (back pain)
Neurogenic pain
-Disk herniation
-Nerve compression

It is necessary for clinicians to make a rapid assessment of etiology and of severity. The treatment plan for a clinician may include medications, including opiates, surgery, or other options.

Chronic pain is long-term pain classified as acute, moderate, and severe. It is often differentiated as malignant or non-malignant pain. Chronic pain is often described as gnawing, aching, and diffuse and is more gradual in onset and cessation than acute pain, which can also be simultaneously superimposed on top of the former. It can vary in intensity, may remit briefly, and has definite impact psychologically and socially. The treatment for such pain is often successful with traditional pharmacologic measures; however, often less traditional drugs and even non-pharmacologic therapies are necessary to achieve relief.

Case Scenario

Adam Fendius, BSc (Hons), MBBS, FRCA, DipIMC (RCSED), DipHEP

Kevin, a 24-year-old man who has recently purchased a brand new motorcycle, is out testing its capability on the highway. Having reached a speed of 50 mph he fails to notice oil on the road and hits the patch. He loses control of the motorcycle and collides with a tree. His helmet saves his life and he is brought to the emergency department, conscious, but very distressed at the loss of his new prized possession and his pain. The ambulance crew report states that there was no loss of consciousness. The patient is complaining of severe pain in both of his legs, his left shoulder, and his right hand. He is on a backboard and his vital signs are stable.

What are this man's likely injuries?
Motorcyclists are prone to head injuries, although it appears in this instance that Kevin is lucky to not have sustained any. The nature of the impact makes him prone to a number of other injuries. His pain is suggestive of possible fractures of femur, humerus, clavicle, and right hand.

What is your best first-line treatment for this man's pain, and how will you deliver it?
Patients who are severely distressed after acute trauma will need reassurance that their injuries are being looked after. This should be delivered in a clear, direct, and open manner and in a calm, reassuring tone of voice. **Intravenous analgesia is initially the most appropriate route. Gastric absorption is unreliable in the setting of acute pain and intravenous analgesia has the benefit of more predictable pharmacokinetics.** It would be prudent to avoid increasing gastric content, especially if he is to require surgery.

Opioid-based analgesia, preferably hydromorphone or morphine, are first-line drugs in acute trauma. Ketorolac does have opioid sparing effect, but its use by intravenous route might not be ideal in this situation as there could be co-existing hypovolemia with attendant risk of renal damage. In addition, ketorolac can interfere with platelet function, increasing the risk of bleeding from the fractures and other associated injuries, some of which might not be very evident at the time of initial assessment.

Could you cite any diagnostic problems associated with using opioids in this instance?
If there is associated head injury, then opioids can interfere with the neurological assessment, producing sedation, emesis, and miosis. However, effective pain relief is important in this situation and CT scan of the brain can easily be undertaken to assess the patient in case of neurological deterioration.

How will you achieve adequate analgesia?
At presentation he is likely to require an initial bolus of 5–10 mg morphine or 0.5–1 mg hydromorphone IV, followed by boluses of 2 mg morphine or 0.2–0.4 mg hydromorphone every 2–5 min, titrated against his pain and respiratory rate. If fentanyl is chosen as an analgesic, an initial bolus of 25–50 mcg could be used, followed by 25–50 mcg boluses every 5 min, titrated to effect.

The patient's condition has stabilized. He has a full trauma series of radiographs, which show that there is no obvious C-spine injury. Limb radiographs show bilateral femoral shaft fractures and some minor fractures of the right-hand phalanges with no angulations or rotation.

The orthopedic team feels that given his stable condition he should be transferred to the operating room for the fixation of his femoral fractures. His C-spine and thoracic spine are further imaged using CT, and no evidence of fractures is found. His C-spine is cleared on the basis of clinical and radiological findings. He has no evidence of internal bleeding. A log roll with the femurs splinted reveals no spinal tenderness and there is no sign of neurological injury.

You accept the surgeon's request for early fixation of fractures and leave emergency department to get the OR ready. An hour later you are requested to return urgently and assess Kevin as he has become less responsive and started to vomit. You immediately return to the emergency department. Kevin is now drowsy and not obeying vernal commands, but he is still able to locate pain. His respiratory rate is about 8, and both of his pupils are pinpoint but reactive to light.

What are the possible causes of Kevin's deterioration? How will you confirm your diagnosis?
There are two possibilities. One is an unidentified head injury such as a fresh/undiagnosed intracranial event (bleed or edema). This is unlikely as the CT scan of brain is normal. The other is an opioid overdose. You will have to follow *Airway, Breathing, Circulation* (ABCs) protocol. Kevin is easily arousable and he is maintaining his airway spontaneously. Oxygen saturation is 99% with an oxygen supplement of 4 L through a facemask. He has normal blood pressure, warm extremities, and a normal capillary refill time. His respiratory rate increases in rate and depth when he is awakened by verbal command. You go through the drug chart and note that he has been given 2 mg of hydromorphone. All the present clinical features are most likely due to an opioid overdose.

How will you confirm the diagnosis of opioid overdose?
Opioid overdose can be reversed with naloxone, an opioid antagonist. But this is not without risk as this will reverse both opioid-induced analgesia along with side effects. This can be overcome by slowly titrating the dose of naloxone to the desired effect. Moreover, the duration of action of naloxone is much shorter than hydromorphone, leading on to re-narcotization once naloxone wears off. The solution to this issue is using a naloxone as an infusion.

In the present situation administration of naloxone is indicated prior to considering a re-scan. You administer naloxone slowly and carefully and Kevin becomes more awake, his respiratory rate improves, and he is not complaining of any excessive pain. For nausea you administer an anti-emetic.

Kevin is now comfortable and you take him to the OR and administer a general anesthetic. You carefully titrate a few more doses of hydromorphone for intraoperative analgesia. He undergoes successful fixation of his fractures. At the end of the operation, you request the surgeon to infiltrate bupivacaine into the surgical wounds with an aim to reduce postoperative pain and hence the analgesic requirement.

What is your choice of postoperative analgesia?
Administration of an opioid (morphine/hydromorphone/fentanyl) using a PCA pump can be used for adequate pain relief without the risk of respiratory depression. Supplemental oxygen is an added safety measure. Acetaminophen can be prescribed

at regular intervals for opioid sparing and thereby reduce the potential side effects. Addition of a laxative can reduce opioid-induced constipation. Nausea and vomiting can be countered with an anti-emetic.

References

Abram SE, ed. Pain medicine. The requisites in anesthesiology. Philadelphia, PA: Mosby; 2006.

Ballantyne JC, Fishman SM, Abdi S, eds. The Massachusetts General Hospital handbook of pain management. Philadelphia, PA: Lippincott, Williams and Wilkins; 2009.

Hardman JG, Limbird LE, Gilman AG, eds. Goodman and Gilman's the pharmacological basis of therapeutics. 10th ed. New York, NY: McGraw Hill; 2009.

Krantz MJ, Martin J, Stimmel B. QTc interval screening in methadone treatment. Ann Intern Med. 2009;150(6):387–395.

Marcus DA, ed. Chronic pain: a primary care guide to practical management. New Jersey: Humana Press; 2005.

Melzack R, Wall PD, eds. Handbook of pain management: a clinical companion to Wall and Melzack's textbook of pain. London: Churchill-Livingstone; 2003.

Ries R, Fiellin D, Miller S, Saitz R, eds. Principles of addiction medicine. 4th ed. Philadelphia, PA: Lippincott, Williams and Wilkins; 2009.

Savage SR, Joranson DE, Covington ED, et al. Definitions related to the medical use of opioids – evolution of universal agreement. JPSM 2003;26(1):655–67.

Thorn CF, Klein TE, Altman RB. Codeine and morphine pathway. Pharmacogenet Genomics. 2009;19(7):556–8.

Tollison CD, Satterthwaite JR, Tollison JW, eds. Practical pain management. 3rd ed. Philadelphia, PA: Lippincott, Williams and Wilkins; 2002.

Warfield CA, Bajwa ZH, eds. Principles and practice of pain medicine. 2nd ed. New York, NY: McGraw-Hill; 2004.

Chapter 9

Nonopioid Analgesics in Pain Management

Jack M. Berger, MS, MD, PhD and Shaaron Zaghi, MD

Introduction

Since patients rarely present with pure nociceptive pain (i.e., pain caused by activity in the neural pathways in response to damaging or potentially damaging stimuli) or neuropathic pain (i.e., pain initiated by a primary lesion or dysfunction in the nervous system), but rather suffer a mixed pain syndrome (i.e., pain caused by a combination of both the primary injury and secondary effects), a rational polypharmacy approach that targets key peripheral and central pain mechanisms and modulating pathways may yield the best outcomes (Management of Chronic Pain Syndromes 2005).

Opioids are the closest drugs we currently have to ideal analgesics. They exhibit no ceiling effect and can produce profound analgesia by progressive dose escalation. They are the most effective agents for the relief of any type of acute pain because of their predictable dose-dependent response. Opioids have no significant long-term organ toxicity and can be used for years (Zuckerman and Ferrante 1998).

However, since opioids are poorly effective in neuropathic pain states, other agents that either produce analgesia or can be used as adjuvants to enhance the analgesia of the opioids are often necessary. And since inflammation is a major source for activation of nociceptors, anti-inflammatory agents are an important nonopioid class of analgesics.

It is therefore important to understand how the processes contributing to pain generation [i.e., the inflammatory cascade, irritable peripheral nociceptors, and localized central nervous system (CNS) dysfunction] converge to influence the functional status of the patient. Later in this chapter we will consider agents that treat medical comorbidities and psychological factors that also influence the pain experience.

Inflammation

"Inflammation is a local, protective response to microbial invasion or tissue injury. It must be fine-tuned and regulated precisely because deficiencies or excesses of the inflammatory response cause morbidity and shorten lifespan (Libby 2002)." The anti-inflammatory medications used in pain management can be divided into two main categories. The first is the nonsteroidal anti-inflammatory and the second is the glucocorticoid steroid medications. The nonsteroidal anti-inflammatories can be further divided into two groups, the

N. Vadivelu et al. (eds.), *Essentials of Pain Management*,
DOI 10.1007/978-0-387-87579-8_9, © Springer Science+Business Media, LLC 2011

Table 9.1 Common oral nonsteroidal anti-inflammatory drugs (NSAIDs) by chemical class.

Propionic acids	Salicylates	Fenamates	Oxicams	Acidic acids	Benzine-acidic acid
Ibuprofen (Motrin®) 200, 400, 600, 800 mg	Aspirin 325 mg	Meclofenamate sodium (Meclomen®) 50, 100 mg	Piroxicam (Feldene®) 10, 20 mg	Tolmetin sodium (Tolectin®/DS) 200, 400 mg	Diclofenac sodium Voltaren® (25, 50, 75 mg Voltaren® XR 100 mg
Naproxen (Naprosyn®) 250, 375, 500 mg	Diflunisal (Dolobid®) 250, 500 mg			Indomethacin (Indocin®) 25, 50, 75 mg (Indocin® SR)	
Fenoprofen calcium (Nalfon®) 200, 300, 600 mg	Salicylsalicylic acid Disalcid® 500, 750 mg			Sulindac (Clinoril®) 150, 200 mg	
Ketoprofen (Orudis®) 50, 75 mg	Choline magnesium trisalicylate Trilisate® 500, 750 mg				

Adapted from Insel (1996).

nonspecific, nonsteroidal anti-inflammatories (NSAIDs) and the specific cyclooxygenase-2 inhibitors (COXibs).

To understand the analgesic effects of the NSAIDs it is necessary to look first at the beneficial effects of the enzyme cyclooxygenase-1 (COX-1) on converting arachidonic acid to various prostaglandins. These prostaglandins are necessary for maintaining good renal blood flow, adequate glomerular filtration rate, and homeostasis of potassium and sodium retention through appropriate secretions of renin, aldosterone, and antidiuretic hormone (ADH).

When the conversion of arachidonic acid to prostaglandins is inhibited by NSAID inhibition of COX-1, then the kidney comes under risk and loses its ability to regulate salt and water balance. This detrimental effect of NSAIDs on the kidney is potentiated by renal hypoperfusion states (Miyoshi 2001).

All NSAIDs can result in renal insufficiency, and with the exception of salicylsalicylic acid and choline magnesium trisalicylate, for which the risk is less, they can inhibit platelet aggregation and cause dyspepsia and gastric ulceration by virtue of the "constitutive" effects of COX-1 (Morrison et al. 2001, Gilron et al. 2003).

The gastrointestinal effects of the NSAIDs can be modulated by the simultaneous administration of a proton inhibitor medication. However, when combined with acetaminophen, this protective effect may be lost (Rahme et al. 2008). The common NSAIDs are nonspecific because they have variable effects on blockade of COX-1 and COX-2. The most common oral NSAIDs used in clinical practice are shown in Table 9.1.

Many patients use NSAIDs in combination with acetaminophen. In a Canadian study of nearly 650,000 elderly patients being prescribed traditional NSAIDs with or without a proton pump inhibitor (PPI), acetaminophen with or without a PPI, or NSAID and acetaminophen together with or without a PPI, it was found that when given together, an NSAID plus acetaminophen increased the risk of GI bleeding even with the addition of a PPI. Patients must therefore be warned about the combined use of NSAIDs and acetaminophen that can be purchased over the counter.

However, the "inducible" effects of COX-2 on conversion of arachidonic acid to prostaglandin E-2 lead to inflammation and pain. This elevation is primarily due to upregulation of interleukin-1ß. Blockade of the action of COX-2 reduces inflammation and pain without affecting the good effects of the prostaglandins that are COX-1 dependent (Gajraj 2003, Gilron et al. 2003). In the presence of inflammation, COX-2 can be found elevated in the CNS, the spinal cord, and the brain (Samad et al. 2001). Antagonists of interleukin-1β or blocking COX-2 both lead to antinociception (Samad et al. 2001).

There is a ceiling dose effect to all of the NSAIDs, above which no further analgesia is obtained; although the dose may vary, it usually falls below the maximal recommended dose of the manufacturer (Jacox et al. 1994). In general, for elderly patients, agents with short half-lives (e.g., ibuprofen) are most appropriate; for patients with a history of dyspepsia, ulcer disease, or bleeding diatheses, either salicylsalicylic acid or choline magnesium trisalicylate should be used if a traditional NSAID is indicated (Morrison et al. 2001). NSAIDs can be combined with opioids to enhance analgesia.

Parenteral NSAIDs

Parenteral NSAIDs (e.g., ketorolac) are being used increasingly for postoperative pain as sole analgesic agents and in conjunction with opioids as opioid-sparing agents (Cepeda et al. 2005). The efficacy of ketorolac, currently the only available parenteral NSAID in the United States, has been well established with 30 mg being equianalgesic with 10 mg of parenteral morphine for acute pain (Cepeda et al. 2005). When used together, there was a significant reduction of adverse side effects of opioids due to a significant reduction in morphine requirements.

Intravenous ketorolac has been shown to reduce opioid requirements for knee and hip replacement surgery by 35–44% and by 50–75% for thoracotomy and upper abdominal surgery (Etches et al. 1995, Stouten et al. 1992). While ketorolac can reduce opioid requirements, it is not potent enough to be used as a sole analgesic after major surgery such as intra-abdominal surgery (Cepeda et al. 1995).

Peak analgesia from ketorolac is typically seen 1–2 h after administration, and the half-life is approximately 6 h, although it may be prolonged in patients with reduced renal function or in the elderly. The manufacturer's recommended dose for elderly individuals or those with renal insufficiency is 15 mg every 6 h following a 30 mg loading dose, and doses as low as 10 mg have been found to significantly reduce opioid requirements and provide analgesia equivalent to 10 mg of intravenous morphine (Ready et al. 1994).

Ketorolac has a side effect profile similar to that of other NSAIDs. There appears to be a significantly increased risk of gastrointestinal bleeding in the elderly, particularly with high doses and with duration of use of more than 5 days (Strom et al. 1996, Camu 1996, Maliekal and Elboim 1995). However, when used in doses of 15 mg or less q6h for less than 3 days, toxicity seems to be minimal.

Current evidence indicates that a variety of agents have synergistic effects when added to local anesthetics, and there is evidence that the improvement in analgesia is, at least partially, through a local rather than a central mechanism. The results of the review by Brill and Plaza suggest that clonidine (an α-2 adrenergic agonist) and ketorolac, when administered intra-articularly after arthroscopic knee surgery, may reduce postoperative pain (Brill and Plaza 2004).

Parecoxib is a specific COX-2 inhibitor that is available in Europe for intravenous administration. In a study of parecoxib 40 mg IV administered on induction of general anesthesia, and then q12h for 24 h, improved postoperative analgesia without increased bleeding for total hip arthroplasty was observed. Again, it is well known that COX-2 is responsible for the synthesis of prostaglandins, which sensitize the nociceptor and act as excitatory neuromediators in the CNS and in the periphery (Gajraj 2003, Martinez et al. 2007).

In another study, parecoxib was found to be an effective analgesic in acute pain at 20 or 40 mg over placebo given either intravenously or intramuscularly. The number needed to treat (NNT) for parecoxib 20 mg IV for at least 50% pain relief over 6 h was 3.0 and for 40 mg was 2.2 (Kranke et al. 2004). This compares favorably with other analgesics like morphine 10 mg where the NNT was 3, ibuprofen 400 mg where the NNT was 2.7, and acetaminophen 1,000 mg where the NNT was 4.6 (Hyllested et al. 2002). The NNT is the number of patients needed to treat with the medication and dose to produce 50% pain relief in one of the patients. Therefore the lower the NNT, the more effective is the drug.

In direct comparison of 4 mg of intravenous morphine with 30 mg of intravenous ketorolac and 20 mg of intravenous Paracoxib, the times to remedication were 3 h for morphine versus 5.5 h for both ketorolac and parecoxib at the specified doses (Barton et al. 2002).

Symptomatic hepatic effects attributable to therapeutic use of most NSAIDs are extremely rare and usually mild except in overdosage of acetaminophen where fatal hepatic necrosis can occur. There is no clearly established explanation for why some compounds are more hepatotoxic than others. It is possible that some compounds undergo oxidation, probably to the phenylic ring structure, yielding highly reactive metabolites. Compounds that cause mild hepatic damage, such as diclofenac and bromfenac, may produce some reactive epoxides during biotransformation (Insel 1996).

Impairment of wound healing has been attributed to the use of NSAIDs in the postoperative period. Studies have shown that there was no effect on epidermal wound healing with selective COX-2 and nonselective COX inhibitors in a mouse model. The authors propose that this was probably due to redundant mechanisms for wound repair, most of which are not influenced by the COX-2 inhibitors (Hardy et al. 2003).

Power indicates in his review article that the data are conflicting with respect to bone healing and nonunion when these agents are used in orthopedic procedures (Power 2005), but much of the adverse data comes from animal studies which may not have clinical significance in humans (Gerstenfeld et al. 2003, Harder and An 2003). Short-term use of COX-2-specific inhibitors may play an important role in preventive analgesia for postoperative pain management (Martinez et al. 2007, McCrory and Lindahl 2002).

It is important to remember that COX-2-specific inhibitors do not affect platelet aggregation and therefore may pose a risk for myocardial infarction (MI) if low-dose aspirin therapy is discontinued (Gajraj 2003, Martinez et al. 2007). Since low-dose aspirin is increasingly being used for cardioprotection, it is important to note that coadministration of selective COX-2 inhibitors does not alter this protective effect (Jones and Power 2005). It has recently been shown that celecoxib (Celebrex®, Pfizer, New York, NY) does not appear to be associated with an increased risk of serious cardiovascular thromboembolic events and it is the only remaining oral COX-2 inhibitor available in the United States (White et al. 2002). It could therefore be used as a preoperative medication and continued postoperatively through healing if the patient is able to take oral medications and does not have an allergy to sulfa-containing medications.

A complete review of the cardiac and stroke risks of the NSAIDs and COXibs appears in the journal *Circulation* authored by Antman et al. (2007). Current evidence indicates that selective COX-2 inhibitors have important adverse cardiovascular effects that include increased risk for myocardial infarction, stroke, heart failure, and hypertension. The risk for these adverse effects is likely greatest in patients with a prior history of or at high risk for cardiovascular disease. In these patients, use of COX-2 inhibitors for pain relief should be limited to patients for whom there are no appropriate alternatives and then only in the lowest dose and for the shortest duration necessary. More long-term data are needed to fully evaluate the extent to which these important adverse cardiovascular effects may be offset by other beneficial effects of these medications. More data are also needed on the cardiovascular safety of conventional NSAIDs. Until such data are available, the use of any COX inhibitor, including over-the-counter NSAIDs, for long periods of time should only be considered in consultation with a physician (Antman et al. 2007). It is therefore important to weigh the benefit of the COX-2 inhibitor versus its risk in utilizing this class of medication.

Acetaminophen is an outlier of the NSAIDs and is considered by some to be a cyclooxygenase-3 inhibitor (COX-3). COX, the key enzyme in prostaglandin formation, is an important pharmacologic target. The antithrombotic effect of acetylsalicylic acid is caused by irreversible inhibition of COX-1, constitutively expressed in platelets, whereas the analgesic effect of NSAIDs is mediated through inhibition of COX-2, induced during inflammation. The main mechanism of action of acetaminophen is inhibition of prostaglandin synthesis in the central nervous system, the recently characterized COX-3 being a possible target (Munsterhjelm et al. 2005).

However, acetaminophen also has peripheral COX-1-inhibiting properties. Normal platelet function is dependent on the production of proaggregatory thromboxane A2 (TxA2) through COX-1, and acetaminophen has been shown to inhibit platelet function both in vitro and in high intravenous doses in vivo. However, oral administration of conventional doses (approximately 1 g) of acetaminophen does not alter platelet function (Munsterhjelm et al. 2005).

Acetaminophen is widely used for postoperative analgesia, although the optimal dose is debatable. In pediatric patients, no analgesic ceiling effect was detected when acetaminophen was administered rectally in doses up to 60 mg/kg. However, high doses of acetaminophen may alter platelet function through peripheral COX-1 inhibition (Munsterhjelm et al. 2005).

The plasma concentration of acetaminophen required for optimal analgesia is not known. Antipyretic properties of acetaminophen are evident in the plasma concentration range of 10–20 mg/l. This concentration or higher was observed 10 min after infusion with all doses tested, but after 90 min, plasma acetaminophen concentration remained significantly above 10 mg/l only with doses higher than 15 mg/kg. Optimal analgesia may require higher concentrations than antipyresis in adults, but this topic is controversial (Beck et al. 2000, Hahn et al. 2003).

When acetaminophen was administered rectally in children, a linearly increasing morphine-sparing effect was achieved with doses up to 60 mg/kg (Korpela et al. 1999).

Considering that the site of action of acetaminophen is mainly in the central nervous system, a high peak plasma concentration may be important. This could explain why 1 g intravenous acetaminophen has been found more effective in relieving pain than the same dose given orally (Munsterhjelm et al. 2005).

After major surgery, the morphine-sparing effect of acetaminophen, NSAIDs, and COX-2 inhibitors is quantifiable and is, with specific regimens, considerable. Despite this, the combination of a single nonopioid analgesic with morphine PCA offers no (acetaminophen), unclear (COX-2 inhibitors), or only little (NSAIDs) advantage over morphine PCA alone. The combination of several nonopioid analgesics, however, may produce an additive or even synergistic effect. Optimal multimodal postoperative analgesia regimens should be identified in randomized and well-designed, large studies (Elia et al. 2005).

Issioui and associates concluded from their study that oral premedication with a combination of celecoxib (200 mg) and acetaminophen (2,000 mg) was highly effective in decreasing postoperative pain and improving patient satisfaction after ambulatory ear, nose, and throat (ENT) surgery (Issioui et al. 2002). Patients' satisfaction with their postoperative pain management was also improved with celecoxib alone; however, the numbers needed to treat (NNT) to achieve this improvement were larger than with the celecoxib–acetaminophen combination. In this outpatient surgery population, celecoxib (200 mg) or acetaminophen (2 g) alone was not significantly more effective than a placebo in reducing postoperative pain when administered orally before surgery. But, together they were synergistically effective (Issioui et al. 2002).

Steroid Anti-inflammatory Medications
Corticosteroids
There are two types of corticosteroids used in clinical practice:

(1) Glucocorticoids which act to suppress the inflammatory response.
(2) Mineralocorticoids which modify salt and water balance.

Only those steroids with a large anti-inflammatory activity (glucocorticoids) and a low water balance (mineralocorticoids) are useful in pain management (Li et al. 2007, Rumunstad and Audun 2007).

Steroid preparations used as injectables (Benzon et al. 2007) for epidural, intra-articular, periarticular, and intramuscular administration include methylprednisolone acetate, triamcinalone acetonide, triamcinalone diacetate, betamethasone, and dexamethasone. These drugs are discussed in detail below.

Methylprednisolone Acetate (Depo-Medrol®)
Depo-Medrol® (Pfizer, New York, NY) is a high-potency steroid with high glucocorticoid effects and low mineralocorticoid effects. The preparation when injected provides for a slow release of the active steroid to the target site. Controversy occurred over its use in epidural steroid injections with respect to the occurrence of arrachnoiditis and other neurologic injuries when it was accidentally injected intrathecally (Bernat et al. 1976). However, there are other studies of deliberate intrathecal injection of Depo-Medrol® without neurotoxicity (Kotani et al. 2000).

What is clear however is that there is a potential for intravascular injection with the use of any particulate steroid which can lead to arteriole occlusion and stroke. Cervical transforaminal epidural steroid injections, for example, are now discouraged (Rathmell et al. 2000, Cousins 2000).

Triamcinalone Acetonide (Kenalog®)

Kenalog® (Bristol-Meyers Squibb, New York, NY) is also a high-potency glucocorticoid with low mineralocorticoid effect. Triamcinolone acetonide does not contain polyethylene glycol. It can be used as effectively as Depo-Medrol® (Bristol-Meyers Squibb, New York, NY) for epidural injections, zygopophyseal joint (facet joint) injections, or intra-articular injections.

Triamcinalone Diacetate (Aristocort®)

Aristocort® (Pfizer, New York, NY) is also a high-potency glucocorticoid with low mineralocorticoid effects.

Betamethasone (Celestone®)

Celestone® (Schering-Plough, Kennilworth, NJ) has the highest glucocorticoid potency and although it is a "depo"-type injectate, it has the least particulate material in the preparation of these agents.

Dexamethasone (Decadron®)

Decadron® (Merck, Whitehouse Station, NJ) is the next highest in glucocorticoid potency; it is a clear liquid and so does not offer a sustained effect after injection, and it is usually used for intravenous administration to reduce edema.

In a prospective, randomized study, Pobereskin and Sneyd compared postoperative pain scores, morphine consumption, and length of stay in 95 adults who underwent elective lumbar spine surgery via a posterior incision (Pobereskin and Sneyd 2000). Immediately prior to closure, the wound was irrigated with triamcinalone 40, 20, or 0 mg. Visual analogue scale pain scores at 24 h after surgery were median 12, 15, and 33 mm for patients receiving triamcinalone 40, 20 mg, or no steroid, respectively ($P < 0.0005$, Kruskal–Wallis test). Total morphine usage after 24 h was 26, 27, and 43 mg for the same groups ($P < 0.001$, Kruskal–Wallis test). The proportion of patients discharged from the hospital on the first day after surgery was 83.9, 77.4, and 54.8% for patients receiving triamcinalone 40, 20 mg, and no steroid, respectively ($P < 0.028$, chi-squared test). The investigators concluded that extradural triamcinalone reduces pain after lumbar spine surgery and reduces time to discharge from hospital (Pobereskin and Sneyd 2000).

One of the potential problems with corticosteroids is that they markedly affect most aspects of wound healing. When corticosteroids are administered early after injury, high corticosteroid levels delay the appearance of inflammatory cells and fibroblasts, the deposition of ground substance and collagen, regenerating capillaries, contraction, and epithelial migration (Ehrlich and Hunt 2000, Wicke et al. 2000, Witte and Barbul 1997).

Durmus and his associates studied the effects of single-dose dexamethasone 1 mg/kg on wound healing in a prospective, randomized, experimental animal model (Durmus et al. 2003). The authors state that the wound-healing process has been conveniently divided into three phases – inflammatory, proliferative, and remodeling. However, the process is continuous, and phases overlap (Durmus et al. 2003). Therefore, the conceptual distinction between phases serves only as an outline to discuss events that occur during wound repair. The presence of more mature capillary vessels in the vicinity of a wound allows for better nutrition, and this phenomenon, combined with a large amount of collagen fiber, is directly related to a more adequate wound-healing process (Drucker et al. 1998).

Angiogenesis is a dynamic process during wound healing, as the fibrin clot is replaced by blood vessel-rich granulation tissue and is subsequently replaced by a collagenous scar with much less mature vessels (Clark et al. 1982, Welch et al. 1990, Durmus et al. 2003). In their study, Durmus et al. reported significantly more inflammatory cells and vascularity in the dexamethasone group. The presence of significant inflammatory cells and vascularity in the dexamethasone group compared with the control group might be related to delayed inflammatory and proliferation phases. Increased collagenization and epithelization with fewer inflammatory cells and less vascularity provided evidence of repletion of granulation tissue to collagenous scar in the control group because rat wound healing was rapid (Durmus et al. 2003). This study has shown that dexamethasone at 1 mg/kg doses may have negative effects on wound healing. These investigators state that further experiments with dexamethasone at different doses will be required to substantiate the dose-related effects (Durmus et al. 2003).

Although dexamethasone is a cost-effective antiemetic and has been widely used, the delayed wound-healing process suggests that dexamethasone should be avoided in patients with poorly healing wounds or leg ulcers, or when fast healing is essential. In such patients, retinoic acid administration added to the treatment protocol may improve the healing process. In a study by Wicke et al., retinoic acid significantly increased the hydroxyproline content toward normal levels in approximately 80% of controls at day 17 (Wicke et al. 2000). Further studies should be performed after a single-dose dexamethasone administration to determine the effects of retinoic acid on wound healing. It must be remembered that steroids and retinoic acid have regulatory effects for the synthesis of collagen, even in the early phase of wound healing (Witte and Barbul 1997).

Kingery et al. demonstrated that methylprednisolone, when administered by continuous infusion, has antihyperalgesic effects in a complex regional pain syndrome type II (CRPS) model based on sciatic nerve transection (Kingery et al. 2001). In addition, continuous methylprednisolone infusion partially reversed nerve injury-evoked fos expression in the dorsal horns, suggesting that glucocorticoids can inhibit the spinal neuron hyperactivity induced by chronic sciatic nerve transection (Kingery et al. 2001). Finally, no changes were observed in spinal substance P or NK1 immunoreactivity after chronic methylprednisolone infusion, suggesting that depletion of this neuropeptide or its receptor does not contribute to the antihyperalgesic actions of methylprednisolone (Kingery et al. 2001).

Oral steroids are often used in pain management for multiple purposes. Acute inflammatory flare-ups such as radiculitis or acute herpes zoster are often treated with a limited course of oral steroids, methylprednisolone (Medrol® dose pack, Pfizer, New York, NY). Oral steroids have long been used for treatment of patients with collagen vascular diseases, rheumatologic diseases, and pain of arthritis. Recently, Chang et al. studied the use of oral steroids for the treatment of carpal tunnel syndrome and found long-term benefit that could avoid surgery in some patients (Chang et al. 2002).

Of course one must be careful in prescribing oral steroids to patients who are immuno-compromised. However, the use of a course of oral steroids in acute herpes zoster is not contraindicated, because this is a reactivation infection which is IgG mediated, not IgM mediated and is therefore not suppressed by steroids (Toliver et al. 1997, Pardo et al. 1997).

Anticonvulsants in Pain Management

Actions of Anticonvulsants in Pain Therapy

Neuropathic pain, a form of chronic pain caused by injury to or disease of the peripheral or central nervous system, is a formidable therapeutic challenge to clinicians because it does not respond well to traditional pain therapies. Knowledge about the pathogenesis of neuro-pathic pain has grown significantly over the past two decades. Basic research with animal and human models of neuropathic pain has shown that a number of pathophysiological and bio-chemical changes take place in the nervous system as a result of an insult (Tremont-Lukats et al. 2000). This property of the nervous system to adapt morphologically and functionally to external stimuli is known as neuroplasticity and plays a crucial role in the onset and main-tenance of pain symptoms. Many similarities between the pathophysiological phenomena observed in some epilepsy models and in neuropathic pain models justify the rationale for use of anticonvulsant drugs in the symptomatic management of neuropathic pain disorders (Tremont-Lukats et al. 2000).

Carbamazepine (Tegretol®, Novartis, East Hannover, NJ), a tricyclic imipramine intro-duced in 1961, was the first anticonvulsant studied in clinical trials and probably alleviates pain by decreasing conductance in Na^+ channels and inhibiting ectopic discharges. Results from clinical trials have been positive in the treatment of trigeminal neuralgia, painful diabetic neuropathy, and postherpetic neuralgia (Tremont-Lukats et al. 2000). Today, however, it is only used in trigeminal neuralgia when used for management of pain because of significant side effects (rash, reduced white blood cell count, ataxia, dizziness, nausea, folate deficiency, hyponatremia) and the need to monitor liver function and blood count (Zakrzewska 1995).

Phenytoin (Dilantin®, Pfizer, New York, NY), also an older agent, is available for intra-venous administration and oral use. Like carbamazepine it requires careful monitoring of therapeutic level. It has limited use today in pain management. However, it can be used in a neuropathic pain crisis to provide some sustained relief as demonstrated by McCleane who found that intravenous phenytoin 15 mg/kg infused over 2 h could provide up to 7 days of pain reduction (McCleane 1999).

The availability of newer anticonvulsants tested in higher-quality clinical trials has marked a new era in the treatment of neuropathic pain. Today, gabapentin (Neurontin®, Pfizer, New York, NY) and pregabalin (Lyrica®, Pfizer, New York, NY) have become the first-line anticonvulsants used in pain management. Considerable research has defined the mechanisms by which these agents produce antinociception. The drugs bind to the A-2D subunit of the presynaptic voltage-gated calcium channel on C-nociceptor fibers entering the spinal cord, preventing calcium entry into the cell, thus preventing the fusion of the neuro-transmitter releasing vesicles to the cell membrane which is necessary for the release of the neurotransmitters into the synapse (Dahl et al. 2004). In a large meta-analysis study, both gabapentin and pregabalin have been found to have significant preoperative preventive anal-gesic effects as well as significant postoperative analgesic effects (Tippana et al. 2007). Their use in a preoperative preventive analgesic regimen followed by continued use through the immediate postoperative period and through the healing process including physical therapy has been found to provide significant benefit and reduce opioid requirements (Tippana et al. 2007).

Gabapentin and now pregabalin have shown clear efficacy in the treatment of chronic neuropathic pain syndromes, specifically for the treatment of painful diabetic neuropathy and postherpetic neuralgia, and in conditions such as fibromyalgia. Based on the positive results of these studies and their favorable adverse effect profiles, gabapentin and pregabalin should be considered as first-line choices of therapy for neuropathic pain (Freynhagen et al. 2005).

Because lower dosages can be used to treat neuropathic pain, it is likely that pregabalin will be associated with fewer dose-related adverse events (Freynhagen et al. 2005). Part of the reason why pregabalin requires lower dosages is that it has a much higher bioavailability (90 versus 33–66%) and is rapidly absorbed (peak: 1 h). Also, plasma concentrations increase linearly with increasing dose (Wesche and Bockbrader 2005), which is not true with gabapentin. Gabapentin is slowly absorbed (peak: 3–4 h postdose) and more importantly, plasma concentrations have been found to have a nonlinear relationship to increasing doses (Wesche and Bockbrader 2005).

Tarride et al. estimated analgesic outcomes in patients with painful diabetic peripheral neuropathy or postherpetic neuralgia receiving pregabalin versus gabapentin (Tarride et al. 2006). They developed a model to estimate the impact on analgesic outcomes of treatment with pregabalin (375 mg/day) versus gabapentin (1,200 mg/day and 1,800 mg/day) in a hypothetical cohort of 1,000 patients with diabetic peripheral neuropathy or postherpetic neuralgia. Targeted outcomes included the mean number of days with no or mild pain (score <3), and days with at least a 30–50% reduction in pain intensity. The study concluded that pregabalin may provide better analgesic outcomes than gabapentin over a 12-week period (Tarride et al. 2006).

Turan et al. compared the effectiveness of patient-controlled postoperative epidural analgesia with and without supplementation with oral gabapentin on the quality of postoperative pain relief delivered by patient-controlled epidural analgesia in patients undergoing general anesthesia (Turan et al. 2006). The authors have described the efficacy of gabapentin in postoperative pain previously, but this is the first investigation elucidating its effects on postoperative epidural analgesia (Turan et al. 2006).

In a placebo-controlled, double-blind study, they demonstrated that gabapentin 1,200 mg, administered before and for 2 days after surgery, was associated with a significant reduction in the requirement for patient-controlled epidural analgesia and escape analgesia. Furthermore, there was a statistical and clinically significant improvement in postoperative pain scores and patient satisfaction with less postoperative motor block. The study was well designed and involved 40 patients undergoing surgery to the lower extremities (scar revision and/or skin grafting). There was a significant increase in the incidence of dizziness (35 versus 5%) and a nonsignificant increase in somnolence (25 versus 10%). However, the occurrence of these recognized side effects of gabapentin was not reflected in overall patient satisfaction with postoperative pain relief; this was significantly superior in the gabapentin group (Turan et al. 2006).

Another anticonvulsant that has gained popularity in modern pain management is topiramate (Topamax®, Ortho-McNeil-Janssen, New Brunswick, NJ). It has gained significant popularity in migraine headache management, and it has the advantage of not causing weight gain which is a side effect of not only the anticonvulsants but also the antidepressants used in pain management. It appears to have Na$^+$ channel blocker, gamma aminobutyric acid (GABA) modulation effects.

The efficacy of topiramate in migraine prevention (prophylaxis) was established in two multicenter, randomized, double-blind, placebo-controlled, pivotal trials. Topiramate has received regulatory approval for use in adults for migraine prophylaxis (prevention) in the United States and numerous other countries, including France, Ireland, Switzerland, Brazil, Taiwan, Spain, and Australia. Treatment with 100 or 200 mg per day of topiramate was associated with significant reductions in the frequency of migraine headaches, number of migraine days, and use of acute medications. No increase in efficacy has been observed between 100 and 200 mg per day of topiramate (Silberstein 2005, Management of Chronic Pain Syndromes 2005).

Based on efficacy and tolerability, 100 mg per day of topiramate should be the initial target dose for most patients. The most common adverse events were paresthesia, fatigue, decreased appetite, nausea, diarrhea, weight decrease, and taste perversion. Topiramate is a first-line migraine-preventive drug and should especially be considered as a preferred treatment for all patients who are concerned about gaining weight, who are currently overweight, or who have coexisting epilepsy (Turan et al. 2006, Management of Chronic Pain Syndromes 2005).

Lamotrigine (Lomictal$^®$, Glaxo Smith Kline, Philadelphia, PA) is another anticonvulsant used frequently in pain management. Central poststroke pain (CPSP) is usually difficult to treat. Amitriptyline (a tricyclic antidepressant), the only oral preparation shown to be effective in a randomized controlled trial, is often associated with a range of side effects related to the many mechanisms of actions of tricyclic antidepressants.

Therefore, Vestergaard et al. investigated the effect of lamotrigine, a drug that reduces neuronal hyperexcitability, on poststroke pain. Thirty consecutive patients with CPSP (median age 59 years), with median pain durations of 2.0 years, range 0.3–12 years, participated in a randomized, double-blind, placebo-controlled crossover study (Vestergaard et al. 2001). The study consisted of two 8-week treatment periods separated by 2 weeks of washout. The primary endpoint was the median value of the mean daily pain score during the last week of treatment while treated with 200 mg/day lamotrigine. Secondary endpoints were median pain scores while on lamotrigine 25, 50, and 100 mg/day; a global pain score; assessment of evoked pain; areas of spontaneous pain; and allodynia/dysesthesia (Vestergaard et al. 2001). The authors found that lamotrigine 200 mg/day reduced the median pain score to 5, compared to 7, during placebo (p5 = 0.01) in the intent-to-treat population of 27 patients. No significant effect was obtained at lower doses. Twelve patients (44%) responded to the treatment. There was a uniform tendency to reduction of all secondary outcome measures, but lamotrigine only had significant effects on some of the secondary outcome measures (Vestergaard et al. 2001).

Lamotrigine was well tolerated with few and transient side effects. Two mild rashes occurred during lamotrigine treatment, one causing withdrawal from study. The authors concluded that oral lamotrigine 200 mg daily is a well-tolerated and moderately effective treatment for central poststroke pain. Lamotrigine may be an alternative to tricyclic antidepressants in the treatment of CPSP (Vestergaard et al. 2001).

Clonazepam (Klonopin$^®$, Roche Laboratories, Nutley, NJ) has been used in the treatment of trigeminal neuralgia since 1975 (Caccia 1975). It appears to be more effective as an adjunct to the other anticonvulsants when used in pain management. It appears particularly helpful in cases where pain is episodic and "lancinating" in nature. After oral ingestion, clonazepam is well absorbed and reaches maximum blood levels in 1–2 h. It is about 80% protein bound in the blood (Zakrzewska 1995).

Valproic acid, sodium valproate (Depakote®, Abbott Laboratories, Abbot Park, IL), is the only antiepileptic drug approved by the Food and Drug Administration (FDA) for migraine prevention. The mainstay of migraine treatment is pharmacotherapy. There have been numerous medications used to prevent migraine headaches, including β-blockers, calcium channel blockers, anticonvulsants, and nonsteroidal anti-inflammatory drugs. Newer antiepileptics, including gabapentin, pregabalin, and topiramate, are being evaluated for their role in preventive therapy. The mechanism of action of antiepileptics is not fully understood, but they all share a common role in enhancing GAMA-mediated inhibition (Corbo 2003).

Depakote has no specific advantage over gabapentin or pregabalin in the treatment of other neuropathic pain syndromes and has more side effects such as irritability, restlessness, nausea, gastric irritation, and weight gain and has been associated with hepatic failure in younger patients (Zakrzewska 1995).

Antidepressants

Antidepressant drugs are used in the treatment of patients with chronic pain. Pain is an unpleasant phenomenon and is often linked with depression. The observation that antidepressant drugs are beneficial, even in the absence of depression, suggests that these drugs could have intrinsic analgesic activity independent of their antidepressive effects (Feinmann 1985). The analgesic effects tend to be independent of the doses of heterocyclic antidepressants used for analgesia, as they are less than those considered effective in the treatment of depression (Egbunike and Chaffee 1990).

Almost all norepinephrine-containing terminals in the dorsal horn of the spinal cord are supraspinal in origin. Baba et al. studied the mechanism of descending pain-control pathways and how they inhibit nociceptive transmission at the spinal level (Baba et al. 2000). They proposed that activation of noradrenergic descending systems releases norepinephrine, which can directly hyperpolarize a proportion of the substantia gelatinosa (SG) neurons that may be excitatory interneurons in the pain pathway (postsynaptic inhibition) (Baba et al. 2000).

Alternatively, norepinephrine could depolarize inhibitory interneurons that contain GABA, glycine, or other inhibitory peptides. Iontophoretic application of norepinephrine near nociceptive dorsal horn neurons generally inhibits background activity of these cells and the responsiveness to excitatory amino acids (Baba et al. 2000). This inhibition most likely results from α-2-receptor activation, which increases K^+ conductance, thereby evoking a membrane hyperpolarization.

However, norepinephrine (and brain stem stimulation) has also been reported to produce excitatory effects. The neurons excited by iontophoretically applied norepinephrine and electrical stimulation of the periaqueductal gray were low-threshold cells, possibly inhibitory interneurons that synapse onto high-threshold and wide-dynamic-range neurons (Baba et al. 2000).

Antidepressants, such as amitriptyline, nortriptyline, imipramine, doxepin, trimipramine, and trazadone, have been used to treat diabetic neuropathy, postherpetic neuralgia, headache, arthritis, chronic back pain, cancer pain, facial pain, and phantom limb. Many of the antidepressants currently available have marked anticholinergic activity, which can cause dry mouth, visual disturbance, constipation, difficulty in micturition, and alterations in heart rate. Rani et al. compared amitriptyline to fluoxetine selective serotonin reuptake inhibitor (SSRI) as analgesic adjuvants in the treatment of rheumatic pain. Fluoxetine was more effective after 4 weeks with fewer side effects, especially autonomic side effects (Rani et al. 1996).

In recent years, tricyclic antidepressant drugs have experienced resurgence in their use as valuable pharmacological tools in the treatment of pain. Along with the evolution in our understanding of their analgesic mechanisms of action, there have been concurrent breakthroughs regarding their indications for use and modes of administration. The mechanisms of the antinociceptive effects of the antidepressant drugs were reviewed by Cohen and Abdi (2001). Antidepressants that have been used in pain management are list below along with starting doses and tolerability (Management of Chronic Pain Syndromes 2005).

Tricyclic Antidepressants

Examples of least anticholinergic tricyclic antidepressants (TCAs) include amitriptyline 10–25 mg qhs and desipramine 10–25 mg qhs.

Best tolerated TCAs are desipramine 10–25 mg qhs, imipramine 10–25 mg/day, and nortriptyline 10–25 mg/day. Finally, the TCA that produces significant sedation is doxipin 25 mg qhs.

Nontricyclic antidepressants that have both serotonin and norepinephrine reuptake inhibition effects (norepinephrine reuptake inhibition is necessary for pain modulation) are venlafaxine (Effexor®, Pfizer, New York, NY) ≥150 mg for norepinephrine, duloxetine (Cymbalta®, Eli Lily, Indianapolis, IN) 30 mg/day advancing to 60–120 mg/day, bupropion (Wellbutrin®, Glaxo-Smith-Kline, Philadelphia, PA) SR 150–300 mg/day, and trazadone (Deseryl®, Bristol-Myers-Squibb, New York, NY) 50–300 mg/day (avoid in men due to risk of priapism) (Management of Chronic Pain Syndromes 2005).

The advantage of duloxetine is its lack of side effects and rapid onset of action, within a few days instead of weeks. Goldstein et al. (2005) studied the efficacy and safety of duloxetine, a balanced and potent dual reuptake inhibitor of serotonin and norepinephrine, in the management of diabetic peripheral neuropathic pain (Goldstein et al. 2005). Serotonin and norepinephrine are thought to inhibit pain via descending pain pathways. In a 12-week, multicenter, double-blind study, 457 patients experiencing pain due to polyneuropathy caused by Type 1 or Type 2 diabetes mellitus were randomly assigned to treatment with duloxetine 20 mg/day (20 mg QD), 60 mg/day (60 mg QD), 120 mg/day (60 mg BID), or placebo. The diagnosis was confirmed by a score of at least 3 on the Michigan Neuropathy Screening Instrument. The primary efficacy measure was the weekly mean score of the 24-h Average Pain Score (APS), which was rated on an 11-point (0–10) Likert scale (no pain to worst possible pain) and computed from diary scores between two site visits (Goldstein et al. 2005). Duloxetine 60 and 120 mg/day demonstrated statistically significant greater improvement compared with placebo on the 24-h APS, beginning 1 week after randomization and continuing through the 12-week trial. Duloxetine also separated from placebo on nearly all the secondary measures including health-related outcome measures. Significantly more patients in all three active-treatment groups achieved a 50% reduction in the 24-h APS compared with placebo. Duloxetine treatment was considered to be safe and well tolerated with less than 20% discontinuation due to adverse events. The authors concluded that Duloxetine at 60 and 120 mg/day was safe and effective in the management of diabetic peripheral neuropathic pain (Goldstein et al. 2005).

Bupropion (Wellbutrin®, Zyban®, Glaxo Smith Kline, New York, NY) is an atypical antidepressant that acts as a norepinephrine and dopamine reuptake inhibitor, and nicotinic antagonist (Slemmer et al. 2000, Fryer and Lukas 1999). Bupropion belongs to the chemical class of aminoketones and is similar in structure to the stimulant cathinone, to the anorectic diethylpropion, and to phenethylamines in general.

Bupropion lowers seizure threshold, but at the recommended dose the risk of seizures is comparable to that observed for other antidepressants. Bupropion is an effective antidepressant on its own but it is particularly popular as an add-on medication in the cases of incomplete response to the first-line SSRI antidepressant (Zisook et al. 2006).

In contrast to many psychiatric drugs, including nearly all antidepressants, bupropion does not cause weight gain or sexual dysfunction (Clayton 2003). It is helpful in patients with a history of prior substance abuse since it has dopamine reuptake inhibition in addition to norepinephrine reuptake effects (Slemmer et al. 2000, Fryer and Lukas 1999).

Dopamine is the neurotransmitter associated with the "pleasure system" of the brain. It provides feelings of enjoyment and reinforcement to motivate us to continue certain activities. Dopamine was originally known as the "reward chemical" because it is released during rewarding activities such as food and sex – this neurotransmitter is primarily involved in regulation of attention, motivation, pleasure, and reward. Lack of dopamine is associated with decreased ability to experience pleasure, decreased motivation, decreased attention, and cognitive slowing.

Very few agents with dopamine activity have been developed to date. Prodopaminergic agents represent a potential for treatment breakthrough for major depressive disorders, and agents with prodopaminergic activity may possess efficacy and tolerability advantages over traditional 5HT-selective agents (Zisook et al. 2006). To date, there are no specific studies indicating advantages of Buprion over other antidepressants in the treatment of pain. However, in this author's experience it seems to be a good adjunct in patients who have a history of substance abuse as an adjunct to their other medications.

Specific Serotonin Reuptake Inhibitors (SSRIs)

Although fluoxetine (an SSRI) was shown to be as effective as amitriptyline in the control of rheumatic pain (Rani et al. 1996), the SRRIs generally are not effective in pain other than for their antidepressant effects. Yet, Prozac® (Eli Lily, Indianapolis, IN), Zoloft® (Pfizer, New York, NY), Lexapro® (Forest Pharmaceuticals, New York, NY), etc. are frequently used as adjuncts to other adjuvants in the treatment of chronic pain conditions. And as indicated previously, bupropion may also be helpful in the polypharmaceutical approach to pain management.

Local Anesthetics

Lidocaine is reported to have significant analgesic effects that are distinct from those produced by morphine (Wu et al. 2002). In this randomized double-blind, active-placebo-controlled, crossover trial, the authors demonstrated that stump pain was diminished both by morphine and by lidocaine while phantom pain was diminished only by morphine. These observations suggest that the mechanisms and pharmacological sensitivity of phantom and stump pains differ. Stump pain may be predominantly peripherally mediated via a mechanism involving sodium channels, while phantom pain may involve both peripheral and central mechanisms (Wu et al. 2002). Despite the observed efficacy, the drugs tested did not eliminate pain completely, suggesting that these patients may require multimodal therapy, and that future analgesic studies in this area should be expanded to include neuraxial opioids, anticonvulsants, and antidepressants to the currently tested drugs.

Abram and Yaksh in another animal model demonstrated that systemic local anesthetics can affect the behavioral responses to noxious stimulation by two distinct mechanisms (Abram and Yaksh 1994). While they are capable of blocking nociceptor-induced spinal sensitization, they do so incompletely and only at blood levels that are close to those associated with symptoms of toxicity. They also appear to have no effect on previously established spinal hypersensitivity. Therefore, it appears likely that the predominant effect of systemic lidocaine on neuropathic pain is through suppression of spontaneous impulse generation arising from injured nerve segments or associated dorsal root ganglia (Abram and Yaksh 1994).

Lidocaine is available as a 5% transdermal patch which is applied for 12 h per day and is approved for use in postherpetic neuralgia after the skin lesions have healed and the skin is intact. It can produce 30–40% reduction in pain in some patients. Although there are no controlled studies, some physicians are prescribing these patches for pain other than postherpetic neuralgia and the patients do get relief (e.g., low back pain and wrist pain). Galer reported in March 2005 at the American Pain Society annual meeting that his data strongly suggest that the patch (currently approved in the United States for treating postherpetic neuralgia) was as effective as celecoxib for reducing daily pain intensity in patients with osteoarthritis of the knee (Galer 2005).

Mexilitine [Mexitil® (Boehr Ingelheim Pharmaceuticals, Ridgefield, CT) 150 mg advancing to qid dosing] is a cardiac antiarrhythmic drug which is a lidocaine analogue available in oral form (Management of Chronic Pain Syndromes 2005). For cardiac arrhythmias, both mexilitine and lidocaine decrease ventricular irritability, stabilize the Purkinje fiber system, and decrease circuit reentry arrhythmias. It is this sodium channel interaction that likely reduced the neural activity in studies of neuroma-generated nerve pain (Chabal et al. 1989).

N-Methyl-D-Aspartate Receptor Blocking Agents

The N-methyl-D-aspartate (NMDA) receptor and its activation is intimately involved in the pathological processes of wind-up, central sensitization, hyperalgesia, allodynea, and reduced opioid effectiveness (tolerance) (Dickenson 1994). Unfortunately, there are few NMDA receptor antagonists available to us clinically.

Recent advances in the understanding of postoperative pain have demonstrated its association with sensitization of the CNS which clinically elicits pain hypersensitivity. NMDA receptors play a major role in synaptic plasticity and are specifically implicated in CNS facilitation of pain processing. Therefore, NMDA receptor antagonists, and specifically ketamine, have been employed in clinical practice at subanesthetic (i.e., low) doses to exert a specific NMDA blockade and hence modulate central sensitization induced both by the incision and tissue damage and by perioperative analgesics such as opioids (Kock and Lavand'homme 2007).

Ketamine is probably the best known agent which is used primarily as an intravenous anesthetic. In subanesthetic doses it has been shown to inhibit or reverse acute opioid tolerance and can enhance opioid analgesia (Ellers et al. 2001). It has also been successfully used combined with morphine in PCA to decrease opioid requirements (Svedicic et al. 2003).

Dextromethorphan is an antitussive found in many cough medications. However it has been found to have antinociceptive effects and can attenuate acute pain sensation through antagonistic effects on the NMDA receptor (Weinbrown et al. 2000). It is available in oral form; however, at doses necessary to produce adequate pain relief (up to 100 mg qid) it can be too sedating and poorly tolerated by patients at that dose.

Skeletal Muscle Relaxants

Health care providers prescribe skeletal muscle relaxants for a variety of indications. However, the comparative efficacy of these drugs is not well known. Skeletal muscle relaxants consist of both antispasticity and antispasmodic agents, a distinction that prescribers often overlook. The antispasticity agents – baclofen, tizanidine, dantrolene, and diazepam – aid in improving muscle hypertonicity and involuntary jerks. Antispasmodic agents, such as cyclobenzaprine, are primarily used to treat musculoskeletal conditions. Much of the evidence from clinical trials regarding skeletal muscle relaxants is limited because of poor methodological design, insensitive assessment methods, and small numbers of patients. Although trial results seem to support the use of these agents for their respective indications, efficacy data from comparator trials did not particularly favor one skeletal muscle relaxant over another. Therefore, the choice of a skeletal muscle relaxant should be based on its adverse-effect profile, tolerability, and cost (See and Ginzburg 2008).

Spasm is defined as an involuntary and abnormal muscle contraction and therefore encompasses multiple different subtypes of involuntary muscle activity. After acute musculoskeletal injury, the most common type of involuntary muscle activity found is spasm from segmental reflex activity resulting in increased muscle contraction in an effort to splint and protect injured tissues (Clawson 2001). Antispasticity and antispasmodic agents are often used in conjunction with the other nonopioid analgesics and with opioids for pain with a component of muscle spasm.

As reviewed by Chou et al., skeletal muscle relaxants are a heterogeneous group of medications used to treat two different types of underlying conditions: spasticity from upper motor neuron syndromes and muscular pain or spasms from peripheral musculoskeletal conditions (Chou et al. 2004). Although widely used for these indications, there appear to be gaps in our understanding of the comparative efficacy and safety of different skeletal muscle relaxants.

Chou et al. systematically reviewed the evidence for the comparative efficacy and safety of skeletal muscle relaxants for spasticity and musculoskeletal conditions (Chou et al. 2004). They used randomized trials, observational studies, electronic databases, reference lists, and pharmaceutical company submissions. Searches were performed through January 2003. The validity of each included study was assessed using a data abstraction form and predefined criteria. An overall grade was allocated for the body of evidence for each key question. A total of 101 randomized trials were included in this review. No randomized trial was rated good quality, and there was little evidence of rigorous adverse event assessment in included trials or observational studies (Chou et al. 2004). They concluded that there was fair evidence that baclofen, tizanidine, and dantrolene were effective compared to placebo in patients with spasticity (primarily multiple sclerosis). There was fair evidence that baclofen and tizanidine were roughly equivalent for efficacy in patients with spasticity, but insufficient evidence to determine the efficacy of dantrolene compared to baclofen or tizanidine. There was fair evidence that although the overall rate of adverse effects between tizanidine and baclofen was similar, tizanidine was associated with more dry mouth and baclofen with more weakness (Chou et al. 2004).

There was fair evidence that cyclobenzaprine, carisoprodol, orphenadrine, and tizanidine were effective compared to placebo in patients with musculoskeletal conditions (primarily acute back or neck pain). Cyclobenzaprine has been evaluated in most clinical trials and has consistently been found to be effective. There are very limited or inconsistent data regarding the effectiveness of metaxalone, methocarbamol, chlorzoxazone, baclofen, or dantrolene compared to placebo in patients with musculoskeletal conditions. There was insufficient evidence to determine the relative efficacy or safety of cyclobenzaprine, carisoprodol, orphenadrine, tizanidine, metaxalone, methocarbamol, and chlorzoxazone. Dantrolene and, to a lesser degree chlorzoxazone, have been associated with rare serious hepatotoxicity (Chou et al. 2004).

Antispasticity Agents

Baclofen is a GABA receptor antagonist and is believed to work through descending pain modulation in the central nervous system. It works best for pain associated with spasticity. It is available for oral as well as intrathecal (Lioresal®, Novartis, East Hanover, NJ) administration. Intrathecally, it is administered via a continuous implanted pump and is very effective in cases of severe spasticity such as cerebral palsy or multiple sclerosis (Bowery et al. 1980, Albright et al. 1993).

The oral tablets of 5 or 10 mg are titrated slowly to effect increasing every 3 days until therapeutic benefit is reached or overwhelming side effects occur. Sedation, dizziness, weakness, hypotension, nausea, respiratory depression, and constipation may occur; the drug must be discontinued by slow taper. The maximum dose is 80 mg/day orally, and the withdrawal syndrome consists of hallucinations or even seizures. Care must be taken in renal failure patients and elevations of alkaline phosphatase and aspirate aminotransferase (AST) levels may occur. Baclofen (Lioresal®) – 5 mg tid to 15 mg tid.

Dantrolene is a powerful muscle relaxant which is used in the treatment of malignant hyperthermia as an intravenous agent. Dantrolene, unlike other antispasm muscle relaxants, acts peripherally instead of centrally by inhibiting the release of calcium ions from the sarcoplasmic reticulum (Max and Gilron 2001). Orally, it is titrated as 10 or 25 mg qd × 7 days, then 25 mg tid × 7 days, then 50 mg tid × 7 days. It should be discontinued if no benefit is observed after 45 days. It does have a black box warning about possible nonfatal or even fatal hepatic failure.

Diazepam (Valium®, Roche Laboratories, Nutley, NJ) has been used for many years as a muscle relaxant, often prescribed after whiplash injuries. In adults, 2–10 mg tid–qid can be prescribed. However it carries all of the problems of the benzodiazepines such as abuse potential as a "tranquilizer" or anxiolytic agent. Patients may experience dizziness, drowsiness, and confusion possibly with memory difficulty at higher doses. It has active metabolites which can significantly extend the half-life up to 100 h. Again, it should be avoided in patients with renal insufficiency or hepatic impairment.

Tizanidine (Zanaflex®, Acorda Therapeutics, Hawthorne, NY) is an α-2 adrenergic agonist like clonidine and works through central modulation. Side effects like hypotension, sedation, asthenia, and dry mouth (dose related) can be significant and so very low doses should be started initially. This may be even less than 0.5 mg. The dose can be gradually increased to a maximum of 36 mg/day. It may cause elevated liver function studies or even hepatotoxicity. Dosages need to start small, 1–2 mg qhs, further titrated to 4–8 mg qhs and 2–4 mg bid (Mclain 2002).

Antispasmodic Agents

Cyclobenzaprine (Flexeril®, Ortho-McNeil-Janssen, New Brunswick, NJ), 5 mg tid; may increase to 10 mg tid. Anticholinergic effects (drowsiness, urinary retention, dry mouth): avoid in elderly; QT prolongation: avoid in patients with arrhythmias, cardiac conduction disturbances, heart block, heart failure, or recent myocardial infarction; may raise intraocular pressure: avoid in patients with glaucoma; elimination half-life ~18 h in young subjects, ~33 h in elderly, and ~46 h in patients with hepatic impairment.

Carisoprodol (Soma®, Wallace Laboratories, Abbot Park, IL) 350 mg qid, is not recommended in children under 12 years of age; drowsiness; can cause psychological and physical dependence, withdrawal symptoms can occur with discontinuation; excessive use, overdose, or withdrawal may precipitate seizures; reports describe idiosyncratic or allergy-type reactions after first dose (mental status changes, transient quadriplegia, fever, angioneurotic edema, asthmatic episodes) metabolized to meprobamate, a barbiturate and so there is a significant risk of dependency. Rapid cessation can lead to delayed seizure when patients are taking higher doses.

In this author's experience, a patient who was taking six Soma® per day was admitted to the hospital for surgery and her Soma medication was not restarted after surgery. On her 5th postoperative day, she had a seizure which was originally attributed to the antibiotics. It is easy to lose track of long-term medications when patients are hospitalized.

Chlorzoxazone (Paraflex®, Ortho-McNeil-Janssen, New Brunswick, NJ) 250–750 mg tid or qid, causes dizziness and drowsiness, rare cases of hepatotoxicity, gastrointestinal irritation, and rare cases of gastrointestinal bleeding; may cause red or orange urine; avoid in patients with liver impairment.

Metaxalone (Skelaxin®, Myung Moon Pharm, Korea) 800 mg tid–qid. Not recommended in children <12 years; do not use in patients with renal or hepatic failure or a history of anemia; dizziness and drowsiness may occur, and in rare cases leukopenia or hemolytic anemia may result.

Methocarbamol (Robaxin®, Schwarz Pharma, Mequon, WI) 1,500 mg qid for 72 h then 1,000 mg qid. Available as an injectable but should not be injected in patients with renal failure; may cause brown-to-black or green discoloration of urine; may impair mental status; may exacerbate symptoms of myasthenia gravis.

Orphenadrine (Norflex®, 3 M Pharmaceuticals, St. Paul, MN) 100 mg bid has anticholinergic effects such as drowsiness, urinary retention, and dry mouth. This drug should be avoided in the elderly; it may raise intraocular pressure and therefore must be avoided in patients with glaucoma. Orphenadrine is associated with gastrointestinal disturbances. Its elimination half-life is 13–20 h, and elimination is extended when use is prolonged. Finally, orphenadrine should be avoided in patients with cardiospasm or myasthenia gravis, and is generally contraindicated in duodenal or pyloric obstruction or stenosing peptic ulcers.

Amphetamines

The use of amphetamines or other stimulants as adjuvant medications can be tempting when treating chronic pain patients, especially high-dose therapy patients in whom side effects such as sedation can become more prevalent. In terminal cancer patients, the use of amphetamines as adjuncts is even more pressing because of the emphasis on side effect reduction and improvement in the patient's quality of life in their remaining months.

Although one would think that there would be many studies looking at amphetamines to mitigate opioid-induced sedation, in fact there are only a few randomized, double-blinded, placebo-controlled, clinical trials (Wilwerding et al. 1995). In one such study conducted in patients with terminal cancer (Bruera et al. 1986), patients were given mazindol or placebo for 1 week and then switched to the other treatment/placebo arm. During the study period there were no differences in patient sedation as primarily measured by the number of hours slept, but the mazindol-treated group had much higher prevalence of side effects such as anxiety, nausea, and sweating.

Another similar study (Bruera et al. 1992) included terminal cancer patients on continuous intravenous opioid infusions. The patients were double-blinded and randomized to a 3-day treatment course of methylphenidate versus placebo. The patients were then evaluated every 6 h for markers of sedation including drowsiness, confusion, and cognitive function. After 3 days of treatment, reports for all three endpoints were improved with drowsiness (8 versus 35%), confusion (8 versus 22%), and cognitive function (25 versus 1%) in the methylphenidate versus placebo groups, respectively.

There are obvious limitations that preclude applying these outcomes in favor of chronic amphetamine use to counteract opioid sedation (Max and Gilron 2001). In prescribing amphetamines, one has to remember that these are controlled drugs with a high potential for abuse and diversion (Hertz and Knight 2006). Chronic amphetamine use runs its own risk with cardiopulmonary and central nervous system effects as well as the development of tolerance. Hence, alternate drug strategies to mitigate sedation such as evaluation and treatment for other causes of sedation such as anemia, endocrinopathies, or depression should be undertaken. Simple medication changes such as changing to sustained release opioid medication may also help as these formulations are less associated with sedation.

Benzodiazepines

Benzodiazepines are drugs used to treat a variety of painful and nonpainful conditions, in particular benzodiazepines provide for a degree of flexibility in the route of administration not seen in many other analgesic drug classes. Benzodiazepines work by potentiating the GABA receptor–ligand complex (Johnston 2005). In the practice of pain medicine, benzodiazepines have been researched as possible treatment for anxiety, as muscle relaxants, and as potential sole analgesics.

Benzodiazepines have long been prescribed as treatments for anxiety despite the American Psychiatric Association (1998) and the National Institute of Health (National Institute for Health and Clinical Excellence 2004) guidelines stating that SSRI/serotonin norepinephrine reuptake inhibitor (SNRI) and cognitive behavioral therapy are much more efficacious. These guidelines advise that benzodiazepines can still be used as abortive anxiolytics, but their utility needs to be counterbalanced by their potential for abuse and lack of antidepressant properties.

Another usage for benzodiazepines has been for a wide array of myofascial diseases. While there are several studies that demonstrate benzodiazepines are better than placebo, for short-term low back muscle spasm, the data are not favorable when benzodiazepines are compared to other medications for lumbar muscle spasm. Joint practice guidelines for acute and chronic low back pain written by the American Pain Society and the American College of Physicians discouraged the use of benzodiazepines in favor of other medications (Chou and Huffman 2007). Controlled studies using benzodiazepines have been done in pain states like CTTH and TMJ (List et al. 2003) which support its use, but even then benzodiazepines are reserved for a select set of patients that have failed better established modalities.

The studies investigating if benzodiazepines could function as pure analgesics have generally not been favorable. Early studies demonstrated mixed findings, but it was unclear from these studies if the benzodiazepines were controlling the patients' pain or anxiety. More recent studies have shown more definitively that benzodiazepines do not inherently have analgesic potential. Randomized, blinded, placebo-controlled trials using lorazepam showed no difference in analgesia in neuropathic pain states like postherpetic neuralgia, trigeminal neuralgia, or diabetic peripheral neuropathy (Hempenstall et al. 2005).

Pain physicians need to be aware of the side effects of benzodiazepines, including hypoventilation and sedation that is synergistic with other centrally acting depressant medication. Withdrawal symptoms include autonomic hyperactivity, but unlike opioid withdrawal, benzodiazepine withdrawal can be life threatening. On a societal level, benzodiazepines remain only second to opioids as a favorite drug of abuse and diversion. One study showed that 20% of adult detoxification program admissions were because of benzodiazepine, but more worrisome is the rate of abuse in the adolescent population where benzodiazepines were responsible for 40% of adolescent detoxification admissions (O'Brien 2005).

In summary, other than for short-term use for acute low back muscle spasm or short-term anxiolytic therapy while awaiting for other modalities to work [i.e., SNRI and cognitive behavior therapy (CBT)], or for select refractory myofascial disease states, there is an unfavorable risk–benefit profile to support the widespread general use of benzodiazepines as adjuvant analgesics in chronic pain management (Max and Gilron 2001).

Cannabinoids in Pain Therapy

Cannabinoids have been used historically to alleviate the pain from migraines, cramps, nausea, and vomiting and to support appetite stimulation (Fontelles et al. 2008). Interest in the development of cannabinoid analgesics was not pursued like it was with opium derivatives until the 1960s when THC was pharmacologically isolated. Cannabinoid pharmacology and intracellular pathways were elucidated in the 1990s when the endogenous receptor was cloned, and endogenous ligands called "endocannabinoids" were discovered. These initial studies demonstrated that cannabinoids act at several different sites with two subtypes CB1 and CB2 being expressed in the supraspinal, intrinsic interspinal, DRG, and peripheral nervous systems (Guindon and Hohmann 2009). CB1 is reported to play a role in neuromodulation and analgesia, while CB2 has been more specifically characterized as an immunomodulator (Pertwee 2005). Interestingly, unlike other neurotransmitters, endo-cannabinoids are synthesized on demand from arachidonic acid precursors and then released into the synaptic cleft. The basic science data have helped researchers develop cannabinoid derivatives that retain their analgesic nature but reduce the psychotropic effects.

Animal studies have shown promise with cannabinoids reversing hyperalgesia from induced neuropathy models, including models of sciatic nerve compression, chemotherapy-induced neuropathy, and diabetic neuropathy. Although these animal models for neuro-pathic pain are robust and reproducible, neuropathic pain states in the human are much harder to reproduce because they often are caused by more than one etiology.

Application of cannabinoid analgesia in human studies is made even harder because many studies conducted in humans lack strict inclusion criteria which can underestimate a more pronounced efficacy of cannabinoid in possible patient subgroups. Second, those studies that do show efficacy are often carried out in small groups, have no placebo arm, or reach nonsignificant endpoints. One randomized crossover, double-blind study comparing the analgesic effects of nabilone, a synthetic cannabinoid, and dihydrocodeine in diabetic neu-ropathy patients showed near equal efficacy in analgesia between the two drugs but nabilone had a much higher side effect profile. A meta-analysis of nine trials with 222 patients did not show that cannabinoids were more effective than codeine in controlling pain and authors did not encourage widespread use of cannabinoid derivates (Campbell et al. 2001).

In select subgroups, the data supporting cannabinoid therapy are much stronger. There were several case reports in the multiple sclerosis literature utilizing synthetic cannabinoids to improve objective mobility and pain, but it was not until a 3-month duration, placebo-controlled, randomized, double-blinded, large multicenter trial conducted by Zajicek et al. (2003) who demonstrated this more conclusively. Interestingly, the study was continued as open label which showed continued reduction in painful muscle spasticity over a 1-year period (Zajicek et al. 2005). In fibromyalgia, a double-blind, randomized, placebo-controlled trial of 40 patients with fibromyalgia and short (4 weeks) treatment phase showed significant 20% reduction on visual analog scale (VAS) fibromyalgia impact questionnaire reduction and reduction in anxiety (Skrabek et al. 2007).

Side effects which are most commonly reported include dysphoria, reduction in con-centration, motor in-coordination, nausea, and dizziness. Drug development has attempted to derive a synthetic cannabinoid that is approximately 90% less psychoactive than phytocannabinoids. Studies investigating dependence and tolerance to cannabinoids are equivocal.

Currently, cannabinoid derivates include tetrahydrocannabinol, cannabidiol, as well as Sativex® (G. W. Pharmaceuticals, Salisbury, UK) – all have indications for neuropathic pain from multiple sclerosis and cancer pain. A formulation called Nabilone® (Valiant Pharmaceuticals, Costa Mesa, CA) is approved by the FDA for chemotherapy associated with refractory nausea and vomiting, but pain physicians are using it off-label for pain therapy (Berlach et al. 2006).

Therefore, after extensive research elucidating the pharmacodynamics of the cannabinoid system, and further preclinical animal models showing that cannabinoid therapy can help in animal models of neuropathy, there is still a shortcoming of well-controlled clinical studies demonstrating efficacy for common neuropathic syndromes, that preclude the widespread use of cannabinoid therapy.

Barbiturates

Barbiturates are medicines that act on the central nervous system and cause drowsiness. Also known as sedative-hypnotic drugs, barbiturates make people very relaxed, calm, and sleepy. Because of these properties they have been used as "sleeping pills" and tranquilizers. A major property however is their ability to control seizures through their depressant effect on the CNS (Hobbs et al. 1996).

The ultra-short-acting barbiturates produce anesthesia within about 1 min after intravenous administration. Those in current medical use are the Schedule IV drug methohexital (Brevital®, King Pharmaceuticals Inc., Bristol, TN) and the Schedule III drugs thiamyl (Surital®, Pfizer, New York, NY) and thiopental (Pentothal®, Hospira, Lake Forest, IL). Barbiturate abusers prefer the Schedule II short-acting and intermediate-acting barbiturates that include amobarbital (Amytal®), pentobarbital (Nembutal®, Ovation Pharmaceuticals, Deefield, IL), secobarbital (Seconal®, Eli Lily, Indianapolis, IN), and tuinal (an amobarbital/secobarbital combination product). Other short- and intermediate-acting barbiturates are in Schedule III and include butalbital (Fiorina®, Novartis, East Hannover, NJ), butabarbital (Butisol®, Meda Pharmaceutical, Somerset, NJ), talbutal (Lotusate®, Sanofi-Aventis, Bridgewater, NJ), and aprobarbital (Alurate®, Roche Pharmaceuticals, Nutley, NJ). After oral administration, the onset of action is from 15 to 40 min, and the effects last up to 6 h. These drugs are primarily used for insomnia and preoperative sedation. Veterinarians use pentobarbital for anesthesia and euthanasia (Hobbs et al. 1996).

Long-acting barbiturates include phenobarbital (Luminal®, Hospira Inc., Lake Forest, IL) and mephobarbital (Mebaral®, Ovation Pharm, Deerfield, IL), both of which are in Schedule IV. Effects of these drugs are realized in about 1 h and last for about 12 h and are used primarily for daytime sedation and the treatment of seizure disorders (Hobbs et al. 1996).

While barbiturates were once used commonly as premedication for surgical patients or sleep aids, other more suitable drugs are now being used. In pain management, the use of barbiturates as antianxiety medication has also been replaced by more suitable drugs (benzodiazepines) (Hobbs et al. 1996). However, in spite of the fact that we do not use this class of drug commonly in pain management, patients may come to the pain clinic having been prescribed these medications for many years by their primary care physician and so it behooves us to review their properties briefly.

Because barbiturates work on the CNS, they may add to the effects of alcohol and other drugs that slow the central nervous system, such as antihistamines, cold medicine, allergy medicine, sleep aids, other medicines for seizures, tranquilizers, some pain relievers, and muscle relaxants. They may also add to the effects of anesthetics, including those used for dental procedures (Brevital®). The combined effects of barbiturates and alcohol or other CNS depressants can lead to unconsciousness, respiratory depression, or even death (Hobbs et al. 1996).

Signs of barbiturate overdose include:
• severe drowsiness
• breathing problems
• slurred speech
• staggering

- slow heartbeat
- severe confusion
- severe weakness

Barbiturates may change the results of certain medical tests and may cause physical or mental dependence when taken over long periods.

Withdrawal symptoms, such as anxiety, nausea or vomiting, trembling, sleep problems, or convulsions, may occur if these medications are stopped abruptly after prolonged use. The withdrawal symptoms may be delayed even for several weeks depending on the dosage that had been employed and therefore any weaning schedule from barbiturate medication must be 4–6 weeks and cannot be accomplished rapidly.

Children may be especially sensitive to barbiturates. This may increase the chance of side effects such as unusual excitement. Older people may also be more sensitive and the barbiturates may be more likely to cause confusion, depression, or unusual agitation. These effects are also more likely in patients who are severely ill.

Interactions

Birth control pills may not work properly when taken while barbiturates are being taken. Blood thinners, adrenocorticoids (cortisone-like medicines), and other antiseizure medicines such as valproic acid (Depakote® and Depakene®) and carbamazepine (Tegretol®) may interact with the barbiturates. Porphyria is a serious medical condition that can be initiated by the barbiturates (Hobbs et al. 1996).

Summary

It is clear that there are many adjuvants and nonopioid analgesics available to physicians for the treatment of pain and that polypharmacy in pain management is more likely to be the rule rather than the exception. Combining multiple agents that inhibit the pain transmission system at different levels is more likely to have success than any single agent alone and may allow for lower doses of each agent so as to reduce potential adverse or side effects. Combining agents that have NMDA receptor blocking action, Mu opioid agonist action, tetrodotoxin resistance (TTXr) sodium channel blockers, SNRI, neuronal calcium channel blockade, and anti-inflammatory actions can all contribute to central nervous system protection. Combining oral gabapentin (Neurontin®) 300–1,200 mg (Dirks et al. 2002, Gilron 2002, Matthews and Dickerson 2002, Hayashida et al. 2008, Begon et al. 2002) or pregabalin 75–150 mg (Lyrica®), and clonidine 0.2 mg along with acetaminophen 1,000 mg, and a COX-2 inhibitor (celecoxib 200 mg) (Celebrex®) preoperatively, and then continuing postoperatively with the antineuropathic regimen of gabapentin or pregabalin (100–300 mg tid or 50 mg tid, respectively) (Begon et al. 2002) along with an appropriate opioid, anti-inflammatory, and antidepressant (for SNRI action) until wound healing has occurred could potentially reduce or eliminate the development of chronic pain after surgery. On this basis we can begin to target polypharmacy to help the brain to modulate neuropathic pain (Weissman and Haddox 1989). This is similar to the multimodal therapeutic recommendations of Power (2005).

Case Scenario

Sreekumar Kunnumpurath, MBBS, MD, FCARCSI, FRCA, FFPMRCA

Lee is a 53-year-old teacher who is scheduled for an elective right inguinal herniorrhaphy. You are the anesthesiologist responsible for the anesthetic management of this patient. You met him in the preassessment clinic, took a detailed history, and performed clinical examination. Lee has a very healthy lifestyle; he does not smoke or drink alcohol, works out in the gym every day, and does not eat junk food. The only significant medical history includes mild childhood asthma and chicken pox at the age of 14. Lee mentions that he wants to avoid "drugs" such as morphine, as he fears that he might get addicted to them. The underlying reason for this fear is that his younger brother was addicted to heroin and died of a drug overdose. He is looking forward to your expert advice so that he can avoid as many "drugs" as possible during his stay in the hospital.

Outline your anesthetic plan for Lee.
Since herniorrhaphy is a relatively superficial surgery, the intraoperative and postoperative pain management is not particularly challenging. It is usually undertaken as a day case surgery. However, the specific wish of Lee to avoid opioids altogether could sometimes prove difficult. It is worth reasoning with him that the risk of using a short- or ultra-short-acting opioid in the perioperative period could make his recovery smoother and more pleasant.

Lee is adamant that he should not have any opioids whatever happens and he is willing to accept the limitations that his wish might impose on the anesthetic management. You explain that pain from hernia surgery could be controlled with a multimodal approach to pain management, and opioids can be avoided. Nonopioid options include local anesthetic infiltration of the wound, acetaminophen, and nonsteroidal anti-inflammatory drugs such as ketorolac. Ketorolac has the advantage of parenteral administration, whereas celecoxib is given orally. A neuraxial block either alone or in combination with a general anesthetic is another option but a spinal or an epidural could potentially delay his discharge from the hospital.

Hernia surgery can at times involve bowel resection, leading to increased pain perception and analgesic requirement. Of course, analgesic requirement can vary widely among individual patients.

From the given history, do you think you can safely use nonsteroidal anti-inflammatory drugs?
NSAIDs have several potential side effects, including precipitating an acute asthmatic attack and gastrointestinal bleeding. Lee has a history of childhood asthma, and therefore it is essential to find out whether he can take NSAIDs without the risk of inducing a bronchospasm. Lee states that he can take ibuprofen and aspirin and these medications do not make him wheezy. In fact, he has not had an asthma attack since the age of 18. During the conversation, he asks whether there is any medication that he can take before surgery to reduce postoperative pain. He has heard about chronic pain resulting from "cutting

of nerves during surgery." He tells you that he has read an article on the Internet about "preemptive analgesia."

What medication can you prescribe for this purpose?
There is some evidence to show that preoperative administration of gabapentin can preemptively reduce postoperative pain. It is also claimed to reduce the incidence of developing postoperative neuropathic pain. Lee finally undergoes surgery under general anesthesia, combined with an inguinal block by the surgeon and ketorolac. The surgeon offers to infiltrate the surrounding tissue with an extra dose of local anesthetic. He also receives gabapentin. Lee is now in the recovery room and is pain-free while recovering from general anesthesia. To add to this preemptive and post-operative analgesia, an ultrasound guided continuous trans abdominal plane block (TAP) with a continuous catheter could be placed at the end of the case. A continuous infusion of local (e.g., 0.2% Ropivacaine) anesthetic delivered between the internal oblique and transverse abdominis muscles on the operative can be initiated with the help of an elastomeric pump designed for home infusion. The infusion catheter would be removed by the patient at home after 2–3 days. This should provide excellent pain control in addition to the anti-inflammatory, gabapentin, and acetaminophen regimen. He is discharged home with acetaminophen and ibuprofen. He is advised to take these medications regularly for about 5 days and as needed afterward.

Two months later Lee is referred to you by his surgeon because he is experiencing a burning pain sensation in the area of his previous hernia repair. Lee tells you that the pain is in fact "shooting and burning" in nature and radiates to his back.

Describe your management?
First, you need to determine the precise nature of pain, including site, character, and radiation, as well as precipitating and relieving factors. Then, you undertake a detailed physical examination. You note that the surgical wound has healed well and there is a fine thin scar. However, it is tender to palpation. You also note that the skin is red and hyperalgesic over the area extending from the scar to his back – corresponding to the T10 dermatome on the right side. You can see partially healed small blisters as well. His white cell count is elevated and there is lymphocytosis.

What is the possible diagnosis? How would you treat this condition?
The most likely diagnosis is herpes zoster, though it is less commonly seen over the lumbar dermatomes. Treatment includes administration of antiviral agents (acyclovir) and analgesics. A wide range of drugs have been used to treat the neuropathic pain, including tricyclic antidepressants, capsaicin, anticonvulsants, local anesthetics, and steroids. TENS is also an option. Opioids can be useful but your patient refuses them, as before.

Since herpes zoster is a reactivation infection, it is IgG mediated immunity which is not inhibited by steroids. If noted in the first few days after the outbreak of the lesions, steroids can be very helpful either as an epidural injection at the involved dermatome, or subcutaneous injection with local anesthetic under the lesioned area. Another approach for this level would be a paravertebral catheter with the infusion of local anesthetic via a home pump for several days to help with pain control.

References

Abram S, Yaksh T. Systemic lidocaine blocks nerve injury-induced hyperalgesia and nociceptor-driven spinal sensitization in the rat. Anesthesiology 1994;80:383–91.

Albright A, Barron W, Fasick M, et al. Continuous intrathecal baclofen infusion for spasticity of cerebral origin. JAMA 1993;270(20):2475–7.

American Psychiatric Association. Practice guideline for the treatment of patients with panic disorder. Am J Psychiatry 1998;155(suppl 5):1–34.

Antman E, Bennett J, Daugherty A, et al. Use of nonsteroidal anti-inflammatory drugs: an update for clinicians: a scientific statement from the American Heart Association. Circulation 2007;115:1634–42.

Baba H, Shimoji K, Yoshimura M. Facilitates inhibitory transmission in substantia gelatinosa of adult rat spinal cord (Part 1): Effects on axon terminals of GABAergic and glycinergic. Anesthesiology 2000;92:473–84.

Barton S, Langeland F, Snabes M, et al. Efficacy and safety of intravenous parecoxib sodium in relieving acute postoperative pain following gynecologic laparotomy surgery. Anesthesiology 2002;97:306–14.

Beck DH, Schenk MR, Hagemann K, Doepfmer UR, Kox WJ. The pharmacokinetics and analgesic efficacy of larger dose rectal acetaminophen (40 mg/kg) in adults: a double-blinded, randomized study. Anesth Analg. 2000;90:431–6.

Begon S, Pickering G, Eschalier A, Dubray C. Magnesium increases morphine analgesic effect in different experimental models of pain. Anesthesiology 2002;96(3):627–32.

Benzon H, Teng-Leong C, McCarthy R, Benzon H. Comparison of the particulate sizes of different steroids and effect of dilution: a review of the relative neurotoxicities of the steroids. Anesthesiology 2007;106:331–8.

Berlach DM, Shir Y, Ware MA. Experience with the synthetic cannabinoid nabilone in chronic noncancer pain. Pain Med. 2006 Jan–Feb;7(1):25–9.

Bernat J, Sandowsky C, Vincent F, Nordgren R, Margolis G. Sclerosing spinal pachymeningitis: a complication of intrathecal administration of Depo-Medrol® for multiple sclerosis. J Neurol Neurosurg Psychiatry. 1976;39:1124–8.

Bowery N, Hill D, Hudson A, et al. (-)Baclofen decreases neurotransmitter release in the mammalian CNS by an action at a novel GABA receptor. Nature 1980;283(5742):92–4.

Brill S, Plaza M. Non-narcotic adjuvants may improve the duration and quality of analgesia after knee arthroscopy: a brief review. Can J Anesth. 2004;10:975–8.

Bruera E, Carraro S, Roca E, Barugel M, Chacon R. Double-blind evaluation of the effects of mazindol on pain, depression, anxiety, appetite, and activity in terminal cancer patients. Cancer Treat Rep. 1986 Feb;70(2):295–8.

Bruera E, Fainsinger R, MacEachern T, Hanson J. The use of methylphenidate in patients with incident cancer pain receiving regular opiates. A preliminary report. Pain 1992 Jul;50(1):75-7.

Caccia M. Clonazepam in facial neuralgia and cluster headaches: clinical and electrophysiological study. Eur Neurol. 1975;13:560-3.

Campbell FA, Tramèr MR, Carroll D, et al. Are cannabinoids an effective and safe treatment option in the management of pain? A qualitative systematic review. BMJ 2001 Jul 7;323(7303):13-6. Review. PMID: 11440935.

Camu F, Lauwers MH, Vandersberghe C. Side effects of NSAIDs and dosing recommendations for ketorolac. Acta Anaesthesiol Belg. 1996;47:143-49.

Cepeda M, Carr D, Miranda N, et al. Comparison of morphine, ketorolac, and their combination for postoperative pain, results from a large, randomized double-blind trial. Anesthesiology 2005;103:1225-32.

Cepeda S, Vargas L, Ortegon G, et al. Comparative analgesic efficacy of patient-controlled analgesia with ketorolac versus morphine after elective intraabdominal operations. Anesth Analg. 1995;80:1150-53.

Chabal C, Russell L, Burchiel K. The effect of intravenous lidocaine, tocainide, and mexilitine on spontaneously active fibers originating in rat sciatic neuromas. Pain 1989;38:333-8.

Chang M, Ger L, Hsieh P, Huang S. A randomised clinical trial of oral steroids in the treatment of carpal tunnel syndrome: a long term follow up. J Neurol Neurosurg Psychiatry. 2002;73:710-4.

Chou R, Huffman LH. Medications for acute and chronic low back pain: a review of the evidence for an American Pain Society/American College of Physicians clinical practice guideline. American Pain Society; American College of Physicians. Ann Intern Med. 2007;147(7):505-14.

Chou R, Peterson K, Helfand M. Comparative efficacy and safety of skeletal muscle relaxants for spasticity and musculoskeletal conditions: a systematic review. J Pain Symptom Manage. 2004 Aug;28(2):140-75.

Clark RA, Lanigan JM, DellaPelle P, et al. Fibronectin and fibrin provide a provisional matrix for epidermal cell migration during wound reepithelization. J Invest Dermatol. 1982;79:264-9.

Clawson D. Treatment of acute musculoskeletal pain. In: Loeser J, Chief editor, Chapter 31 in Bonica's Management of Pain. 3rd ed. Philadelphia, PA: Lippincott Williams & Wilkins; 2001.

Clayton A. Antidepressant-associated sexual dysfunction: A potentially avoidable therapeutic challenge. Primary Psychiatry 2003;10(1):55-61.

Cohen, S, Abdi S. New developments in the use of tricyclic antidepressants for the management of pain [Review Article]. Curr Opin Anaesthesiol. 2001;14(5):505-511.

Goldstein D, Lu Y, Detke M, et al. Duloxetine vs. placebo in patients with painful diabetic neuropathy. Pain 2005;116(1):109–18.

Corbo J. The role of anticonvulsants in preventive migraine therapy. Curr Pain Headache Rep. 2003;7(7):63–6.

Cousins M. An additional dimension to the efficacy of epidural steroids. Anesthesiology 2000;93:565.

Dahl JB, Mathiesen O, Moniche S. Protective premedication: an option with gabapentin and related drugs? A review of gabapentin and pregabalin in the treatment of post-operative pain. Acta Anaesthesiol Scand 2004;48:1130–36.

Devlin JW, Roberts RJ. Pharmacology of commonly used analgesics and sedatives in the ICU: benzodiazepines, propofol, and opioids. Crit Care Clin. 2009 Jul;25(3):431–49, vii. Review. PMID: 19576523 [PubMed – indexed for MEDLINE].

Dickenson A. NMDA receptor antagonists as analgesics. In: Fields H, Liebeskind J, editors, Chapter 11 in Pharmacological approaches to the treatment of chronic pain: new concepts and critical issues. Progress in pain research and management. Vol. 1. Seattle, WA: IASP Press; 1994. pp. 173–87.

Dirks J, Fredensborg B, Christensen D, et al. A Randomized study of the effects of single-dose Gabapentin versus placebo on postoperative pain and morphine consumption after mastectomy. Anesthesiology 2002;97(3):560–4.

Drucker M, Cardenas E, Azitri P, Valenzuela A. Experimental studies on effect of lidocaine on wound healing. World J Surg 1998;22:394–8.

Durmus M, Karaaslan E, Ozturk E, et al. The effects of single-dose dexamethasone on wound healing in rats. Anesth Analg. 2003;97:1377–80.

Egbunike I, Chaffee B. Antidepressants in the management of chronic pain syndromes. Pharmacotherapy 1990;10:262–70.

Ehrlich H, Hunt T. Effects of cortisone and vitamin A on wound healing. Ann Surg. 1968;167:324–8

Elia, N, Lysakowski C, Tramèr M. Does multimodal analgesia with acetaminophen, non-steroidal anti-inflammatory drugs, or selective cyclooxygenase-2 inhibitors and patient-controlled analgesia morphine offer advantages over morphine alone? A meta-analyses of randomized trials. Anesthesiology 2005;103:1296–304.

Ellers H, Phillip L, Bickler P, et al. The reversal of fentanyl-induced tolerance by administration of "small-dose" Ketamine. Anesth Analg. 2001;93:213–214.

Etches RC, Warriner CB, Badner N, et al. Continuous intravenous administration of ketoro-lac reduces pain and morphine consumption after total hip or knee arthroplasty. Anesth Analg. 1995;81:1175–1180.

Feinmann C. Pain relief by antidepressants, possible modes of action. Pain 1985;23:1–8.

Fontelles M, Martín I, García CG. Role of cannabinoids in the management of neuropathic pain. CNS Drugs 2008;22(8):645–53.

Freynhagen R, Strojek K, Griesing T, et al. Efficacy of pregabalin in neuropathic pain evalu-ated in a 12-week, randomised, double-blind, multicentre, placebo-controlled trial of flexible- and fixed-dose regimens. Pain 2005;115(3):254–63.

Fryer J, Lukas R. Noncompetitive functional inhibition at diverse, human nicotinic acetyl-choline receptor subtypes by bupropion, phencyclidine, and ibogaine. J Pharmacol Exp Ther. 1999;288(6):88–92.

Gajraj N. Cyclooxygenase-2 inhibitors: review article. Anesth Analg. 2003;96:1720–38.

Galer B. Lidocaine patch may equal coxibs for knee OA pain relief. In: Presented at the 24th Annual Scientific Meeting of the American Pain Society, March 30–April 2, 2005 Boston, MA; abstract 771.

Gerstenfeld L, Thiede M, Seibert K, et al. Differential inhibition of fracture healing by non-selective and cyclooxygenase-2 selective non steroidal anti-inflammatory drugs. J Orthop Res. 2003;21:670–5.

Gilron I. Is gabapentin a "broad-spectrum" analgesic? Editorial, Anesthesiology 2002;97(3):537–8.

Gilron I, Milne B, Hong M. Cyclooxygenase-2 inhibitors in postoperative pain management; current evidence and future directions. Anesthesiology 2003;99:1198–2008.

Guindon J, Hohmann AG, The endocannabinoid system and pain. CNS Neurol Disord Drug Targets. 2009 Oct 19;19839937.

Hahn TW, Mogensen T, Lund C, et al. Analgesic effect of i.v. paracetamol: Possible ceiling effect of paracetamol in postoperative pain. Acta Anaesthesiol Scand 2003;47:138–45.

Harder A, An Y. The mechanism of the inhibitory effects of non steroidal anti-inflammatory drugs on bone healing: a concise review. J Clin Pharmacol. 2003;43:807–15.

Hardy MM, et al. Selective cyclooxygenase-2 inhibition does not alter keratinocyte wound responses in the mouse epidermis after abrasion. J Pharmacol Exp Ther. 2003;304:959–67.

Hayashida K, Hideaki O, Kunie N, Eisenach J. Gabapentin acts within the locus coeruleus to alleviate neuropathic pain. Anesthesiology 2008;109(6):1077–84.

Hempenstall K, Nurmikko TJ, Johnson RW, A'Hern RP, Rice AS. Analgesic therapy in posttherpetic neuralgia: a quantitative systematic review. PLoS Med. 2005 Jul;2(7):e164. Epub 2005 Jul 26. Review. PMID: 16013891 [PubMed – indexed for MEDLINE].

Hertz JA, Knight JR. Prescription drug misuse: a growing national problem. Adolesc Med Clin. 2006;17(3):751–69; abstract xiii. Review. PMID: 17030290 [PubMed – indexed for MEDLINE].

Hobbs WR, Rall TW, Verdoorn TA. Hypnotics and sedatives; ethanol. In: Hardman JG, Limbird LE, editors in chief, Chapter 17 in Goodman & Gillman's pharmacologic basis of therapeutics. 9th ed. New York, NY: McGraw-Hill; 1996. pp. 361–98.

Hyllested M, Jones S, Pedersen J, Kehlet H. Comparative effect of paracetamol, NSAIDs or their combination in postoperative pain management: a qualitative review. Br J Anesth 2002;88:199–214.

Insel P. Analgesic-antipyretic and anti-inflammatory agents and drugs employed in the treatment of gout. In: Hardman J, Limbird L, editors in chief, Chapter 27 in Goodman & Gilman's the pharmacological basis of therapeutics. 9th ed. New York, NY: McGraw-Hill; 1996. pp. 617–58.

Issioui T, Klein K, White P, et al. Efficacy of premedication with celecoxib and acetaminophen in preventing pain after otolaryngologic surgery. Anesth Analg. 2002;94:1188–1193.

Jacox A, Carr DB, Payne R, et al. Management of cancer pain. Clinical Practice Guideline No. 9. AHCPR Publication No. 94-0592. Rockville, MD: Agency for Health Care Policy and Research, U.S. Department of Health and Human Services, Public Health Service; 1994, p. 257.

Johnston GA. GABA(A) receptor channel pharmacology. Curr Pharm Des. 2005;11(15):1867–85. Review. PMID: 15974965 [PubMed – indexed for MEDLINE].

Jones S, Power I. Postoperative NSAIDs and COX-2 inhibitors: cardiovascular risks and benefits, editorial. Br J Anaesth. 2005;95:281–4.

Kingery W, Agashe G, Sawamura S, et al. Glucocorticoid inhibition of neuropathic hyperalgesia and spinal fos expression. Anesth Analg. 2001;92:476–82.

Kock M, Lavand'homme P. The clinical role of NMDA receptor antagonists for the treatment of postoperative pain. Best Pract Res Clin Anaesthesiol. 2007;21(1):85–98.

Korpela R, Korvenoja P, Meretoja OA. Morphine-sparing effect of acetaminophen in pediatric day-case surgery. Anesthesiology 1999;91:442–7.

Kotani N, Kushikata T, Hashimoto H, et al. Intrathecal methylprednisolone for intractable postherpetic neuralgia. N Engl J Med. 2000;343:1514–9.

Kranke P, Morin A, Roewer N, Leopold H. Patients' global evaluation of analgesia and safety of injected parecoxib for postoperative pain: A quantitative systematic review. Anesth Analg 2004;99:797–806.

Li W, Xiew W, Strong J, Zhang J. Systemic anti-inflammatory corticosteroid reduces mechanical pain behavior, sympathetic sprouting, and elevation of proinflammatory cytokines in a rat model of neuropathic pain. Anesthesiology 2007;107(3):469–77.

Libby P. Inflammation in atherosclerosis. Nature 2002;420:868–74.

List T, Axelsson S, Leijon G, Orofac J. Pharmacologic interventions in the treatment of temporomandibular disorders, atypical facial pain, and burning mouth syndrome. A qualitative systematic review. Pain 2003 Fall;17(4):301–10. Review. PMID: 14737874 [PubMed – indexed for MEDLINE].

Littrell R, Hayes L, Stillner V. Carisoprodol: a new and cautious perspective on an old agent. South Am Med J. 1993;86:753–6.

Maliekal J, Elboim CM. Gastrointestinal complications associated with intramuscular ketorolac tromethamine therapy in the elderly. Ann Pharmacother 1995;29:698–701.

Management of Chronic Pain Syndromes: Issues and Interventions. A CME program of the American Academy of Pain Medicine, Pain Med. 2005;6:S1–S21.

Martinez V, et al. The influence of timing of administration on the analgesic efficacy of paracoxib in orthopedic surgery. Anesth Analg. 2007;104:1521–7.

Matthews E, Dickerson A. A combination of Gabapentin and morphine mediates enhanced inhibitory effects on dorsal horn neuronal responses in a rat model of neuropathy. Anesthesiology 2002;96(3):633–40.

Max M, Gilron I. Antidepressants, muscle relaxants, and N-Methyl-D-Aspartate receptor antagonists. In: Loeser J, chief editor, Chapter 85 in Bonica's management of pain. 3rd ed. Philadelphia, PA: Lippencott Williams & Wilkins; 2001. pp. 1710–26.

McCleane GJ. Intravenous infusion of phenytoin relieves neuropathic pain: a randomized, double blinded, placebo-controlled crossover study. Anesth Analg. 1999;89:985–8.

McCrory C, Lindahl S. Cyclooxygenase inhibition for postoperative analgesia. Anesth Analg. 2002;95:169–76.

McLain D. An open label dose finding trial of Tizanidine [Zanaflex®] for treatment of Fibromyalgia. J Musculoskelet Pain 2002;10(4):7–18.

Miyoshi HR. Systemic nonopioid analgesics. In: Loeser J, Butler S, Chapman C, Turk D, editors, Chapter 83 in Bonica's management of pain. 3rd ed. Philadelphia, PA: Lippincott Williams & Wilkins; 2001. pp. 1667–81.

Morrison R, Carney M, Manfredi P. Pain management. In: Rosenthal RA, Zenilman ME, Katlic MR, editors, Chapter 12 in Principles and practice of geriatric surgery. New York, NY: Springer; 2001:160–171.

Munsterhjelm E, Munsterhjelm N, Niemi T, et al. Dose-dependent inhibition of platelet function by acetaminophen in healthy volunteers. Anesthesiology 2005;103:712–7.

National Institute for Health and Clinical Excellence. Management of anxiety (panic disorder with or without agoraphobia, and generalized anxiety disorder) in adults in primary, secondary and community care. London: NICE guidelines 2004 (amended 2007). http://www.nice.org.uk/Guidance/CG22.

O'Brien CP. Benzodiazepine use, abuse, and dependence. J Clin Psychiatry 2005;66(suppl 2):28–33. Review. PMID: 15762817.

Pardo ES, Berger JM, Toliver KT. Post herpetic neuralgia. Semin Anesth. 1997;16(2):132–135.

Pertwee RG. Pharmacological actions of cannabinoids. Handb Exp Pharmacol. 2005;(168):1–51, 16596770.

Pobereskin, L, Sneyd J. Does wound irrigation with triamcinalone reduce pain after surgery to the lumbar spine? Br J Anaesth. 2000;84:731–4.

Power I. Recent advances in postoperative pain therapy. Br J Anesth. 2005;95(1):43–51.

Rahme E, Barkam A, Nedjar H, et al. Hospitalizations for upper and lower GI events associated with traditional NSAIDs and acetaminophen among elderly in Quebec, Canada. Am J Gastroenterol. 2008;103(4):872–82.

Rani P, Naidu M, Prasad V, et al. An evaluation of antidepressants in rheumatic pain conditions. Anesth Analg. 1996;83:371–5.

Rathmell J, Aprill C, Bogduk N. Cervical transforaminal injection of steroids. Anesthesiology 2004;100:1595–600.

Ready L, Brown C, Stahlgren L, et al. Evaluation of intravenous ketarolac administered by bolus or infusion for treatment of post-op pain: a double-blind placebo-controlled multicenter study. Anesthesiology 1994;80:1277–86.

Rumunstad L, Audun S. Glucocorticoids for acute and persistent postoperative neuropathic pain. Anesthesiology 2007;107(3):371–3.

Samad T, Moore K, Sapirstein A, et al. Interleukin-1[beta]-mediated induction of Cox-2 in the CNS contributes to inflammatory pain hypersensitivity. Nature 2001;410 (6827):471–75.

See S, Ginzburg R. Skeletal muscle relaxants. Pharmacotherapy 2008;28(2):207–213.

Silberstein S. Topiramate in migraine prevention headache. J Head Face Pain. 2005;45(s1):S57–S65 Published Online: Apr 2005.

Skrabek RQ, Galimova L, Ethans K, Perry DJ. Nabilone for the treatment of pain in fibromyalgia. Pain 2008 Feb;9(2):164–73. Epub 2007 Nov 5. PMID: 17974490.

Slemmer J, Martin R, Damaj M. Bupropion is a nicotinic antagonist. J Pharmacol Exp Ther. 2000;295(1):321–7.

Stouten E, Armbuster S, Houmes R, et al. Comparison of ketorolac and morphine for post operative pain after major surgery. Acta Anesthesiol Scand 1992;336:716–721.

Strom BL, Berlin JA, Kinman JL, et al. Parenteral ketorolac and risk of gastrointestinal and operative site bleeding: a postmarketing surveillance study. JAMA 1996;275:376–382.

Svedicic G, Gentilini A, Eichenberger U, et al. Combinations of Morphine with Ketamine for patient-controlled analgesia-A new optimization method. Anesthesiology 2003;98(5): 1195–205.

Tarride J-E, Gordon A, Vera-Llonch M, et al. Cost-effectiveness of pregabalin for the management of neuropathic pain associated with diabetic peripheral neuropathy and postherpetic neuralgia: a Canadian perspective. J Clinthera 2006;28(11):1922–34.

Tippana E, Hamunen K, Kontinen V, Kalso E, Do surgical patients benefit from perioperative Gabapentin/Pregabalin? A systematic review of efficacy and safety. Anesth Analg. 2007;104:1545–56.

Toliver, KT, Berger JM, Pardo ES. Review of Herpes Zoster. Semin Anesth. 1997;16(2): 127–131.

Tremont-Lukats I, Megeff C, Backonja M. Anticonvulsants for neuropathic pain syndromes: mechanisms of action and place in therapy drugs: review article. Drugs 2000;60(5):1029–52.

Turan A, Kaya G, Karamanlio B, et al. Effect of oral gabapentin on postoperative epidural analgesia. Br J Anaesth. 2006;96:242–6.

Vestergaard K, Andersen G, Gottrup H, et al. Lamotrigine for central poststroke pain: a randomized controlled trial . Neurology 2001;56:184–90.

Weinbrown A, Rudick V, Paret G, Ben-Abraham R. The role of dextromethorphan in pain control: review article. Can J Anesth. 2000;47:585–96.

Weissman D, Haddox J. Opioid pseudoaddiction: an iatrogenic syndrome. Pain 1989;36: 363–6.

Welch MP, Odland GF, Clark RA. Temporal relationships of F-actin bundle formation, collagen and fibronectin assembly, and fibronectin receptor expression to wound contraction. J Cell Biol. 1990;110:133–45.

Wesche D, Bockbrader H. A pharmacokinetic comparison of pregabalin and gabapentin. J Pain 2005;6(3):S29–S29.

White W, Faich G, Whelton A, et al. Comparison of thromboembolic events in patients treated with Celecoxib, a cyclooxygenase-2 specific inhibitor, versus ibuprofen or diclofenac. Am J Cardiol. 2002;89:425–30.

Wicke C, Halliday B, Allen D, et al. Effects of steroids and retinoids on wound healing. Arch Surg. 2000;135:1265–70.

Wilwerding MB, Loprinzi CL, Mailliard JA, et al. A randomized, crossover evaluation of methylphenidate in cancer patients receiving strong narcotics. Support Care Cancer 1995 Mar;3(2):135–8. PMID: 7539701.

Witte MB, Barbul A. Wound healing. Surg Clin North Am 1997;77:509–28.

Wu CL, Tella P, Staats PS, et al. Analgesic effects of intravenous lidocaine and morphine on postamputation pain. Anesthesiology 2002;96:841–8.

Zajicek J, Fox P, Sanders H, et al. Cannabinoids for treatment of spasticity and other symptoms related to multiple sclerosis (CAMS study): multicentre randomized placebo-controlled trial. UK MS Research Group. Lancet 2003 Nov 8;362(9395):1517–26. PMID: 14615106.

Zajicek JP, Sanders HP, Wright DE, et al. Cannabinoids in multiple sclerosis (CAMS) study: safety and efficacy data for 12 months follow up. J Neurol Neurosurg Psychiatry. 2005 Dec;76(12):1664–9. PMID: 16291891.

Zakrzewska J. Major problems in neurology 28: trigeminal neuralgia. London: W.B. Saunders; 1995.

Zisook S, Rush A, Haight B, et al. Use of bupropion in combination with serotonin reuptake inhibitors. Biol Psychiatry 2006;59(3):203–10.

Zuckerman L, Ferrante FM. Nonopioid and opioid analgesics. In: Asburn M, Rice L, editors, Chapter 8 in The management of pain. New York, NY: Churchill Livingstone; 1998. pp. 111–40.

Chapter 10

Alternative and Herbal Pharmaceuticals

Alan D. Kaye, MD, PhD, Muhammad Anwar, MD, and Amir Baluch, MD

Introduction

The use of alternative medicines such as minerals, vitamins, and herbal products has increased dramatically in recent years. Reasons for such an increase in prevalence include anecdotal reports on efficacy, impressive advertisement, lower cost of products compared to prescription medications, and ease of attainment of the supplements. Regardless of the reasons, it is important that physicians, particularly the pain practitioner be cognizant of the effects of these agents, whether beneficial or harmful.

Minerals

Calcium

It may be reasonable for patients to supplement their diet with calcium, as calcium deficiency is a common finding and our typical diet does not adequately keep pace with daily calcium loss (Thys-Jacobs et al. 1998). Many women supplement with calcium to improve symptoms associated with premenstrual syndrome and premature bone breakdown (McCarron and Hatton 1996).

Calcium may interfere with a host of commonly used drugs. The pain practitioner must be aware of patients with cardiac problems who may be taking calcium channel blockers or β-blockers. The effects of calcium channel blockers may be affected by calcium supplementation, as calcium has been shown to antagonize the effects of verapamil (Bar-Or 1981). In fact, calcium has recently been used in the successful management of calcium channel blocker overdose (Durward 2003). Calcium supplementation may also decrease levels of β-blockers, leading to a greater chronotropic and inotropic presentation than one would expect (Kirch et al. 1981).

Thiazide diuretics have been shown to increase serum calcium concentrations, possibly leading to hypercalcemia due to increased reabsorption of calcium in the kidneys. Dysrhythmias may occur in patients taking digitalis and calcium together. The antibiotic effect of tetracyclines and quinolone and pharmacological blood levels of bisphosphonates and levothyroxine may be decreased with calcium supplementation. These medications should not be taken within 2 h of calcium intake (Hendler and Rorvik 2001, Minerals 2000).

N. Vadivelu et al. (eds.), *Essentials of Pain Management,*
DOI 10.1007/978-0-387-87579-8_10, © Springer Science+Business Media, LLC 2011

Calcium supplementation may also affect the choice of anesthesia used in operative procedures. Recent data suggest that the use of propofol may have a protective effect on erythrocytes in patients with elevated levels of calcium (Zhang and Yao 2001). Documenting the use of calcium by patients preoperatively may prevent many of these drug interactions.

Chromium

Chromium is an essential nutrient involved in metabolism of carbohydrates and lipids. Recently chromium has received attention from consumers in the belief that it may improve glucose tolerance in diabetics, reduce body fat, and reduce atherosclerotic formation. These purported effects stem from chromium's effect on insulin resistance. However, the evidence regarding its use for insulin resistance and mildly impaired glucose tolerance is inconclusive (Anderson et al. 1991, Uusitupa et al. 1992, Bahijri 2000, Urmila et al. 2004).

A double-blind trial with 180 patients concluded that high doses of chromium supplementation (1,000 mg) may have beneficial effects on hemoglobin A1c, insulin, cholesterol, and overall glucose control in type 2 diabetics (Anderson et al. 1997). The pain practitioner should consider asking any diabetics if they supplement with chromium in an attempt to attain these effects. Because of chromium's effects on insulin resistance and impaired glucose control, some patients will supplement with this mineral for preventing risk of cardiovascular disease. Human studies have shown decreased total cholesterol and triglyceride levels in elderly patients taking 200 μg twice per day (Rabinovitz et al. 2004).

Chromium is generally well tolerated; however, some patients may experience nervous system symptoms such as perceptual, cognitive, and motor dysfunction with doses as low as 200–400 μg (Fox and Sabovic 1998). In addition, toxicity has been reported with chromium consumption. In one case a woman developed anemia, thrombocytopenia, hemolysis, weight loss, and liver and renal toxicity when attempting to lose weight with 1,200–2,400 μg of chromium picolinate. These problems resolved after discontinuation of chromium ingestion (Cerulli et al. 1998). A lower dose of only 600 μg was demonstrated to have resulted in interstitial nephritis in another female patient (Wasser et al. 1997).

Magnesium

Magnesium plays many important roles in structure, function, and metabolism and is involved in numerous essential physiologic reactions in the human body. Supplemental magnesium has been used extensively by patients for cardiovascular disease, diabetes, osteoporosis, asthma, and migraines, although most individuals consume adequate levels in their diet (Institute of Medicine 2001). Patients with a history of these illnesses may be supplementing with magnesium and therefore should be questioned.

The most obvious pain-related consideration in treating a patient taking magnesium supplements has to do with its effect on muscle relaxants in the operating room. The mineral can potentiate the effects of non-depolarizing skeletal muscle relaxants such as tubocurarine. Therefore, it may be advisable to ask patients about their magnesium usage preoperatively to avoid complications during certain interventional procedures performed in the operating room (Hendler and Rorvik 2001).

It should be noted that when caring for obstetrical patients (typically out of the realm of pain practitioners), one must be aware of the effects of magnesium sulfate in the patient undergoing cesarean section. Literature suggests that the duration of action of relaxant anesthetics, such as mivacurium, may be affected by subtherapeutic serum magnesium levels (Hodgson et al. 1998).

Magnesium may also interfere with the absorption of antibiotics such as tetracyclines, fluoroquinolones, nitrofurantoins, penicillamine, angiotensin-converting enzyme (ACE) inhibitors, phenytoin, and histamine (H2) blockers. Absorption problems can be ameliorated by not taking doses of magnesium within 2 h from these other medications (Tatro 1999, Shiba et al. 1995, Naggar and Khalil 1979, Osman et al. 1983). The mineral may also make oral hypoglycemics, specifically sulfonylureas, more effective when used, thus increasing the risk of hypoglycemic episodes (Kivisto and Neuvonen 1992).

Iron

In both developed and underdeveloped countries, iron deficiency is the most common nutrient deficiency. Worldwide, at least 700 million individuals have iron deficiency anemia (Shils et al. 1999). More than just a constituent of hemoglobin and myoglobin, iron is a key component in nearly every living organism and in humans is associated with hundreds of enzymes and other protein structures. People have been supplemented with iron in order to increase treatment of iron deficiency anemia, alleviate poor cognitive function in children, increase athletic performance, and suppress restless legs syndrome (RLS).

High concentrations of iron in the blood may worsen neuronal injury secondary to cerebral ischemia (Davolos et al. 2000). Increased iron levels during pregnancy may lead to preterm delivery and neonatal asphyxia (Lao et al. 2000). These complications may occur even with normal iron intake if the patient also takes vitamin C, as high doses of the vitamin can increase iron absorption (Siegenberg et al. 1991).

Iron may inhibit absorption of many drugs including levodopa, methyldopa, carbidopa, penicillamine, thyroid hormone, captopril, and antibiotics in the quinolone and tetracycline family (Lehto et al. 1994, Campbell and Hasinoff 1991, Heinrich 1974, Osman et al. 1983, Campbell et al. 1992). Some medications may decrease iron absorption and lead to decreased therapeutic levels of the mineral. These include antacids, H2 receptor antagonists, proton pump inhibitors, and cholestyramine resin (Hendler and Rorvik 2001, Minerals 2000). Oral iron should not be given within 2 h of other pharmaceuticals to avoid alterations in drug or mineral absorption.

Selenium

Selenium, an essential trace element, functions in a variety of enzyme-dependent pathways, especially those utilizing selenoproteins. Much of its supplemental efficacy is due to its antioxidant properties. Glutathione peroxidase incorporates this mineral at its active site, and as dietary selenium intake decreases, glutathione levels drop (Ursini et al. 1999).

Patients supplement with selenium for a variety of reasons, most notably a supposed improvement in immune status. Elderly patients may be inclined to supplement with selenium for this reason.

Toxicity with selenium supplementation begins at intake greater than 750 μg/day and may manifest as garlic-like breath, loss of hair and fingernails, gastrointestinal distress, or central nervous system changes (Patterson and Levander 1997, Fan and Kizer 1990). Few interactions with other pharmacological agents have been found (Hendler and Rorvik 2001).

Zinc

Zinc deficiency was first described in 1961, when it was found to be associated with "adolescent nutritional dwarfism" in the Middle East (Prasad et al. 1961). Deficiency of this mineral is thought to be quite common in infants, adolescents, women, and elderly (Sandstead 1995, Goldenberg et al. 1995, Ma and Betts 2000, Prasad 1996). The most well-known use for zinc supplementation is in treatment of the common cold caused principally by the rhinovirus.

Patients self-medicating with zinc supplements may inadvertently overmedicate themselves with zinc. Signs of zinc toxicity include anemia, neutropenia, cardiac abnormalities, unfavorable lipid profiles, impaired immune function, acute pancreatitis, and copper deficiency (Bratman and Girman 2003, Mikszewski et al. 2003).

Zinc supplements may interfere with the absorption of antibiotics such as tetracyclines, fluoroquinolones, and penicillamine (Bratman and Girman 2003). Zinc should not be ingested within 2 h of antibiotics (Minerals 2000).

Vitamins
Vitamin A

The term "vitamin A" refers to a large number of related compounds: preformed retinol (an alcohol) and retinal (an aldehyde). Vitamin A deficiency is common in teenagers, in lower socioeconomic groups, and in developing countries (Combs 1998). Furthermore, some studies indicate that diabetic patients are at an increased risk for vitamin A deficiency (Queiroz et al. 2000). This deficiency may manifest as night blindness, immune deterioration, birth defects, or decreased red blood cell production (Higdon 2003). Purported therapeutic uses for vitamin A include diseases of the skin, acute promyelocytic leukemia, and viral infections.

Retinoids have been used as pharmacologic agents to treat disorders of the skin. Psoriasis, acne, and rosacea have been treated with natural or synthetic retinoids. Moreover, retinoids are effective in treating symptoms associated with congenital keratinization disorder syndromes. Therapeutic effects stem from its antineoplastic activity (Brzezinska-Wcislo et al. 2004). Patients suffering from these illnesses may be supplementing with vitamin A and their dosages should be explored.

Vitamin A may increase anticoagulant effects of warfarin (Harris 1995). This interaction could increase the risk of bleeding complication in these patients. Bleeding complications may therefore be avoided by informing the patient about this effect preoperatively.

Excess vitamin A intake during pregnancy, as well as deficiency, may lead to birth defects. For this reason, pregnant woman who are not vitamin A deficient should not consume more than 2,600 IU/day of supplemental retinol (Binkley and Krueger 2000).

Patients using isotretinoin and pregnant women taking valproic acid are likewise at increased risk for vitamin A toxicity (Higdon 2003, Nau et al. 1995). Finally, alcohol consumption decreases the liver toxicity threshold for vitamin A, thereby narrowing its therapeutic window in alcoholics (Leo and Lieber 1999).

Vitamin B$_{12}$

Vitamin B$_{12}$, the largest and most complex of all vitamins, is unique in that it contains cobalt, a metal ion. B$_{12}$ deficiency may affect up to 10–15% of people over the age of 60 (Baik and Russel 1999). B$_{12}$ deficiency manifests as pernicious anemia. This syndrome includes a megaloblastic anemia as well as neurologic symptoms. The neurologic manifestations result from degeneration of the lateral and posterior spinal columns and include symmetrical paresthesia with loss of proprioception and vibratory sensation, especially involving the lower extremities (Higdon 2003).

The most documented use of vitamin B_{12} is in the treatment of pernicious anemia. Many of the neurological, cutaneous, and thrombotic clinical manifestations have been successfully treated with oral or intramuscular cyanocobalamin (Loikili et al. 2004).

A commonly used anesthetic, nitrous oxide, inhibits both vitamin B_{12}-dependent enzymes and may produce clinical features of deficiency such as megaloblastic anemia and neuropathy. Some experts believe that vitamin B_{12} deficiency should be ruled out before the use of nitrous oxide since many elderly patients will present to the operating room with deficiency (Baik and Russel 1999, Weimann 2003).

The drugs colchicines, metformin, phenformin, and zidovudine (AZT) may decrease the levels of vitamin B_{12} in a patient (Webb et al. 1968, Adams et al. 1983, Flippo and Holder 1993, Baum et al. 1991). Histamine-2 receptor blockers and proton pump inhibitors may decrease absorption of vitamin B_{12} from food, but not absorption from dietary supplements (Marcuard et al. 1994, Streeter et al. 1982, Aymard et al. 1988).

Vitamin C

Ascorbic acid, also known as vitamin C, is an essential water-soluble vitamin. The symptoms of scurvy, which include bleeding and easy bruising, can be prevented with as little as 10 mg of vitamin C due to its association with collagen, but it can also be used to prevent a host of other disease processes (Sauberlich 1997).

Numerous people supplement their diet with vitamin C in order to prevent infection from viruses responsible for the common cold, yet research reviews over the last 20 years conclude that there is no significant impact on the incidence of infection (Hemila 1997). However, there are a few studies that show that certain groups of people who are susceptible to low dietary intake of vitamin C, such as marathon runners, may be less susceptible when supplementation is used. Furthermore, vitamin C may decrease the duration or severity of colds via an antihistamine effect when taken in large doses (Johnston et al. 1992).

There is some evidence that patients taking vitamin C supplements may have a reduced anticoagulant effect from warfarin or heparin. Increased doses of these anticoagulants might be advised to achieve therapeutic levels (Rosenthal 1971, Harris 1995). It is recommended that patients on anticoagulation therapy should limit vitamin C intake to 1 g/day. As always, the precise dosage regimen must be monitored by the appropriate lab studies. Since high doses may also interfere with certain laboratory tests such as serum bilirubin, creatinine, and stool guaiac assay, it is crucial to inquire about any over-the-counter supplementation with the vitamin (Hendler and Rorvik 2001). There is evidence that vitamin C may increase the inotropic effect of dobutamine in patients with abnormal left ventricular function. Infusion of vitamin C into individuals with normal heart function was shown to increase contractility of the left ventricle (Mak and Newton 2001). High doses of vitamin C may increase acetaminophen levels, while aspirin and oral contraceptives may lower serum levels of vitamin C (Houston and Levy 1976, Molloy and Wilson 1980, Rivers and Devine 1972).

Vitamin D

Vitamin D deficiency does occur in the elderly and shows increased incidence in people who live in northern latitudes (Utiger 1998, Semba et al. 2000). The main function of this vitamin is in calcium homeostasis.

Individuals with osteoporosis frequently have a deficiency in vitamin D (Mezquita-Raya et al. 2001). With increasing age, vitamin D and calcium metabolism increase the risk of deficiency. Studies show a clear benefit of vitamin D and calcium supplementation in older postmenopausal women. Supplementation results in increased bone density, decreased bone turnover, and decreased non-vertebral fractures as well as decreases in fall risk and body sway (Malabanan and Holick 2003).

Hypervitaminosis D can occur with high doses of the vitamin. Symptoms include nausea, vomiting, loss of appetite, polydipsia, polyuria, itching, muscular weakness, joint pain, and in severe cases may lead to coma and death (Higdon 2003). In order to prevent the syndrome, the Food and Nutrition Board has set an upper limit of supplementation at 2,000 IU/day for adults (Food and Nutrition Board 1997).

The cardiac patient taking calcium channel blockers may present to the operating room while taking supplemental vitamin D and calcium. The combination of vitamin D and calcium may interfere with calcium channel blockers by antagonizing its effect. Hypercalcemia exacerbates arrhythmias in patients taking digitalis. A state of hypercalcemia may be induced by the concomitant use of thiazide diuretics with vitamin D which may lead to these complications. Conversely, anticonvulsants, cholesterol-lowering medications, and the fat substitute olestra may decrease the absorption of vitamin D (Vitamins 2000).

Vitamin E

Antioxidant properties define the primary function of vitamin E. Dietary deficiency is quite prevalent even in the developed world; therefore supplementation is reasonable (Ford and Sowell 1999).

The pain practitioner must be keenly aware of vitamin E supplementation as it may increase the effects of anticoagulant and antiplatelet drugs. Concomitant use of vitamin E with these drugs may increase the risk of hemorrhage (Liede et al. 1998). Further, preliminary evidence suggests that type 2 diabetics may have an increased risk of hypoglycemia since vitamin E may enhance insulin sensitivity, and therefore adjustment of oral hypoglycemics would be advisable (Paolisso et al. 1993a, b). Cholestyramine, colestipol, isoniazid, mineral oil, orlistat, sucralfate, and the fat substitute olestra may possibly decrease the absorption of vitamin E, leading to decreased levels in the serum (Hendler and Rorvik 2001).

Folate

Folic acid and folate have been used interchangeably, although the most stable form that is used by the human body is folic acid. This water-soluble, B-complex vitamin occurs naturally in foods and in metabolically active forms (Food and Nutrition Board 1998). Since 1998, the fortification of cereal with folate has decreased the prevalence of folate deficiency significantly (Cembrowski et al. 1999). Excess folate intake has not been associated with any significant adverse effects.

Patients taking large amounts of non-steroidal antiinflammatory drugs (NSAIDs) such as aspirin or ibuprofen experience interference in folate metabolism, although regular use shows no significant changes. Patients suffering from seizures that use phenytoin for therapy may report decrease in seizure threshold when taking folate supplements (Lewis et al. 1995). The body's ability to absorb or utilize folate may be decreased if taking nitrous oxide, antacids, bile acid sequestrants, H2 blockers, certain anticonvulsants, and high-dose triamterene. Supplementation of folic acid may also correct for megaloblastic anemia due to B_{12} deficiency, but the neurological damage will not be prevented. In these cases, one must be careful to pinpoint the true cause of the anemia to prevent neurological complications (Queiroz et al. 2000).

Herbals

Saw Palmetto

Saw palmetto is used mainly for treatment of benign prostatic hyperplasia with free fatty acids and sterols being the main components (Hughes et al. 2004). Despite an uncertain mechanism, the literature does demonstrate antagonism at the androgen receptor for dihydrotestosterone and 5α-reductase enzyme (Hughes et al. 2004). Though prostate size and prostate-specific antigen level are not decreased by saw palmetto, biopsies have demonstrated decreases in transitional zone epithelia in prostates of men treated with this agent compared to placebo (Hughes et al. 2004). When compared with finasteride, a 5α-reductase inhibitor, saw palmetto use resulted in fewer side effects and increased urine flow (Hughes et al. 2004). However, a study of patients with prostatitis/chronic pelvic pain syndrome that evaluated the safety and efficacy of saw palmetto compared to finasteride reported that at the end of the investigation, more patients opted to continue finasteride treatment rather than saw palmetto treatment. The researchers found that in patients with the studied condition, saw palmetto had no appreciable long-term improvement and, with the exception of voiding, patients on finasteride experienced significant improvement in all other analyzed parameters (Kaplan et al. 2004).

Adverse reactions to saw palmetto are rare but there are reports of mild gastrointestinal symptoms and headaches (Hughes et al. 2004). Results of a recent investigation indicated that recommended doses of saw palmetto are not likely to alter the pharmacokinetics of coadministered medications dependent on the cytochrome P-450 isoenzyme CYP2D6 or CYP3A4, such as dextromethorphan and alprazolam (Markowitz et al. 2003). Further, there are few herbal–drug interactions in the literature regarding saw palmetto, but, as always, care and responsibility should be exercised when taking this agent (Hughes et al. 2004).

St. John's Wort

St. John's wort is used to treat anxiety, mild-to-moderate depression, and sleep-related disorders (Hughes et al. 2004, Kaye et al. 2000). Other uses have included treatment of cancer, fibrositis, headache, obsessive–compulsive disorder, and sciatica (Jellin et al. 2002). Active compounds in the agent include the naphthodihydrodianthrones, hypericin, and pseudohypericin, the flavonoids, quercitin, rutin, and hypericin, and the xanthones (Hughes et al. 2004, Leak 1999).

It is thought that extracts of St. John's wort, such as WS 5570, are widely used to treat mild-to-moderate depression (Hostanska et al. 2002, Lecrubier 2002). Such extracts are standardized based on their hypericin content and have demonstrated an effectiveness superior to placebo and potentially as great as selective serotonin reuptake inhibitors and low-dose tricyclic antidepressants (Jellin 2002).

The exact mechanism of action of St. John's wort remains controversial. This herbal substance demonstrates irreversible inhibition of monoamine oxidase in vitro, but such inhibition has yet to be observed in vivo (Staffeldt et al. 1994). In the feline lung vasculature, St. John's wort exhibited a vasodepressor effect that was mediated or modulated by both a GABA receptor and an L-type calcium channel-sensitive mechanism (Hoover et al. in press). Studies performed in vitro have demonstrated γ-aminobutyric acid (GABA) receptor inhibition by hypericum. This finding may indicate that a GABA inhibitory mechanism is responsible for the antidepressant effect (Cott 1997, Cott and Misra 1998). However, another theorized pathway includes inhibition of serotonin, dopamine, and norepinephrine reuptake in the central nervous system, thus making its mechanism of action somewhat similar to traditionally used antidepressant medications (Hughes et al. 2004).

Regarding side effects, St. John's wort is typically well tolerated (Hughes et al. 2004). Associated side effects may include photosensitivity, restlessness, dry mouth, dizziness, fatigue, constipation, and nausea (Hughes et al. 2004, Kaye et al. 2007) (see Table 10.1). Other noteworthy side effects of St. John's wort include its induction of the cytochrome P-450 system (CYP34A), thus affecting serum levels of cyclosporine in patients after organ transplantation, and the potential threat of serotonergic syndrome in patients concurrently taking prescription antidepressants, a common class of agents prescribed by pain practitioners (Hughes et al. 2004). The serotonergic syndrome is characterized by hypertonicity,

Table 10.1 Herbal agents, potential side effects, and anesthesia considerations.

Herbal agents	Potential side effects	Anesthesia considerations
Echinacea	Unpleasant taste, tachyphylaxis, affects cytochrome P-450 enzyme, hepatotoxicity	Can potentiate barbiturate toxicity
Ephedra (ma huang)	Hypertension, tachycardia, cardiomyopathy, stroke, cardiac arrhythmias	Can interact with anesthetics, i.e., halothane, and cause cardiac dysrhythmias
Feverfew	Aphthous ulcers, gastrointestinal irritability, headache	Can increase risk of intraoperative hemodynamic instability
Garlic	Halitosis, increases in bleeding time, hypotension, affects cytochrome P-450 enzyme	Can increase risk of intraoperative hemodynamic instability
Ginger	Increases in bleeding time	Can increase risk of intraoperative hemodynamic instability
Ginkgo biloba	Platelet dysfunction	Can increase perioperative bleeding tendencies and decrease effectiveness of intravenous barbiturates
Ginseng	Hypertension, increases in bleeding time, hypoglycemia, insomnia, vomiting, epistaxis	Can increase risk of intraoperative hemodynamic instability
Kava kava	Dermopathy, affects cytochrome P-450 enzyme, hepatotoxicity	Can potentiate the effect of barbiturates/benzodiazepines resulting in excessive sedation
St. John's wort	Dry mouth, dizziness, affects cytochrome P-450 enzyme, constipation, nausea, serotonergic syndrome	Pseudoephedrine, MAOIs, SSRIs should be avoided

MAOIs = monoamine oxidase inhibitors, SSRIs = selective serotonin reuptake inhibitors.
Modified from Kaye (2000).

myoclonus, autonomic dysfunction, hallucinosis, tremors, hyperthermia, and potentially death (Ness et al. 1999, Czekalla et al. 1997). Specifically, use of St. John's wort is not recommended with photosensitization drugs such as tetracyclines, antidepressants such as monoamine oxidase inhibitors and SSRIs, and β-sympathomimetics such as ephedra and pseudoephedrine hydrochloride. Finally, there is little-to-no data regarding the potential anesthetic–St. John's wort interactions; however, there have been anecdotal unpublished reports of meperidine–St. John's wort-induced serotonergic crisis.

Echinacea

Echinacea is part of the daisy family found throughout North America. There are nine species of *Echinacea* in total and the medicinal preparations are derived from three of these: *Echinacea purpurea* (purple coneflower), *Echinacea pallida* (pale purple coneflower), and *Echinacea angustifolia* (narrow leaved coneflower) (Ness et al. 1999, Bauer and Khan 1985, Melchart et al. 1998). *Echinacea* is recommended as a prophylactic and treatment substance for upper respiratory infections. However, data are insufficient at present to support the former (Hughes et al. 2004). It has alkylamide and polysaccharide substance which possess significant in vitro and in vivo immunostimulation properties due to enhanced phagocytosis and nonspecific T-cell stimulation (Grimm and Muller 1999).

The consumption of *Echinacea* at the onset of symptoms has been clinically shown to decrease both the severity and duration of the cold and flu. Employing quantitative polymerase chain reaction (PCR) to identify in vivo alterations in the expression of immunomodulatory genes in response to *Echinacea* has been performed (Randolph et al. 2003). Investigations conducted on in vivo gene expression within peripheral leukocytes were evaluated in six healthy non-smoking subjects. Blood samples were obtained at baseline and on subsequent days following consumption of a commercially blended *Echinacea* product. The overall gene expression pattern between 48 h and 12 days after taking *Echinacea* was consistent with an antiinflammatory response. The expression of interleukin-1β, intracellular adhesion molecule, tumor necrosis factor-α, and interleukin-8 was modestly depressed up through day 5 and returned to baseline by day 12. Further, the expression of interferon-α consistently increased through day 12, thus indicating an antiviral response. Therefore, initial data yielded a gene expression response pattern consistent with the ability of *Echinacea* to decrease both the intensity and duration of cold and flu symptoms (Randolph et al. 2003).

Aside from the effects of *Echinacea* on innate immunity, few studies are available that have examined the ability for enhancement of humoral immunity. Although, a study using female Swiss mice as the model found support for the use of *E. purpurea*, as suggested by anecdotal reports, and demonstrated potential enhancement of humoral immune responses, in addition to innate immune responses (Freier et al. 2003). However, it is important to note that the use of *E. purpurea*, as dosed in one study, was not effective in treating upper respiratory tract infections and related symptoms in pediatric patients, aged 2–11. Further, the consumption of *E. purpurea* was associated with an increased risk of rash (Taylor et al. 2003).

Regarding side effects, *Echinacea* is often well tolerated with the most common side effect being its unpleasant taste (Hughes et al. 2004, Parnham 1996). Extended use of *Echinacea* for more than 2 months may lead to tachyphylaxis (Blumenthal et al. 1998). Anaphylaxis has also been reported with a single dose of this herbal agent (Ness et al. 1999). Further, *Echinacea* use has been associated with hepatotoxicity if taken with hepatotoxic agents including anabolic steroids, amiodarone, ketoconazole, and methotrexate (Miller 1998). Further, flavonoids from *E. purpurea* can affect the hepatic cytochrome P-450 and sulfotransferase systems (Eaton et al. 1996, Schubert et al. 1995). For example, one investigation found that *Echinacea* decreased the oral clearance of substrates of the cytochrome P-450 1A2 system but not the oral clearance of substrates of the 2C9 and 2D6 isoenzymes in vivo. The herbal also selectively modulates the activity of the cytochrome P-450 P3A isoenzyme at both hepatic and intestinal sites. The researchers, therefore, urged caution when *Echinacea* is combined with medications dependent upon the cytochrome P-450 3A or 1A2 systems for elimination (Gorski et al. 2004). Drug levels may become elevated with concomitant use of *Echinacea*. Some drugs that are metabolized by the cytochrome P-450 3A enzyme include lovastatin, clarithromycin, cyclosporine, diltiazem, estrogens, indinavir, triazolam, and numerous others. Taking midazolam and *Echinacea* together seems to increase levels of the sedative (Gorski et al. 2004). Finally, *Echinacea* use should exceed 4 weeks and it should not be used in patients with systemic or autoimmune disorders, patients who are pregnant, or patients who are immunocompromised (Hughes et al. 2004, Bordia 1978).

The immunostimulatory effects of *Echinacea* may antagonize the immunosuppressive actions of corticosteroids and cyclosporine (Chavez and Chavez 1998). *Echinacea* may also lead to inhibition of the hepatic microsomal enzyme system and as such its use with drugs such as phenobarbital, phenytoin, and rifampin, which are metabolized by these enzymes, should be avoided as toxicity may result.

Feverfew

Feverfew is used to treat headache, fever, menstrual abnormalities, and prevent migraines (Jellin et al. 2003). The name is derived from the Latin word febrifugia, which means "fever reducer (Kaye et al. 2000)." Although feverfew is commonly used for migraine headaches, the literature is inconclusive regarding its efficacy (Murphy et al. 1988, De Weerdt et al. 1996). In a study reviewing evidence from double-blind randomized controlled trials of the clinical efficacy of feverfew versus placebo for migraine prophylaxis, investigators found insufficient evidence to suggest a benefit of feverfew over placebo for the prevention of migraine (Pittler and Ernst 2004). As with most herbal compounds, analyses of feverfew-based products have yielded significant variations in the parthenolide contents, which are believed to be the active ingredients (Nelson et al. 2002).

Regarding the effects of the antiinflammatory lactone parthenolide, a German study indicated that parthenolide may support T-cell survival by down-regulating the CD95 system. The CD95 system is a critical component of the apoptotic or programmed cell death pathway of activated T-cells. Further, the authors reported that parthenolide may have therapeutic potential as an antiapoptotic substance blocking the activation-induced cell death of T cells (Li-Weber et al. 2002).

Feverfew also has demonstrated inhibition of serotonin release from aggregating platelets. This mechanism may be related to the inhibition of arachidonic acid release via a phospholipase pathway (Marles et al. 1992, Fozard 1985, Makheja and Bailey 1982). It has also been found that feverfew has decreased approximately 86–88% of prostaglandin production without exhibiting inhibition of the cyclooxygenase enzyme (Collier et al. 1980).

Adverse reactions to feverfew include aphthous ulcers, abdominal pain, nausea, and vomiting. A rebound headache may occur with abrupt cessation of this herbal (Jellin et al. 2003,

Kaye et al. 2000). Better tolerance to feverfew has been suggested when compared to conventional migraine medications because in studies feverfew use resulted in no alteration in heart rate, blood pressure, body weight, or blood chemistry like conventional migraine medications (Jellin et al. 2003). A condition known as "post-feverfew syndrome" can occur in long-term users which manifests as fatigue, anxiety, headaches, insomnia, arthralgias, and muscle and joint stiffness (Jellin et al. 2003, Kaye et al. 2000).

Feverfew may inhibit platelet action; therefore, it is reasonable to avoid the concomitant use of this herb in patients taking medications such as, heparin, warfarin, NSAIDs, aspirin, and vitamin E (Heptinstall et al. 1987, Makheja and Bailey 1981). Further, herbs like feverfew can interact with iron preparations, thereby reducing the bioavailability of that substance (Miller 1998).

Ephedra

Since the US government's ban on ephedra-based products, there has been an obvious decline in its prevalent use in that country. However, patients may still present for pain evaluation with a history of use of ephedra or be taking related compounds, many of which are readily available and possess potent dose-dependent increases in heart rate and in blood pressure. Ma huang, an ephedra-based alkaloid, is similar in structure to amphetamines and is traditionally indicated for the treatment of various respiratory disorders such as the flu, common cold, allergies, and bronchitis. Additionally, it is commonly used as an appetite suppressant (Hughes et al. 2004). Ma huang or ephedra acts as a sympathomimetic agent and exhibits potent positive inotropic and chronotropic responses. In addition to its antitussive actions, ephedra may also possess bacteriostatic properties (Kaye et al. 2000). As a cardiovascular and respiratory sympathomimetic, it utilizes an α-adrenergic or β-adrenergic sensitive pathway (Tinkleman and Avner 1977). Recent laboratory data using the cat lung vascular bed indicate that ephedra-mediated pulmonary hypertension is dependent upon $\alpha(1)$-adrenoreceptor sensitive mechanisms (Fields et al. 2003).

The appetite suppressant and metabolic enhancer effects of ma huang made it a potent ingredient of various over-the-counter weight loss compounds. However, even prior to the United States' federal ban on ma huang, many herbal manufacturers were already promoting their ephedra-free supplements due to the numerous reported adverse effects of ephedra.

Dangerous side effects of ma huang administration include systemic hypertension, pulmonary hypertension, tachycardia, cardiomyopathy, cardiac dysrhythmias, myocardial infarction, stroke, seizures, psychosis, and death (Hughes et al. 2004). Many of these complications have been attributed to a lack of standardization in its formulation (Gurley et al. 1998 and MMWR 1996). Prior to the United States' federal ban of ma huang, approximately 16,000 cases of adverse events including 164 deaths had been reported to the United States Food and Drug Administration (FDA) since 1994 (Jurgensen and Stevens 2004). Further, The Bureau of Food and Drug Safety of the Texas Department of Health reported eight ephedra-associated fatalities during a 21-month period between 1993 and 1995; seven of the fatalities secondary to myocardial infarction or stroke (Leak 1999). There have also been a number of large groups of lawsuits for ephedra-linked myocardial infarction, stroke, and pulmonary hypertension in recent years. Patients at highest risk of side effects include those who are pregnant, have hypertension, coronary vascular disease, seizures, glaucoma, anxiety, or mania (Hughes et al. 2004).

The use of ma huang, still available over US borders, is highly relevant to the pain practitioner in the perioperative period. The possibility of hypertension causing myocardial ischemia or stroke needs to be considered. Further, ephedra or similar compounds readily available over the counter can potentially interact with general anesthetic agents, such as halothane, isoflurane, desflurane, or cardiac glycosides, like digitalis, to cause cardiac dysrhythmias. Patients taking ephedra for prolonged periods of time can also deplete their peripheral catecholamine stores. Therefore, under general anesthesia, these patients can potentially experience profound intraoperative hypotension which can be controlled with a direct vasoconstrictor (e.g., phenylephrine) instead of ephedrine. Finally, use of ephedra with phenelzine or other monoamine oxidase inhibitors may result in insomnia, headache, and tremulousness and concurrent use with the obstetric drug oxytocin has been resulted in hypertension (Grontved and Hentzer 1986).

Ginger

Ginger has been used for the treatment of nausea, vomiting, motion sickness, and vertigo (Kaye et al. 2000). A study of the effects of ginger on subjects with vertigo found that no subjects experienced nausea after caloric stimulation of the vestibular system, in contrast to those treated with placebo (Grontved and Hentzer 1986). It is postulated that ginger may be superior to dimenhydrinate in decreasing motion sickness (Holtmann et al. 1989). For vomiting episodes, this herbal has also been effective in decreasing symptoms associated with hyperemesis gravidarum (Fischer-Rasmussen et al. 1990).

The effect of ginger on the clotting pathway has also been investigated. Ginger has exhibited potent inhibition of thromboxane synthetase and this effect results in an increased bleeding time, which can potentially cause morbidity if an interventional pain procedure is performed (Backon 1986). The ability of ginger constituents and related substances to inhibit arachidonic acid-induced platelet activation in human whole blood has also been investigated. The data from that study revealed that ginger compounds and derivatives are more potent antiplatelet agents than aspirin under conditions employed in the study. Paradol, a constituent of ginger, was identified as the most potent antiplatelet aggregation agent and cyclooxygenase-1 (COX-1) inhibitor (Nurtjahja-Tjendraputra et al. 2003). In another study, administration of ginger has also resulted in decreases in blood pressure, serum cholesterol, and serum triglycerides in diabetic rats (Akhani et al. 2004). Thus, further investigation into these effects in this disease is warranted.

Adverse effects of ginger include bleeding dysfunction and its use is contraindicated in patients with coagulation abnormalities or those on anticoagulant medications such as nonsteroidal antiinflammatory drugs (NSAIDs), aspirin, warfarin, and heparin (Kaye et al. 2000). Ginger may increase bleeding risk, enhance barbiturate effects, and, as a result of an inotropic effect, interfere with cardiac medications. Large quantities of ginger may also cause cardiac arrhythmias and central nervous system depression (Jellin et al. 1993).

Garlic

Garlic's use is prevalent and is available in powdered, dried, and fresh forms (Hughes et al. 2004). Allicin, the main active ingredient in garlic, contains sulfur and crushing the clove activates the enzyme allinase, thus facilitating the conversion of alliin to allicin (Ness et al. 1999).

Recommended uses for garlic have focused on treating hypercholesterolemia, hypertension, and cardiovascular disease and studies have targeted its hypocholesterolemic and vasodilatory activity (Hughes et al. 2004, Jain et al. 1993, Silagy and Neil 1994, Neil et al. 1996, Berthold et al. 1998, Cooperative group 1986). Investigations have found that garlic may lead to inhibition of the 3-hydroxy-3-methyl-glutaryl-CoA (HMG-CoA) reductase and 14α-demethylase enzyme systems thereby exerting a lipid-reducing effect (Hughes et al. 2004). Garlic may also be used for its antiplatelet, antioxidant, and fibrinolytic actions (Neil et al. 1996, Reuter 1995, Beaglehole 1996). There is minimal data present to support the use of garlic for hypertension, as its depressor effects on systolic and diastolic blood pressure appear to range from minimal to modest (Hughes et al. 2004, Ness et al. 1999).

Chronic oral use of garlic has been reported to augment the endogenous antioxidants of the heart (Kaye et al. 1995). A recent study hypothesized that garlic-induced cardiac antioxidants may provide protection against acute adriamycin-induced cardiotoxicity. Using the rat model, researchers discovered an increase in oxidative stress as evidenced by a significant increase in myocardial thiobarbituric acid reactive substances (TBARS) and a decrease in myocardial superoxide dismutase (SOD), catalase, and glutathione peroxidase activity in the adriamycin group. However, in the garlic-treated rats, the increase in myocardial TBARS and a decrease in endogenous antioxidants by adriamycin were significantly attenuated. Therefore, one may conclude that garlic administration may help prevent this form of drug-induced cardiotoxicity (Mukherjee et al. 2003). The effects of allicin in the feline and rat lung vasculature have also been studied. Allicin has shown significant vasodepressor activity in the pulmonary vascular bed of the rat and cat (Kaye et al. 1995). Further, although allicin has been found to lower blood pressure, insulin, and triglycerides levels in fructose-fed rats, it has also been considered important to investigate its effect on the weight of animals.

Recent data indicate that garlic may be an effective treatment against methicillin-resistant *Staphylococcus aureus* (MRSA) infection. In a study using mice, investigators demonstrated that the garlic extracts, diallyl sulfide and diallyl disulfide, showed protective qualities against MRSA infection. Such conclusions, coupled with further investigation, may result in the use of such extracts in MRSA infection treatment (Tsao et al. 2003).

Side effects of garlic are minimal, with odor and gastrointestinal discomfort being the most commonly reported (Hughes et al. 2004). Induction of the cytochrome P-450 system may occur as evidenced by reduction of serum levels of one medication (Hughes et al. 2004). Pain practitioners must be aware that garlic may augment the effects of warfarin, heparin, and aspirin and may result in an abnormal bleeding time. This effect can result in increased risk of perioperative hemorrhage or catastrophic hematoma on interventional pain procedures (Bordia 1978).

Ginkgo biloba

There are many active components present in *Ginkgo*, including the flavinoid glycosides and terpenoids. The flavinoids have demonstrated antioxidant activity while the terpenoids have shown antagonism to platelet action (Hughes et al. 2004). *Ginkgo* has been used to treat intermittent claudication, vertigo, and enhance memory (Leak 1999). Subjects using this herbal have reported decreased pain in the affected lower extremities and increased symptom-free distance in ambulation. In addition to inhibiting platelet-activating factor, *Ginkgo* may also mediate nitric oxide release and decrease inflammation (Hughes et al. 2004, Bauer 1984,

Peters et al. 1998, Braquet 1985, Braquet and Bourgain 1987, Marcocci 1997, Kobuchi et al. 1997).

To evaluate the efficacy of *Ginkgo* on dementia, a double-blind and placebo-controlled randomized trial using the extract EGB761 was performed. It was found that EGB761 had the potential to stabilize and modestly improve cognitive performance and social functioning (Hughes et al. 2004, LeBars et al. 1997). In addition, the improvement in cognition was comparable to the effect of donezepil on dementia (Hughes et al. 2004). This effect on cognition function and memory may be related to activation of cholinergic neurotransmitters. It is important to note, however, that data are inconclusive regarding the ability of this herbal to improve memory in subjects without dementia (Hughes et al. 2004).

Although the pathogenesis of acute pancreatitis is not well understood, there are numerous data that suggest a role for oxygen-free radicals in the progression and complications of pancreatitis. The effects of EGB761 have shown a positive effect on acute pancreatitis and this effect may be linked to a free radical scavenger effect by *Ginkgo* (Zeybek et al. 2003).

Ginkgo is generally well tolerated in healthy adults for about 6 months (Hughes et al. 2004). However, aside from the mild gastrointestinal distress, the potential of *Ginkgo* on antiplatelet-activating factor has resulted in *G. biloba*-induced spontaneous hyphema (bleeding from iris the anterior chamber of the eye), spontaneous bilateral subdural hematomas, and subarachnoid hemorrhage (Hughes et al. 2004, Kaye et al. 2000, Rosenblatt and Mindel 1997, Rowin and Lewis 1996, Gilbert 1997, Vale 1998). Therefore, the use of anticoagulants and *Ginkgo* should be strictly monitored and possibly avoided when patients are scheduled for interventional pain procedures (Hughes et al. 2004).

Regarding the effects of *Ginkgo* on pharmacokinetics, an open-labeled and randomized crossover trial was conducted on healthy human volunteers to determine if *Ginkgo* alters the pharmacokinetics of digoxin. The investigators found that the concurrent use of orally administered *Ginkgo* and digoxin did not seem to have a significant effect on the pharmacokinetics of digoxin in healthy volunteers (Mauro et al. 2003). Therefore, one may conclude that concurrent use of *G. biloba* with aspirin, NSAIDs, warfarin, and heparin is not recommended as *Ginkgo* may increase the potential for bleeding in these patients. It is also advisable to avoid use of *Ginkgo* with anticonvulsant drugs such as carbamazepine, phenytoin, and phenobarbital as the herbal may decrease the effectiveness of these medications (Miller 1998). Concurrent use of *Ginkgo* and tricyclic antidepressants is also not advised because of the potential to lower the seizure threshold in these patients (Miller 1998).

Kava Kava

Kava kava, an extract of the *Piper methysticum* plant, is employed for its proposed anxiolytic, antiepileptic, antidepressant, antipsychotic, and sedative properties (Nowakowska et al. 1998, Skidmore-Roth 2001, Uebelhack et al. 1998). Some of the active ingredients of kava kava include the lactones or pyrones, kawain, methysticin, dihydrokawain, and dihydromethysticin (Jellin et al. 2002, Volz and Kieser 1997). Kava extracts available commercially are usually found to contain approximately 30–70% kava lactones (Jellin et al. 2002).

The extract WS 1490 has been investigated to determine its effectiveness in the treatment of anxiety (Volz and Kieser 1997). WS 1490 has been shown to be effective in anxiety disorders as a treatment alternative to benzodiazepines and tricyclic antidepressants and reported not to have the problems associated with those two classes of drugs (Volz and Kieser 1997).

However, therapeutic effect may take up to 4 weeks and data have indicated treatment for 1–8 weeks to obtain significant improvement (Jellin et al. 2002, Forget et al. 2000).

Although the exact mechanism of kava kava's effects on the central nervous system is largely unknown, the pyrones have demonstrated competitive inhibition of the monoamine oxidase B enzyme (Jellin et al. 2002). Inhibition of this enzyme may result in the psychotropic effects related to kava kava use as this enzyme is responsible for the breakdown of amines that play a role in psychoses (Seitz et al. 1997).

Regarding adverse effects, patients who experience hepatic adverse reactions are known as "poor metabolizers." Typically, these patients have a deficiency in the cytochrome P-450 2D6 isoenzyme (Jellin et al. 2002). Therefore, it is recommended that patients who use kava kava receive routine liver function tests to monitor the development of hepatotoxicity (Jellin et al. 2002). Furthermore, there have been 24 documented cases of hepatotoxicity following the use of kava kava and, in some cases, death or liver transplant occurred after 1–3 months of use (Jellin et al. 2002). In countries such as Germany and Australia, kava kava use for longer than 3 months is not recommended (Forget et al. 2000). Other side effects of kava kava use include visual changes, a pellagra-like syndrome with characteristic ichthyosiform dermopathy, and hallucinations (Jellin et al. 2002, Winslow and Kroll 1998, Garner and Klinger 1985).

Regarding drug interactions, kava kava may react adversely with the benzodiazepine alprazolam, other central nervous system depressants, statins, alcohol, and levodopa, consequently resulting in excessive sedation among other side effects; therefore the supplement should be avoided in those patients with endogenous depression (Jellin et al. 2002, Jellin et al. 1990, Jamieson and Duffield 1990, Gruenwald et al. 1998). Finally, kava kava may also affect platelets in an antithrombotic fashion by inhibiting cyclooxygenase and, thus, attenuating thromboxane production (Jellin et al. 2002). Pain relief mechanisms utilized by the herbal may be similar to local anesthetic responses and could be dependent on a non-opiate sensitive pathway (Jamieson and Duffield 1990, Singh 1983).

Ginseng

There are three main groups of ginseng that are classified based on their geographic origin (Hughes et al. 2004). These are Asian ginseng, American ginseng, and Siberian ginseng, with the pharmacologically active ingredient in ginseng being ginsenosides (Hughes et al. 2004, Leak 1999, Kaye et al. 2000). Asian and American ginsengs have been used to increase resistance to environmental stress, promote diuresis, stimulate the immune system, and aid digestion (Ng et al. 1987, Jellin et al. 2003). Further, while Asian ginseng has shown promise in improving cognition when combined with the herbal agent *Ginkgo*, American ginseng has been studied for its potential to stimulate human tumor necrosis factor-α (TNF-α) production in cultured human white blood cells (Jellin et al. 2003, Zhou and Kitts 2002). American ginseng may also possess hypoglycemic activity (Jie et al. 1984, Sotaniemi et al. 1995). Such effects have been observed in both normal and diabetic subjects and may be attributed to ginseng components, specifically ginsenoside Rb2 and panaxans I, J, K, and L (Yokozawa et al. 1985, Oshima et al. 1985, Konno et al. 1985, Konno et al. 1984, Tokmoda et al. 1984).

Typically ginseng is well tolerated, but side effects such as bleeding abnormalities secondary to antiplatelet effects, headache, vomiting, Stevens-Johnson syndrome, epistaxis, and hypertension have been reported (Baldwin 1986, Hammond and Whitworth 1981, Dega et al. 1996, Greenspan 1983, Hopkins et al. 1988, Palmer et al. 1978, Kuo et al. 1990)

Table 10.2 Herbal medications associated with bleeding abnormalities.

Bilberry
Bromelain
Chamomile
Dandelion root
Dong quai
Fenugreek
Feverfew
Fish oil
Flaxseed oil
Garlic
Ginger
Ginkgo biloba
Ginseng
Grape seed extract
Horse chestnut
Kava kava
Meadowsweet
Motherwort
Red clover
Tamarind
Turmeric
Willow

(see Table 10.2). Drug interactions between Asian ginseng and calcium channel blockers, warfarin, phenelzine, and digoxin have also been noted (Hughes et al. 2004). It may be advisable that ginseng be avoided by interventional pain patients on anticoagulant medications such as warfarin, heparin, aspirin, and NSAIDs. Further, because of ginseng's association with hypertension and the deleterious outcomes linked to chronic hypertension, the pain practitioner should be aware of whom and for how long patients may have been taking this herbal product. Since many agents can cause generalized vasodilation, hemodynamic lability may be seen.

Regarding ginseng's interaction with antidepressants such as monoamine oxidase inhibitors, concurrent use of ginseng with phenelzine sulfate should be avoided as manic episodes have been reported with routine use of both (Shader and Greenblatt 1985, Jones and Runikis 1987). Finally, as a result of ginseng's potential to cause decreased blood glucose levels, it should be used cautiously in diabetic patients on insulin or other oral hypoglycemic agents and blood glucose levels should be monitored.

Cloves

Cloves, also known as clove oil, have been used orally for stomach upset, for its antiplatelet effect, and as an expectorant. Cloves may also be used topically for pain relief from mouth and throat inflammation as well as athlete's foot. Its constituent, eugenol, has long been used topically for toothache, but the FDA has classified this drug into category III, meaning there is inadequate data to support efficacy (Covington et al. 1996). More evidence is necessary to rate clove for this purpose.

Topically, clove can cause tissue irritation and in some people even allergic dermatitis (Kanerva et al. 1996). Moreover, repeated oral application may result in gingival damage and skin and mucous membrane irritation (Covington et al. 1996, Robbers and Tyler 1999).

The eugenol constituent in clove may theoretically increase the risk of bleeding in some people who are concomitantly using herbs such as garlic, ginger, *Ginkgo*, and white willow bark (Chen et al. 1996). Likewise, patients taking antiplatelet agents such as aspirin, clopidogrel, dipyridamole, ticlopidine, heparin, and warfarin may also experience an increased risk of bleeding.

Black Pepper

Black pepper, also known as *Piper nigrum*, has been used to treat upset stomach, bronchitis, and even cancer. Some have used black pepper to treat pain associated with neuralgia and skin irritation when used topically and may also possess antimicrobial and diuretic properties (Leung and Foster 1996, Gruenwald et al. 1998). The putative compounds include volatile oils (sabinene, limonene, caryophyllene, β-pinene, α-pinenes), acid amines (e.g., piperines), and fatty acids.

The compound is not without side effects. Eye contact may lead to redness and/or swelling. Large amounts have even been reported to cause death secondary to aspiration (Cohle et al. 1988).

Black pepper may decrease the activity of the CYP3A4 enzyme, thereby increasing levels of drugs such as phenytoin, propranolol, and theophylline metabolized by the enzyme. The piperine constituent of pepper seems to inhibit CYP3A4 in vitro (Bhardwaj et al. 2002). Other drugs that may be affected include calcium channel blockers, chemotherapeutic agents, antifungals, glucocorticoids, cisapride, alfentanil, fentanyl, losartan, fluoxetine, midazolam, omeprazole, and ondansetron. Caution is advised if patients are taking these drugs concomitantly as their doses may need to be decreased.

Capsicum annuum

Capsicum annuum, also known as Cayenne pepper, has been used orally for upset stomach, toothache, poor circulation, fever, hyperlipidemia, and heart disease prevention. *Capsicum* can be used topically to treat pain associated with osteoarthritis, shingles, rheumatoid arthritis, post-herpetic neuralgia, trigeminal neuralgia, diabetic neuropathy, fibromyalgia, and back pain. Others have used *Capsicum* for relief of muscle spasms and even as a gargle for laryngitis (Covington et al. 1996, Mason et al. 2004, Gagnier et al. 2007, McCarty et al. 1994).

Capsaicinoids, carotenoids, flavonoids, and steroid saponins are the putative compounds involved. The mechanism of action involves the binding of nociceptors in the skin, which initially causes neuronal excitation and heightened sensitivity (itching, burning) followed by cutaneous vasodilation. Selective stimulation of afferent C fibers, which act as thermoreceptors and nociceptors, and release of substance P, a sensory neurotransmitter that mediates pain, are purported to be implicated. Furthermore, this excitatory period is followed by a refractory period with reduced sensitivity, possibly due to desensitization secondary to substance P depletion (Mason et al. 2004, Surh and Lee 1996, Bortolotti et al. 2002). Cough, dyspnea, nasal congestion, and eye irritation may occur through stimulation of unmyelinated slow C-fibers of the sensory nervous system (Millqvist 2000).

About 10% of patients who use capsaicin topically discontinue its use secondary to adverse effects such as burning, stinging, and erythema (Mason et al. 2004). Exacerbation of ACE inhibitor cough has been reported in patients using topical capsaicin and taking ACE inhibitors (Hakas 1990). Skin contact with fresh capsicum fruit can cause irritation or contact dermatitis (Williams et al. 1995). Furthermore, concomitant use of herbs and supplements (garlic, ginseng, *Ginkgo*, cloves) may increase the risk of bleeding by decreasing platelet aggregation.

White Willow Bark

From the family of salicylates, white willow bark is used to treat headache, mild feverish colds, influenza, muscle and joint pain caused by inflammation, arthritic conditions, and systemic connective tissue disorders. Preliminary research suggests that willow bark extracts have analgesic, antiinflammatory, and antipyretic effects (Fiebich and Chrubasik 2004).

Evidence demonstrates that willow bark extract providing 120–240 mg of the salicin constituent daily can reduce low back pain in some patients with the higher concentration being more effective. Of note, it may take up to 1 week for significant relief (Chrubasik et al. 2000). Salicin's therapeutic had in fact been reported to be comparable to rofecoxib (Vioxx – now discontinued) for low back pain (Chrubasik et al. 2001).

Research is conflicting concerning white willow barks efficacy on osteoarthritis, with some studies suggesting a moderate analgesic effect while others consider it similar to placebo (Schmid et al. 2001, Biegert et al. 2004). More studies must be conducted to identify its use in these conditions.

Flavonoids, tannins, and salicylates are attributed to the antiinflammatory, antipyretic, and antiuricosuric activities of white willow bark. Salicin is eventually metabolized to salicylic acid, which then shares the same metabolic pathway as aspirin (Schmid et al. 2001).

An ethanolic extract of willow bark seems to inhibit COX-2 indirectly by mediating prostaglandin release, while other constituents of white willow bark may have lipoxygenase-inhibiting and antioxidant properties that could contribute to analgesia (Chrubasik et al. 2000). Moreover, other literature suggests that they may also prevent prostaglandin and cytokine release (Fiebich and Chrubasik 2004).

Willow bark inhibits platelet aggregation, but to a lesser degree than aspirin (Krivoy et al. 2001), thus, concomitant use with other herbals such as *Ginkgo*, ginseng, garlic, or cloves may increase the risk of bleeding, as will use with anticoagulants and antiplatelet drugs.

Devil's Claw

Devil's claw has been used to treat pain symptoms from osteoarthritis, rheumatoid arthritis, gout, myalgia, fibrositis, lumbago, tendonitis, pleuritic chest pain, and gastrointestinal upset. The active constituent, harpagoside, seems to reduce nonspecific low back pain when used in a dose range from 50 to 100 mg. In fact, its use in this range has been compared to 12.5 mg of the discontinued drug, rofecoxib (Chrubasik et al. 2002, Gagnier et al. 2004, Chrubasik et al. 2005). Additionally, oral dosing of devil's claw either alone or in combination with NSAIDs may lessen pain associated with osteoarthritis (Chantre et al. 2000, Chrubasik et al.

2002, Wegener and Lupke 2003) and may even need lower doses of NSAIDs to achieve the same level of pain relief (Chantre et al. 2000). More evidence is needed to substantiate its use or disuse for rheumatoid arthritis-related pain although preliminary data suggest it may be ineffective (Grahame and Robinson 1981).

Besides containing harpagoside, Devil's claw contains iridoid glycoside constituents and procumbide that add to its effect, as well as phenylethanol derivatives acteoside (verbascoside) and isoacteoside, and the oligosaccharide stachyose (Fiebich et al. 2001). The iridoid glycoside constituents seem to provide an antiinflammatory effect (Chantre et al. 2000). Current evidence implies that harpagoside inhibits both the cyclooxygenase and lipoxygenase inflammatory pathways (Chrubasik et al. 2000). Devil's claw seems to inhibit only COX-2, not COX-1, and also inhibits the inflammation-modulating enzyme nitric oxide synthetase (Jang et al. 2003). An increased synthesis and release of tumor necrosis factor (TNF)-α by compounds other than harpagoside aid in the antiinflammatory effect; however, research in humans shows no effect of devil's claw on the arachidonic acid pathway (Moussard et al. 1992).

The most commonly reported side effect of devil's claw is diarrhea, but the supplement is generally well tolerated (Chantre et al. 2000). Other generalized complaints include nausea, vomiting, and abdominal pain, headache, tinnitus, anorexia, and loss of taste. Some people have experienced dysmenorrhea and hemodynamic instability (Chrubasik et al. 2002).

Possible drug interactions may stem from devil's claw ability to inhibit cytochrome P-450 2C9 (CYP2C9), although the effect has not been reported in humans (Unger and Frank 2004). The pain physician should be advised that drugs metabolized by CYP2C9 such as NSAIDs; meloxicam (Mobic); piroxicam (Feldene); celecoxib (Celebrex); amitriptyline (Elavil); warfarin (Coumadin); glipizide (Glucotrol); losartan (Cozaar); and others may need to be reduced or even eliminated.

Boswellia

Boswellia, also known as Indian Frankincense, has been used to manage pain associated with osteoarthritis, rheumatoid arthritis (RA), rheumatism, bursitis, and tendonitis. Non-pain-related uses include ulcerative colitis, dyspepsia, asthma, allergic rhinitis, sore throat, syphilis, pimples, and cancer.

There is preliminary evidence that taking Indian Frankincense extract orally might reduce osteoarthritis symptoms such as knee pain and swelling (Kimmatkar et al. 2003), while its use in rheumatoid arthritis is controversial. More evidence is needed for use of boswellia in both these conditions.

The principle constituents, boswellic acid and α-boswellic and β-boswellic acids, come from the resin. These constituents have antiinflammatory properties (Ammon et al. 1993) that aid in pain management with arthritic patients, but not all extracts of Indian Frankincense extracts show antiarthritis, antiinflammatory, or antipyretic effects (Kimmatkar et al. 2003). The mechanism behind boswellic acids comes from inhibition of 5-lipoxygenase and leukotriene synthesis, along with the inhibition of leukocyte elastase. Some have suggested that the acids may have disease-modifying effects, thereby decreasing glycosaminoglycan degradation and cartilage damage. *Boswellia* seems to decrease production of antibodies and cell-mediated immunity (Kimmatkar et al. 2003, Liu et al. 2002).

Side effects include gastrointestinal upset such as epigastric pain, nausea, and diarrhea, while topical use may cause contact dermatitis (Kimmatkar et al. 2003, Acebo et al. 2004). Not enough studies have been done to comment on pharmacologic interactions with other drugs.

Summary

The growing use of alternative medicines such as minerals, vitamins, and herbals in the world warrants a more comprehensive understanding of these agents by the medical community. It is important for the pain practitioner to recognize certain facts regarding these supplements. For example, there are about 1,300 g of calcium in a 70-kg adult and the mineral magnesium activates approximately 300 enzyme systems in the human body; most of these systems involved in energy metabolism (Kaye and Grogono 2000). Aside from these, the pain practitioner must appreciate the effect of these supplements on such functions on a regular basis as well as during various operative procedures. As demonstrated in this chapter, the use of these compounds may prove beneficial for some patients, but result in alterations in normal physiologic functions in others, thus potentially resulting in deleterious consequences. Moreover, in our own survey, in patients undergoing operative surgery, including interventional pain procedures, approximately one in three patients takes some form of herbal supplement although 70% of these patients did not admit to its use during routine questioning (Kaye et al. 2004). For this reason, these agents, in addition to all other medications taken by the patient, should be screened for by medical practitioners vigorously, in particular pain practitioners, as some of these compounds may interact with chosen anesthetics during the stages of anesthesia or can affect treatment or even worse cause harm to the patient. In this regard, education of patients regarding the serious potential supplement–supplement and drug–supplement interactions should be an integral component of pain assessment and ongoing pain management. Currently the American Society of Anesthesiologists (ASA) suggests that all herbal medications should be discontinued 2–3 weeks before an elective surgical procedure. If the patient is not sure of the contents of the herbal medicine, he or she should be urged to bring the container so that the pain practitioner/anesthesiologist can review the contents of the herb or preparation (Kaye et al. 2004).

Due to current lax regulations in some countries, some of these agents are poorly categorized and standardized, thus resulting in a high risk of adverse effects when used by an uninformed or misinformed public. Within the last few decades, hundreds of deaths have been linked to the use of these agents, specifically the herbals. Given that the FDA considers herbals as foods and that this industry has developed into a multibillion dollar business, it is imperative for the pain practitioner to have a basic understanding of issues related to the over 29,000 supplements and herbal-related agents available without prescription in the United States. Worldwide there are varying levels of scrutiny and protection for consumers. Data also suggest that less than 1% of adverse effects associated with herbals are reported in the United States. In general, whether the patient is taking minerals, vitamins, and/or herbals, one thing is for certain: an open line of communication between pain physician and patient should exist regarding all of these agents. This communication is essential to ensure quality patient treatment, a stable and secure rapport, and a properly informed and educated general public. Though only recently being taught in many medical schools, pain practitioners will be well advised to gain a solid foundation in this most important and relevant topic.

Case Scenario

Alan D Kaye, MD, PhD, Muhummad Anwar, MD, and Amir Baluch, MD

Barbara is a 52-year-old woman with back pain due to a paracentral disk herniation. She is referred to your pain clinic for an L4/5 epidural steroid injection. She has tried various treatments in the past including physiotherapy, TENS, yoga, and homeopathy, all without much benefit. She was advised to undergo surgery, but states that she is too afraid and wants to explore other options first. Finally, she has opted to try the epidural injection for the relief of her symptoms. On initial review of her home medications, she states that she is taking irbesartan for hypertension, levothyroxine for hypothyroidism, and tramadol and tylenol for lower back and leg pain. On review of systems, she notes that she has been feeling weak and having pain radiating down both legs. Her physical examination shows bilateral positive straight leg raise test (likely due to herniated lumbar disk). During your interview, you note that her breath smells of garlic. You quiz her if besides the medicines she has noted she is taking any herbals or vitamin supplements. She answers that she is actually taking three different vitamin supplements: a multivitamin, calcium, and selenium.

Can you correlate the smell of garlic with her medications?
This could be an indication of selenium toxicity. Toxicity with selenium supplementation begins at intake greater than 750 μg/day and may manifest as garlic-like breath, loss of hair and fingernails, gastrointestinal distress, or central nervous system changes.

How would the above information modify your further interview?
A. You should try to get a detailed history of her current medications including the dose and duration of treatment. You have to examine all her prescriptions and food supplements. A detailed clinical examination is mandatory. You should contact her primary care physician for any missing information.

Your inquisitiveness reveals that she is currently on several herbals including **saw palmetto, garlic,** and *Ginkgo biloba.*

When would you proceed with the epidural injection?
Her procedure should be delayed for approximately 3 weeks to ensure that all of the herbals are out of her system. She is counseled that the calcium supplement may affect her levothyroxine and a new thyroid panel is ordered.

The following month she returns to your clinic after an uneventful epidural steroid injection under fluoroscopy, with good result. She was told to take her calcium supplement 4 h before or after taking her levothyroxine to minimize a drug interaction. She now reports having more energy and concentration. You ask her to continue to take acetaminophen and tramadol for back pain if it returns.

Two years later Barbara appears in your clinic. Now she is complaining of jaundice, generalized weakness, and abdominal bloating. On review of medications she states that she is taking the same medications prescribed over the past 2 years. She suspects that her jaundice is due to the medications that you have prescribed.

What is your explanation?

Significant acetaminophen overdose can lead to liver failure. An infective etiology is also possible. With the background history of herbal medications, you will have to review her medications again. Physical examination needs to be undertaken and appropriate investigations ordered. When pressed, Barbara confides that 7 weeks earlier, she was at a vitamin store and bought kava for her muscle spasms and occasional agitation.

A liver panel shows significant abnormality and she is referred to a hepatologist. She is diagnosed with acute liver failure and eventually placed on a waiting list for a liver transplant. Upon review of the literature, you noted that there is a link between kava and liver toxicity including hepatitis, cirrhosis, and liver failure. Existing literature also notes that there is no safe dose of kava, as there is no method to assess which individuals will have severe adverse reactions.

References

Acebo E, Raton JA, Sautua S, et al. Allergic contact dermatitis from *Boswellia serrata* extract in a naturopathic cream. Contact Dermat. 2004;51:91–2.

Adams JF, Clark JS, Ireland JT, et al. Malabsorption of vitamin B12 and intrinsic factor secretion during biguanide therapy. Diabetologia 1983;24:16–8.

Akhani SP, Vishwakarma SL, Goyal RK. Anti-diabetic activity of *Zingiber officinale* in streptozotocin-induced type I diabetic rats. J Pharm Pharmacol. 2004;56:101–5.

Ammon HP, Safayhi H, Mack T, Sabieraj J. Mechanism of antiinflammatory actions of curcumine and boswellic acids. J Ethnopharmacol. 1993;38:1139.

Anderson RA, Cheng N, Bryden NA, et al. Elevated intakes of supplemental chromium improve glucose and insulin variables in individuals with type 2 diabetes. Diabetes 1997;46:1786–91.

Anderson RA, Polansky MM, Bryden NA, et al. Supplemental-chromium effects on glucose, insulin, glucagons, and urinary chromium losses in subjects consuming controlled low-chromium diets. Am J Clin Nutr. 1991;54:909–16.

Aymard JP, Aymard B, Netter P, et al. Haematological adverse effects of histamine H2-receptor antagonists. Med Toxicol Adverse Drug Exp. 1988;3:430–48.

Backon J. Ginger: inhibition of thromboxane synthetase and stimulation of prostacyclin: relevance for medicine and psychiatry. Med Hypoth. 1986;20:271–8.

Bahijri SM. Effect of chromium supplementation on glucose tolerance and lipid profile. Saudi Med J. 2000;21:45–50.

Baik HW, Russel RM. Vitamin B12 deficiency in the elderly. Annu Rev Nutr. 1999;19:357–77.

Baldwin CA, Anderson LA, Phillipson JD, et al. What pharmacists should know about feverfew. J Pharm Pharmacol. 1987;239:237–8.

Baldwin CA. What pharmacists should know about ginseng. Pharm J. 1986;237:583–6.

Bar-Or D, Gasiel Y. Calcium and calciferol antagonize effect of verapamil in atrial fibrillation. Br Med J (Clin Res Ed). 1981;282:1585–6.

Bauer R, Khan IA. Structure and stereochemistry of new sesquiterpene esters from *E. purpurea*. Helv Chim Acta. 1985;68:2355–8.

Bauer U. 6-Month double-blind randomized clinical trial of *Ginkgo biloba* extract versus placebo in two parallel groups in patients suffering from peripheral arterial insufficiency. Arz-neimittelforschung 1984;34:716–20.

Baum MK, Javier JJ, Mantero-Atienza E, et al. Zidovudine-associated adverse reactions in a longitudinal study of asymptomatic HIV-1-infected homosexual males. J Acquir Immune Defic Syndr 1991;4:1218–26.

Beaglehole R. Garlic for flavor, not cardioprotection. Lancet 1996;348:1186–7.

Berthold HK, Sudhop T, von Bergmann K. Effect of a garlic oil preparation on serum lipoproteins and cholesterol metabolism: a randomized controlled trial. JAMA 1998;279:1900–2.

Bhardwaj RK, Glaeser H, Becquemont L, et al. Piperine, a major constituent of black pepper, inhibits human P-glycoprotein and CYP3A4. J Pharmacol Exp Ther. 2002;302:645–50.

Biegert C, Wagner I, Ludtke R, et al. Efficacy and safety of willow bark extract in the treatment of osteoarthritis and rheumatoid arthritis: results of 2 randomized double-blind controlled trials. J Rheumatol. 2004;31:2121–30.

Binkley N, Krueger D. Hypervitaminosis A and bone. Nutr Rev. 2000;58(5):138–44.

Blumenthal M, Gruenwald J, Hall T, et al, eds. German Commission E monographs: therapeutic monographs on medicinal plants for human use. Austin: American Botanical Council; 1998.

Bordia A. Effect of garlic on human platelet aggregation in vitro. Atherosclerosis 1978;30:355–360.

Bortolotti M, Coccia G, Grossi G, Miglioli M. The treatment of functional dyspepsia with red pepper. Aliment Pharmacol Ther. 2002;16:1075–82.

Braquet P, Bourgain RH. Anti-anaphylactic properties of BN 52021: a potent platelet activating factor antagonist. Adv Exp Med Biol. 1987;215:215–33.

Braquet P. BN 52021 and related compounds: a new series of highly specific PAF-acether receptor antagonists isolated from *Ginkgo biloba*. Blood Vessels 1985;16:559–572.

Bratman S, Girman AM. Handbook of herbs and supplements and their therapeutic uses. St. Louis, MO: Mosby; 2003.

Brzezinska-Wcislo L, Pierzchala E, Kaminska-Budzinska G, et al. The use of retinoids in dermatology [Polish]. Wiad Lek 2004;57(1–2):63–69.

Campbell NR, Hasinoff BB, Stalts H, et al. Ferrous sulfate reduces thyroxine efficacy in patients with hypothyroidism. Ann Intern Med. 1992;117:1010–1013.

Campbell NR, Hasinoff BB. Iron supplements: a common cause of drug interactions. Br J Clin Pharmacol. 1991;31:251–5.

Cembrowski GS, Zhang MM, Prosser CI, et al. Folate is not what it is cracked up to be. Arch Intern Med. 1999;159:2747–8.

Cerulli J, Grabe DW, Gauthier I, et al. Chromium picolinate toxicity. Ann Pharmacother. 1998;32:428–31.

Chantre P, Cappelaere A, Leblan D, et al. Efficacy and tolerance or *Harpagophytum procumbens* versus diacerhein in treatment of osteoarthritis. Phytomedicine 2000;7:177–84.

Chen SJ, Wang MH, Chen IJ. Antiplatelet and calcium inhibitory properties of eugenol and sodium eugenol acetate. Gen Pharmacol. 1996;27:629–33.

Chrubasik S, Eisenberg E, Balan E, et al. Treatment of low back pain exacerbations with willow bark extract: a randomized double-blind study. Am J Med. 2000;109:9–14.

Chrubasik S, Kunzel O, Model A, et al. Treatment of low back pain with a herbal or synthetic anti-rheumatic: a randomized controlled study. Willow bark extract for low back pain. Rheumatology 2001;40:1388–93.

Chrubasik S, Kunzel O, Thanner J, et al. A 1-year follow-up after a pilot study with doloteffin for low back pain. Phytomedicine 2005;12:1–9.

Chrubasik S, Sporer F, Dillmann-Marschner R, et al. Physicochemical properties of harpagoside and its in vitro release from *Harpagophytum procumbens* extract tablets. Phytomedicine 2000;6:469–73.

Chrubasik S, Thanner J, Kunzel O, et al. Comparison of outcome measures during treatment with the proprietary *Harpagophytum* extract doloteffin in patients with pain in the lower back, knee or hip. Phytomedicine 2002;9:181–94.

Cohle SD, Trestrail JD III, Graham MA, et al. Fatal pepper aspiration. Am J Dis Child. 1988;142:633–6.

Collier HO, Butt NM, McDonald-Gibson WJ, et al. Extract of feverfew inhibits prostaglandins biosynthesis. Lancet 1980;2:922–923.

Combs GF. The vitamins: fundamental aspects in nutrition and health. 2nd ed. San Diego, CA: Academic; 1998. pp. 5–6.

Cooperative Group for Essential Oil of Garlic. The effect of essential oil of garlic on hyperlipidemia and platelet aggregation: an analysis of 308 cases. J Tradit Chin Med. 1986; 6:117–20.

Cott J, Misra R. Medicinal plants: a potential source for new psychotherapeutic drugs. In: Kanba S, Richelson E, editos. Herbal medicines for neuropsychiatric diseases: current developments and research. Philadelphia, PA: Brunner/Mazel & Tokyo: Seiwa Shoten; 1999. pp. 51–70.

Cott JM. In vitro receptor binding and enzyme inhibition by *Hypericum perforatum* extract. Pharmacopsychiatry 1997;30:108–12.

Covington TR, et al. Handbook of nonprescription drugs. 11th ed. Washington, DC: American Pharmaceutical Association; 1996.

Czekalla J, Gastpar M, Hubner WD, et al. The effect of hypericum extract on cardiac conduction as seen in the electrocardiogram compared to that of imipramine. Pharmacopsychiatry 1997;30:86–8.

De Weerdt C, Bootsma H, Hendricks H. Herbal medicines in migraine prevention: randomized double-blind, placebo-controlled crossover trial of a feverfew preparation. Physomedicine 1996;3:225–30.

Dega H, Laporte J, Frances C, et al. Ginseng a cause of Steven-Johnson syndrome [letter]? Lancet 1996;347:1344.

Durward A. Guerguerian AM. Lefebvre M. Shemie SD. Massive diltiazem overdose treated with extracorporeal membrane oxygenation. [Case Reports. Journal Article] Pediatr Crit Care Med. 2003;4(3):372–6.

Eaton EA, Walle UK, Lewis AJ, et al. Flavinoids, potent inhibitors of the human form of phenolsulfotransferase : potential role in drug metabolism and chemoprevention. Drug Met Disp. 1996;24:232–237.

Fan AM, Kizer KW. Selenium: nutritional, toxicologic, and clinical aspects. West J Med. 1990;153:160–7.

Fiebich BL, Chrubasik S. Effects of an ethanolic salix extract on the release of selected inflammatory mediators in vitro. Phytomedicine 2004;11:135–8.

Fiebich BL, Heinrich M, Hiller KO, Kammerer N. Inhibition of TNF-alpha synthesis in LPS-stimulated primary human monocytes by *Harpagophytum* extract SteiHap 69. Phytomedicine 2001;8:28–30.

Fields AM, Kaye AD, Richards TA, et al. Pulmonary vascular responses to ma huang extract. J Altern Complement Med. 2003;9:727–33.

Fischer-Rasmussen W, Kjaer SK, Dahl C, et al. Ginger treatment of hyperemesis gravidarum. Eur J Obstet Gyn Rep Biol. 1990;38:19–24.

Flippo TS, Holder WD Jr. Neurologic degeneration associated with nitrous oxide anesthesia in patients with vitamin B12 deficiency. Arch Surg. 1993;128:1391–5.

Food and Nutrition Board, Institute of Medicine. Folic acid. Dietary reference intakes: thiamin, riboflavin, niacin, vitamin B-6, vitamin B-12, pantothenic acid, biotin, and choline. Washington, DC: National Academy Press, 1998; pp. 193–305.

Food and Nutrition Board, Institute of Medicine. Vitamin D. Dietary reference intakes: calcium, phosphorus, magnesium, vitamin D, and fluoride. Washington, DC: National Academy Press, 1997; pp. 250–87.

Ford ES, Sowell A. Serum alpha-tocopherol status in the United States population: findings from the Third National Health and Nutrition Examination Survey. Am J Epidemiol. 1999;150:290–300.

Forget L, Goldrosen J, Hart JA, et al, eds. Herbal companion to AHFS DI. Bethesda, MD: American Society of Health-System Pharmacists, Inc.; 2000.

Fox GN, Sabovic Z. Chromium picolinate supplementation for diabetes mellitus. J Fam Pract. 1998;46(1):83–86.

Fozard JR. 5-Hydroxytryptamine in the pathophysiology of migraine. In: Bevan JA, editor. Vascular neuroeffector mechanisms. Amsterdam: Elsevier; 1985. pp. 321–8.

Freier DO, Wright K, Klein K, et al. Enhancement of the humoral immune response by *Echinacea purpurea* in female Swiss mice. Immunopharmacol Immunotoxicol. 2003;25:551–60.

Gagnier JJ, Chrubasik S, Manheimer E. *Harpagophytum procumbens* for osteoarthritis and low back pain: a systematic review. BMC Complement Altern Med. 2004;4:13.

Gagnier JJ, van Tulder MW, Berman B, Bombardier C. Herbal medicine for low back pain. A Cochrane Rev. Spine 2007;32:82–92.

Garner LF, Klinger JD. Some visual effects caused by the beverage kava. J Ethnopharm. 1985;13:307–311.

Gilbert GJ. *Ginkgo biloba* [commentary]. Neurology 1997;48:1137.

Goldenberg RL, Tamura T, Neggers Y, et al. The effect of zinc supplementation on pregnancy outcome. JAMA 1995;274:463–468.

Gorski JC, Huang SM, Pinto A, et al. The effect of echinacea (*Echinacea purpurea* root) on cytochrome P450 activity in vivo. Clin Pharmacol Ther. 2004;75:89–100.

Chavez ML, Chavez PI. *Echinacea*. Hosp Pharm. 1998;33:180–188.

Grahame R, Robinson BV. Devils's claw (*Harpagophytum procumbens*): pharmacological and clinical studies. Ann Rheum Dis. 1981;40:632.

Greenspan EM. Ginseng and vaginal bleeding [letter]. JAMA 1983;249:2018.

Grimm W, Muller HH. A randomized controlled trial of the effect of fluid extract of *Echinacea purpurea* on the incidence and severity of colds and respiratory infections. Am J Med. 1999;106:138–43.

Grontved A, Hentzer E. Vertigo-reducing effect of ginger root. J Otolaryngol. 1986;48:282–6.

Gruenwald J, Brendler T, Jaenicke C, et al. PDR for herbal medicines. 1st ed. Montvale, NJ: Medical Economics Company; 1998. pp. 826–7.

Gruenwald J, Brendler T, Jaenicke C, et al. PDR for herbal medicines. 1st ed. Montvale, NJ: Medical Economics Company; 1998. pp. 1043–5.

Gurley BJ, Gardner SF, White LM, et al. Ephedrine pharmacokinetics after ingestion of nutritional supplements containing *Ephedra sinica* (ma huang). Ther Drug Monit. 1998;20: 439–45.

Hakas JF Jr. Topical capsaicin induces cough in patient receiving ACE inhibitor. Ann Allergy 1990;65:322–3.

Hammond TG, Whitworth JA. Adverse reactions to ginseng [letter]. Med J Aust. 1981;1:492.

Harris JE. Interaction of dietary factors with oral anticoagulants: review and applications. J Am Diet Assoc. 1995;95:580–4.

Heinrich HC, Oppitz KH, Gabbe EE. Inhibition of iron absorption in man by tetracycline [German]. Klin Wochenschr. 1974;52:493–8.

Hemila H. Vitamin C intake and susceptibility to the common cold. Br J Nutr. 1997;77(1): 59–72.

Hendler SS, Rorvik DR, eds. PDR for nutritional supplements. Montvale, NJ: Medical Exonomics Company; 2001.

Heptinstall S, Groenwegen WA, Spangenberg P, et al. Extracts of feverfew may inhibit platelet behavior neutralization of sulphydryl groups. J Pharm Pharmacol. 1987;39:459–65.

Makheja AN, Bailey J. The active principle in feverfew [letter]. Lancet 1981;2:1054.

Higdon, J. An evidence-based approach to vitamins and minerals. New York, NY: Thieme Medical Publishers; 2003. pp. 148–56.

Hodgson RE, Rout CC, Rocke DA, Louw NJ. Mivacurium for caesarean section in hypertensive parturients receiving magnesium sulphate therapy. Int J Obstet Anesth. 1998;7(1):12–7.

Holtmann S, Clarke AH, Scherer H, et al. The anti-motion sickness mechanism of ginger. Acta Otolaryngol (Stockh) 1989;108:168–74.

Hoover J, Kaye AD, Ibrahim IN, Fields AM, Richards T. Analysis of responses to St. Johns' Wort in the feline pulmonary vascular bed. J Herb Pharmacol. 2004;4(3):47–62.

Hopkins MP, Androff L, Benninghoff AS, et al. Ginseng face cream and unexpected vaginal bleeding. Am J Obs Gyn. 1988;159:1121–2.

Hostanska K, Reichling J, Bommer S, et al. Aqueous ethanolic extract of St. John's wort (*Hypericum perforatum* l.) induces growth inhibition and apoptosis in human malignant cells in vitro. Pharmazie 2002;57:323–31.

Houston JB, Levy G. Drug biotransformation interactions in man. VI. Acetaminophen and ascorbic acid. J Pharm Sci. 1976;65:1218–21.

Hughes EF, Jacobs BP, Berman BM. Complementary and alternative medicine. In: Tierney Jr LM, McPhee SJ, Papadakis MA, editors. Current medical diagnosis and treatment. New York, NY: Lange Medical Books/McGraw-Hill; 2004. pp. 1681–703.

Institute of Medicine. Dietary reference intakes for calcium, phosphorus, magnesium, vitamin D and fluoride. Washington, DC: National Academy Press; 2001.

Jain AK, Vargas R, Gotzowsky S, et al. Can garlic reduce levels of serum lipids? A controlled clinical study. Am J Med. 1993;94:632–5.

Jamieson DD, Duffield PH. Positive interaction of ethanol and kava resin in mice. Clin Exp Pharm Physiol. 1990;17:509–14.

Jamieson DD, Duffield PH. The antinociceptive actions of kava components in mice. Clin Exp Pharm Physiol. 1990;17:495–507.

Jang MH, Lim S, Han SM, et al. *Harpagophytum procumbens* suppresses lipopolysaccharide-stimulated expressions of cyclooxygenase-2 and inducible nitric oxide synthase in fibroblast cell line L929. J Pharmacol Sci. 2003;93:367–71.

Jellin JM, Batz F, Hitchens K, et al, eds. Ginger. Natural medicines: comprehensive database. 2nd ed. Stockton, CA: Therapeutic Research Faculty; 1999. pp. 416–8.

Jellin JM, Gregory PJ, Batz F, et al, eds. Feverfew. Natural medicines: comprehensive database. 5th ed. Stockton, CA: Therapeutic Research Faculty; 2003. pp. 541–3.

Jellin JM, Gregory PJ, Batz F, et al, eds. Ginseng, American, Ginseng, Panax. Natural medicines: comprehensive database. 5th ed. Stockton, CA: Therapeutic Research Faculty; 2003. pp. 614–9.

Jellin JM, Gregory PJ, Batz F, et al, eds. Kava. Natural medicines: comprehensive database. 4th ed. Stockton, CA: Therapeutic Research Faculty; 2002. pp. 759–61.

Jellin JM, Gregory PJ, Batz F, et al, eds. Kava. Natural medicines: comprehensive database. 5th ed. Stockton, CA: Therapeutic Research Faculty; 2003. pp. 788–91.

Jellin JM, Gregory PJ, Batz F, et al, eds. St. John's Wort. Natural medicines: comprehensive database. 4th ed. Stockton, CA: Therapeutic Research Faculty; 2002. pp. 1180–4.

Jie YH, Cammisuli S, Baggiolini M, et al. Immunomodulatory effects of panax ginseng: CA Meyer in the mouse. Agents Actions Suppl. 1984;15:386–91.

Johnston CS, Martin LJ, Cai X. Antihistamine effect of supplemental ascorbic acid and neutrophil chemotaxis. J Am Coll Nutr. 1992;11(2):172–6.

Jones BD, Runikis AM. Interactions of ginseng with phenelzine. J Clin Psychopharm 1987;7:201–2.

Jurgensen K, Stevens C, eds. Finally, a ban on ephedra. USA Today Newspaper. Moon CA (pub), April 13, 2004, p. 22A.

Kanerva L, Estlander T, Jolanki R. Occupational allergic contact dermatitis from spices. Contact Dermat. 1996;35:157–62.

Kaplan SA, Volpe MA, Te AE. Prospective, 1-year trial using saw palmetto versus finasteride in the treatment of category III prostatitis/chronic pelvic pain syndrome. J Urol. 2004;171:284–8.

Kaye AD, Clarke RC, Sabar R, et al. Herbal medicines: current trends in anesthesiology practice – a hospital survey. J Clin Anesth. 2000;12(6):468–71.

Kaye AD, Grogono AW. Fluid and electrolyte physiology. In: Miller RD, Cucchiara RF, Miller ED Jr, et al, editors. Anesthesia. Vol. 1. 5th ed. Philadelphia, PA: Churchill Livingstone; 2000. pp. 1586–612.

Kaye AD, Kucera I, Sabar R. Perioperative anesthesia clinical considerations of alternative medicines. Anesthesiol Clin North Am. 2004;22(1):125–39.

Kaye AD, Nossaman BD, Ibrahim IN, et al. Analysis of responses of allicin, a compound from garlic, in the pulmonary vascular bed of the cat and in the rat. Eur J Pharmacol. 1995;276: 21–6.

Kaye AD, Sabar R, Vig S, et al. Nutraceuticals – current concepts and the role of the anesthesiologist. Am J Anesthesiol. 2000;27:467–71.

Kimmatkar N, Thawani V, Hingorani L, et al. Efficacy and tolerability of *Boswellia serrata* extract in treatment of osteoarthritis of knee – a randomized double blind placebo controlled trial. Phytomedicine 2003;10:3–7.

Kirch W, Schafer-Korting M, Axthelm T, et al. Interaction of atenolol with furosemide and calcium and aluminum salts. Clin Pharmacol Ther. 1981;30:429–35.

Kivisto KT, Neuvonen PJ. Effect of magnesium hydroxide on the absorption and efficacy of tolbutamide and chlorpropamide. Eur J Clin Pharmacol. 1992;42:675–9.

Kobuchi H, Ldroy-Lefaix MT, Christen Y, et al. *Ginkgo biloba* extract (Egb 761): inhibitory effect on nitric oxide production in macrophage cell line RAW 264.7. Biochem Pharmacol. 1997;53:897–903.

Konno C, Murakami M, Oshima Y, et al. Isolation and hypoglycemic activity of panaxans Q, R, S, T and U, glycans of panax ginseng roots. J Ethnopharm. 1985;14:69–74.

Konno C, Sugiyama K, Oshima Y, et al. Isolation and hypoglycemic activity of panaxans A, B, C, D and E glycans of panax ginseng roots. Planta Med. 1984;50:436–8.

Krivoy N, Pavlotzky E, Chrubasik S, et al. Effect of salicis cortex extract on human platelet aggregation. Planta Med. 2001;67:209–12.

Kuo SC, Teng CM, Lee JG, et al. Antiplatelet components in panax ginseng. Planta Med. 1990;56:164–7.

Lao TT, Tam K, Chan LY. Third trimester iron status and pregnancy outcome in non-anemic women; pregnancy unfavourably affected by maternal iron excess. Hum Reprod. 2000;15:1843–8.

Leak JA. Herbal medicine: is it an alternative or an unknown? A brief review of popular herbals used by patients in a pain and symptom management practice setting. Cur Rev Pain 1999;3:226–236.

LeBars PL, Katz MM, Berman N, et al. A placebo controlled, double-blind, randomized trial of an extract of *Ginkgo biloba* for dementia. JAMA 1997;278:1327–32.

Lecrubier Y, Clerc G, Didi R, et al. Efficacy of St. John's wort extract WS 5570 in major depression: a double-blind, placebo-controlled trial. Am J Psychiatry. 2002;159:1361–6.

Lehto P, Kivisto KT, Neuvonen PJ. The effect of ferrous sulphate on the absorption of norfloxacin, ciprofloxacin and ofloxacin. Br J Clin Pharmacol. 1994;37:82–5.

Leo MA, Lieber CS. Alcohol, vitamin A, and beta-carotene: adverse interactins, including hepatotoxicity and carcinogenicity. Am J Clin Nutr. 1999;69(6):1071–85.

Leung AY, Foster S. Encyclopedia of common natural ingredients used in food, drugs and cosmetics. 2nd ed. New York, NY: Wiley; 1996.

Lewis DP, Van Dyke DC, Willhite LA, et al. Phenytoin–folic acid interaction. Ann Pharmacother. 1995;29:726–35.

Liede KE, Haukka JK, Saxen LM, et al. Increased tendency towards gingival bleeding caused by joint effect of alpha-tocopherol supplementation and acetylsalicylic acid. Ann Med. 1998;30:542–6.

Liu JJ, Nilsson A, Oredsson S, et al. Boswellic acids trigger apoptosis via a pathway dependent on caspase-8 activation but independent on Fas/Fas ligand interaction in colon cancer HT-29 cells. Carcinogenesis 2002;23:2087–93.

Li-Weber M, Giaisi M, Baumann S, et al. The anti-inflammatory sesquiterpene lactone parthenolide suppresses CD95-mediated activation-induced-cell-death in T-cells. Cell Death Differ. 2002;9:1256–65.

Loikili NG, Noel E. Blaison G, et al. Update of pernicious anemia. A retrospective study of 49 cases] [French] Rev Med Intern. 2004;25(8):556–61.

Ma J, Betts NM. Zinc and copper intakes and their major food sources for older adults in the 1994–96 continuing survey of food intakes by individuals (CSFII). J Nutr. 2000; 130:2838–43.

Mak S, Newton GE. Vitamin C augments the inotropic response to dobutamine in humans with normal left ventricular function. Circulation 2001;103:826–30.

Makheja AN, Bailey JM. A platelet phospholipase inhibitor from the medicinal herb feverfew (*Tanacetum parthenium*). Prostaglandins Leukot Med. 1982;8:653–60.

Malabanan AO, Holick MF. Vitamin D and bone health in postmenopausal women. J Womens Health (Larchmt). 2003;12(2):151–6.

Marcocci L. The nitric oxide scavenging properties of *Ginkgo biloba* extract Egb761: inhibitory effect on nitric oxide production in the macrophage cell line RAW 264.7. Biochem Pharmacol. 1997;53:897–903.

Marcuard SP, Albernaz L, Khazanie PG. Omeprazole therapy causes malabsorption of cyanocobalamin (vitamin B12). Ann Intern Med. 1994;120:211–5.

Markowitz JS, Donovan JL, Devane CL, et al. Multiple doses of saw palmetto (*Serenoa repens*) did not alter cytochrome P450 2D6 and 3A4 activity in normal volunteers. Clin Pharmacol Ther. 2003;74:536–42.

Marles RJ, Kaminski J, Arnason JT, et al. A bioassay of inhibition of serotonin release from bovine platelets. J Nat Prod. 1992;55:1044–56.

Mason L, Moore RA, Derry S, et al. Systematic review of topical capsaicin for the treatment of chronic pain. BMJ 2004;328:991.

Mauro VF, Mauro LS, Kleshinski JF, et al. Impact of *Ginkgo biloba* on the pharmacokinetics of digoxin. Am J Ther. 2003;10:247–51.

McCarron DA, Hatton D. Dietary calcium and lower blood pressure: we can all benefit. JAMA 1996;275:1128–9.

McCarty DJ, Csuka M, McCarthy G, et al. Treatment of pain due to fibromyalgia with topical capsaicin: a pilot study. Semin Arthr Rheum. 1994;23:41–7.

Melchart D, Walther E, Linde K, et al. *Echinacea* root extracts for the prevention of upper respiratory tract infections: a double-blind, placebo-controlled, randomized trial. Arch Fam Med. 1998;7:541–5.

Mezquita-Raya P, Munoz-Torres M, De Dios Luna J, et al. Relation between vitamin D insufficiency, bone density, and bone metabolism in healthy postmenopausal women. J Bone Miner Res. 2001;16:1408–15.

Mikszewski JS, Saunders HM, Hess RS. Zinc-associated acute pancreatitis in a dog. J Small Anim Pract. 2003;44(4):177–80.

Miller LG. Herbal medicinals. Arch Intern Med. 1998;158:2200–11.

Millqvist E. Cough provocation with capsaicin is an objective way to test sensory hyperreactivity in patients with asthma-like symptoms. Allergy 2000;55:546–50.

Minerals. Drugs facts and comparisons. Facts and comparisons. St. Louis, MO: 2000.

MMWR Morb Mortal Wkly Rep 1996;45:689–93.

Molloy TP, Wilson CW. Protein-binding of ascorbic acid. 2. Interaction with acetyl-salicylic acid. Int J Vitam Nutr Res. 1980;50:387–92.

Moussard C, Alber D, Toubin MM, et al. A drug used in traditional medicine, Harpagophytum procumbens: no evidence for NSAID-like effect on whole blood eicosanoid production in human. Prostaglandins Leukot Essent Fatty Acids. 1992;46:283–6.

Mukherjee S, Banerjee SK, Maulik M, et al. Protection against acute adriamycin-induced cardiotoxicity by garlic: role of endogenous antioxidants and inhibition of TNF-alpha expression. BMC Pharmacol. 2003;3:16.

Murphy J, Heptinstall S, Mitchell JR, et al. Randomized double-blind, placebo-controlled trial of feverfew in migraine prevention. Lancet 1988;2:189–192.

Naggar VF, Khalil SA. Effect of magnesium trisilicate on nitrofurantoin absorption. Clin Pharmacol Ther. 1979;25:857–63.

Nau H, Tzimas G, Mondry M, et al. Antiepileptic drugs alter endogenous retinoid concentrations: a possible mechanism of teratogenesis of anticonvulsant therapy. Life Sci. 1995;57:53–60.

Neil HAW, Silagy CA, Lancaster T, et al. Garlic powder in the treatment of moderate hyperlipidemia: a controlled trial and meta-analysis. J R Coll Physician. 1996;30:329–34.

Nelson MH, Cobb SE, Shelton J. Variations in parthenolide content and daily dose of feverfew products. Am J Health Syst Pharm. 2002;59:1527–31.

Ness J, Sherman FT, Pan CX. Alternative medicine: what the data say about common herbal therapies. Geriatrics 1999;54:33–43.

Ng TB, Li WW, Yeung HW. Effects of ginsenosides, lectins and *Momordica charantia* insulin like peptide on corticosterone production by isolated rat adrenal cells. J Ethnopharm. 1987;21:21–9.

Nowakowska E, Ostrowicz A, Chodera A. Kava-kava preparations-alternative anxiolytics. Pol Merkuriusz Lek. 1998;4:179–80.

Nurtjahja-Tjendraputra E, Ammit AJ, Roufogalis BD, et al. Effective anti-platelet and COX-1 enzyme inhibitors from pungent constituents of ginger. Thromb Res. 2003; 111:259–65.

Oshima Y, Kkonno C, Hikono H. Isolation and hypoglycemic activity of panaxans I, J, K and L, glycans of panax ginseng roots. J Ethnopharm. 1985;14:255–9.

Osman MA, Patel RB, Schuna A, et al. Reduction in oral penicillamine absorption by food, antacid, and ferrous sulfate. Clin Pharmacol Ther. 1983;33:465–70.

Palmer BV, Montgomery AC, Monterio JC, et al. Ginseng and mastalgia. BMJ 1978;1:1284.

Paolisso G, D'Amore A, Galzerano D, et al. Daily vitamin E supplements improve metabolic control but not insulin secretion in elderly type II diabetic patients. Diabetes Care 1993a;16:1433–7.

Paolisso G, D'Amore A, Giugliano D, et al. Pharmacologic doses of vitamin E improve insulin action in healthy subjects and non-insulin-dependent diabetic patients. Am J Clin Nutr. 1993b;57:650–6.

Parnham MJ. Benefit–risk assessment of the squeezed sap of the purple coneflower (*E. purpurea*) for long term oral immunostimulation. Phytomedicine 1996;3:95–102.

Patterson BH, Levander OA. Naturally occurring selenium compounds in cancer chemoprevention trials: a workship summary. Cancer Epidemiol Biomarkers Prev. 1997;6:63–9.

Peters H, Kieser M, Holscher U. Demonstration of the efficacy of *Ginkgo biloba* special extract EGB 761 on intermittent claudication – a placebo controlled, double-blind multicenter trial. Vasa 1998;27:106–10.

Pittler M, Ernst E. Feverfew for preventing migraine. Cochrane Database Syst Rev. 2004;1:CD002286.

Prasad AS, Halsted JA, Nadimi M. Syndrome of iron deficiency anemia, hepatosplenomegaly, hypogonadism, dwarfism, and geophagia. Am J Med. 1961;31:532–46.

Prasad AS. Zinc deficiency in women, infants, and children. J Am Coll Nutr. 1996;15:113–20.

Queiroz E, Ramalho A, Saunders C, et al. Vitamin A status in diabetic children. Diabetes Nutr Metab. 2000;13(5):298–9.

Rabinovitz H, Friedensohn A, Leibovitz A, et al. Effect of chromium supplementation on blood glucose and lipid levels in type 2 diabetes mellitus elderly patients. Int J Vitam Nutr Res. 2004;74(3):178–82.

Randolph RK, Gellenbeck K, Stonebrook K, et al. Regulation of human immune gene expression as influenced by a commercial blended *Echinacea* product: preliminary studies. Exp Biol Med (Maywood). 2003;228:1051–6.

Reuter HD. *Allium sativum* and *Allium ursinum*, part 2: pharmacology and medicinal applications. Phytomedicine 1995;2:73–91.

Rivers JM, Devine MM. Plasma ascorbic acid concentrations and oral contraceptives. Am J Clin Nutr. 1972;25:684–9.

Robbers JE, Tyler VE. Tyler's herbs of choice: the therapeutic use of phytomedicinals. New York, NY: The Haworth Herbal Press; 1999.

Rosenblatt M, Mindel J. Spontaneous hyphema associated with ingestion of *Ginkgo biloba* extract [letter]. NEJM 1997;336:1108.

Rosenthal G. Interaction of ascorbic acid and warfarin [letter]. JAMA 1971;215:1671.

Rowin J, Lewis SL. Spontaneous bilateral subdural hematomas associated with chronic *Ginkgo biloba* ingestion have also occurred. Neurology 1996;46:1775–6.

Sandstead HH. Is zinc deficiency a public health problem? Nutrition 1995;11:87–92.

Sauberlich HE. A history of scurvy and vitamin C. In: Packer L, Fuchs J, editors. Vitamin C in health and disease. New York, NY: Marcel Decker; 1997. pp. 1–24.

Schmid B, Kotter I, Heide L. Pharmacokinetics of salicin after oral administration of a standardised willow bark extract. Eur J Clin Pharmacol. 2001;57:387–91.

Schmid B, Ludtke R, Selbmann HK, et al. Efficacy and tolerability of a standardized willow bark extract in patients with osteoarthritis: randomized placebo-controlled, double blind clinical trial. Phytother Res. 2001;15:344–50.

Schubert W, Eriksson U, Edgar B, et al. Flavonoids in grapefruit juice inhibit the in-vitro hepatic metabolism of 17 beta-estradiol. Eur J Drug Metab Pharmacokinet. 1995; 20:219–24.

Seitz U, Schule A, Gleitz J. [3H]-Monoamine uptake inhibition properties of kava pyrones. Planta Med. 1997;63:548–9.

Semba RD, Garrett E, Johnson BA, et al. Vitamin D deficiency among older women with and without disability. Am J Clin Nutr. 2000;72:1529–34.

Shader RI, Greenblatt DJ. Phenelzine and the dream machine-ramblings and reflections [editorial]. J Clin Psychopharmacol. 1985;5:65.

Shiba K, Sakamoto M, Nakazawa Y, et al. Effects of antacid on absorption and excretion of new quinolones. Drugs 1995;49(suppl 2):360–361.

Shils ME, Olson JA, Shike M, eds. Modern nutrition in health and disease. 9th ed. Baltimore, MD: Williams and Wilkins; 1999, p. 210, 860, 1422, 1424, 1772.

Davolos A, Castillo J, Marrugat J, et al. Body iron stores and early neurologic deterioration in acute cerebral infarction. Neurology 2000;54:1568–74.

Shinde Urmila A, Sharma G, Xu Yan J, et al. Anti-diabetic activity and mechanism of action of chromium chloride. Exp Clin Endocrinol Diabetes. 2004;112(5):248–52.

Siegenberg D, Baynes RD, Bothwell TH, et al. Ascorbic acid prevents the dose-dependent inhibitory effects of polyphenols and phytates on nonheme-iron absorption. Am J Clin Nutr. 1991;53:537–41.

Silagy CA, Neil HAW. A meta-analysis of the effect of garlic on blood pressure. J Hypertension. 1994;12:463–68.

Singh YN. Effects of kava on neuromuscular transmission and muscular contractility. J Ethnopharm. 1983;7:267–76.

Skidmore-Roth L. Kava. Mosby's handbook of herbs and natural supplements. St. Louis, MO: Mosby-Harcourt Health Sciences; 2001. pp. 486–90.

Sotaniemi EA, Haapakkoski E, Rautio A, et al. Ginseng therapy in non-insulin dependent diabetic patients. Diabetes Care 1995;18:1373–5.

Staffeldt B, Kerb R, Brockmoller J, et al. Pharmacokinetics of hypericin and pseudohypericin after local intake of the *Hypericum perforatum* extract LI160 in healthy volunteers. J Geriatr Psych Neurol. 1994;7:S47–S53.

Streeter AM, Goulston KJ, Bathur FA, et al. Cimetidine and malabsorption of cobalamin. Dig Dis Sci. 1982;27:13–6.

Surh YJ, Lee SS. Capsaicin in hot chili pepper: carcinogen, co-carcinogen or anticarcinogen? Food Chem Toxicol. 1996;34:313–6.

Tatro D, ed. A to Z drug facts. St. Louis, MO: Facts and Comparisons; 1999.

Taylor JA, Weber W, Standish L, et al. Efficacy and safety of *Echinacea* in treating upper respiratory tract infections in children: a randomized controlled trial. JAMA 2003;290: 2824–30.

Thys-Jacobs S, Starkey P, Bernstein D, et al. Calcium carbonate and the premenstrual syndrome: effects on premenstrual and menstrual symptoms. Premenstrual Syndrome Study Group. Am J Obstet Gynecol. 1998;179:444–52.

Tinkleman DG, Avner SE. Ephedrine therapy in asthmatic children. Clinical tolerance and absence of side effects. JAMA 1977;237:553–7.

Tokmoda M, Shimada K, Konno M, et al. Partial structure of panax A: a hypoglycemic glycan of panax ginseng roots. Planta Med. 1984;50:436–8.

Tsao SM, Hsu CC, Yin MC. Garlic extract and two diallyl sulphides inhibit methicillin-resistant *Staphylococcus aureus* infection in BALB/cA mice. J Antimicrob Chemother. 2003;52:974–80.

Uebelhack R, Franke L, Schewe HJ. Inhibition of platelet MAO-B by kava pyrone-enriched extract from *Piper methysticum* Forster (kava-kava). Pharmacopsychiatry 1998;31:187–92.

Unger M, Frank A. Simultaneous determination of the inhibitory potency of herbal extracts on the activity of six major cytochrome P450 enzymes using liquid chromatography/mass spectrometry and automated online extraction. Rapid Commun Mass Spectrom. 2004;18:2273–81.

Ursini F, Heim S, Kiess M, et al. Dual function of the selenoprotein PHGPx during sperm maturation. Science 1999;285(5432):1393–6.

Utiger R. The need for more vitamin D. N Engl J Med. 1998;338:828–9.

Uusitupa MI, Mykkanen L, Siitonen O, et al. Chromium supplementation in impaired glucose tolerance of elderly: effects on blood glucose, plasma insulin, C-peptide and lipid levels. Br J Nutr. 1992;68:209–16.

Vale S. Subarachnoid hemorrhage associated with *Ginkgo biloba* [letter]. Lancet 1998;352:36.

Vitamins. Drug facts and comparisons. St. Louis, MO: Facts and Comparisons; 2000. pp. 6–33.

Volz HP, Kieser M. Kava-kava extract WS 1490 versus placebo in anxiety disorders a randomized placebo-controlled 25-week outpatient trial. Pharmacopsychiatry 1997;30:1–5.

Wasser WG, Feldman NS, D'Agati VD. Chronic renal failure after ingestion of over-the-counter chromium picolinate [letter]. Ann Intern Med. 1997;126:410.

Webb DI, Chodos RB, Mahar CQ, et al. Mechanism of vitamin B12 malabsorption in patients receiving colchicines. N Engl J Med. 1968;279:845–50.

Wegener T, Lupke NP. Treatment of patients with arthrosis of hip or knee with an aqueous extract of devil's claw (*Harpagophytum procumbens* DC). Phytother Res. 2003;17:1165–72.

Weimann J. Toxicity of nitrous oxide. Best Pract Res Clin Anaesthesiol. 2003;17(1):47–61.

Williams SR, Clark RF, Dunford JV. Contact dermatitis associated with capsaicin: Hunan hand syndrome. Ann Emerg Med. 1995;25:713–5.

Winslow LC, Kroll DJ. Herbs as medicines. Arch Intern Med. 1998;158:2192–9.

Yokozawa T, Kobayashi T, Oura H, et al. Studies on the mechanism of hypoglycemic activity of ginsenoside-Rb2 in streptozotocin-diabetic rats. Chem Pharm Bull. 1985;33:869–72.

Zeybek N, Gorgulu S, Yagci G, et al. The effects of *Ginkgo biloba* extract (EGb 761) on experimental acute pancreatitis. J Surg Res. 2003;115:286–93.

Zhang S. Yao S. The protective effect of propofol on erythrocytes during cardiopulmonary bypass. [Clinical Trial. Journal Article. Randomized Controlled Trial]. J Tongji Med Univ. 2001;21(1):65–7.

Zhou DL, Kitts DD. Peripheral blood mononuclear cell production of TNF-alpha in response to North American ginseng stimulation. Can J Physiol Pharmacol. 2002;80:1030–3.

Chapter 11

Importance of Placebo Effect in Pain Management

Charles Brown, MD and Paul J. Christo, MD

Introduction

The word placebo is derived from the Latin verb "to please" and, as early as 1811, appeared in the Hooper's Medical Dictionary as a medical treatment aimed at pleasing – a placebo was defined as "an epithet given to any medication adopted more to please than to benefit the patient (Hooper 1817)." In the modern day era, Tilburt et al. refer to the placebo effect as "positive clinical outcomes caused by a treatment that is not attributable to its known physical properties or mechanism of action (Tilburt et al. 2008)."

Despite the lack of specific action of the placebo on the condition being treated, the placebo often provides benefit. In 1955, Henry Beecher, the first chairman of anesthesia at Massachusetts General Hospital, published a seminal article, "The Powerful Placebo," in which he observed a high rate of response to placebo administration. In this article, he observed, "It is evident that placebos have a high degree of therapeutic effectiveness in treating subjective responses, decided improvement, interpreted under the unknown technique as a real therapeutic effect, being produced in $35.2 \pm 2.2\%$ of cases (Beecher 1955)." Beecher observed this high degree of therapeutic effectiveness across a variety of clinical conditions, the breadth of which has been confirmed in subsequent scientific trials (Table 11.1). Since its publication, Beecher's article has become one of the most cited analyses of the powerful therapeutic effect of the placebo.

In recent years, however, the magnitude of the placebo effect has been questioned. Even the results of Beecher's landmark article have been criticized because none of the studies he referenced was properly controlled. In fact, recent reviewers have concluded that in fact no evidence of placebo effect could be found in any of the original studies cited by him (Kiene 1997). Nevertheless, the use of the placebo continues to be ubiquitous in clinical medicine today, both as a clinical intervention and as a research tool.

Mechanism for the Placebo Effect

Several theories have been proposed for the mechanism of the placebo effect.

N. Vadivelu et al. (eds.), *Essentials of Pain Management*,
DOI 10.1007/978-0-387-87579-8_11, © Springer Science+Business Media, LLC 2011

Table 11.1 **Partial list of conditions in which the placebo effect has been shown to be effective.**

ADHD
Anxiety
Asthma
BPH
Chronic fatigue
Crohn's disease
Depression
Epilepsy
Erectile dysfunction
Ulcers
Headache
CHF
Hypertension
Nausea
Pain
Parkinson's
Psoriatic arthritis
Reflux
Ulcerative colitis
Multiple sclerosis

ADHD = attention-deficit hyperactivity disorder,
BPH = benign prostatic hyperplasia,
CHF = congestive heart failure.

Cognitive Theory (Expectation Theory)

The cognitive theory states that patient expectations are critical in the placebo response. The administration of a placebo creates an expectation of a certain response, and the expectation of this response creates a biological effect. The mechanisms whereby expectancies might produce biological effects are many. They include (1) a reduction in anxiety which could aid immune system functioning, (2) changes in cognition or coping mechanisms, or (3) changes in behavior that would improve health outcomes (Stewart-Williams and Podd 2004). Patient expectations can be quite specific, and studies have shown that expectations of pain relief in particular body parts lead to the expected effect in that body part alone (Benedetti et al. 1999, Montgomery and Kirsch 1996).

Conditioning Theory

The classic example of conditioning theory is the Pavlovian experiment on dogs, in which administration of food was paired with the ringing of a bell. Over time, the ringing of the bell alone would produce salivation in the dogs. In this experiment, a neutral stimulus (the bell) paired with an unconditional stimulus (food) elicited an unconditioned response (salivation). Over time, the neutral stimulus alone elicited a response similar to the unconditional response and became a conditioned stimulus capable of eliciting a conditioned response (salivation). With respect to the placebo effect, the placebo drug represents the conditioned stimulus, and the beneficial effect is the conditioned response.

The biological effects of conditioning can be profound and varied. For instance, in 1975, Ader and Cohen showed that a flavoring agent administered with an immunosuppressant produced profound immune suppression. After conditioning, the administration of the flavoring agent alone decreased the immune response (Ader and Cohen 1975). In 1973, Laska and Sunshine demonstrated a similar conditioning response to pain medication. In their study, patients were first given analgesics at different strengths, and subjects experienced pain relief in proportion to the strength of pain medication administered. Later, patients were instead given a placebo medication. Those patients who had experienced greater pain relief from the higher strength analgesic during the first arm of the study reported greater pain relief with the administration of the placebo. In effect, the patients' prior analgesic experience predicted the efficacy of the placebo (Laska and Sunshine 1973).

Endogenous Opioids
The transmission of endogenous opioids may be responsible for placebo analgesia by fostering pain suppression. Using molecular imaging techniques, Zubieta et al. examined the activity of the endogenous opioid system in patients with chronic pain. They found that placebo agents could activate regional opioid neurotransmission, and this activation correlated with lower pain ratings (Zubieta et al. 2005). To further test this mechanism, Levine et al. examined whether an opioid antagonist, naloxone, could block placebo-induced pain relief. They found that among the subset of patients whose pain improved with placebo administration, the added administration of naloxone inhibited the pain relief (Levine et al. 1978). This suggests that placebo-induced analgesia was mediated by the release of endogenous opioids.

Placebo Characteristics
Active Agents and Specific Therapeutic Benefit
The specific therapeutic benefit of an active agent is the difference in efficacy between an active agent and a placebo. The overall clinical benefit of the active agent is therefore the sum of the benefit from the specific therapeutic effect of the active agent and the benefit from the placebo effect. Because of this, active agents will usually have an efficacy greater than that of a placebo.

The Response to Placebo
In his landmark paper on the power of the placebo, Beecher found that the number of patients who responded to a placebo varied between 15 and 53% (Beecher 1955). Other investigators examining such various diseases as headaches, low back pain, and angina have even reported response rates higher than 50%. The oft-cited statement that the response rate to placebo is 30% likely derives from the average of Beecher's original observations.

These figures, however, represent the average of many individual placebo responses and do not indicate how each member of the group responds. One might imagine all members of the group responding equally well or in contrast, some members responding extremely well, and other members not responding at all, with a group response average of 30%. Levine et al. demonstrated this concept in a study of pain following tooth extraction. When given placebo medication, he found that 39% of the patients had some response to the placebo while 61% had no response at all (Levine et al. 1979). Thus, he was able to categorize individual patients as "placebo responders" or "placebo non-responders."

Predicting which individuals would respond to placebo administration becomes important, but this information is difficult to identify. Various studies have determined that intelligence or susceptibility poorly predicts the response to placebo. Furthermore, gender has been shown to be a poor predictor of placebo response, and there have been varied results in attempting to link personality traits with placebo response. In addition, people who respond to placebo in one setting may not respond in another setting (Oken 2008, Harrington 1997). However, adherence to a placebo regimen has been shown to be predictive of high placebo response (Horwitz et al. 1990).

Perceived Effects and True Effects from Placebo Agents

In quantifying the placebo effect during a clinical trial, it is important to understand that this effect is composed of multiple components. To better understand these components, consider a clinical trial that compares three groups of patients: those treated with an active agent, those treated with a placebo agent, and those receiving no treatment. As discussed earlier, the specific therapeutic benefit of the active drug is the difference in efficacy between the active drug and the placebo. Similarly, the specific effect of the placebo is the difference in efficacy between the placebo group and the untreated group. This specific effect of the placebo itself is called the "true placebo effect." In contrast, the overall efficacy of the placebo is defined as the "perceived placebo effect (Ernst and Resch 1995)."

The increased efficacy seen in the perceived placebo effect compared to that measured in the true placebo effect results from several factors. First, the symptoms of a disease may change over time, so the natural history of the disease itself may contribute to the perceived placebo effect. For instance, it is well known that acute episodes of low back pain often significantly resolve within 4–6 weeks. A clinical trial comparing an active agent against a placebo during this time period would demonstrate a large perceived placebo effect, when in fact the improvement in clinical symptoms would likely be expected from understanding that acute low back pain is usually self-resolving.

A second contributor to the perceived placebo effect is the change over time in measured symptoms of a disease due to biologic fluctuation. In fact, many biologic variables such as temperature, blood pressure, and heart rate fluctuate around a mean value, and over time these values will show statistical regression to the mean value. Clinical trials will often enroll patients above a defined measured variable, such as a blood pressure. A certain percentage of patients with high blood pressure at the time of enrollment will often have mean blood pressures that are much lower than the cutoff, but are selected into the trial because of the biologic variability. Over time, the measured blood pressure will show regression to the mean and contribute to the perceived placebo benefit.

Finally, the perceived placebo benefit is potentially increased by any beneficial factor that would change over the course of the clinical trial. For instance, the skill of an individual doctor might increase over time in a way that lessens disease progression. Similarly, characteristics of the patient might change over time. For example, a patient with "white coat hypertension" might become more comfortable after repeated office visits over the course of a trial, with a subsequent decline in measured blood pressure. Each of these examples would contribute to the perceived placebo effect, but would not affect the true placebo effect (Ernst and Resch 1995).

Nocebo Effect

In addition to beneficial side effects from the placebo, patients may also experience unwanted side effects such as headache, fatigue, or drowsiness. These harmful effects are termed nocebo effects. In 2002, Barsky et al. conducted a literature search of articles related to non-specific medication side effects, and they identified several factors associated with increased nocebo effect. These factors included patient expectation of adverse effects before beginning therapy, prior experiences of medication consumption leading to adverse symptoms, psychological co-morbidity such as depression or anxiety, and other situational factors. Patients who suffer from chronic pain are often characterized by several of these factors and are thereby at increased risk for nocebo effects (Barsky et al. 2002).

Placebo Sag

After patients have experienced numerous treatment failures, they often exhibit a decrease in placebo response rate. This phenomenon is termed placebo sag and is frequently seen in chronic pain patients who have failed numerous therapies. Conversely, in patients who have had treatment successes, the placebo effect may be enhanced with further intervention. Over time, the placebo sag often proves particularly problematic in chronic pain patients because the overall effect of therapeutic medicines declines when the non-specific placebo component of the therapy inevitably sags.

Placebos and Procedures

The placebo response can also be evident with procedures and medical devices. A particularly powerful example of the effect of placebo was published in the *New England Journal of Medicine* in 1959. For the 20 years prior to this article, angina had been treated by ligation of the internal mammary artery, under the assumption that blood flow to the myocardium could be increased. However, Cobb et al. showed that patients who were anesthetized and received sham incisions fared just as well as those with the real procedure. In fact, studies showed that both interventions could produce significant (70%) decrease in angina and increase in exercise tolerance (Cobb et al. 1959). This study conclusively demonstrated that procedures could have a powerful placebo effect.

On occasion, the placebo effect from an invasive procedure can be even more powerful than the placebo effect from medication. In 2006, Kaptchuk et al. examined the effects of sham acupuncture compared to a sham pill on patients with arm pain due to repetitive stress injury. They found that over the course of the trial, improvement in pain score and symptom severity scale increased in the group receiving sham acupuncture more than in the group receiving the sham pill (Kaptchuk et al. 2006).

Active Placebo

Although placebo agents are often chosen in blinded clinical trials because they do not have clinical effects, patients may be able to differentiate placebo from active drug and thereby unblind the study. To make this awareness difficult, active placebos may be used. An active placebo is a drug that has no effect on the condition being treated but does simulate medical therapy, often through other side effects. For instance, consider a trial investigating chemotherapeutic agents, which often have known side effects of nausea and vomiting. An active agent would have no specific therapeutic effect on the patient's cancer, but would provoke nausea and vomiting.

The Placebo as a Therapeutic Intervention

Employing the placebo effect as a therapeutic intervention is controversial. Some clinicians argue that the benefits of the placebo effect might be quite useful in treating patients with conditions that are refractory to standard medical therapy. Others argue that the use of a placebo in the guise of therapy is deceptive, unethical practice and undermines the physician–patient relationship of trust.

Nevertheless, it appears that nationwide the practice of prescribing placebo treatments is quite pervasive. In 2009, Tilburt et al. published the results of a survey of 1200 internists and rheumatologists in the United States regarding their attitudes toward placebo therapy (Tilburt et al. 2008). Over 60% of respondents agreed that it is permissible to prescribe placebo therapy primarily to promote patients' expectations. When then queried if this permissive attitude toward prescribing placebo treatment applied to clinical practice, almost half of all respondents stated that they had recommended placebo treatment for patients at least once in the past year. Moreover, when placebo treatments were prescribed, 68% of prescribers described the proposed therapy as "medicine not typically used for your condition but might benefit you."

Interestingly, the authors found that the type of placebo prescribed was varied, but that purely inert substances such as sugar pills or saline were prescribed less than 5% of the time. The most frequently prescribed placebo treatments included multivitamins and over-the-counter analgesics. Alarmingly, more than one-quarter of prescribed placebo treatments were sedatives or antibiotics – medicines with potentially deleterious effects. Thus, practice patterns alone suggest that using the placebo effect as a therapeutic intervention is quite widespread.

Given the ubiquitous nature of placebo treatment in clinical practice, determining the beneficial effect of this form of therapy is paramount. Clearly this task is difficult. As noted earlier, since the publication of Beecher's landmark article, "The Powerful Placebo," the placebo effect has been reported to be effective in 30–40% of cases. However, differentiating the improvement in a clinical condition due to the placebo itself, as opposed to improvement due to the natural course of the disease or other factors, is challenging.

In 2001, Hrobjartsson et al. attempted to answer the question of whether placebo treatment conferred therapeutic benefit by systematically reviewing 130 clinical trials in which patients were assigned to either placebo or no treatment. They looked at the difference in outcome between the placebo and the no-treatment groups, rather than looking at the effect of the intervention arm of each trial. The underlying disease processes in each trial were diverse and involved 40 clinical conditions, such as asthma, schizophrenia, and chronic pain syndromes. In their analysis, they found no significant placebo effect in trials with binary outcomes, either subjective or objectively measured, nor in trials with continuous, objective outcomes. However, they did find a significant difference in trials with continuous subjective outcomes and in trials where pain was investigated (Hróbjartsson and Gøtzsche 2001). The authors acknowledged several limitations to their study, including the inability to blind the untreated group, the effects of reporting bias, and the inability to assess the effects of the physician–patient relationship independent from the placebo itself. Moreover, critics contend that the ability to find a placebo effect in subgroup analysis was limited due to sample size, and in fact, the authors did show statistical significance of the placebo effect in one important group – chronic pain patients. Critics also report that some of the referenced trials were methodologically poor or were studying serious conditions, whose outcomes may have masked any placebo effect (Bailar 2001). However, in general the authors make a powerful argument that the clinical effect of placebo therapy may be less impressive than generally thought.

The questionable efficacy of the placebo effect must be considered when deciding whether the benefits outweigh the risks of placebo therapy. As previously mentioned, some placebo therapy may cause deleterious effects, such as a sedative prescription leading to delirium, respiratory compromise, and addiction, or inappropriate antibiotic therapy leading to further antibiotic resistance. Yet, other risks of placebo therapy may be more subtle though just as dangerous. In an accompanying editorial, Bailar writes with respect to placebos that "they may divert patients from seeking more effective treatments, they may mask symptoms that need attention, they may add to the cost of treatment. . .this deception may damage the doctor patient relationship in subtle ways (Bailar 2001)."

The Placebo and Clinical Trials

Placebos have been commonly used in clinical trials in an attempt to understand specific effects of a drug or intervention on a clinical condition. Typical study designs include open-label study, single-blinded study, double-blinded study, and crossover study (Table 11.2).

Table 11.2 Examples of research study designs.

Study design	Explanation
Open label	The patient and physician know what therapy the patient is receiving
Single blinded	Although the physician knows what therapy each patient is receiving, the patients are unaware
Double blinded	Both the patient and the physician are unaware of what therapy the patient is receiving
Crossover	The patient receives both the placebo and the active therapy in a sequential, blinded fashion

However, allowing patients to receive inert agents during a placebo-controlled trial has been controversial, especially when patients who are treated with placebo forgo effective therapy.

In 2001, Emanuel et al. argued that two polarized schools of thought have emerged to guide ethical decision-making in placebo-controlled trials (Emanuel et al. 2001). The first school of thought argues that no drug should be approved unless it demonstrates superior efficacy compared to the placebo or no treatment. They argue that trials using standard therapy as the control are often methodologically flawed, due to such factors as variable responses to drugs, high rates of spontaneous improvements, and large placebo effect even with standard therapy. This school of thought values the scientific rigor of placebo-controlled trials and argues that no drug should be approved unless it is shown to be effective in comparison to placebo.

The second school of thought argues that the current therapy for a particular condition must always act as the control group in a clinical trial if it is effective. Furthermore, they argue that withholding active treatment from the control group is unethical. Using this logic, new drugs would be tested only compared to standard therapies, not to placebo. This school of thought is supported by language within the Declaration of Helsinki, a set of ethical principles for human experimentation developed by the World Medical Association. Within this document it states, "The benefits, risks, burdens, and effectiveness of a new method should be tested against those of the best current prophylactic, diagnostic, and therapeutic methods. This does not exclude the use of the placebo, or no treatment, in studies where no proven prophylactic, diagnostic, or therapeutic method exists (World Medical Association Declaration 2000)."

However, Emanuel et al. highlight several problems with the mandated use of active controls in every clinical trial. In some cases, the discomfort or harm suffered by a patient is relatively minor and an inert placebo would cause little harm, and so forcing a clinical trial using standard therapy would not be ethically necessary. For instance, the use of a sugar pill as the control instead of celecoxib in a trial exploring treatments for chronic low back pain would not cause undue and irreparable harm. Furthermore, patients receiving placebo therapy do receive clinical attention, and this may lead to clinical improvement irrespective of the efficacy of any pharmacologic intervention. Finally, they argue that clinical trials comparing an investigational drug against standard therapy require a larger number of participants than trials using placebo. This arises because the difference in clinical effect is likely larger in the placebo-controlled trial, so researchers need a fewer number of patients in order to demonstrate a difference. In effect, a greater number of patients would be exposed to known or unknown harmful side effects of a drug in a trial using standard therapy as a control.

Consequently, an emerging consensus opinion suggests that placebo-controlled trials may be conducted ethically with certain caveats and protections in place – such as rigorous oversight and observation, exclusion of patients at increased risk for harm, limitation of the placebo period to the minimum required, and clear disclosure to the participants. In spite of this, Huston et al. feel that proponents of the policy proposed by the Helsinki Document have trouble accepting these arguments altogether or any ethical justifications for placebo-controlled trials (Huston et al. 2001). However, they also concede that proven treatment would be withheld in both placebo arms and investigational drug arms, and sometimes patients in placebo arms fare better than those patients who did not enroll in the trial at all.

In evaluating the ethics of placebo-controlled trials, placebo surgery deserves special consideration. In 1959, Cobb et al. showed no improvement in angina symptoms from ligation of the internal mammary artery when compared to sham operations. Since then, ethicists have debated whether the risks of placebo surgery outweigh the benefits. In a 2002 article in the *New England Journal of Medicine*, Horng et al. argue that trials involving placebo-controlled surgery can and must fulfill three criteria in order to be considered ethical: the trials must minimize the risk of the procedure and demonstrate that the control for the placebo surgery is necessary for validity of the test; the trials must justify the risks by showing that the risks of the placebo arm are minimal; finally, the trials must demonstrate that adequate informed consent has been obtained (Horng et al. 2002). Placebo-controlled surgeries have met and continue to meet these criteria.

Conclusion

The placebo effect can be profound. As a clinician, it is important to recognize the power of this effect, both in clinical practice and as a comparison group in controlled trials. The fiduciary trust that connects patients to their doctors demands that all clinicians consider placebo in a way that furthers the well-being of each individual patient.

Case Scenario

Charles Brown, MD and Paul J. Christo, MD

After injuring his back from lifting a piece of furniture, James, a 42-year-old man, is urged to take a multivitamin by his primary care doctor following a clinic appointment. Although the patient does not believe that the multivitamin will help, he reports a 50% pain relief in his follow-up visit 4 weeks later. The patient attributes this reduction to the multivitamin.

What could be the best possible explanation for the pain reduction?
The decrease in pain was likely due to the natural history of lower back pain: within 4–6 weeks, the symptoms from acute-onset back pain often resolve spontaneously. The perceived "placebo effect" accounts for improvements due to the natural history of the disease. The true placebo effect is the specific difference in effect observed in a trial of multivitamins for back pain patients, with some patients taking no medication and some patients taking multivitamins. This would control for any resolution of symptoms due to disease improvement. The specific therapeutic effect of the drug did not account for the observed degree of pain relief, since there is little evidence or biologic plausibility that vitamins could decrease back pain in such a short time.

Which theory of placebo action would best explain any pain relief that he experiences due to the placebo effect?
The cognitive theory of the placebo effect states that the expectations of the patient play an important role in the efficacy of the placebo, which is applicable to James. The conditioning theory would be applicable if he had previously experienced success with neuraxial blocks and subsequently responded favorably to the current procedure because of his previous successes. The endogenous opioid theory could explain his pain relief, but it is not the best answer.

Several weeks later, James develops postherpetic neuralgia and is prescribed a lidocaine patch. He is now complaining of nausea and vomiting, in addition to a moderate fatigue.

Which effect would best describe his symptoms?
The patient is suffering from a nocebo effect from the lidocaine patch: these symptoms are probably not related to the specific pharmaceutical action of the lidocaine

patch itself. If these effects helped to decrease his pain, the effects would be considered specific therapeutic drug effects or placebo effects. However, since the effects are undesirable, they are either side effects from the medication (not a choice) or nocebo effects.

Ten years later, James develops hypertension and stable angina which are well controlled with lisinopril and metoprolol and sees you regularly to manage his conditions. He would like you to consider him for a placebo-controlled clinical trial for angina. When he is not compliant with his medication regimen, his anginal symptoms escalate. As part of the trial, he would need to stop his current medication regimen.

Which consideration would make it unethical for James to participate in the trial?
When conducting a placebo-controlled trial, it is important to ensure that several ethical considerations are fulfilled. In this case, the patient suffers from unstable angina when his medications are discontinued. **Therefore, the risk to the patient would be high, and enrolling him in placebo-controlled trial and discontinuing his medications would not be ethical.** Clearly, there is a scientific rationale for improving the care of angina, and there is nothing in the vignette to suggest that the patient could not be monitored closely or would not be able to give informed consent.

References

Ader R, Cohen N. Behaviorally conditioned immunosuppression. Psychosom Med. 1975;37:333–40.

Bailar, JC. The powerful placebo and the Wizard of Oz. NEJM 2001;344:1630–2.

Barsky AJ, Saintfort R, Rogers MP, Borus JF. Nonspecific medication side effects and the nocebo phenomenon. JAMA 2002;287:622–7.

Beecher HK. The powerful placebo. JAMA 1955;159:1602–6.

Benedetti F, Arduino C, Amanzio M. Somatotopic activation of opioid systems by target-directed expectations of analgesia. J Neurosci. 1999;19:3639–48.

Cobb L, et al. An evaluation of internal mammary artery ligation by a double-blind technique. NEJM 1959;260:1115–8.

Emanuel, et al. The ethics of placebo controlled trials—a middle ground. NEJM 2001;345:915–9.

Ernst E, Resch KL. Concept of true and perceived placebo effects. BMJ 1995;311:551–3.

Harrington A. Introduction. In: Harrington A, editor. The placebo effect. Cambridge, MA: Harvard University Press; 1997. pp. 1–11.

Hooper R. A new medical dictionary. Philadelphia, PA: M. Carey and Son, Benjamin Warner, and Edward Parker; 1817.

Horng S et al. Is placebo surgery unethical? NEJM 2002;347;137–9.

Horwitz RI, Viscoli CM, Berkman L, Donaldson RM, Horwitz S, Murray CJ, et al. Treatment adherence and risk of death after a myocardial infarction. Lancet 1990;336:542–5.

Hróbjartsson A, Gøtzsche PC. Is the placebo powerless? An analysis of clinical trials comparing placebo treatment with no treatment. NEJM 2001;344:1594–602.

Huston P et al. Withholding proven treatment in clinical research. NEJM 2001;345;912–4.

Kaptchuk TJ et al. Sham device v inert pill: randomized controlled trial of two placebo treatments. BMJ 2006;332:391–7.

Kiene GS. The powerful placebo effect: fact or fiction? J Clin Epidemiol. 1997;50:1311–8.

Laska E, Sunshine A. Anticipation of analgesia: a placebo effect. Headache 1973;13:1–11.

Levine JD, Gordon NC, Bornstein JC, Fields HL. Role of pain in placebo analgesia. Proc Natl Acad Sci USA 1979;76:3528–31.

Levine JD, Gordon NC, Fields HL. The mechanism of placebo analgesia. Lancet 1978;2:654–7.

Montgomery G, Kirsch I. Mechanisms of placebo pain reduction: an empirical investigation. Psychol Sci. 1996;7:174–6.

Oken BS. Placebo effects: clinical aspects and neurobiology. Brain 2008;131:2812–23.

Stewart-Williams S, Podd J. The placebo effect: dissolving the expectancy versus conditioning debate. Psychol Bull. 2004;130:324–40.

Tilburt JC, et al. Prescribing placebo treatments: results of national survey of US internists and rheumatologists. BMJ 2008;337:1938.

World Medical Association Declaration of Helsinki: ethical principles for medical research involving human subjects. Edinburgh, Scotland: World Medical Association; October 2000.

Zubieta J, Bueller JA, Jackson LR, Scott DJ, Xu Y, Koeppe RA, Nicols TE, Stohler CS. Placebo effects mediated by endogenous opioid activity on opioid receptors. J Neurosci. 2005;25:7754–62.

Section V

Non-pharmacologic Management of Pain

Chapter 12

Psychological and Psychosocial Evaluation of the Chronic Pain Patient

Raphael J. Leo, MA, MD, Wendy J. Quinton, PhD, and Michael H. Ebert, MD

Introduction

Pain is among the most common and disabling chronic health problems in the United States (Health United States 2006). The ubiquity of chronic, non-malignant pain and the complexities encountered with its management have prompted efforts to establish theoretical models to unveil, and otherwise explicate, factors other than those which are purely physical/sensory that contribute to the perception of pain and its associated impairments. One such model, the biopsychosocial model (Engel 1980), has gained significant appeal, emphasizing the bidirectional influences of psychological states and social/environmental factors with medical disorders and their associated symptoms, including pain. Rather than dichotomizing between physical and psychological origins, the biopsychosocial perspective maintains that the experience of pain, one's presentation, and response to treatment are determined by the interaction of biological factors, the patient's psychological makeup, the presence of psychological comorbidities, and the extent of social support and extenuating environmental circumstances (Gallagher 1999, Leo 2007).

The experience of pain is multidimensional (Loeser 1982). First, there is nociception, i.e., a sensory component of the pain experience relying on the transfer of information from receptors in the periphery through nerves to the central nervous system (CNS). The second dimension involves an appraisal of the nociceptive information that the person labels as "pain." Next, there is an emotional reaction to the sensory experience, i.e., dysphoria, anxiety, hopelessness, and the appraisal that the discomfort is associated with suffering. The final, i.e., social, dimension consists of the behaviors displayed by the patient in response to the unpleasant experience. These behaviors convey to others how much distress is experienced and can be verbal, paraverbal (moaning), or non-verbal (guarding of an affected limb, splinting, wearing a neck brace, taking medication, reclining).

It has long been observed that differences exist in perceived pain severity and perceived level of impairment among individuals with comparable disease. Two individuals with similar objective clinical findings can present with very different qualitative reports of pain severity and perceived disability. For example, in one scenario, two individuals may report divergent pain severity despite comparable illness and longitudinal clinical courses, e.g., one rated as an 4 out of possible 10 and the other as a 9 out of possible 10 on a numeric pain rating scale. Conversely, consider another hypothetical scenario in which two individuals report the same pain severity, e.g., rated as an 8 out of possible 10. Despite the fact that they both invoke the same numeric rating, one cannot assume that the subjective experience of the pain is the same for both of these persons. One of the hypothetical patients may have less anxiety but greater physical discomfort than the other patient. Consequently, these scenarios illustrate that pain cannot be construed solely as a sensory experience. Instead, one's perception of pain intensity is also influenced by cognitive, affective, and social variables.

The range of biopsychosocial factors relevant to a particular patient can change throughout the various phases of pain response (Gatchel 1991). Acute and subacute pain, such as pain associated with trauma, injury, and surgery, has important adaptive and survival value. Under such circumstances, the pain signals the need for and prompts the individual to engage in some activity to remove the damaging situation to prevent further injury, tend to the injury, and seek recuperation. By contrast, chronic pain, e.g., back pain, headache, rheumatic disease, abdominal pain, neuropathies, temporomandibular pain, has little or no adaptive value, can become pathologic, and can cause dysfunction, e.g., taking on a life of its own.

Unlike patients with acute pain, those for whom pain persists are beset with multiple psychosocial stressors and sequelae. Psychological and social covariates start to play a more significant role in the overall pain experience for those with subacute and chronic pain (Banks and Kerns 1996). It is not uncommon for patients to become preoccupied with pain and perceived disability. The stress of unrelenting pain can unearth a variety of premorbid, semidormant characteristics and aspects of personality (Dersh et al. 2002), affecting mood, thought patterns, perceptions, and coping abilities. Psychological vulnerabilities may develop into psychiatric disorders. Activities and interests may be avoided due to fear of increasing pain or furthering injury, and thus interpersonal relationships and vocational endeavors may be profoundly affected. The patient may experience impatience with treatment measures, intolerance for adverse effects, and lack of follow through with rehabilitative efforts.

Neuromatrix Theory and the Biopsychosocial Model

Advances in the neuroscience of pain processing have provided support for the role of higher brain centers, i.e., those responsible for emotion and cognition, in influencing pain transmission from the periphery (Melzack 1999), lending support for the biopsychosocial approach. Abandoning the archaic Cartesian viewpoint of the brain as a passive recipient of pain information from the periphery, the neuromatrix model acknowledges that the brain is dynamically involved in the processing (inhibition, modulation, or excitation) of pain. This is thought to involve the sensory, thalamic, limbic, hypothalamic–pituitary axis (HPA), and cortical pathways (Melzack 1999, Rome and Rome 2000) (Fig. 12.1).

Normally, physical and/or psychological stress triggers mechanisms to attempt to restore homeostasis. When stress persists (e.g., in the form of ongoing pain, psychological distress, inadequate coping with environmental stressors, and persisting depression), multiple processes are set in motion that exceed the delicately balanced regulatory homeostatic mechanisms initially intended to effectively manage stress, and instead generate destructive processes perpetuating pain. Several lines of research have pointed to plausible mechanisms underlying the reciprocal relationships between pain, affective distress, and stress:

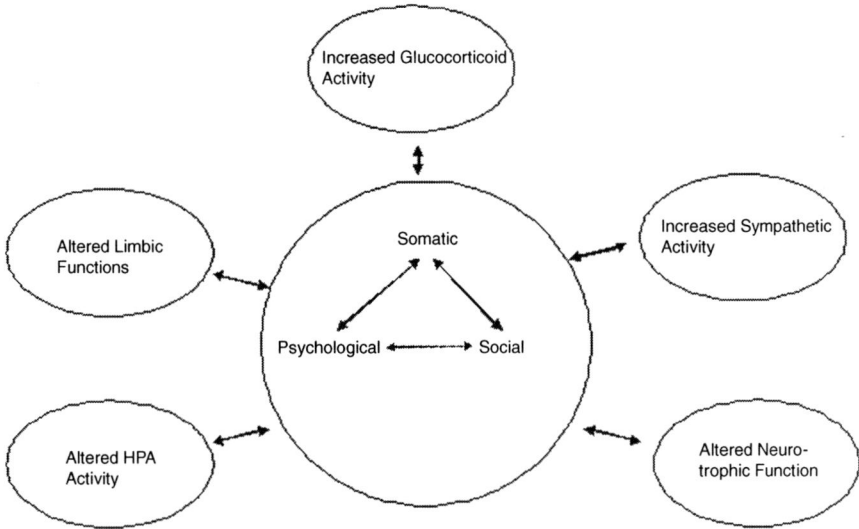

Figure 12.1   The neuromatrix model and biopsychosocial paradigm. Adapted from Melzack (1999).

- The amygdala, a limbic structure, acts as the interface between pain and emotional states; chronic negative affective states can influence the amygdala to enhance the response to pain (Neugebauer et al. 2004).
- Stress, depression, and pain can produce dysregulation of the HPA, increasing systemic sympathetic tone in the body as a whole. This, in turn, has multiple influences including activation of macrophages and heightened cortisol secretion.
  - Activation of macrophages results in the release of pro-inflammatory cytokines (leading to the lowering of pain thresholds and reductions of monoamine release)
  - Systemically, glucocorticoids can produce diffuse effects, including bone demineralization, muscle atrophy, and immune dysregulation all of which have the propensity to enhance pain and injury and thereby increasing the potential for pain. Centrally, the actions of glucocorticoid excess can interfere with serotonin and norepinephrine monoamine neurotransmission, neurotransmitters implicated in the modulation of pain information emanating from the periphery. The net effect is to disinhibit potential pro-algesic pain information relayed from the periphery.
- Stress and pain can alter the mechanisms by which the brain functions in its own maintenance (Duman and Monteggia 2006, Duric and McCarson 2005). Presumably through heightened glucocorticoid activity, stress and pain can alter the expression of neurotrophic factors, e.g., brain-derived neurotrophic factor (BDNF), reducing dendritic branching within hippocampal structures and predisposing one toward depression. Down-regulation of BDNF is preventable with antidepressant medication and, in the course of depression treatment, antidepressants can restore normal serum BDNF levels (Gonul et al. 2005).

In the composite, such evidence, and related emerging research, lends support for theoretical conceptualizations such as that of the biopsychosocial approach. Together, these lines of evidence begin to delineate the complex interactions of CNS mechanisms involved in pain and emotional processing, stress regulation, and cognitive processing.

Comprehensive Pain Assessment

Ongoing physician–patient communication is essential to the assessment of chronic pain and its biopsychosocial correlates. Comprehensive assessment requires a patient interview, physical examination, diagnostic testing when indicated, and prudent use of standardized scales and psychometric inventories. Recognizing that the chronic pain experience can be a dynamic process, the multiple objectives of assessment strategies include:

- establishing an accurate diagnosis of the underlying conditions(s) causing/exacerbating pain;
- clarification of the often uniquely individualized elements of the biopsychosocial aspects of the patient's pain experiences;
- development of a comprehensive treatment plan, and determination over the course of treatment when refinement and modification of those treatment strategies will be required;
- identification of objective and quantifiable outcome criteria against which the efficacy of implemented treatment strategies can be gauged;
- provision of the patient with an educational framework within which he/she can come to understand the interrelatedness of the biopsychosocial components of pain, the gamut of treatment approaches available, and the treatment options that are being implemented.

Biological Component

Initially, it becomes essential to obtain a detailed history of the characteristics of the pain. Toward this end, the physician must inquire into the onset of the pain, its quality or characteristics, its location, its duration, and temporal course and factors that precipitate, aggravate, and those that alleviate the discomfort (Table 12.1). Consideration must be given to the treatments and diagnostic assessments that had been undertaken previously and the perceived effectiveness of previous treatment interventions.

Rating the severity of pain can be a useful parameter upon which to rely to track responsiveness to implemented treatment strategies. As described in the introduction of this chapter, ratings of pain intensity should never be treated as a standalone measure as pain ratings can be influenced by psychosocial distress. Most commonly, an 11-point numeric rating scale (NRS), rated from $0 =$ no pain to $10 =$ worst pain possible, is employed. Alternative pain intensity measures include the visual analog scale (VAS) and the verbal rating scale (VRS). The VAS is composed of a 10-cm line with the anchors "no pain" and "pain as bad as it could be." (The patient is asked to place a mark on the line in a position that best reflects his/her pain intensity; a score is derived by measuring the distance from the "no pain" end of the line.) This instrument may be slightly more cumbersome than the NRS, but it can be an effective tool for use with patients who have a difficult time providing a numerical rating for their pain. The VRS includes a list of pain descriptors ordered by level of intensity; patients are asked to select the descriptor that best indicates their pain (the corresponding score indicates pain intensity). This measure is easy to administer and score, but it can be difficult for people with language difficulties. Each of the aforementioned instruments is a valid measure

Table 12.1 Biological component of chronic pain assessment.

Location:
Have the patient identify the specific physical area(s) where the pain is felt and related radiation patterns
Onset:
Have the patient describe when and how the pain started, e.g., precipitating injury or inciting events
Pattern:
Have the patient describe the current frequency of pain, how long it lasts, and whether it has changed over time
Intensity of the pain:
Have the patient rate the pain severity; useful anchors include current pain, pain at its worst, pain at its best, and on average
Description of pain:
Have the patient describe how the pain feels, whether it is superficial or deep, constant or intermittent, and whether it fluctuates in intensity. Encourage a description of associated symptoms, e.g., including nausea, vomiting, weakness, or confusion
Aggravating and relieving factors:
Have the patient describe those factors that increase or decrease the experience of pain, e.g., sitting, lying down, standing, heat, cold, exercises, or particular movements

of pain intensity and has demonstrated sensitivity to change in the context of pain treatment (Jensen and Karoly 2001).

Psychological Component

The clinician should carefully inquire into the relationship of cognitive, emotional, and psychological states to subjective pain complaints and exacerbations. In the course of prior treatment, patients may have been made to feel that their pain complaints have been dismissed as being "all in their head." In addition, patients with chronic pain may well fear that attention that is paid to psychological factors may detract from physical aspects of treatment. Accordingly, inquiry should be conducted in a manner that does not trigger defensiveness. An explanation of the biopsychosocial model and multifactorial relationships between pain and psychological factors may help to reassure the patient and allay fears. Such communication may also serve to lay the foundation in establishing the patient's expectations that treatment directed at psychological factors can contribute to pain-mitigating effects and vice versa.

The essential components of the psychological variables related to pain are summarized in Table 12.2. It is important that clinicians assess the effect of pain on the patient's psychological functioning. Psychological functioning includes concentration, motivation or energy, and emotions such as depression or anxiety. It is imperative to recognize that transient subsyndromal emotional and cognitive reactions to life events, e.g., sadness, anger, and fear, as well as the emotional distress accompanying psychiatric disorders (discussed below) are germane to the psychological component of chronic pain assessment. Because these items are interrelated, there will be considerable overlap and bidirectional influences between pain and one's moods, cognitive appraisals, and coping strategies.

Attention should be paid to the patient's beliefs about the meaning of the pain, expectations about future pain, and interpretation of the impact the pain on one's functioning. Negative pain-related cognitions, e.g., catastrophizing, helplessness, and lack of perceived

Table 12.2 Psychological component of chronic pain assessment.

Mood:
Have the patient describe one's mood experienced most days in recent weeks; whether this is a departure from one's customary mood or distinctly different from baseline
Affect:
Have the patient describe emotional reactions to pain; whether there is a relationship between day-to-day emotions and subsequent pain severity
Cognition:
Have the patient describe how one interprets/understands the meaning of the pain; how incapacitated or disabled one is perceived to be; and the expectations the patient harbors about future pain and incapacitation. Does the patient express futility or despair? If so, is the patient hopeless? Suicidal?
Coping:
Have the patient describe how s/he reacts when pain is experienced, e.g., do they avoid activities? Focus on the pain? Expect the worst? Become overwhelmed with fear?
What is done to cope with pain and unpleasant emotions, e.g., distraction, relaxation, praying, hoping?
What means does the patient have to self-soothe and secure needed support?

control over pain and related stressors, are robust predictors of pain and disability and significantly impede one's adaptation in the face of chronic painful conditions (Keefe et al. 2005, Sullivan et al. 2001). Such cognitions can feed and even serve as ineffective coping strategies by reducing self-efficacy, draining one's support systems, and accentuating unpleasant emotional states (e.g., anger, anxiety, depression), which may result in adverse influences exceeding those of other variables, e.g., biomechanical deformities and pathophysiological disease status (Hagglund et al. 1989, Parker et al. 1988, Vlaeyen 1991, Young 1992).

Identification of problematic emotions and cognitive patterns should prompt an inquiry into the coping strategies used by the individual to self-soothe, reduce distress, and modulate unpleasant states. Coping with a chronic illness requires the individual to adopt new strategies for coping with pain and other unpleasant symptoms. To do so effectively, patients need to believe that they possess the repertoire of skills necessary and develop confidence in their ability to efficaciously implement those strategies. Patients invoking active coping strategies, i.e., activity, exercise, distraction, and other measures in which one takes control over one's pain management, experience improved adjustment, functioning, and less depression and disability than individuals relying on passive coping strategies, i.e., strategies that abdicate responsibility for pain management such as resting, reliance on analgesics, and deferring to physicians (Jensen et al. 1991).

Social Component
Lastly, it is important to assess the impact of pain on the patient's social functioning. Assessment into the patient's social functioning is broad-based and would necessitate inquiry into the impact of pain on lifestyle, personal relationships, work or school, activities of daily living (ADLs), and instrumental activities of daily living (IADLs) (Table 12.3). Inquiry should be focused on what the patient is able to do and what activities are avoided due to the pain. It is pertinent to assess the patient's general life satisfaction, e.g., how free time is spent and pursuit of interests; along with the economic impact of pain by inquiring into restriction in the types of work activity and job loss, the resultant restrictions in income, financial

Table 12.3 Social component of chronic pain assessment.

Adaptation and function:
Have the patient describe the extent to which one is capable of managing ADLs, e.g., bathing, grooming, dressing, and toileting, and IADLs, e.g., meal preparation, payment of bills, laundry, house cleaning, use of public transportation, and driving
Vocational:
Have the patient describe how work/academic pursuits are affected, e.g., restriction in work activity or job loss; if unemployed, how one is supported
Economic:
Have the patient describe whether there has been reduction in income, financial hardships imposed my medical treatment, and the impact on family/others with who one resides
Recreational and life satisfaction:
Have the patient describe what is done to derive pleasure; what hobbies and interests have been given up due to pain, what is maintained despite the pain; and how satisfying life is despite pain
Social support network:
Have the patient describe the impact of pain on relationships; the accessibility and availability of significant persons in the patient's life; and capacity for intimacy, sexuality, and shared experiences with friends/family
Legal issues:
Have the patient describe whether there are pending legal issues, e.g., litigation related to injuries, workers' compensation, and social security disability claims

hardships imposed by medical treatment, concerns over the accessibility and cost of medical care, whether litigation related to the cause of pain is pending, and whether applications for disability are under review.

It is helpful to identify the significant persons in the patient's life and how pain has influenced relationships with those persons, e.g., changes in role responsibilities within the home can strain relationships. Given that interpersonal relationships are bidirectional, it is equally important to ascertain the extent to which one's adaptation in the context of pain may be shaped or reinforced by the responses of others in one's life (Turk and Okifuji 2002). The clinician needs to listen for elements that suggest the patient assumes an "invalid role" in all or some aspects of life and assess the function that role serves for the patient.

Careful histories of alcohol and drug use are also imperative. This may be predictive of future risks of addiction and may assist in determining what types of medical and pharmacologic approaches best suit the patients' needs.

Multidimensional Pain Assessment Instruments

The measures reviewed here are not intended to reflect a full accounting of all of the multidimensional instruments available. Instead, the goal is to provide the reader with a sampling of some of the more widely used measures of domains pertinent to the assessment of the patient with chronic pain (Table 12.4). The selection of assessment inventories should be based upon its practical utility, so that the clinician can yield insights into factors contributing to and underlying the patient's condition.

Comorbid Psychiatric Conditions

Chronic pain is not a unitary condition, rarely presenting alone. There is an extensive epidemiological literature that supports the high prevalence of primary psychiatric disorders among persons with chronic pain. It is prudent, therefore, in the assessment of patients with chronic pain that one considers an extensive array of psychiatric comorbidities and that

Table 12.4 Multidimensional pain assessments.

Brief pain inventory
Originally developed in the assessment of pain severity and pain-related life interference among patients with cancer, this scale has increasingly been employed among patients with non-malignant pain. It is used to monitor response to treatment interventions (Cleeland and Ryan 1994).

Coping strategies questionnaire
Assesses one's repertoire of coping strategies to deal with chronic pain; may predict the level of activity, physical impairment, and psychological functioning associated with pain (Rosenstiel and Keefe 1983).

Fear-avoidance beliefs questionnaire
Assesses beliefs characterized by danger, threat, or harm associated with pain. The degree to which patients assign threat to activities may limit their participation in, and lead to avoidance of, activities related to work (Waddell et al. 1993).

McGill pain questionnaire
Assesses the features of pain severity and intensity. Allows patients to qualify pain in emotional, cognitive, evaluative, and sensory terms (Melzack 1975).

Medical outcomes study short-form health survey – (SF-36)
Developed as a general measure of one's perceived health status, can be used to assess bodily pain; physical, emotional, and social functioning; and mental health (Ware and Sherbourne 1992).

Minnesota multiphasic personality inventory-2
Comprises 567 true–false items that are used to derive scores on 10 clinical scales and 3 validity scales; employed to assess the psychological functioning of patients with pain (Hathaway et al. 1989).

Multidimensional pain inventory
Assessment of one's appraisals of pain, its impact on functioning, and perceived responses of others in response to pain (Kerns et al. 1985).

Pain disability index
Comprises measures of disability, pain, and impact on activities of daily living; however, the instrument can be lengthy which may preclude using this instrument regularly in clinical practice (Tait et al. 1987).

Survey of pain attitudes (SOPA)
Assesses the patient's beliefs and attitudes about pain, including perceived control over pain, perceived disability, need for avoidance of activity to prevent harm, and solicitousness (Jensen et al. 1987).

psychiatric treatment is secured whenever appropriate. The most commonly cited disorders are those which are outlined below; diagnosis of these conditions among persons with chronic pain requires the use of a clinical interview to assure that several specific criteria as established in the Diagnostic and Statistical Manual of Mental Disorders (American Psychiatric Association 2000) are met. Structured psychiatric interviews and diagnostic decision trees have been developed for facilitating reliable and valid diagnosis.

Depression

Depression prevalence rates among patients with chronic pain are substantially higher than those in the general population, with reported prevalence rates of depression ranging from as low as 10% to as high as 100% (Banks and Kerns 1996, Romano and Turner 1985). Estimates vary depending on the variety of pain conditions examined, whether patients were sampled from clinical or community settings and the methodologies employed to diagnose depression. Nonetheless, depression constitutes a common psychiatric comorbidity among patients with chronic pain (Fishbain 1999, Koenig and Clark 1996).

Although much of the data suggest that chronic pain predisposes patients to depression (Fishbain et al. 1997), some longitudinal studies suggest that depression predicts future pain. For example, a 10-year study of industrial workers revealed that depression predicted the development of subsequent low back pain and other musculoskeletal impairments (Leino and Magni 1993) and in another 5-year follow-up survey, subjective assessments of depression predicted the development of fibromyalgia (Forseth et al. 1999).

As alluded to previously in the description of the neuromatrix theory, emerging evidence has suggested putative neurobiological mediators of the relationship between pain and depression (Blackburn-Munro and Blackburn-Munro 2001, Nestler et al. 2002, Raison et al. 2006). Given that there are common underlying substrates for these conditions, it is unsurprising that they co-occur at such high rates.

Depression among persons with chronic pain may result in perpetuation of pain, increasing the number, severity, and duration of physical symptoms, and enhancing subjective assessments of pain-related disability, e.g., higher unemployment rates (Bairs et al. 2003, Burns et al. 1998). Additionally, comorbid depression can impede treatment efforts (Haythornthwaite et al. 1991). Depression is associated with poor prognosis among patients with pain (Bair et al. 2003), influencing adaptation to illness and quality of life. Health risk behaviors are often associated with depression, e.g., cigarette smoking, overeating, and decreased physical activity, complicating the functional disability of patients with pain. Furthermore, depression is associated with higher non-adherence rates than that of non-depressed patients, undermining rehabilitative efforts and increasing health care utilization (DiMatteo et al. 2000). Treatment of depression, therefore, is a necessary component to multimodal treatment approaches to address pain; when effectively treated, patients experience dramatically less interference from pain (Lin et al. 2003).

Anxiety

The coprevalence of pain and anxiety has been supported in the literature, with rates as high or perhaps greater than that for depression (Roy-Byrne et al. 2008). Research suggests a relationship between anxiety states and arthritic conditions (McWilliams et al. 2003), atypical chest pain (Katerndahl 2004), migraine (Swartz et al. 2000), back pain (McWilliams et al. 2004), and fibromyalgia (Cohen et al. 2002). In a cross-sectional study of chronic pain patients, the tendency toward worry was significantly associated with long-term suffering related to pain (Lackner and Quigley 2005). The presence of comorbid anxiety may lead to hyperarousal and increased vigilance for pain and somatic concerns. Anxiety may influence the emotional valence associated with somatic sensations and an increased proclivity to misinterpret somatic experiences (Derakshan and Eysenck 1997, van der Kolk et al. 1996).

In a survey of a nationally representative sample, panic attacks and generalized anxiety disorder were more than two times as likely to be present among patients endorsing back pain or arthritis and almost four times as likely in those endorsing migraine as compared to a control group without pain. Strikingly, rates of diagnosable clinical depression were notably lower, observed at a rate of 1.5–2 times among those with pain as compared to controls (McWilliams et al. 2004).

Commonly encountered anxiety disorders include generalized anxiety disorder, panic disorder, social anxiety disorder, and posttraumatic stress disorder (PTSD) (Gureje et al. 2008). PTSD is associated with chronic somatic pain in several studies, particularly among military veterans with chronic pain and among chronic pain patients whose pain developed after a work injury or motor vehicle accident (Asmundson et al. 2002).

Like depression, the presence of an anxiety disorder can predict poor outcomes for patients with chronic pain (Roy-Byrne et al. 2008). Fears related to precipitating pain can lead to restriction of movement and avoidance of activity thereby contributing to deconditioning and muscle weakness and undermining rehabilitative measures such as physical therapy (Vlaeyen et al. 1995). The treatment of comorbid anxiety may serve to supplement preventive pain treatment measures, e.g., with migraine (Breslau and Davis 1993), and enhances rehabilitative measures; thus, it is a necessary component of comprehensive pain treatment.

Sleep Disorders

Sleep disturbances are common among patients with a variety of pain disorders (Moldofsky 2001); patients may report difficulty falling asleep, frequent awakenings and disrupted sleep, decreased total sleep time, and daytime fatigue. The etiology is likely to be multifactorial, including disruptions due to pain itself, comorbid psychiatric disturbances, effects of pain medications, lack of aerobic exercise, and behavioral conditioning due to protracted reclining and daytime napping (Cohen et al. 2000). Protracted sleep deprivation can increase pain severity (Moldofsky and Scarisbrick 1976) and can predispose patients to additional medical complications, e.g., impaired immune functioning, weight gain, and insulin resistance/diabetes (Irwin et al. 1996, Knutson et al. 2007). Interventions can include (a) patient education and training in the development of appropriate sleep hygiene techniques; (b) use of long-acting analgesics to reduce sleep-interfering effects of pain; (c) prudent use of non-benzodiazepine sedatives, e.g., zolpidem; (d) judicious use of adjuvant co-analgesics, e.g., antidepressants and anticonvulsants required for certain pain states can be useful in augmenting sleep potential due to their sedating effects; and (e) careful patient selection for possible stimulant use to reduce excess daytime sedation associated with opioid analgesics.

Substance Abuse and Dependence

Reported rates of substance abuse or dependence among patients with chronic pain have been higher than those in the general population (Brown et al. 1996). For most, the substance use disorder preceded the onset of the pain disorder (Brown et al. 1996). In fact, a preexisting substance use disorder may have predisposed the individual to accidents and physical trauma, some of which may evolve into chronic pain syndromes (Polatin et al. 1993).

Of particular concern is the relationship of opioid dependence to chronic pain. It is arguable that signs of physiological dependence, i.e., demonstration of tolerance to the effects of opioids or the precipitation of withdrawal with abrupt medication cessation, would naturally result from the chronic administration of opioid analgesics and otherwise do not signal psychological dependence that accompanies dependence or addiction. Instead, psychological signs of dependence would be reflective in behaviors suggesting a loss of control over the use of opioids, e.g., using more of the opioid than intended; using the agent to acquire effects apart from analgesia, e.g., emotional effects; going to inordinate lengths to acquire, use, or recover from the opioids; and using the agent to the point of, and despite, inducing deleterious effects. Behaviors suggestive of loss of control, and therefore dependence, include lying, seeking additional prescriptions from other doctors, using street drugs, escalating doses beyond prescribed levels, seeking early refills, and manipulative behaviors displayed with the intended purpose of obtaining narcotic analgesics.

Although chronic pain patients may be vulnerable to developing new substance use disorders in the course of treatment (Dersh et al. 2002, Brown et al. 1996, Dunbar and Katz 1996), investigations assessing the presence of opioid dependence in chronic pain patients have reported contradictory conclusions. Some contend that this is an extraordinarily rare event (Zenz et al. 1992) whereas other investigators have found high rates of opioid dependence in chronic pain populations (Ives et al. 2006, Wu et al. 2006). Risk factors for opioid dependence include a prior history of substance abuse; prior physical/sexual abuse; major depression, anxiety disorders, and personality disorders (Dersh et al. 2002, Ives et al., Fishbain et al. 1998). Opioids have been a predominant focus; however, several other agents used in pain treatment are likewise prone to abuse and dependence; including the muscle relaxant carisoprodol; ketamine; ergot alkaloids and barbiturates employed in migraine treatment; and benzodiazepines.

Although challenging, effective pain management should never be withheld because of an abuse/addiction history. Effective treatment may require use of an array of pain-reducing approaches, e.g., use of adjunctive agents, or those with low abuse potential, physical, and psychological therapies, as well as participation in concurrent substance abuse treatment programs.

Treatment of pain in patients with opioid dependence can be particularly challenging, however. In fact, some evidence points to the fact that opioid dependence can enhance sensitivity to pain, i.e., opioid-induced hyperalgesia (Chang et al. 2007). Patients on long-term methadone maintenance have been shown to have less tolerance for experimentally induced pain (Doverty et al. 2001). Ongoing opioid consumption can set off a cascade of cellular responses and neurophysiologic mechanisms that enhance pain sensitivity (White 2004), e.g., increasing the production and activity of neuropeptides such as dynorphin (Vanderah et al. 2001), cholecystokinin (Xie et al. 2005), and substance P (King et al. 2005). Activation of glial cells producing inflammatory cytokines also results in amplified pain (Watkins et al. 2007).

In some cases, detoxification from the substance(s) upon which one is dependent, e.g., alcohol, may be required before the initiation of treatment. The substances abused may be employed to self-medicate one's psychological distress, necessitating psychological along with prudent psychopharmacologic interventions.

Treatment Approaches

Utilizing the biopsychosocial approach to comprehensive assessment, it may then be possible to develop, implement, and refine treatment strategies that are contoured to the unique and individualized needs of the chronic pain patient. This section will survey the use of psychotherapeutic and psychopharmacologic approaches for the patient with chronic pain.

Ultimately, treatment objectives include alleviation of subjectively perceived discomfort and improvement of the patient's functional capacity. Assessing the patient's goals related to pain will necessarily help guide the pain management plan. Areas for improvement may be reduction of pain to levels that the patient would find tolerable, acquiring comfortable and consistent sleep, comfortable movement, and/or a return to specific activities. The goals of the patient may be divergent from those of the clinician. Failure to identify and address such disparate goals may interfere with establishment of a therapeutic alliance, adherence, and treatment success.

Psychotherapy

There are multiple psychotherapy approaches to assist the patient with chronic, non-malignant pain; however, the approach that has received the most empirical attention in terms of its applicability to pain treatment has been cognitive behavioral therapy (CBT). This section will primarily focus on a description of the CBT paradigm, its goals, and the research on its uses in pain management.

Fundamentally, the basic assumption of CBT is that although one cannot always control or avoid distressing experiences or life events, one can nonetheless, through the acquisition and implementation of certain requisite skills, almost always exert some control over how much suffering and life disruption that those events produce. For example, it is assumed that the pain is not responsible for causing the patient to be inactive, socially withdrawn, isolated, or less capable of deriving pleasure in life. Rather, these behavior patterns evolve from beliefs that the patient harbors when one becomes convinced that s/he is physically disabled. Therefore, CBT is a time-limited treatment approach directed at assisting patients in acquiring skills including (a) the identification of thoughts, feelings, and behaviors that predispose one to suffering; (b) the modification of those maladaptive thoughts, feelings, and behaviors; and (c) fostering the development of adaptive problem solving and effective coping strategies. Ultimately, the goals are to reduce physical and psychological distress and enhance quality of life, despite having a chronic painful condition.

In initial sessions, the therapist gathers information to elicit an understanding of the patient's perception of the pain; appraisals of current life situations; beliefs about one's life, relationships, and the future; and current coping measures the individual employs. Homework assignments are assigned to the patient, in which the patient is asked to log pain ratings, environmental events and associated thoughts, feelings, and behaviors. With information gleaned from these assignments, the therapist attempts to educate the patient about the temporal patterns influencing perceived pain severity and the resultant impact on one's mood and functioning.

The focus shifts in subsequent sessions to a collaborative process whereby the therapist enlists the patient in an assessment of the accuracy and overall usefulness of one's beliefs and identifies maladaptive and distorted thoughts that may lead the patient to avoid activities and to experience negative feelings, such as depression, anxiety, and anger. Patients are encouraged to reappraise irrational and self-defeating thoughts and reframe them, replacing them with those that are more rational and objective, a process referred to as cognitive restructuring.

Simultaneously, the patient and therapist undertake the process of coping skills training. Using data from homework assignments completed by the patient and issues discussed in sessions, the therapist and patient attempt to identify situations that are likely to tax coping abilities, assess the utility of the existing strategies, develop alternatives when existing strategies fail to produce relief, and rehearse newly developed coping strategies when those situations re-occur. The patient may be instructed on modalities to instill a sense of control over pain and adverse life events including progressive muscle relaxation and deep breathing exercises. Together, the therapist and patient work to implement alternate ways of looking at one's condition, one's life, and one's future, cultivating a repertoire of skills to enhance adapting to the challenges one faces and at the same time re-introducing behaviors that allow one to derive pleasure and self-efficacy.

Consistent with the neuromatrix theory, the presumption is that as a result of cognitive restructuring and coping skills training, patients will experience less physiological arousal and less intense pain. In a study employing positron emission tomography, improvement in symptoms following CBT treatment was found to correspond with changes in baseline limbic activity, i.e., in the amygdala and anterior cingulate cortex (Lackner et al. 2006). Although the sample size was small and solely consisted of patients with chronic irritable bowel syndrome (IBS), the preliminary evidence gleaned from this investigation suggests that CBT may have a role in modification of brain circuitry in a manner that decreases painful symptoms, specifically by altering the activity of those brain areas mediating both pain perception and emotional self-regulation.

CBT has been used as a treatment for a diverse array of chronic pain problems, having been applied to patients with headache (Andrasik 2007, Campbell et al. 2009); facial pain, e.g., temporomandibular disorders (TMD) (Dworkin et al. 2002, Dworkin et al. 1994, Turner et al. 2005, Turner et al. 2006); osteoarthritis and rheumatoid arthritis (Keefe et al. 2005, Astin et al. 2002); fibromyalgia (Goldenberg et al. 2004); and low back pain (Hoffman et al. 2007, Henschke et al. 2010). Across conditions, i.e., grouping different pain conditions together, CBT has been shown to significantly reduce pain severity and increase coping and social role functioning compared to wait-listed control conditions (Morley et al. 1999). Further, after reviewing the evidence across a number of painful medical conditions, a National Institutes of Health (NIH) technology conference concluded that there was moderate evidence to support the use of CBT in reducing chronic pain (NIH Technology Assessment Panel 1996).

A few caveats are worth noting, however. First, the benefits of CBT have not been consistently demonstrated within specific painful conditions. For example, contradictory evidence and differences in sets of studies being compared have led to disagreements among empirical reviews regarding the treatment value of CBT in fibromyalgia (Goldenberg et al. 2004, Bradley et al. 2003). Second, the results of trials assessing the benefits of CBT vary depending upon the control groups to which CBT-treated patients are compared. For example, among IBS patients, CBT has been shown to be superior to inactive wait-listed controls but it has not been shown to be consistently effective in IBS when compared to active attention-placebo controls (Blanchard 2005). Third, assessments of CBT effectiveness may vary depending upon the outcome (dependent variables) assessed. This was highlighted in studies assessing CBT use in the treatment of patients with low back pain. Evidence stemming from meta-analyses and systematic reviews suggested that CBT resulted in significantly lower back pain intensity but no difference in health-related quality of life (Albert 1999) or vocational functioning (Alaranta et al. 1994, Scheer et al. 1997) when compared to wait-listed controls. Lastly, the efficacy of CBT has not been systematically investigated in a variety of other chronic pain conditions, e.g., interstitial cystitis, chronic pelvic pain, or neuropathy. Studies that have investigated the role of CBT or related psychotherapeutic approaches in these pain disorders (Albert 1999, Chaiken et al. 1993, Ehde and Jensen 2004, Evans et al. 2003, Farquhar et al. 1989, Norrbrink et al. 2006, Webster and Brennan 1995) are too few in number and/or of insufficient methodological quality, preventing definitive conclusions from being drawn.

Although it is not feasible to provide an exhaustive overview of alternate psychotherapy approaches useful in pain management here, the reader should recognize that several other therapeutic approaches likewise demonstrate promise as adjunctive treatment interventions (Leo 2007). The selection of psychotherapy modality would therefore depend upon the particular patient's needs, the commitment to pursue psychotherapy and the training/skills of the psychiatrists, and other available mental health practitioners enlisted in the care of the patient with pain. Briefly, some of these approaches can include:

- Interpersonal Psychotherapy (Weissman et al. 2000) for individuals experiencing marked difficulties in role transitions or relationship difficulties
- Couples/marital and family therapies
- Behavioral (operant conditioning techniques) used to modify entrenched pain-associated behavior patterns, e.g., excess reclining and avoidance of activity, through modification of environmental contingencies and reinforcements (Sanders 2003)
- Biofeedback, hypnosis, and mindfulness therapy, which attempt to reduce distress, facilitate relaxation, and reduce physiological states linked with the genesis and perpetuation of pain, and thereby modify one's experience of pain and imparts a sense of mastery over pain

Psychopharmacology

An extensive array of psychopharmacologic agents is available for use in a number of painful conditions. Empirical investigations of the utility of these psychoactive agents as adjuncts in chronic non-malignant pain management have largely focused on antidepressants and anticonvulsants. The following overview will delineate the range of psychopharmacological approaches available to address pain and related psychological comorbidities, although the emphasis will be placed on the role of antidepressants and anticonvulsants.

Antidepressants

Several meta-analyses and evidence-based reviews suggest that antidepressants are useful in mitigating pain associated with neuropathy (Collins et al. 2000, Saarto and Wiffen 2007), headache (Tomkins et al. 2001), fibromyalgia (Arnold et al. 2000, O'Malley et al. 2000), and irritable bowel syndrome (Jackson et al. 2000, Lesbros-Pantoflickova et al. 2004). Although antidepressants are advocated for use in other chronic pain syndromes, e.g., rheumatologic pain conditions, chronic pelvic pain, interstitial cystitis, and oro-facial pain (Kelada and Jones 2007, Onghena and Van Houdenhove 1992, Reiter 1998), these assertions are not often based on a solid foundation of empirical work. In fact, in some of these conditions, e.g., chronic pelvic pain and interstitial cystitis, there are few randomized controlled trials with small sample sizes upon which such recommendations are based (Onghena and Van Houdenhove 1992, Sharav et al. 1987, Stones et al. 2007, Van Ophoven et al. 2004).

The pain-mitigating effects of antidepressants are thought to involve a number of neuro-modulatory influences within the CNS. Analgesia produced by antidepressants is thought to be primarily mediated by enhancing the inhibitory neurotransmitters (e.g., noradren-ergic (NE) and serotonergic (5-HT)) present within descending pain-mediating pathways extending down the spinal cord from axons emanating from the dorsolateral pontomesen-cephalic tegmentum and rostral ventromedial medulla (Fields and Basbaum 1999, Yokogawa et al. 2002). Additional putative analgesic effects of antidepressants may be mediated by the: (i) reduction in the synthesis and release of pain-promoting neurotransmitters, e.g., gluta-mate in the spinal cord (Kawasaki et al. 2003), (ii) antagonism of N-methyl-D-aspartate (NMDA) receptor effects, (iii) blockade of sodium channels with resultant diminution of painful afferent inputs from the peripheral and central nervous systems (Gerner et al. 2001),

(iv) augmentation of opioid effects within the CNS (Lee and Spencer 1980, Taiwo et al. 1985), and lastly (v) reduction of the extent of limbic output, which might otherwise contribute to depression and anxiety that exacerbate underlying pain.

Evidence gathered from clinical trials and meta-analyses suggests that antidepressants influencing both NE and 5-HT transmission exert analgesic effects that are greater than those antidepressants with more specific effects, e.g., influencing 5-HT re-uptake or NE re-uptake alone (Lynch 2001, Max 1994, Max et al. 1992, McQuay et al. 1996, Mochizucki 2004, Sussman 2003). As a class, the selective serotonin re-uptake inhibitors (SSRIs) have not been demonstrated to be as consistently analgesic as the tricyclic antidepressants (TCAs) or serotonin–norepinephrine re-uptake inhibitors (SNRIs), possibly related to the 5-HT selectivity of the SSRIs (Lynch 2001, Sindrup and Jensen 1999). The major antidepressant classes used in pain management are summarized in Table 12.5.

Other Antidepressants

Although less extensively studied than the previously mentioned antidepressants, there are some data suggesting the potential utility of bupropion, nefazodone, trazodone, and mirtazapine for selected pain states (Ansari 2000, Bendtsen and Jensen 2004, Samborski et al. 2004, Saper et al. 2001, Semenchuk and Davis 2000, Ventafridda et al. 1988). Given the limited number of randomized controlled trials and small sample sizes, definitive statements regarding the utility of these agents and the generalizability of results are not possible.

Anticonvulsant Drugs

Anticonvulsant drugs (ACDs) have efficacy in mitigating neuropathic pain, including trigeminal neuralgia and phantom limb pain (McQuay et al. 1995), as well as migraine (Pappagallo 2003, Snow et al. 2002). As with the antidepressants, analgesic differences exist among the ACDs with regard to utility across types of pain conditions. Carbamazepine is Food and Drug Administration (FDA)-approved for the treatment of trigeminal neuralgia; gabapentin, for treatment of postherpetic neuralgia; pregabalin, for postherpetic neuralgia, diabetic neuropathy, and fibromyalgia (Crofford et al. 2005); and divalproex sodium and topiramate have both been indicated for migraine prophylaxis.

Although the neuromodulatory mechanisms underlying analgesia produced by ACDs are varied, the mechanisms of action are thought to influence several of the physiologic processes contributing to neural hyperexcitability predisposing patients to central sensitization and chronic pain. The precise mechanisms of action of ACDs remain uncertain. The principal proposed mechanism of action for both pregabalin and gabapentin is the interaction with the alpha 2-delta subunit of L-type voltage-regulated calcium channels thought to influence central pro-neuropathic processes, i.e., glutamate release (Frampton and Scott 2004, Guay 2003, Vinik 2005). Other mechanisms of action are presumed to involve enhanced gamma-aminobutyric acid inhibition (valproate, topiramate) or a stabilizing effect on neuronal cell membranes via inhibition of voltage-gated sodium channels (carbamazepine). The net effects of these presumed mechanisms are believed to mediate inhibition of pain pathways within the CNS, e.g., reducing the ability of neurons to fire at high frequency (Chong and Smith 2000).

Evidence has been limited with regard to the relative effectiveness of ACDs. For example, one systematic review demonstrated that although gabapentin was effective in treating postherpetic and diabetic neuropathy, it did not appear to be superior to carbamazepine. There were, however, no direct comparisons between these two drugs (Wiffen et al. 2009).

Table 12.5 Major antidepressant classes used in pain management.

Tricyclic antidepressants (TCAs)	
	General uses: neuropathic pain, headache, poststroke pain, thalamic pain, fibromyalgia, irritable bowel (diarrhea type), and chronic pelvic pain with or without comorbid depression/anxiety *Pain-related FDA approvals:* none available for any of the TCAs *Standard dosage:* initiate with 10 mg daily at bedtime. Increase the dosage gradually (e.g., by 10 mg weekly), to achieve desired pain-mitigating and antidepressant effects until side effects supervene. Analgesic doses are often considerably lower than those required for antidepressant efficacy, e.g., 75–150 mg/d for amitriptyline; 25–350 mg/d for imipramine; and 10–75 mg/d for nortriptyline *Main side effects:* anticholinergic side effects, drowsiness, insomnia, agitation, and cardiac arrhythmia *Drug interactions:* TCAs should not be used with monoamine oxidase inhibitors; can accentuate CNS sedative effects when combined with alcohol, benzodiazepines, and barbiturates
Serotonin–norepinephrine re-uptake inhibitors (SNRIs)	
	General uses: neuropathic pain and fibromyalgia *Pain-related FDA approvals:* duloxetine has received FDA approval for treatment of diabetic neuropathy and fibromyalgia. Milnacipran has received FDA approval for treatment of patients with fibromyalgia *Standard dosage:* milnacipran: 100–200 mg/d; duloxetine: 60–120 mg/d; venlafaxine: 15–225 mg/d *Main side effects:* nausea, dry mouth, nervousness, constipation, somnolence, and elevations in diastolic blood pressure *Drug interactions:* SNRIs should not be used with monoamine oxidase inhibitors or thioridazine
Serotonin selective re-uptake inhibitors (SSRIs)	
	General uses: data are limited; paroxetine and citalopram may be effective in alleviating symptoms of diabetic neuropathy and fluoxetine may be useful in fibromyalgia *Pain-related FDA approvals:* none available for any of the SSRIs *Standard dosage:* citalopram: 20–40 mg/d; fluoxetine: 20–80 mg/d; paroxetine: 20–40 mg/d *Main side effects:* nausea, diarrhea, insomnia or sedation, tremors, and sexual dysfunction *Drug interactions:* SSRIs should not be used in conjunction with monoamine oxidase inhibitors, triptans, tramadol, dextromethorphan, or other highly serotonergic agents because of the potential for serotonin syndrome

FDA = Food and Drug Administration; CNS = central nervous system. (Adapted from Leo 2007; Tomkins et al. 2001; Arnold et al. 2000; Lynch 2001; Ansari 2000.)

Emerging evidence suggests the potential analgesic roles of newer ACDs, e.g., lamotrigine, oxcarbazepine, and tiagabine (Pappagallo 2003, Galer 1995, Khoromi et al. 2005, Novak et al. 2001). Although these agents demonstrate some promise with regard to mitigating neuro-pathic states (Remillard 1994, Solaro et al. 2001, Zakrzewska et al. 1997), the utility and safety of several of these agents among chronic pain patients has not been systematically investi-gated. A recent review indicated that for lamotrigine, some evidence existed for efficacy in central poststroke pain and in a subgroup of HIV-related neuropathy. However, no benefit was demonstrated with lamotrigine for diabetic neuropathy, spinal cord injury, or trigeminal neuralgia (Wiffen and Rees 2009).

Adverse effects common to ACDs include sedation, fatigue, gastrointestinal, and motor side effects (tremor, ataxia, and nystagmus). Rash and Stevens-Johnson syndrome are possible with carbamazepine and lamotrigine (Pappagallo 2003). Patients taking gabapentin or pregabalin do not require serum drug, hematologic, electrolyte, or hepatic enzyme monitoring as is often required with other ACDs, e.g., carbamazepine or divalproex sodium. Both gabapentin and pregabalin are eliminated through renal excretion; dose reductions are required in patients with impaired renal function. ACDs can accentuate sedative effects when combined with alcohol, benzodiazepines, or barbiturates. Carbamazepine, oxcarbazepine, phenytoin, and topiramate can reduce the efficacy of oral contraceptives, increasing the risk of pregnancy. Fetal malformations are associated with carbamazepine, valproate, and phenytoin use during pregnancy (Yerby 2000).

Selection of ACD versus Antidepressant Pharmacotherapy

Both antidepressants and ACDs have demonstrated comparable efficacy in a number of chronic pain conditions, e.g., migraine headache and neuropathic pain. In a review of randomized controlled trials in which TCAs and anticonvulsants were employed to treat pain associated with diabetic and postherpetic neuropathies, it was found that at least 50% of pain relief was achieved in two-thirds of the patient episodes treated with anticonvulsants and in half of those treated with antidepressants (Collins et al. 2000, Sindrup and Jensen 1999, McQuay 2002). However, adverse effects were slightly more common with antidepressant use, particularly TCAs, as compared with anticonvulsants (Collins et al. 2000, McQuay 2002).

Selection of medication options for patients needs to be individualized, taking into consideration the tolerability of side effects and safety of use of particular medications in the context of the patient's comorbid medical and psychiatric conditions (Leo 2006). For example, the patient with comorbid depression and/or anxiety might be best managed with selection of an antidepressant. On the other hand, ACDs have mood-stabilizing effects that benefit patients with bipolar disorder, schizoaffective disorder, and impulsivity arising from dementia (Chandramouli 2002, Leo and Narendran 1999); therefore, ACD selection for patients with these conditions would be ideal. Regarding medical comorbidities, there are several factors to consider. Heart block, arrhythmias, or severe cardiac disease prohibit use of TCAs. For patients with renal dysfunction, doses of duloxetine, venlafaxine, carbamazepine, gabapentin, pregabalin, and topiramate would need to be reduced, and if the renal dysfunction is severe enough may preclude use of these agents. For patients with hepatic disease, doses of carbamazepine, duloxetine, and lamotrigine should be reduced. TCAs can conceivably exacerbate encephalopathy associated with hepatic disease.

In the treatment decision algorithm, it is plausible that ACDs could be alternatively employed for patients with persisting pain despite optimal antidepressant use or for whom antidepressant use proved intolerable. Because of the differences in presumed mechanisms of action between ACDs and antidepressants, simultaneous co-administration of antidepressants and ACDs may be useful, capitalizing on complimentary mechanisms of action.

Adjuvant Roles of Other Psychopharmacologic Agents

Benzodiazepines

There is insufficient evidence for meaningful analgesic properties of benzodiazepines in most clinical circumstances (Reddy and Patt 1994). Benzodiazepines have been employed acutely to mitigate pain arising from muscle spasm, e.g., after spinal cord injury. This effect may be due to an indirect effect related to their psychotropic properties, i.e., alleviation of anxiety. The presumption is that reducing patient anxiety attenuates muscle tension and associated musculoskeletal pain.

Other uses for benzodiazepines have included treatment of restless legs syndrome, tension headache, and neuropathy (Bartusch et al. 1996, Bouckoms and Litman 1985, Dellemijn and Fields 1994). Clonazepam and alprazolam might be effective in patients with lancinating neuropathic pain in which allodynia is a prominent feature (Reddy and Patt 1994, Bouckoms and Litman 1985).

Long-term benzodiazepine use among patients with chronic pain is controversial. Benzodiazepines are gamma-aminobutyric acid (GABA) agonists and, as such, can influence 5-HT neurotransmitter release, attenuating opioid analgesia (Nemmani and Mogil 2003), with the potential for increasing pain sensitivity. In addition, protracted benzodiazepine use may be counterproductive. A study of chronic pain patients referred to a tertiary pain center revealed that long-term benzodiazepine use predicted low activity levels, high utilization of ambulatory medical services, and high disability levels (Ciccone et al. 2000). Benefits of benzodiazepine administration must be weighed against potential risks, e.g., the development of memory impairments, gait instability, excess sedation, physical and psychological dependence, and worsening depression (Reddy and Patt 1994).

Histamine Antagonists

Because histamines have been implicated in facilitating inflammatory processes (e.g., prostaglandin production), histamine antagonists would, therefore, be expected to reduce pain mediated by inflammatory processes (Raffa 2001). Diphenhydramine, hydroxyzine hydrochloride, hydroxyzine pamoate, and promethazine are among those that are commonly employed.

Used alone, antihistamines appear to have an analgesic ceiling effect. Histamine antagonists can augment opiate receptor binding of opioid analgesics (Rumore and Schlichting 1986) and therefore are often employed as co-administered adjuvant agents. The failure to observe substantial analgesia from the use of these agents alone, however, has largely restricted the use of histamine antagonists for persons with chronic pain who have other indications. These agents may be particularly useful in patients given their sedative, anti-emetic, antipruritic, and anxiolytic properties. They are generally well tolerated, with few respiratory or gastrointestinal side effects.

N-Methyl-D-Aspartate Antagonists

Research implicates the excitatory neurotransmitter glutamate in the development of central sensitization and the maintenance of chronic pain. Some evidence suggests that N-methyl-D-aspartate (NMDA) antagonists, i.e., dextromethorphan, ketamine, memantine, and amantadine, may have a role in mitigating chronic pain, including neuropathy, chronic phantom pain, fibromyalgia, and in cases of pain associated with spinal cord injury (Fisher et al. 2000, Sang et al. 2002). However, the analgesic effects in various trials have demonstrated inconsistent results (Eisenberg et al. 1998, Enarson et al. 1999).

The side effects associated with the NMDA antagonists include sedation, dry mouth, headache, and constipation; in some cases these effects can be prohibitively severe limiting usefulness (Eide et al. 1994). For example, ketamine is a dissociative anesthetic producing hallucinations, frightening nightmares, and delirium. These effects can be avoided when low doses are employed, e.g., 50–60 mg four to six times daily. The place of ketamine and other NMDA antagonists in the treatment of chronic pain and the effects of long-term use remain unclear (Brown and Krupp 2006, Visser and Schug 2006).

Neuroleptics

There is limited data suggesting the analgesic efficacy of various neuroleptics in chronic pain states; the results of studies assessing the efficacy of these agents in the treatment of different painful conditions are heterogeneous and sample sizes in the randomized double-blind studies were small (Seidel et al. 2009). These agents have been found to be useful in certain cases of neuropathic pain (Gomez-Perez et al. 1985); small clinical case series report that the atypical antipsychotic, olanzapine, was effective in reducing the severity ratings of recurrent migraine and tension headache refractory to other interventions (Silberstein et al. 2000) as well as cancer pain (Fishbain et al. 2004, Khojainova et al. 2002). Given that there is limited data on the efficacy of neuroleptics, an abundance of other analgesic agents from which to choose, and potentially hazardous side effects associated with neuroleptic use (e.g., extrapyramidal side effects and tardive dyskinesia), it may be best to confine the use of neuroleptics to the pain patient who also has delirium and psychosis (Fishbain et al. 2004).

Sympathomimetics/Stimulants

Although the literature is limited by number of subjects, duration, and trial design, there is some evidence to support the use of methylphenidate (5–15 mg two to four times daily), donepezil (5–10 mg daily), and modafinil (200–400 mg daily) for the pharmacologic management of opioid-induced sedation and fatigue (Larijani et al. 2004, Reissig and Rybarczyk 2005). Potential adverse effects can include overstimulation (e.g., anxiety, insomnia, and even paranoia), appetite suppression, exacerbation of motor abnormalities (e.g., tics, dyskinetic movements), and confusion. Contraindications for stimulant use include glaucoma, poorly controlled hypertension, arrhythmias, and cardiovascular disorders, anorexia, seizure disorders, and hyperthyroidism. Methylphenidate is a schedule II medication under federal regulatory control; caution is advised in patients with current or preexisting substance use disorders, especially prior stimulant abuse (e.g., cocaine).

Summary

Effective management of chronic non-malignant pain necessitates the consideration of biological, psychological, and social covariates that influence the experience, presentation, and clinical course of such chronic conditions. Evolving research in neuroscience continues to unravel the physiological substrates for interactions among these factors. Consequently, it is incumbent on the clinician, therefore, to avoid the inclination to dichotomize between physical/sensory aspects of pain and psychosocial factors. A multimodal approach, i.e., employing psychotherapeutic and psychopharmacologic treatments, is necessary to address the complex interactions among the biopsychosocial covariates accompanying pain conditions.

Case Scenario

Raphael J. Leo, MA, MD, Wendy J. Quinton, PhD, and Michael H. Ebert, MD

Anne, a 50-year-old woman with a 20-year history of type 2 diabetes mellitus, has developed diabetic neuropathy. She presents to her primary care provider with sensations of pain alternating with tingling and burning sensations in both hands and feet. Her pain score is 10/10 on most days and the lowest score is 7. The pain has started to affect her sleep and daily activities. She has been taking acetaminophen and ibuprofen without much relief. Following a detailed assessment, the PCP prescribes gabapentin. Two weeks later she returns to the clinic in tears and very upset, complaining that her pain is worse. She believes the medications are not working at all. She mentions that her appetite is reduced.

What should be the further course of management?
Chronic pain and affective illnesses can often co-exist. Lack of sleep, appetite, and failure of medication could be an indication of depression. She requires a detailed psychiatric evaluation.
Further assessment reveals that psychological and psychosocial factors are playing an important role in her pain exacerbation. Anne's husband had to relocate because of job restructuring and the couple moved away from their home, family, and neighbors. She reported that the move proved to be very distressing to her, as she felt isolated from customary supports. Additionally, her son reportedly has a problem with gambling, incurring significant debt. She had given him money to cover his debts, only to realize that he returned to gambling once again. It is striking that even though she admits that she has "a hard time" accepting these events, she could not acknowledge any sort of anger or frustration. When directly asked about her reactions, she avoids the line of inquiry and instead focuses on her pain complaints. In the past year, the severity of pain has been the focus of multiple clinical presentations and consultations. Anne reports that, "The pain is always there and ruins my entire life. There is absolutely nothing that gives me relief." The patterns reflected in these statements signal the presence of catastrophizing, overgeneralizing, and helplessness.

She complains that her husband "is on the computer all day long" and that they have not shared activities together in recent years. She has a hard time making her displeasure known to him or making requests of him to share in activities. She perceives that he has a tendency to disregard her feelings. At such times, she has noted that she is most apt to experience pain exacerbations. She denies any ongoing litigation issues and is not receiving any disability compensation.

Anne endorsed dysphoria and bouts of tearfulness that seem to "overwhelm" her. She acknowledged that she has difficulty sustaining sleep and is often tired during the day. She feels that she has less interest in activities that she would customarily engage in due to her sadness and fatigue. Her appetite has been slightly reduced, although she was unsure if she had sustained significant weight loss. She reports periods of indecision and at times entertains passive thoughts of death. Such thoughts fuel escape fantasies that allow her to distract herself from her sadness, pain, inactivity, and isolation. Despite periods of futility and hopelessness related to pain with associated passive death thoughts, she vehemently denies any suicidal ideas, intent, or plans. She denies any significant alcohol use, illicit substance, and smoking cigarettes. She is advised to continue gabapentin for a total of 30 days.

At a 1-month follow-up appointment Anne reported some improvement in her symptoms, stating that the burning and tingling sensations had lessened allowing her more mobility during the day but that she continued to have paroxysms of pain at night that frequently disturb her sleep. Nonetheless, her pain was still rated as a 6 or 7 out of 10.

How will you assess depression in the clinic?
It could be assessed through clinical interview and use of self-rated questionnaires such as the Hospital Anxiety and Depression scale or Beck Depression Inventory. Often chronic pain and depression can co-exist. Her pain may have been augmented by her dysphoria, isolation, and depressive symptoms. In discussion with her primary care provider and psychiatrist, Anne agreed to add duloxetine to her medication regimen. She was begun on 30 mg daily, which was increased after 10 days, to 60 mg daily.

What are the non-pharmacological strategies that could be beneficial for Anne?
Cognitive Behavioral Therapy, hypnosis and Interpersonal Psychotherapy have been suggested.

She was also enlisted in psychotherapy with a cognitive behavioral focus. The emphasis of therapy was to identify affective states and cognitive distortions that were temporally related to pain exacerbations, develop a repertoire of coping skills to deal with stressors, and effectively express her anger. She was given instruction on self-regulatory approaches, e.g., relaxation techniques and self-hypnosis, to assist her with reducing distress. These measures helped to reduce her pain severity ratings.

Simultaneously, she was enrolled to participate in physical therapy as well as Yoga classes. These measures helped to increase her capacity for activity and physical endurance.

At a 3-month follow-up visit Anne reported the pain as significantly better. Her pain at its worst was rated as a 2 to 3 out of 10. Her mood was improved, and she reported less tearfulness. She was sleeping better and seemed to have more energy to pursue interests. She was even beginning to engage with some of her new neighbors and peers from her Yoga class and had become involved in social engagements that effectively reduced her isolation.

Anne is now able to perform all activities of daily living. In addition, she reported the paroxysms of pain at night have ceased to disturb her sleep and she can't remember the last time she experience that "unbearable" pain.

References

Alaranta H, Rytokoski U, Rissanen A, et al. Intensive physical and psychosocial training program for patients with chronic low back pain. A controlled clinical trial. Spine 1994;19(12):1339–49.

Albert H. Psychosomatic group treatment helps women with chronic pelvic pain. J Psychosom Obstet Gynaecol. 1999;20:216–25.

American Psychiatric Association. Diagnostic and statistical manual of mental disorders, 4th ed. Text Revision. Washington, DC: American Psychiatric Association; 2000.

Andrasik F. What does the evidence show? Efficacy of behavioural treatments for recurrent headaches in adults. Neurol Sci. 2007;28(Suppl 2):70–7.

Ansari A. The efficacy of newer antidepressants in the treatment of chronic pain: a review of current literature. Harv Rev Psychiatry. 2000;7:257–77.

Arnold LM, Keck PE, Welge JA. Antidepressant treatment of fibromyalgia. A meta-analysis and review. Psychosomatics 2000;41(2):104–13.

Asmundson GJ, Coons MJ, Taylor S, Katz J. PTSD and the experience of pain: research and clinical implications of shared vulnerability and mutual maintenance models. Can J Psychiatry. 2002;47(10):930–7.

Astin JA, Beckner W, Soeken K, Hochberg MC, Berman B. Psychological interventions for rheumatoid arthritis: a meta-analysis of randomized controlled trials. Arthritis Rheum. 2002;47:291–302.

Bair MJ, Robinson RL, Katon W, Kroenke K. Depression and pain comorbidity: a literature review. Arch Intern Med. 2003;163(20):2433–45.

Banks SM, Kerns RD. Explaining high rates of depression in chronic pain: a diathesis–stress framework. Psychol Bull. 1996;119:95–10.

Bartusch SL, Sanders BJ, D'Alessio JG, Jernigan JR. Clonazepam for the treatment of lancinating phantom limb pain. Clin J Pain 1996;12(1):59–62.

Bendtsen L, Jensen R. Mirtazapine is effective in the prophylactic treatment of chronic tension-type headache. Neurology 2004;62(10):1706–11.

Blackburn-Munro G, Blackburn-Munro RE. Chronic pain, chronic stress and depression: coincidence or consequence? J Neuroendocrinol. 2001;13(12):1009–23.

Blanchard EB. A critical review of cognitive, behavioral, and cognitive-behavioral therapies for irritable bowel syndrome. J Cogn Psychother. 2005;19(2):101–23.

Bouckoms AJ, Litman RE. Clonazepam in the treatment of neuralgic pain syndrome. Psychosomatics 1985;26:933–936.

Bradley LA, McKendree-Smith NL, Cianfrini LR. Cognitive-behavioral therapy interventions for pain associated with chronic illnesses. Sem Pain Med. 2003;1(2):44–54.

Breslau N, Davis GC. Migraine, physical health and psychiatric disorder: a prospective epidemiology study in young adults. J Psychiatr Res. 1993;27:211–21.

Brown DG, Krupp JJ. N-Methyl-D-aspartate receptor (NMDA) antagonists as potential pain therapeutics. Curr Top Med Chem. 2006;6(8):749–70.

Brown RL, Patterson JJ, Rounds LA, Papasouliotis O. Substance abuse among patients with chronic back pain. J Fam Pract. 1996;43(2):152–60.

Burns JW, Johnson BJ, Mahoney N, Devine J, Pawl R. Cognitive and physical capacity process variables predict long-term outcome after treatment of chronic pain. J Consult Clin Psychol. 1998;66(2):434–9.

Campbell JK, Penzien DB, Wall EM. Evidenced-based guidelines for migraine headache: behavioral and physical treatments. The US Headache Consortium. Available at: http://www.aan.com/professionals/practice/pdfs/gl0089.pdf. Accessed May 2009.

Chaiken DC, Blaivas JG, Blaivas ST. Behavioral therapy for the treatment of refractory interstitial cystitis. J Urol. 1993;149:1445–8.

Chandramouli J. Newer anticonvulsant drugs in neuropathic pain and bipolar disorder. J Pain Palliat Care Pharmacother. 2002;16(4):19–37.

Chang G, Chen L, Mao J. Opioid tolerance and hyperalgesia. Med Clin North Am. 2007;91(2):199–211.

Chong MS, Smith TE. Anticonvulsants for the management of pain. Pain Rev. 2000;7:129–49.

Ciccone DS, Just N, Bandilla EB, Reimer E, Ilbeigi MS, Wu W. Psychological correlates of opioid use in patients with chronic nonmalignant pain: a preliminary test of the downhill spiral hypothesis. J Pain Symptom Manage. 2000;20(3):180–92.

Cleeland CS, Ryan KM. Pain assessment: global use of the Brief Pain Inventory. Ann Acad Med Singapore. 1994;23:129–38.

Cohen H, Neumann L, Haiman Y, Matar MA, Press J, Buskila D. Prevalence of post-traumatic stress disorder in fibromyalgia patients: overlapping syndromes or post-traumatic fibromyalgia syndrome? Semin Arthritis Rheum. 2002;32(1):38–50.

Cohen MJM, Menefee LA, Doghramji K, et al. Sleep in chronic pain: problems and treatments. Int Rev Psychiatry. 2000;12:115–26.

Collins SL, Moore RA, McQuay HJ, Wiffen P. Antidepressants and anticonvulsants for diabetic neuropathy and postherpetic neuralgia: a quantitative systematic review. J Pain Symptom Manage. 2000;20(6):449–58.

Crofford LJ, Rowbotham MC, Mease PJ, et al. Pregabalin for the treatment of fibromyalgia syndrome: results of a randomized, double-blind, placebo-controlled trial. Arthritis Rheum. 2005;52(4):1264–73.

Dellemijn PL, Fields HL. Do benzodiazepines have a role in chronic pain management? Pain 1994;57:137–52.

Derakshan N, Eysenck MW. Interpretive biases for one's own behavior and physiology in high-trait-anxious individuals and repressors. J Pers Soc Psychol. 1997;73:816–25.

Dersh J, Polatin PB, Gatchel RJ. Chronic pain and psychopathology: research findings and theoretical considerations. Psychosom Med. 2002;64:773–86.

DiMatteo MR, Lepper HS, Croghan TW. Depression is a risk factor for noncompliance with medical treatment. Meta-analysis of the effects of anxiety and depression on patient adherence. Arch Intern Med. 2000;160:2101–7.

Doverty M, White JM, Somogyi AA, Bochner F, Ali R, Ling W. Hyperalgesic responses in methadone maintenance patients. Pain 2001;90(1–2):91–6.

Duman RS, Monteggia LM. A neurotrophic model for stress-related mood disorders. Biol Psychiatry. 2006;59:1116–27.

Dunbar SA, Katz NP. Chronic opioid therapy for nonmalignant pain in patients with a history of substance abuse: report of 20 cases. J Pain Symptom Manage. 1996;11(3):163–71.

Duric V, McCarson KE. Hippocampal neurokinin-1 receptor and brain-derived neurotrophic factor gene expression is decreased in rat models of pain and stress. Neuroscience 2005;133:999–1006.

Dworkin SF, Turner JA, Mancl, L, et al. A randomized clinical trial of a tailored comprehensive care treatment program for temporomandibular disorders. J Orofac Pain. 2002;16(4):259–76.

Dworkin SF, Turner JA, Wilson L, et al. Brief group cognitive-behavioral intervention for temporomandibular disorders. Pain 1994;59(2):175–87.

Ehde DM, Jensen MP. Feasibility of a cognitive restructuring intervention for treatment of chronic pain in persons with disabilities. Rehabil Psychol. 2004;49(3):254–8.

Eide PK, Jorum E, Stubhaug A, Bremnes J, Breivik H. Relief of post-herpetic neuralgia with the N-methyl-aspartic acid receptor antagonist ketamine: a double-blind cross-over comparison with morphine and placebo. Pain 1994;58(3):347–54.

Eisenberg E, Kleiser A, Dotort A, et al. The NMDA (N-methyl-D-aspartate) receptor antagonist memantine in the treatment of postherpetic neuralgia: a double-blind, placebo-controlled study. Eur J Pain. 1998;2:321–7.

Enarson MC, Hays H, Woodroffe MA. Clinical experience with oral ketamine. J Pain Symptom Manage. 1999;17:384–6.

Engel GL. The clinical application of the biopsychosocial model. Am J Psychiatry. 1980;137:535–44.

Evans S, Fishman B, Spielman L, Haley A. Randomized trial of cognitive behavior therapy versus supportive psychotherapy for HIV-related peripheral neuropathic pain. Psychosomatics 2003; 44:44–50.

Farquhar CM, Rogers V, Franks S, Pearce S, Wadsworth J, Beard, RW. A randomized controlled trial of medroxyprogesterone acetate and psychotherapy for the treatment of pelvic congestion. Br J Obstet Gynaecol. 1989;96:1153–62.

Fields HL, Basbaum AI. Central nervous system mechanisms of pain modulation, In: Wall PD, Melzack R, editors. Textbook of pain. 4th ed. Edinburgh: Churchill Livingstone; 1999. pp. 309–29.

Fishbain DA, Cutler R, Rosomoff H. Comorbid psychiatric disorders in chronic pain patients. Pain Clin 1998;11:79–87.

Fishbain DA, Cutler R, Rosomoff HL, Rosomoff RS. Chronic pain-associated depression: antecedent or consequence of chronic pain? A review. Clin J Pain. 1997;13:116–37.

Fishbain DA, Cutler RB, Lewis J, Cole B, Rosomoff RS, Rosomoff HL. Do the second-generation "atypical neuroleptics" have analgesic properties? A structured evidence-based review. Pain Med. 2004;5(4):359–65.

Fishbain DA. Approaches to treatment decisions for psychiatric comorbidity in the management of the chronic pain patient. Med Clin North Am. 1999;83:737–60.

Fisher K, Coderre TJ, Hagen NA. Targeting the N-methyl-D-aspartate receptor for chronic pain management: preclinical animal studies, recent clinical experience and future research directions. J Pain Symptom Manage. 2000;20(5):358–73.

Forseth KO, Husby G, Gran JT, Forre O. Prognostic factors for the development of fibromyalgia in women with self-reported musculoskeletal pain. A prospective study. J Rheumatol. 1999;26(11):2458–67.

Frampton JE, Scott LJ. Pregabalin in the treatment of painful diabetic neuropathy. Drugs 2004;64(24):2813–20.

Galer BS. Neuropathic pain of peripheral origin: advances in pharmacologic treatment. Neurology 1995;45(suppl 9):17–25.

Gallagher RM. Treatment planning in pain medicine – integrating medical, physical, and behavioral therapies. Med Clin North Am. 1999;83(3):823–49.

Gatchel RJ. Early development of physical and mental deconditioning in painful spinal disorders. In: Mayer TG, Mooney V, Gatchel RJ, editors. Contemporary conservative care for painful spinal disorders. Philadelphia, PA: Lea & Febiger; 1991. pp. 278–89.

Gerner P, Mujtaba M, Sinnott CJ, Wang GK. Amitriptyline versus bupivacaine in rat sciatic nerve blockade. Anesthesiology 2001;94(4):661–7.

Goldenberg DL, Burckhardt C, Crofford L. Management of fibromyalgia syndrome. JAMA 2004;292(19):2388–95.

Gomez-Perez FJ, Rull JA, Dies H, Rodriquez-Rivera JG, Gonzalez-Barranco J, Lozano-Castaneda O. Nortriptyline and fluphenazine in the symptomatic treatment of diabetic neuropathy: a double-blind cross-over study. Pain 1985;23(4):395–400.

Gonul AS, Akdeniz F, Taneli F, Donat O, Eker C, Vahip S. Effect of treatment on serum brain-derived neurotrophic factor levels in depressed patients. Eur Arch Psychiatry Clin Neurosci. 2005;255:381–6.

Guay DR. Oxcarbazepine, topiramate, zonisamide, and levetiracetam: potential use in neuropathic pain. Am J Geriatr Pharmacother. 2003;1(1):18–37.

Gureje O, Von Korff M, Kola L, et al. The relation between multiple pains and mental disorders: results from the World Mental Health Surveys. Pain 2008;135(1–2): 82–91.

Hagglund KJ, Haley WE, Reveille JD, Alarcon GS. Predicting individual differences in pain and functional impairment among patients with rheumatoid arthritis. Arthritis Rheum. 1989;32:851–8.

Hathaway SR, McKinley JC, Butcher JN, et al. Minnesota multiphasic personality inventory-2: manual for administration. Minneapolis, MN: University of Minnesota Press; 1989.

Haythornthwaite JA, Sieber WJ, Kerns RD. Depression and the chronic pain experience. Pain 1991;46:177–84.

Health United States, 2006 with chartbook on trends in the health of Americans. Hyattsville, MD: National Centers for Health Statistics; 2006. pp. 116–24.

Henschke N, Ostelo RWJG, van Tulder MW, Vlaeyen JWS, Morley S, Assendelft WJJ, Main CJ. Behavioural treatment for chronic low-back pain. Cochrane Database Syst Rev. 2010;(7):CD002014. DOI: 10.1002/14651858.CD002014.pub3. Available from www2. cochrane.org/reviews/en/ab002014.html

Hoffman BM, Papas RK, Chatkoff DK, Kerns RD. Meta-analysis of psychological interventions for chronic low back pain. Health Psychol. 2007;26(1):1–9.

Irwin M, McClintick J, Costlow C, Fortner M, White J, Gillin JC. Partial night sleep deprivation reduces natural killer and cellular immune response in humans. FASEB J. 1996;10(5):643–53.

Ives TJ, Chelminski PR, Hammett-Stabler CA, et al. Predictors of opioid misuse in patients with chronic pain: a prospective cohort study. BMC Health Serv Res. 2006;6:46.

Jackson JL, O'Malley PG, Tomkins G, Balden E, Santoro J, Kroenke K. Treatment of functional gastrointestinal disorders with antidepressant medications: a meta-analysis. Am J Med. 2000;108:65–72.

Jensen MP, Karoly P, Huger R. The development and preliminary validation of an instrument to assess patients' attitudes toward pain. J Psychosom Res. 1987;31(3):393–400.

Jensen MP, Karoly P. Self-report scales and procedures for assessing pain in adults. In: Turk DC, Melzack R, editors. Handbook of pain assessment. 2nd ed. New York, NY: The Guilford Press; 2001. pp. 15–34.

Jensen MP, Turner JA, Romano JM, Karoly P. Coping with chronic pain: a critical review of the literature. Pain 1991;47:249–83.

Katerndahl D. Panic plaques: panic disorder & coronary artery disease in patients with chest pain. J Am Board Fam Pract. 2004;17(2):114–26.

Kawasaki Y, Kumamoto E, Furue H, Yoshimura M. Alpha 2 adrenoceptor-mediated presynaptic inhibition of primary afferent glutamatergic transmission in rat substantia gelatinosa neurons. Anesthesiology 2003;98:682–9.

Keefe FJ, Abernethy AP, Campbell LC. Psychological approaches to understanding and treating disease-related pain. Annu Rev Psychol. 2005;56:601–30.

Kelada E, Jones A. Interstitial cystitis. Arch Gynecol Obstet. 2007;275(4):223–9.

Kerns RD, Turk DC, Rudy TE. The West Haven-Yale Multidimensional Pain Inventory (WHYMPI). Pain 1985;23(4):345–56.

Khojainova N, Santiago-Palma J, Kornick C, Breitbart W, Gonzales GR. Olanzapine in the management of cancer pain. J Pain Symptom Manage. 2002;23(4):346–50.

Khoromi S, Patsalides A, Parada S, Salehi V, Meegan JM, Max MB. Topiramate in chronic lumbar radicular pain. J Pain. 2005;6(12):829–36.

King T, Gardell LR, Wang R, et al. Role of NK-1 neurotransmission in opioid-induced hyperalgesia. Pain 2005;116(3):276–88.

Knutson KL, Spiegel K, Penev P, Van Cauter E. The metabolic consequences of sleep deprivation. Sleep Med Rev. 2007;11(3):163–78.

Koenig TW, Clark MR. Advances in comprehensive pain management. Psychiatr Clin North Am. 1996;19:589–611.

Lackner JM, Lou Coad M, Mertz HR, et al. Cognitive therapy for irritable bowel syndrome is associated with reduced limbic activity, GI symptoms, and anxiety. Behav Res Ther. 2006;44(5):621–38.

Lackner JM, Quigley BM. Pain catastrophizing mediates the relationship between worry and pain suffering in patients with irritable bowel syndrome. Behav Res Ther. 2005;43:943–57.

Larijani GE, Goldberg ME, Hojat M, Khaleghi B, Dunn JB, Marr AT. Modafinil improves recovery after general anesthesia. Anesth Analg. 2004;98(4):976–81.

Lee RL, Spencer PS. Effect of tricyclic antidepressants on analgesic activity in laboratory animals. Postgrad Med J. 1980;56(suppl 1):19–24.

Leino P, Magni G. Depressive and distress symptoms as predictors of low back pain, neck–shoulder pain, and other musculoskeletal morbidity: a 10-year follow-up of metal industry employees. Pain 1993;53:89–94.

Leo RJ, Narendran R. Anticonvulsant use in the treatment of bipolar disorder: a primer for primary care physicians. Primary Care Companion J Clin Psychiatry. 1999;1:74–84.

Leo RJ. Treatment considerations in neuropathic pain. Curr Treat Options Neurol. 2006;8(5):389–400.

Leo RJ. Clinical manual of pain management in psychiatry. Washington, DC: American Psychiatric Publishing, Incorporated; 2007.

Lesbros-Pantoflickova D, Michetti P, Fried M, Beglinger C, Blum AL. Meta-analysis: the treatment of irritable bowel syndrome. Aliment Pharmacol Ther. 2004;20:1253–69.

Lin EHB, Katon W, Von Korff M, et al. Effect of improving depression care on pain and functional outcomes among older adults with arthritis: a randomized controlled trial. JAMA 2003;290(18):2428–34.

Loeser JD. Concepts of pain. In: Stanton-Hicks M, Boas R, eds. Chronic low back pain. New York, NY: Raven; 1982, pp. 145–48.

Lynch ME. Antidepressants as analgesics: a review of randomized controlled trials. J Psychiatry Neurosci. 2001;26(1):30–6.

Max MB, Lynch SA, Muir J, Shoaf SE, Smoller B, Dubner R. Effects of desipramine, amitriptyline, and fluoxetine on pain in diabetic neuropathy. N Engl J Med. 1992;326:1250–6.

Max MB. Treatment of post-herpetic neuralgia: antidepressants. Ann Neurol. 1994;35(suppl):50–3.

McQuay H, Carroll D, Jadad AR, Wiffen P, Moore A. Anticonvulsant drugs for management of pain: a systematic review. Br Med J. 1995;311:1047–52.

McQuay HJ, Tramer M, Nye BA, Carroll D, Wiffen PJ, Moore RA. A systematic review of antidepressants in neuropathic pain. Pain 1996;68:217–27.

McQuay HJ. Neuropathic pain: evidence matters. Eur J Pain. 2002;6(suppl A):11–8.

McWilliams LA, Cox BJ, Enns MW. Mood and anxiety disorders associated with chronic pain: an examination in a nationally representative sample. Pain 2003;106:127–33.

McWilliams LA, Goodwin RD, Cox BJ. Depression and anxiety associated with three pain conditions: results from a nationally representative sample. Pain 2004;111:77–83.

Melzack R. The McGill Pain Questionnaire: major properties and scoring methods. Pain 1975;1:277–99.

Melzack R. From the gate to the neuromatrix. Pain 1999;82(Suppl):S121–6.

Mochizucki D. Serotonin and noradrenaline reuptake inhibitors in animal models of pain. Hum Psychopharmacol Clin Exp. 2004;19(suppl 1):15–9.

Moldofsky H, Scarisbrick P. Introduction of neurasthenic musculoskeletal pain syndrome by selective sleep stage deprivation. Psychosom Med. 1976;38:35–44.

Moldofsky H. Sleep and pain. Sleep Med Rev. 2001;5:387–98.

Morley S, Eccleston C, Williams A. Systematic review and meta-analysis of randomized controlled trials of cognitive behaviour therapy and behaviour therapy for chronic pain in adults, excluding headache. Pain 1999;80:1–13.

Nemmani KVS, Mogil JS. Serotonin–GABA interactions in the modulation of mu- and kappa-opioid analgesia. Neuropharmacology 2003;44:304–10.

Nestler EJ, Barrot M, DiLeone RJ, Eisch AJ, Gold SJ, Monteggia LM. Neurobiology of depression. Neuron 2002;34(1):13–25.

Neugebauer V, Li W, Bird GC, Han JS. The amygdala and persistent pain. Neuroscientist 2004;10(3):221–34.

NIH Technology Assessment Panel on Integration of Behavioral and Relaxation Approaches Into the Treatment of Chronic Pain and Insomnia. Integration of behavioral and relaxation approaches into the treatment of chronic pain and insomnia. JAMA 1996;276(4):313–8.

Norrbrink Budh C, Kowalski J, Lundeberg T. A comprehensive pain management programme comprising educational, cognitive and behavioral interventions for neuropathic pain following spinal cord injury. J Rehabil Med. 2006;38(3):172–80.

Novak V, Kanard R, Kissel JT, Mendell JR. Treatment of painful sensory neuropathy with tiagabine: a pilot study. Clin Auton Res. 2001;11(6):357–61.

O'Malley PG, Balden E, Tomkins G, Santoro J, Kroenke K, Jackson JL. Treatment of fibromyalgia with antidepressants: a meta-analysis. J Gen Intern Med. 2000;15(9):659–66.

Onghena P, Van Houdenhove B. Antidepressant-induced analgesia in chronic non-malignant pain: a meta-analysis of 39 placebo-controlled studies. Pain 1992;49:205–19.

Pappagallo M. Newer antiepileptic drugs: possible uses in the treatment of neuropathic pain and migraine. Clin Ther. 2003;25(10):2506–38.

Parker J, Frank R, Beck N, et al. Pain in rheumatoid arthritis: relationship to demographic, medical, and psychological factors. J Rheumatol. 1988;15(3):433–7.

Polatin PB, Kinney RK, Gatchel RJ, Lillo E, Mayer TG. Psychiatric illness and chronic low-back pain. The mind and the spine—which goes first? Spine 1993;18(1):66–71.

Raffa RB. Antihistamines as analgesics. J Clin Pharm Ther. 2001;26(2):81–85.

Raison CL, Capuron L, Miller AH. Cytokines sing the blues: inflammation and the pathogenesis of depression. Trends Immunol. 2006;27(1):24–31.

Reddy S. Patt RB. The benzodiazepines as adjuvant analgesics. J Pain Symptom Manage. 1994;9(8):510–4.

Reissig JE, Rybarczyk AM. Pharmacologic treatment of opioid-induced sedation in chronic pain. Ann Pharmacother. 2005;39(4):727–31.

Reiter RC. Evidence-based management of chronic pelvic pain. Clin Obstet Gynecol. 1998;41(2):422–35.

Remillard G. Oxcarbazepine and intractable trigeminal neuralgia. Epilepsia 1994;35:528–9.

Romano JM, Turner JA. Chronic pain and depression: does the evidence support a relationship? Psychol Bull. 1985;97:18–34.

Rome HP Jr, Rome JD. Limbically augmented pain syndrome (LAPS): kindling, corticolimbic sensitization, and the convergence of affective and sensory symptoms in chronic pain disorders. Pain Med. 2000;1(1):7–23.

Rosenstiel AK, Keefe FJ. The use of coping strategies in chronic low back pain patients: relationship to patient characteristics and current adjustment. Pain 1983;17:33–44.

Roy-Byrne PP, Davidson KW, Kessler RC, et al. Anxiety disorders and comorbid medical illness. Gen Hosp Psychiatry. 2008;30(3):208–25.

Rumore MM, Schlichting DA. Clinical efficacy of antihistamines as analgesics. Pain 1986;25:7–22.

Saarto T, Wiffen PJ. Antidepressants for neuropathic pain. Cochrane Database of Syst Rev 2007;(4) Art No.: CD005454. doi:10.1002/14651858. CD005454.pub2.

Samborski W, Lezanska-Szpera M, Rybakowski JK. Open trial of mirtazapine in patients with fibromyalgia. Pharmacopsychiatry 2004;37(4):168–70.

Sanders SH. Operant therapy with pain patients: evidence for its effectiveness. In: Lebovits AH, editor. Seminars in pain medicine I. Philadelphia, PA: W.B. Saunders; 2003. pp. 90–8.

Sang CN, Booher S, Gilron I, Parada S, Max MB. Dextromethorphan and memantine in painful diabetic neuropathy and postherpetic neuralgia: efficacy and dose–response trials. Anesthesiology 2002;96(5):1053–61.

Saper JR, Lake AE, Tepper SJ. Nefazodone for chronic daily headache prophylaxis: an open-label study. Headache 2001;41:465–74.

Scheer SJ, Watanabe TK, Radack KL. Randomized controlled trials in industrial low back pain. Part 3. Subacute/chronic pain interventions. Arch Phys Med Rehabil. 1997;78(4): 414–23.

Seidel S, Aigner M, Ossege M, Pernicka E, Wildner B, Sycha T. Antipsychotics for acute and chronic pain in adults. Cochrane Database Syst Rev. 2008;(4):CD004844. DOI: 10.1002/14651858.CD004844.pub2. Available from www2.cochrane.org/reviews/en/ab004844.html

Semenchuk MR, Davis B. Efficacy of sustained-release bupropion in neuropathic pain: an open-label study. Clin J Pain. 2000;16:6–11.

Sharav Y, Singer E, Schmidt E, Dionne RA, Dubner R. The analgesic effect of amitriptyline on chronic facial pain. Pain 1987;31(2):199–209.

Silberstein SD, Young WB, Hopkins MM, et al. Olanzapine in the treatment of refractory migraine and chronic daily headache. Cephalalgia 2000;20:382–3.

Sindrup SH, Jensen TS. Efficacy of pharmacological treatments of neuropathic pain: an update and effect related to mechanism of drug action. Pain 1999;83(3):389–400.

Snow V, Weiss K, Wall EM, Mottur-Pilson C, American Academy of Family Physicians. Pharmacologic management of acute attacks of migraine and prevention of migraine headache. Ann Intern Med. 2002;137(10):840–9.

Solaro C, Uccelli MM, Brichetto G, Gaspperini C, Mancardi G. Topiramate relieves idiopathic and symptomatic trigeminal neuralgia. J Pain Symptom Manage. 2001;21(5):367–8.

Stones W, Cheong YC, Howard FM. Interventions for treating chronic pelvic pain in women. Cochrane Database Syst Rev. 2007;4:CD000387.

Sullivan MJ, Thorn B, Haythornthwaite JA, et al. Theoretical perspectives on the relation between catastrophizing and pain. Clin J Pain. 2001;17(1):52–64.

Sussman N. SNRI's versus SSRI's: mechanisms of action in treating depression and painful physical symptoms. Primary Care Companion J Clin Psychiatry. 2003;5(suppl 7):19–26.

Swartz KL, Pratt LA, Armenian HK, et al. Mental disorders and the incidence of migraine headaches in a community sample: results from the Baltimore Epidemiologic Catchment Area follow-up study. Arch Gen Psychiatry. 2000;57:945–50.

Tait RC, Pollard CA, Margolis RB, Duckro PN. Krause SJ. The Pain Disability index: psychometric and validity data. Arch Phys Med Rehabil. 1987;68(7):438–41.

Taiwo YO, Fabian A, Pazoles CJ, Fields HL. Potentiation of morphine antinociception by monoamine reuptake inhibitors in the rat spinal cord. Pain 1985;21(4):329–337.

Tomkins GE, Jackson JL, O'Malley PG, Balden E, Santoro JE. Treatment of chronic headache with antidepressants: a meta-analysis. Am J Med. 2001;111:54–63.

Turk DC, Okifuji A. Psychological factors in chronic pain: evolution and revolution. J Consult Clin Psychol. 2002;70(3):678–90.

Turner JA, Mancl L, Aaron LA. Brief cognitive-behavioral therapy for temporomandibular disorder pain: effects on daily electronic outcome and process measures. Pain 2005;117:377–87.

Turner JA, Mancl L, Aaron LA. Short- and long-term efficacy of brief cognitive-behavioral therapy for patients with chronic temporomandibular disorder pain: a randomized, controlled trial. Pain 2006;121:181–94.

van der Kolk BA, Pelcovitz D, Roth S, Mandel FS, McFarlane A, Herman JL. Dissociation, somatization, and affect dysregulation: the complexity of adaptation to trauma. Am J Psychiatry. 1996;153(suppl 7):83–93.

Van Ophoven A, Pokupic S, Heinecke A, Hertle L. A prospective, randomised, placebo-controlled, double-blind study of amitriptyline for the treatment of interstitial cystitis. J Urol. 2004;172(2):533–6.

Vanderah TW, Suenaga NM, Ossipov MH, Malan TP Jr, Lai J, Porreca F. Tonic descending facilitation from the rostral ventromedial medulla mediates opioid-induced abnormal pain and antinociceptive tolerance. J Neurosci. 2001;21(1):279–86.

Ventafridda V, Caraceni A, Saita L, et al. Trazodone for deafferentation pain: comparison with amitriptyline. Psychopharmacology (Berl) 1988;95(suppl):S44–9.

Vinik A. Use of antiepileptic drugs in the treatment of chronic painful diabetic neuropathy. J Clin Endocrinol Metab. 2005;90(8):4936–45.

Visser E, Schug SA. The role of ketamine in pain management. Biomed Pharmacother. 2006;60(7):341–8.

Vlaeyen JWS, Kole-Snijders AMJ, Boeren RGB, van Eek H. Fear of movement/(re)injury in chronic low back pain and its relation to behavioral performance. Pain 1995;62(3):363–72.

Vlaeyen JWS. Chronic low back pain: assessment and treatment from a behavioral rehabilitation perspective. Amsterdam: Swets & Zeitlinger; 1991.

Waddell G, Newton M, Henderson I, Somerville D, Main CJ. A Fear-Avoidance Beliefs Questionnaire (FABQ) and the role of fear-avoidance beliefs in chronic low back pain and disability. Pain 1993;52(2):157–68.

Ware JE Jr, Sherbourne CD. The MOS 36-Item Short-Form Health Survey (SF-36). I. Conceptual framework and item selection. Med Care. 1992;30(6):473–83.

Watkins LR, Hutchinson MR, Ledeboer A, Wieseler-Frank J, Milligan ED, Maier SF. Norman Cousins Lecture. Glia as the "bad guys": implications for improving clinical pain control and the clinical utility of opioids. Brain Behav Immun. 2007;21(2):131–46.

Webster DC, Brennan T. Use and effectiveness of psychological self-care strategies for interstitial cystitis. Health Care Women Int. 1995;16:463–75.

Weissman MM, Markowitz JC, Klerman GL. Comprehensive guide to interpersonal psychotherapy. New York, NY: Basic Books; 2000.

White, JM. Pleasure into pain: the consequences of long-term opioid use. Addict Behav. 2004;29(7):1311–24.

Wiffen PJ, Collins S, McQuay HJ, Carroll D, Jadad A, Moore, RA. Anticonvulsant drugs for acute and chronic pain. Cochrane Database Syst Rev. 2010;(1):CD001133. DOI: 10.1002/14651858.CD001133.pub3.

Wiffen PJ, Rees J. Lamotrigine for acute and chronic pain. The Cochrane Collaboration, Cochrane Pain, Palliative and Supportive Care Group. 2009;1.

Wu SM, Compton P, Bolus R, et al. The addiction behaviors checklist: validation of a new clinician-based measure of inappropriate opioid use in chronic pain. J Pain Symptom Manage. 2006;32(4):342–51.

Xie JY, Herman DS, Stiller CO, et al. Cholecystokinin in the rostral ventromedial medulla mediates opioid-induced hyperalgesia and antinociceptive tolerance. J Neurosci. 2005;25(2):409–16.

Yerby MS. Special considerations for women with epilepsy. Pharmacotherapy 2000; 2(suppl 8):159–70.

Yokogawa F, Kiuchi Y, Ishikawa Y, et al. An investigation of monoamine receptors involved in antinociceptive effects of antidepressants. Anesth Analg. 2002;95(1):163–8.

Young LD. Psychological factors in rheumatoid arthritis. J Consult Clin Psychol. 1992;60(4):619–27.

Zakrzewska JM, Chaudhry Z, Nurmikko TJ, Patton DW, Mullens EL. Lamotrigine (lamictal) in refractory trigeminal neuralgia: results from a double-blind placebo controlled crossover trial. Pain 1997;73(2):223–30.

Zenz M, Strumpf M, Tryba M. Long-term oral opioid therapy in patients with chronic nonmalignant pain. J Pain Symptom Manage. 1992;7(2):69–77.

Chapter 13

Interventional Pain Management

Michael A. Cosgrove, MD, David K. Towns, MD, Gilbert J. Fanciullo, MS, MD, and Alan D. Kaye, MD, PhD

Introduction

Invasive procedures performed by the pain management specialist are a mainstay in the diagnosis and treatment of both acute and chronic pain. They range from unguided percutaneous injections with short-acting local anesthetics to neurosurgical operations under computed tomography that permanently alter the anatomy. This chapter provides a description of the most common procedures performed by the pain management specialist, with more detail on the most frequent. The descriptions are not in sufficient enough detail to perform the procedures, and reference should be made to an interventional pain atlas for specifics.

Procedures are usually performed in a dedicated room with nursing staff and monitoring equipment. Imaging equipment, most often fluoroscopy, is used to guide the interventions and add a high level of accuracy. Ultrasound is being utilized more frequently, probably due to its portability and popularity in regional anesthesia. Some patients require sedation, but most procedures can be performed with minimal parenteral medications. Patient participation during some procedures is advantageous. Some of the more invasive require a general operating room and anesthesia, such as intrathecal pumps, spinal cord stimulators, and most of the neurosurgical interventions.

There are many procedures or "blocks" for pre- and postoperative pain that fall into the realm of regional anesthesia that are also utilized in acute and chronic pain management, but the scope of this chapter prevents a detailed description of these blocks. An invaluable resource for these procedures is the New York Society of Regional Anesthesia web site (www.nysora.com). There are also many texts available.

Many of the procedures suffer from a lack of research-based validity due to the difficulty in performing prospective randomized controlled studies. Approval for studies using placebo or sham treatments is difficult to acquire from institutional investigational review boards.

Head and Neck
Supraorbital Nerve Blocks
Indications
This is a useful block for pain after herpes zoster and for supraorbital neuralgia.

N. Vadivelu et al. (eds.), *Essentials of Pain Management*,
DOI 10.1007/978-0-387-87579-8_13, © Springer Science+Business Media, LLC 2011

Anatomy

The supraorbital nerve is a branch of the frontal nerve which enters the orbit via the superior orbital fissure. A smaller branch of the frontal nerve is the supratrochlear nerve.

Technique

To perform this block, the supraorbital notch is identified on the affected side and a 1.5-in. 25-gauge needle is advanced medially at the level of the supraorbital notch to avoid the supraorbital foramen. Depot steroid can be added to the local anesthetic up to 80 mg for the initial block and 40 mg of depot steroid for subsequent blocks. Three cubic centimeters of solution is then injected in a fan-like manner.

Supratrochlear Nerve Blocks
Technique

This block is done lateral to the junction of the bridge of the nose and the supraorbital ridge. A local anesthetic and depot steroid up to 80 mg for the first block and up to 40 mg for blocks thereafter can be used with a 1.5-in. 25-gauge needle. Approximately 3 cc of the solution is injected in a fan-like manner.

Infraorbital Nerve Blocks
Indications

This block can be used to treat pain associated with herpes zoster, facial pain in the supply region of the infraorbital nerve, and infraorbital neuralgias.

Anatomy

The inferior orbital nerve is a branch of the maxillary nerve and enters the orbit via the infraorbital foramen. It innervates the lower eyelid, the upper lip, and the lateral nares. Its superior alveolar branch is a sensory nerve which provides innervation to the upper incisor and canine teeth as well as associated gingivae.

Technique

This block can be done extraorally or intraorally.

(i) The extraoral infraorbital block is performed with a 25-gauge 1.5-in. needle inserted at the level of the infraorbital notch and directed medially to avoid entering the foramen. Along with local anesthetic solution a total of 80 mg of depot steroid can be used for the initial block and 40 mg of depot steroid can be used for subsequent blocks. A total of 3 cc of solution is injected in a fan-like manner.

(ii) The infraoral intraorbital block is done after the administration of topical anesthesia with 10% cocaine or 2% viscous lidocaine given into the mucosa of the alveolar sulcus inferior to the infraorbital foramen. A 25-gauge 1.5-in. needle is directed toward the infraorbital foramen to avoid entering the foramen. Paresthesia may be elicited during the procedure, and local anesthetic and depot steroid can be injected in a manner similar to the extraoral approach.

Complications

The most common complications of the above blocks are hematoma and compression neuropathy.

Auriculotemporal Nerve Blocks

Indications

This block is useful for pain in the areas supplied by the auriculotemporal nerve such as atypical facial pain of the temporomandibular joint, neuralgias after trauma, malignant pain, and acute herpes zoster of the external auditory meatus.

Anatomy

The auriculotemporal nerve is a branch of the mandibular nerve going upward through the parotid gland. It provides sensory innervation to the temporomandibular joint, to the external auditory meatus, and to portions of the pinna of the ear. It continues upward with the temporal artery and provides further sensory innervation to the lateral scalp and the temporal region.

Technique

The temporal artery provides a useful landmark for this block and is identified above the origin of the zygoma of the affected side (Fig. 13.1). A 25-gauge 1.5-in. needle is used to enter this area perpendicularly until the periosteum is reached. A total of 5 cc of solution of the local anesthetic and depot steroid can be injected with 3 cc at this point and another 2 cc in a fan-like fashion with a more cephalad redirection.

Greater Auricular Nerve Blocks

Indications

This block is useful for pain secondary to herpes zoster and for the treatment of painful conditions supplied by the greater auricular nerve.

Anatomy

The greater auricular nerve arises from the ventral rami of the second and the third cervical nerves. It provides sensory innervation to the ear, the skin over the parotid gland, and the external auditory canal.

Technique

The mastoid process is identified on the side of the pain in the area of the greater auricular nerve. After skin preparation at the level of the mastoid process a 22-gauge 1.5-in. needle is inserted and advanced perpendicularly until the periosteum is reached. After aspiration, a total of 5 cc of a solution of local anesthetic and depot steroid is injected. After the first 3 cc of the mixture is given, the needle is redirected medially and the remainder of the 2 cc of solution is injected in a fan-like fashion. As with several of the blocks described above, depot steroid can be used up to 80 mg for the first block with 40 mg used for subsequent blocks.

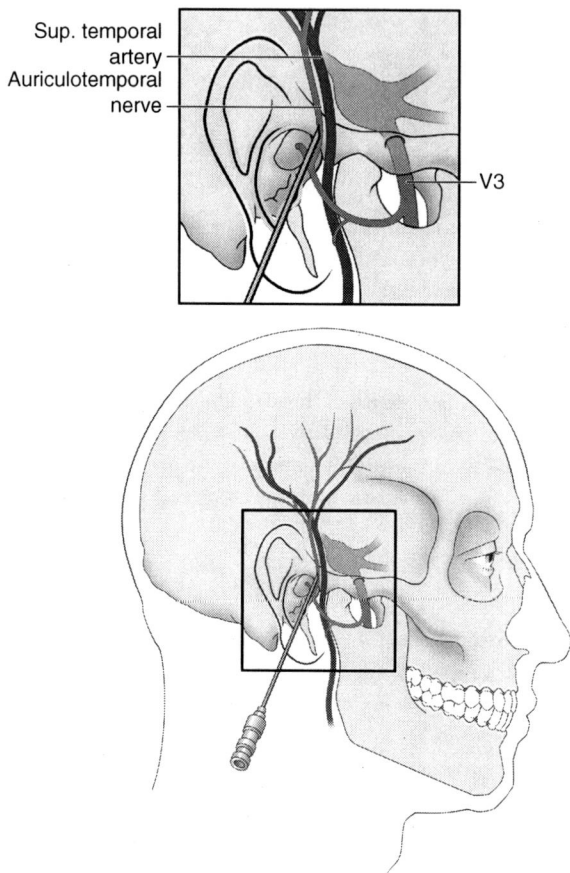

Figure 13.1   Auriculotemporal nerve block.

Inferior Alveolar Nerve Blocks
Indications
The inferior alveolar nerve is a branch of the mandibular nerve and is a useful block to diagnose and treat painful conditions in the areas supplied by the inferior alveolar nerve.

Anatomy
This nerve passes through the mandibular canal and innervates the molars, the premolars, and the associated gingivae. The inferior alveolar nerve gives off two branches: the incisor branch and the mental branch. The mental branch passes through the mental canal.

Technique
To perform this block, the anterior margin of the mandible just before the last molar on the affected side is identified. Topical anesthesia is given over this area with 10% cocaine solution or 2% viscous lidocaine. A 25-gauge 2-in. needle is used to reach the inner surface of the

mandible, and 3–5 cc of local anesthetic with depot steroid is slowly injected. In the case of intractable pain due to malignancy 6.5% aqueous phenol can be used to produce neurolysis.

Mental Nerve Blocks
Anatomy
The mental nerve is a branch of the mandibular nerve and exits the mandible via the mental foramen at the level of the second premolar. Upon exiting it makes a sharp turn upward and provides sensory branches to corresponding oral mucosa, the lower lip, and the chin.

Technique
(i) Extraoral approach for mental nerve block.
   Local anesthetic to the skin is administered after the identification of the mental notch. A 25-gauge 1.5-in. needle is advanced medially at a 15° angle to avoid the foramen, and a total of 3 cc of local anesthetic and depot steroid solution is administered in a fan-like manner. Depot steroid can be used up to 80 mg for the first injection, followed by 40 mg of depot steroid for subsequent injections.
(ii) Intraoral approach for mental nerve block.
   This block requires topical anesthesia with 10% cocaine or 2% viscous lidocaine to be applied to the alveolar sulcus just above the mental foramen after pulling down the lower lip. A 25-gauge 1.5-in. needle is advanced toward the mental foramen and a total of 3 cc of the solution used similar to the mental nerve block done by the extraoral approach.

Trigeminal Ganglion Blocks
Indications
The trigeminal ganglion block is useful in the presence of facial pain and can be used to determine whether the pain is due to somatic or sympathetic causes. It can also be used to treat painful conditions of the region of supply of the trigeminal nerves.

Anatomy
The trigeminal nerve (CNV) is the largest of the cranial nerves and supplies the major sensory innervation to the face. The trigeminal (or Gasserian) ganglion has three sensory divisions: ophthalmic (V1), maxillary (V2), and mandibular (V3). Trigeminal neuralgia, also called *tic douloureux*, may cause excruciating pain in any of the three sensory dermatomes of the ophthalmic (V1), maxillary (V2), or mandibular (V3) branches.

All three branches of cranial nerve V may be blocked at the level of the trigeminal or (Gasserian) ganglion. The maxillary V2 and mandibular V3 branches may be individually blocked in the pterygopalatine fossa and below the zygomatic arch, respectively.

Technique
Trigeminal nerve blockade can be done with a coronoid approach, and the maxillary or the mandibular nerve can be blocked with this approach. The maxillary nerve (V2) is a purely sensory nerve while the mandibular nerve has sensory and motor roots. Usually a 3.5-in. 22-gauge styletted needle is used for this block. The entry point is below the zygomatic arch in the middle of the coronoid notch perpendicular to the skull (Fig. 13.2). The needle is advanced

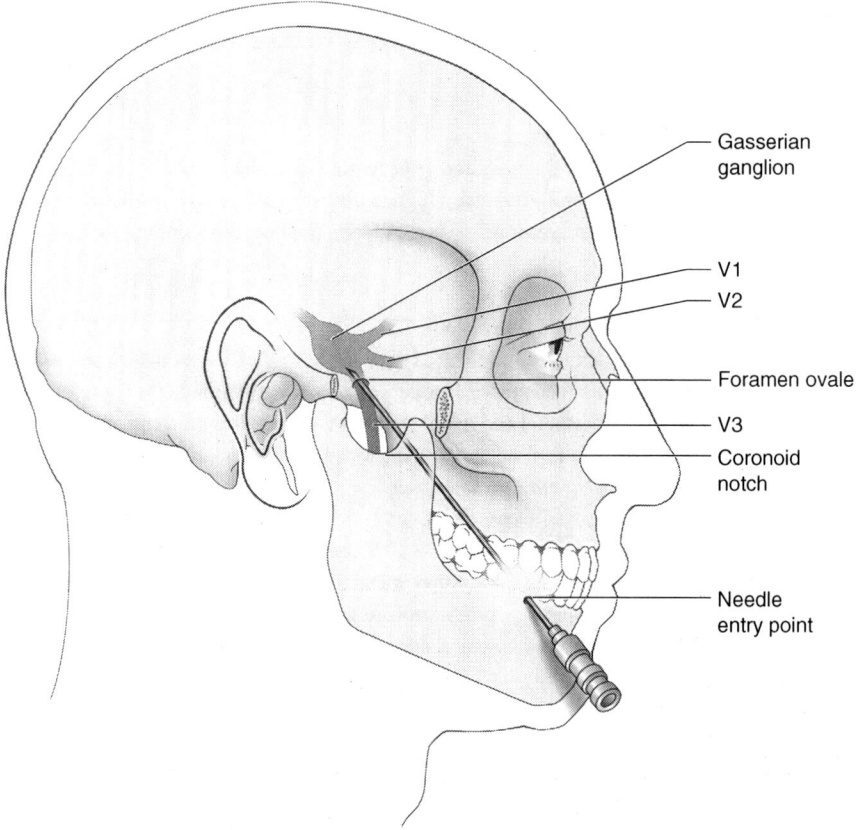

Figure 13.2   Gasserian ganglion block.

until the lateral pterygoid plate is reached. For both maxillary and mandibular nerves to be blocked, 7–8 cc of local anesthetic agent is administered. For selective blockade of the maxillary nerve the needle is redirected anteriorly and superiorly past the anterior margin of the lateral pterygoid plate up to a depth of 1 cm before the administration of 3–5 cc of local anesthetic solution. For selective blockade of the mandibular nerve, the needle is redirected posterior-inferiorly below the inferior margin of the lateral pterygoid plate to a depth of 1 cm before the administration of 3–5 cc of local anesthetic solution.

Complications
A common complication of this block is facial numbness. Some patients may find the resultant facial numbness more unpleasant than the pain from trigeminal neuralgia.

Trigeminal Neurolysis
Indications
Trigeminal neurolysis is performed to treat chronic facial pain. It is most commonly caused by a malignancy that causes the symptoms of trigeminal neuralgia.

Technique

Trigeminal neurolysis can be done using alcohol injection or radiofrequency (RF). Other techniques are less commonly performed today. For trigeminal neurolysis a 13-cm 20-gauge styletted needle is generally used. The needle is placed perpendicular to the pupil of the eye with the eye looking straight in front of the patient and the needle directed toward the external acoustic meatus in a cephalad direction. After touching the base of the skull the needle is withdrawn and redirected posteriorly into the foramen ovale. A free flow of CSF should be observed prior to the injection of a test dose of lidocaine and the administration of contrast medium with fluoroscopic guidance; injection of a neurolytic agent can be then performed.

Sphenopalatine Ganglion Blocks

Indications

Sphenopalatine ganglion (SPG) or Meckel's ganglion blockade has been utilized as a treatment for a variety of pain conditions for over a century. This blockade is especially useful for the treatment of acute attacks of migraine and cluster headaches. Trigeminal neuralgia, atypical facial pain, and cluster and migraine headaches can be treated with this block.

Anatomy

The SPG is located in the pterygopalatine fossa *posterior to the middle nasal turbinate* and has sensory, motor, and autonomic components.

Technique

Transnasal Approach

Intranasal delivery of 4% lidocaine or 2% viscous lidocaine or 10% cocaine in the posterior pharynx superior to the middle turbinate is an effective and noninvasive approach. Cotton-tipped applicators soaked with local anesthetic left in the superior border of the middle turbinate for 20 min is a useful technique via the transnasal approach.

Lateral Approach

This is achieved by the placement of a needle through the coronoid notch. Opening and closing the mouth helps in identifying the area anterior inferior to the acoustic auditory meatus. A 3.5-in., 22-gauge needle through the middle of the coronoid notch is advanced until it touches the lateral pterygoid plate, after which the needle is redirected anterior-superiorly to reach close to the sphenopalatine ganglion. Fluoroscopy or needle stimulation at 50 Hz helps to confirm correct placement of the needle tip. An injection of 2 cc of local anesthetic is usually sufficient.

Greater Palatine Foramen Approach

Sphenopalatine ganglion block can also be performed by the greater palatine foramen approach (Fig. 13.3). This involves the identification of the greater palatine ganglion, which is present on the posterior portion of the hard palate medial to the gum line of the third molar. About 2 cc of local anesthetic is injected 2.5 cm after entering the foramen in a superior posterior fashion at 120° angle.

Radiofrequency lesioning of the sphenopalatine ganglion can be effective in the presence of chronic cluster headache, intractable pain due to cancer, and painful facial neuralgias. This is usually done with the lateral approach. Confirmation by sensory stimulation is first done

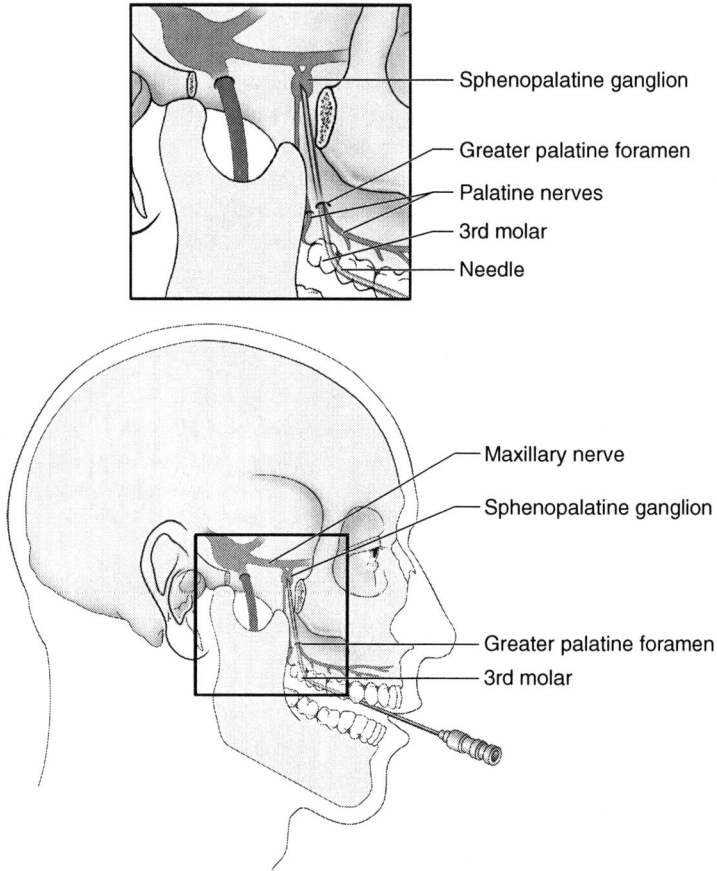

Figure 13.3 Sphenopalatine ganglion block: greater palatine foramen approach.

with 75 pulses with a pulse width of 0.25–0.5 ms, followed by radiofrequency lesioning for 80 s at 80°C.

Complications
Most common complications associated with sphenopalatine ganglion blocks include local anesthetic toxicity, orthostatic hypotension, bradycardia, and epistaxis.

Glossopharyngeal Blocks
Indications
Glossopharyngeal block is useful to provide anesthesia along the distribution of the glossopharyngeal nerve, including pharyngeal mucosa, soft palate, and the posterior third of the tongue region. Thus, glossopharyngeal neuralgia results in pain in the sensory distribution of the ninth cranial nerve, the tongue, the mouth, and the pharynx.

Anatomy

The glossopharyngeal nerve contains motor and sensory fibers with the motor nerve innervating the stylopharyngeus muscle and the sensory portion of the nerve innervating the posterior third of the tongue, the mucous membrane of the mouth and pharynx, and the palatine tonsil. The glossopharyngeal nerve exits from the jugular foramen close to the internal jugular vein and the vagus and the accessory nerves.

Technique

The glossopharyngeal nerve can be blocked from a lateral (extraoral) approach, posterior and inferior to the styloid process (Fig. 13.4). In this approach the midpoint of a line between the mastoid process and the angle of the mandible is accessed with a 1.5-in. 22-gauge needle until the styloid process is reached. The needle is then walked off the styloid process inferiorly, and approximately 7 cc of preservative-free 0.5% lidocaine is injected with 80 mg of depot steroid such as methylprednisolone for the first block and 40 mg of methylprednisolone for

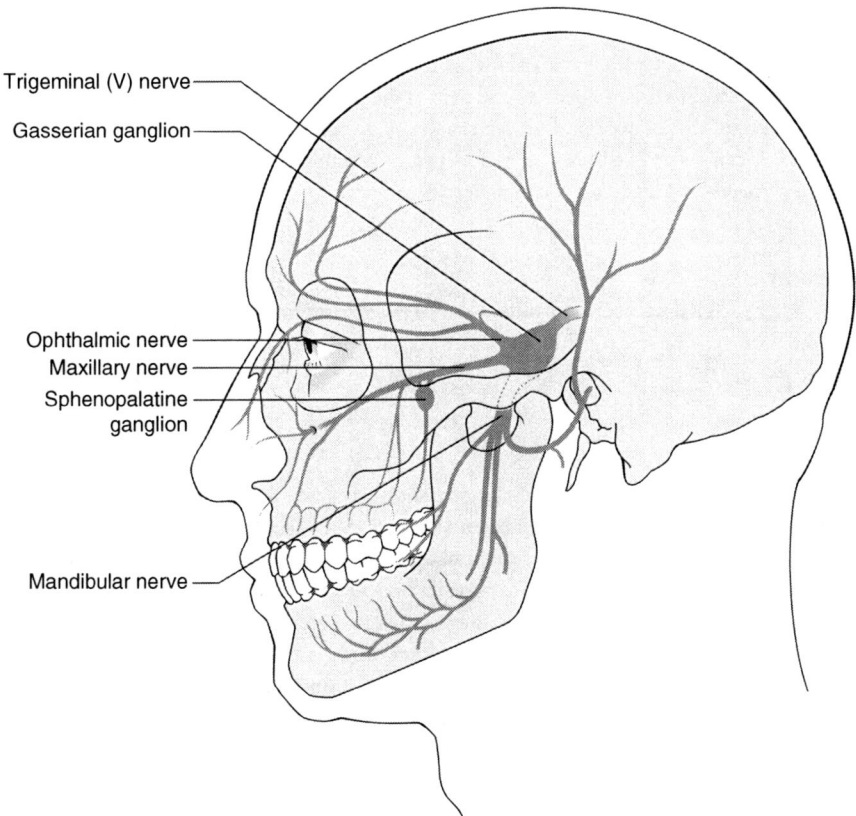

Figure 13.4 Sagittal of head showing major branches of the trigeminal nerve as well as the above-mentioned ganglia.

subsequent blocks. The injection is done slowly after negative aspiration for CSF or blood, and it is always important to inject in incremental doses.

The glossopharyngeal nerve can also be blocked by an intraoral approach. Here, the submucosal area over the medial portion of the palatine tonsil is accessed with a 22-gauge 3.5-in. spinal needle bent at 25°, after anesthetizing the tongue with 2% viscous lidocaine. The mucosa at the lower lateral portion of the posterior tonsillar pillar is entered, and after negative aspiration to blood or CSF, usually 7 cc of preservative-free 0.5% lidocaine combined with 80 mg methylprednisolone for the initial block with 40 mg methylprednisolone for subsequent blocks is injected in incremental doses.

Complications

It must be remembered that the internal carotid artery is posterolateral to the glossopharyngeal nerve when the intraoral approach is used. Nerve damage, intravascular and subarachnoid injection, and worsened pain are all possible complications.

Occipital Blocks
Indications

The occipital block is typically utilized for the treatment of occipital neuralgia. Occipital neuralgia usually manifests as tenderness and pain at the posterior occiput and may be the result of nerve entrapment or neck injuries such as whiplash. Inflammation of the occipital nerves, C2 and C3, can cause headaches as well as precipitate migraines. Occipital neuralgias can affect the greater and the lesser occipital nerves.

Anatomy

The greater occipital nerve arises from the dorsal posterior ramus of the second cervical nerve and the third cervical nerve, while the lesser occipital nerve arises from the ventral rami of the second and the third cervical nerves.

Technique

Injection of local anesthetic can be diagnostic and therapeutic in treating the pain and halting progression of the headache. Addition of a depot steroid may prolong the duration of relief. The injection is usually done in an examination room as fluoroscopic guidance is not required. The approach is to identify the greater occipital protuberance and the mastoid process of the affected side. An imaginary line is drawn between them and divided into thirds. The junction between the medial first and second thirds is the approximate location of the nerve. Palpation of the arterial pulse can help, and if found the injection should be medial to it, but it is not always discernable. The point is usually tender. A fine-gauge needle is then inserted and directed slightly cephalad until bone is contacted. The needle is then withdrawn a few millimeters, aspirated, and then 5 cc of local anesthetic with or without steroid is injected. The *lesser occipital nerve* may be blocked by a similar procedure at the junction of the outer thirds along the same line. The *third occipital nerve* from C3 may be blocked slightly caudal to these in the midline (Rosenberg and Phero 2003, Moore 1965) (Fig. 13.5).

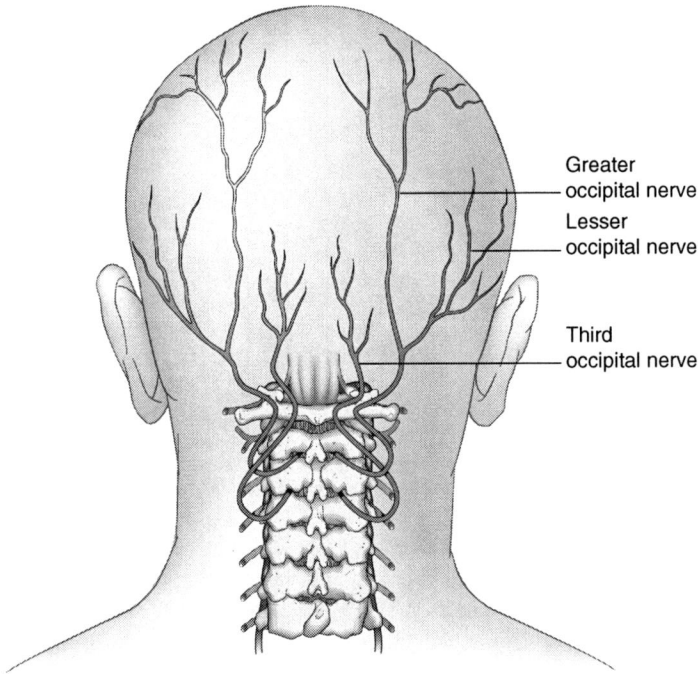

Greater
occipital nerve
Lesser
occipital nerve

Third
occipital nerve

Figure 13.5   Posterior occiput with greater lesser and third occipital nerves identified.

Complications
Complications include subarachnoid block, bleeding, infection, and intravascular or intra-neural injection. Patients with a previous history of posterior cranial surgery can potentially have a higher risk for complications.

Atlanto-occipital Nerve Blocks
Indications
The Atlanto-occipital nerve block can be used to treat pain associated with flexion–extension of the neck. This is the predominant motion between the base of the skull and the first cervical vertebrae. This joint may cause referred pain from the occiput to the base of the neck.

Technique
The block is performed with a 25-gauge 3-in. spinal needle under fluoroscopy in the prone position. Biplanar imaging, viewing the joint from two different axes, is utilized to guide the needle into the joint. Contrast is injected to outline the joint space and check for arterial blush/venous runoff. A combination of local anesthetic and steroid are injected. Complications may include intravascular and subarachnoid injection, as well as intraneu-ral injection. The joint is deeper than the cord at this level, and the vertebral artery, venous vessels, and nerve roots are in close proximity. A similar procedure may be done for the *Atlanto-axial joint*, between the second and the third cervical vertebrae where the predominant motion is rotation (Ogoke 2000) (Fig. 13.6).

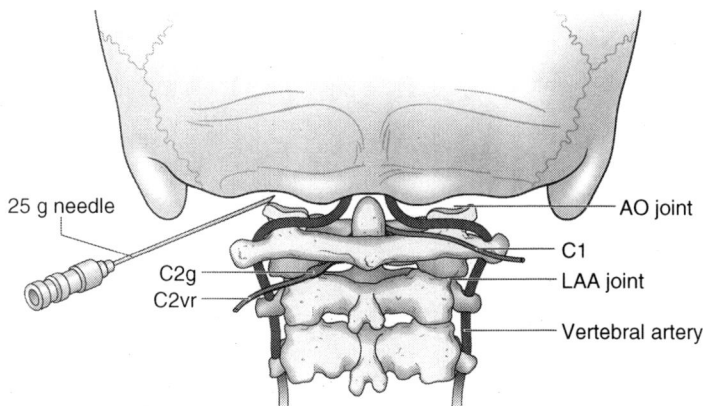

Figure 13.6 Illustration of vertebral anatomy of the bottom of the skull, C1, C2, and C3. C2g = C2 ganglion; C2vr = C2 ventral ramus; AO = atlanto-occipital; LAA = lateral atlanto-axial.

The performance of neural blockade in the head and neck mandates the use of fluoroscopy, dexterity in needle manipulation, and an intricate knowledge of anatomical relationships. Inadvertent subarachnoid or intravascular injection can lead to devastating complications. Diagnostic blocks with short-acting local anesthetic to assess the efficacy usually precede longer lasting treatments such as neurolytic injections and radiofrequency neurolysis. The sensitivity of the area as well as the importance of precise placement sometimes requires deeper anesthesia for the patient.

Facial Nerve Blocks
Indications
Facial nerve block is a useful block for the diagnosis and treatment of a variety of conditions. These include pain associated with Bell's palsy, herpes zoster of the geniculate ganglion also called Ramsay Hunt syndrome, facial spasms in the areas supplied by the facial nerve, and geniculate neuralgia.

Anatomy
The facial nerve arises from the brain stem and has both motor and sensory fibers. The sensory part of the facial nerve is called the nervus intermedius, and it is susceptible to compression, leading to geniculate neuralgia, especially as it exits the pons. It enters the internal auditory meatus and exits the base of the skull through the stylomastoid foramen.

Technique
To perform the block, the anterior border of the mastoid process below the external auditory meatus at the level of the middle of the ramus of the mandible of the affected side is identified. A 22-gauge 1.5-in. needle is inserted perpendicular to the skin until the needle encounters the mastoid bone. The needle is then walked off the mastoid anteriorly to a depth of 0.5 in. After negative aspiration of blood and cerebrospinal fluid, a total of 3–4 cc of local anesthetic is injected slowly in incremental doses along with 80 mg of depot steroid for the initial block.

Superior Cervical Plexus Blocks
Indication

The superior cervical plexus block is utilized for either superficial neck operations or as a supplement for deeper surgical procedures, such as a carotid artery endarterectomy. In many facilities, this type of surgery is only done under a regional approach, with a combination of deep and superficial cervical plexus blocks, to limit the use of shunting and to reduce intraoperative surgical time.

Anatomy

The primary rami of the first, second, third, and fourth cervical nerves form the cervical plexus after dividing into an ascending and descending branches which give fibers to the nerves above and below. This plexus provides both motor and sensory innervation; the most important motor branch is the phrenic nerve. The cervical plexus also provides motor fibers to the spinal accessory nerve and the paravertebral deep muscles of the neck. The cervical plexus provides sensory innervation to the skin of the lower mandible, neck, and supraclavicular fossa, with some sensory fibers joining the greater auricular and lesser auricular nerves. The sensory nerves converge at the midpoint of the sternocleidomastoid muscle at its posterior margin, which is the first point to be identified for the performance of the superior cervical plexus block.

Technique

The injection is done in a fan-like manner with a total of 15 cc of local anesthetic solution injected with a 22-gauge 1.5-in. needle along with 80 mg of depomedrol for the initial injection and 40 mg of depomedrol for subsequent injections. Injection of local anesthetic is done after negative aspiration of blood and CSF. The first 5 cc is injected just behind the sternocleidomastoid muscle at the midline past its posterior border. The next 5 cc is injected in a fan-like fashion along the line passing behind the lobe of the ear, and the remaining 5 cc is injected inferiorly toward the ipsilateral nipple. For surgical anesthesia, only local anesthetics are utilized.

Deep Cervical Plexus Blocks
Indications

Some of the indications for this block include posttraumatic pain, intractable pain secondary to malignancy, and provision of anesthesia for surgeries of the neck requiring muscle relaxation. Surgical anesthesia with a deep cervical nerve block is performed as mentioned above for procedures such as carotid endarterectomy, removal of lesions, and laceration repairs in the areas subserved by the deep cervical plexus.

Anatomy

The deep cervical plexus provides sensory and motor innervation to the neck and is formed by the ventral rami of the first, second, third, and fourth cervical nerves. Each of these nerves then gives off an ascending and a descending branch to the nerves above and below to form the cervical plexus. The most important motor nerve of the cervical plexus is the phrenic nerve.

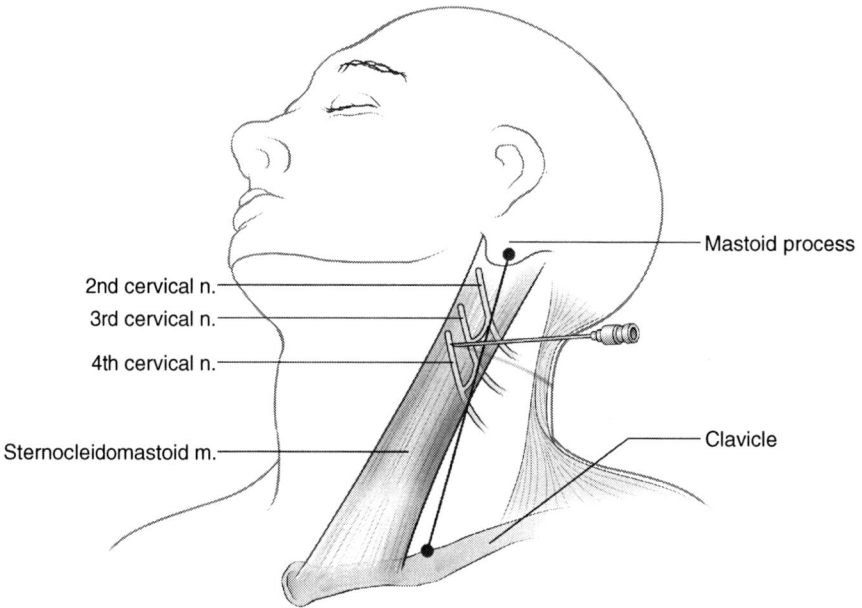

Figure 13.7 Deep cervical plexus block.

Technique

A line is drawn between the mastoid process and the insertion of the sternocleidomastoid muscle at the clavicle (Fig. 13.7). A 22-gauge 1.5-in. needle is used for the block, and a point 2 in. below the mastoid process on the marked line is identified. The needle is inserted about 0.5 in. in front of this point, after appropriate antiseptic preparation of the skin of the entire side of the neck. The needle is advanced up to 1 in. anteriorly and inferiorly until a paresthesia is elicited. After negative aspiration of blood and CSF, a total of 15 cc of local anesthetic solution is injected slowly in incremental doses with 80 mg of depot steroid for the initial block and 40 mg of depot steroid for subsequent blocks, especially for the treatment of painful conditions with an inflammatory component.

Complications

Most common complications include inadvertent injection into the epidural, subdural, intrathecal, and vascular compartments.

Superior Laryngeal Nerve Block
Indications

The superior laryngeal nerve supplies the pharynx and the larynx above the glottis, and its blockade is useful for the diagnosis and treatment of painful conditions in this region. The blockade of this nerve can also serve as an adjunct to topical anesthesia for procedures such as awake fiberoptic intubation, bronchoscopy, laryngoscopy, and transesophageal echocardiography (TEE).

Anatomy

The superior laryngeal nerve is a branch of the vagus nerve with a contribution from the superior cervical ganglion, and it passes the lateral aspect of the hyoid bone. Its internal branch provides sensation to the mucous membranes of the lower portion of the epiglottis, while the external branch provides innervation to the cricothyroid muscle.

Technique

In order to perform the block, a point between the lateral border of the hyoid bone and the upper outer border of the thyroid cartilage is identified. A 25-gauge, 1.5-in. needle is inserted perpendicular to the skin to a depth of about 0.5 cm. After negative aspiration of CSF and blood a total of 2 cc of local anesthetic is injected slowly. If treating painful conditions with an inflammation component, depot steroid (up to 80 mg) can be added for the initial injection and 40 mg added for subsequent injections.

Recurrent Laryngeal Nerve Blocks

Indications

This block is useful for painful conditions below the level of the vocal cords.

Anatomy

The recurrent laryngeal nerve arises from the vagus nerve. The right laryngeal nerve forms as a loop around the innominate artery and then ascends in the lateral groove between the trachea and the esophagus to supply the inferior portion of the larynx. The left recurrent laryngeal nerve forms a loop around the arch of the aorta and then ascends in the lateral groove between the trachea and the esophagus to supply the inferior portion of the larynx.

Technique

To perform the block, the needle entry point is the medial border of the sternocleidomastoid muscle at the level of the first tracheal ring. A 22-gauge 5/8-in. needle is inserted perpendicular to the skin. After inserting the needle to a depth of about 0.5 in., a total of 2 cc of local anesthetic solution is slowly injected. If the block is being done for a painful condition with the presence of inflammation, then 80 mg of depot steroid can be added to the initial injection, followed by 40 mg of depot steroid for each additional injection.

Vagus Nerve Blocks

Indications

Vagus nerve block is useful for patients with vagal neuralgia and when destruction of the nerve is indicated in the presence of intractable pain secondary to malignancy. This block is usually done in aggressive head and neck malignancies.

Anatomy

The vagus nerve has a motor and a sensory component. The motor fibers supply the pharyngeal muscle and the superior and recurrent laryngeal nerves. The sensory fibers supply the mucosa of the larynx below the cords as well as the posterior aspect of the external auditory meatus. The vagus nerve supplies fibers to major intrathoracic viscera such as the heart and the lungs.

Technique

To perform the block, the midpoint of a line between the mastoid process and the angle of the mandible is accessed perpendicular to the skin with a 22-gauge 1.5-in. needle after appropriate preparation of the skin over the area. The styloid process is usually encountered at a depth of 3 cm. The needle is then walked off the styloid process posteroinferiorly. A total of 5 cc of preservative lidocaine 0.5% is injected after negative aspiration of CSF or blood, and 40 mg of methylprednisolone is often given for the initial block.

Complications

The major complications of vagus nerve block are vascular due to the close proximity of the internal jugular vein and the carotid artery. Side effects include dysphonia, difficulty in coughing, and reflex tachycardia.

Spinal Accessory Nerve Blocks
Indications

Spasm of the trapezius and sternocleidomastoid muscle can be relieved with a spinal accessory nerve block.

Anatomy

The spinal root of the nerve provides motor innervation to the superior portion of the sternocleidomastoid muscle and to the upper portion of the trapezius muscle.

Technique

To perform the block, the posterior border of the upper third of the sternocleidomastoid muscle is identified with the raising of the patient's head against resistance. A 1.5-in. needle is used to access this area after appropriate preparation with antiseptic solution in an anterior direction. At a depth of approximately 0.75 in., 10 cc of local anesthetic solution is injected slowly after negative aspiration to CSF or blood. Depot steroid (up to 80 mg) can be added to the local anesthetic solution for the initial block and 40 mg depot steroid for subsequent blocks.

Phrenic Nerve Blocks
Indications

Phrenic nerve block can be used to assist with diagnosis or as a therapeutic modality. Phrenic nerve neurolysis is useful for the treatment of intractable hicupps. Cryoneurolysis, chemical neurolysis, RF lesioning, and surgical resection of the nerve are some of the procedures that can be done to produce neurodestruction of the phrenic nerve.

Anatomy

The primary ventral ramus of the fourth cervical nerve with fibers from the third and fifth cervical nerves forms the phrenic nerve. The phrenic nerve passes between the omohyoid and the sternocleidomastoid muscles inferiorly in close proximity to the subclavian artery and the subclavian vein. The right phrenic nerve gives motor innervation to the right diaphragm after coursing along with the vena cava. The left phrenic nerve follows the course of the vagus nerve to provide motor innervation to the left side of the diaphragm.

Technique

To perform the block, the groove between the posterior border of the sternocleidomastoid muscle and the anterior scalene muscle is identified. One inch above the clavicle at this groove or behind the posterior border of the sternocleidomastoid muscle a 1.5-in. needle is inserted anteriorly after appropriate antiseptic preparation of the skin. After advancing for approximately 1 in. and following negative aspiration of blood or CSF, 10 cc of local anesthetic solution is injected slowly with 80 mg of depot steroid for the initial block and 40 mg of depot steroid for subsequent blocks.

Complications

Potential significant complications include vascular injury and serious fatal complications associated with inadvertent injection into the epidural, the subdural, and the intrathecal spaces. Recurrent laryngeal nerve can often be blocked unintentionally. Close monitoring and recognition of these complications are extremely important.

Thorax

Suprascapular Nerve Blocks

Indications

Suprascapular nerve blocks can be performed for shoulder pain of various etiologies. Pain in these joints may be improved by injection of local anesthetic (LA) and steroid at the suprascapular notch.

Anatomy

The suprascapular nerve provides the predominant amount of sensory innervation to the glenohumeral and acromioclavicular joint.

Technique

Volumes of LA/steroid as high as 10 cc are used. There are several approaches, but common practice is to have the patient sit or lay prone and palpate the spine of the scapula. A line is drawn along it, after which a second line is drawn at the midpoint bisecting it. The needle is inserted 2 cm above the scapular spine on the bisecting line and directed downward into the suprascapular fossa. Bone should be contacted, the syringe aspirated, then injected.

Complications

There is a risk of pneumothorax with improper needle placement (Shanahan et al. 2003).

Intercostal Nerve Blocks

Indications

Intercostal nerve blocks have been used to improve postoperative analgesia as well as treat chronic chest wall pain which may result from thoracotomy, postherpetic neuralgia, chest wall metastasis, and trauma, including rib fracture analgesia.

Anatomy

The intercostal nerves arise from the ventral rami of T1–T11. The intercostal nerves lie just inferior to the intercostal artery and intercostal vein at each space.

Technique

The chest wall can be segmentally anesthetized at the corresponding rib for each thoracic dermatome. Three to five cubic centimeters of LA is injected medial to the posterior axillary line at the inferior border of the rib to cover all three intercostal branches (Fig. 13.8). If the patient is thin, the ribs may be palpated and the procedure completed without fluoroscopy. The needle is advanced to contact the rib and then directed caudally just past the plane of the rib. Aspiration for air and blood is necessary as the needle is next to the neurovascular bundle and above the lung. The local anesthetic is absorbed into circulation very rapidly and provides the largest systemic absorption of any block in the body, and the addition of epinephrine helps prolong the block and decrease the systemic concentration (Fig. 13.9).

Intercostal Nerve Block

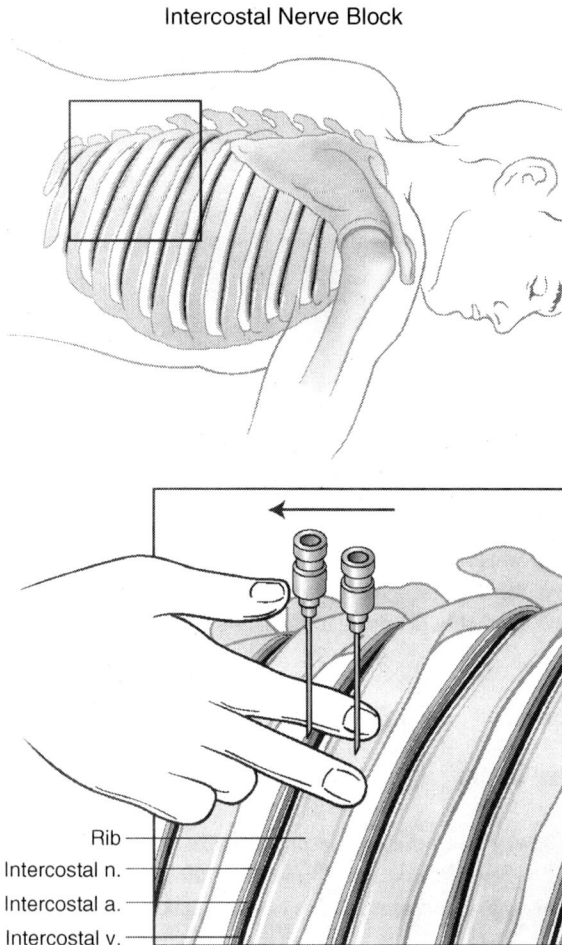

Rib
Intercostal n.
Intercostal a.
Intercostal v.

Figure 13.8   Intercostal nerve block.

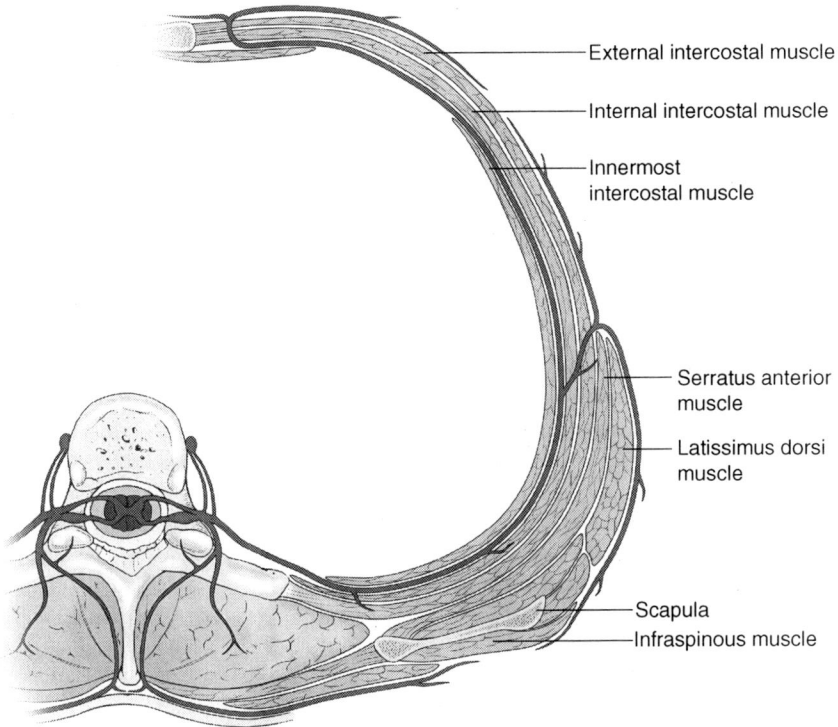

Figure 13.9 Illustration of cross section of thorax showing the four branches of the intercostal nerve.

Thoracic Nerve Radiofrequency Lesioning
Technique

The junction of the posterior axillary line and the rib to be blocked is identified. A 22-gauge 54-mm radiofrequency needle usually equipped with a 4 mm active tip is advanced aiming for the middle of the rib. After encountering the bone the needle is walked off the inferior border of the rib and advanced about 2 mm deeper to be close to the costal groove. First a trial sensory stimulation with 2 V at 50 Hz is performed to ensure that there is a paresthesia along the distribution of the intercostal nerve to be lesioned. A pulsed radiofrequency lesion is then performed by heating at 40–45° for 5 min or alternatively by heating at 49–60° for 90 s.

Complications

Obvious potential complication includes pneumothorax, though data indicate that this is a relatively rare occurrence. It is typically reported at less than 1% with significant pneumothorax reported at approximately 0.1%.

Thoracic Paravertebral Nerve Blocks
Indications
This block is useful for the management of pain in the upper abdominal wall, the chest wall, and the thoracic spine. It is used to control acute pain in conditions such as rib fractures, acute herpes zoster of the thoracic cage, and cancer pain.

Anatomy
The paravertebral nerves exit the intervertebral foramina beneath the transverse process of the vertebrae. The thoracic paravertebral nerve has connections with the thoracic sympathetic chain via the preganglionic white rami communicantes which are myelinated and the unmyelinated gray postganglionic communicantes. Pre- and postganglionic fibers synapse at the level of the thoracic sympathetic ganglia. Sympathetic innervation to the sweat glands, pilomotor muscles of the skin, and the vasculature is by the postganglionic fibers which return to the respective somatic nerves via the gray rami communicantes. The thoracic sympathetic postganglionic fibers also extend over to the cardiac plexus and course up and down the sympathetic trunk, terminating in distant ganglia.

The thoracic paravertebral nerve gives off a recurrent branch to innervate the spinal ligaments, meninges, and respective vertebra. The thoracic paravertebral nerve then divides into an anterior and a posterior branch. The anterior branches go in the inferior aspect of the ribs to become the intercostal nerves which innervate the parietal pleura and the parietal peritoneum. The posterior branch of the paravertebral nerve innervates the facet joint and soft tissues of the back.

Technique
The block is performed with the patient in the prone position. The spinous process of the vertebra above the nerve to be blocked is identified (Fig. 13.10). A 3.5-in. needle is used for the block and is inserted after appropriate antiseptic treatment of the skin immediately below and 1.5 in. lateral to the spinous process. The transverse process should be encountered at a depth approximately 1.5 in. at which point the needle is walked off the inferior aspect of the transverse process and inserted another 0.75 in. deeper until a paresthesia is obtained. After negative aspiration for blood or CSF a total of 5 cc of 1% preservative-free lidocaine solution is injected for pain relief. If there is an inflammatory component then 40 mg of methylprednisolone can be added for the initial block.

Thoracic Sympathetic Ganglion Blocks
Indication
Thoracic sympathetic ganglion block is utilized when a sympathetic mediated pain syndrome involving the thoracic ganglion is suspected. It can be diagnostic and therapeutic.

Technique
With the patient in a prone position, the spinous process of the vertebra just above the nerve to be blocked is identified by palpation. With aseptic technique a 22-gauge 3.5-in. needle is inserted just below and 1.5 in. lateral to the spinous process. The needle is advanced to encounter the transverse process which usually occurs at approximately 1.5 in. after which the needle is walked off the inferior margin of the transverse process to a depth of 1 in. At

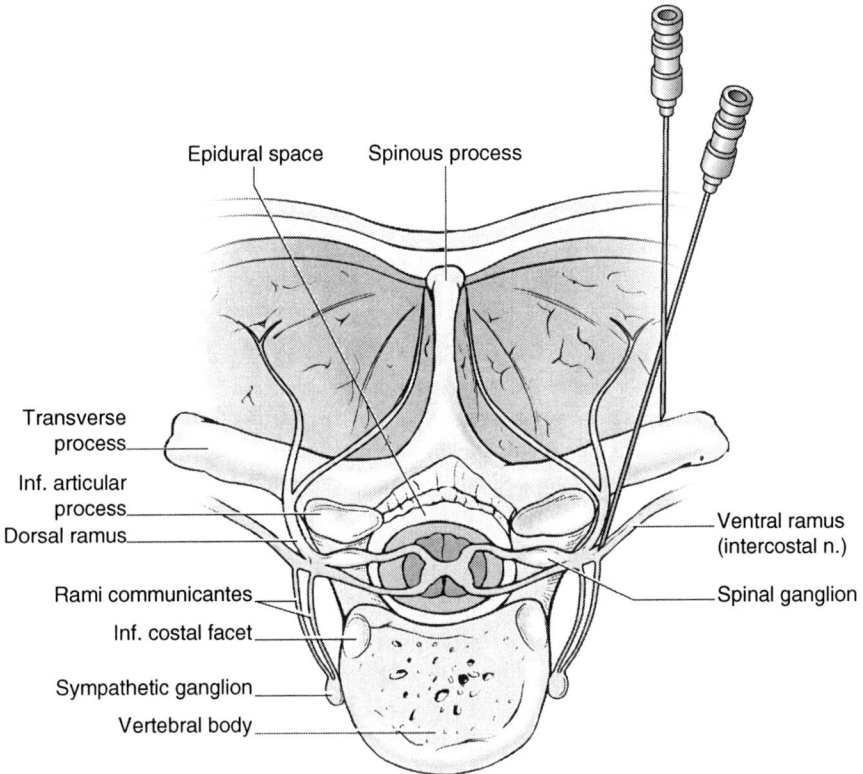

Figure 13.10 Thoracic paravertebral nerve block.

this point it is possible to encounter the corresponding thoracic paravertebral somatic nerve which is close to the thoracic sympathetic ganglion. If there is a paresthesia, it is necessary to withdraw the needle and redirect the needle in a more cephalad fashion, keeping close to the vertebral body to avoid a pneumothorax. Once the needle is in the correct position and after negative aspiration for blood and CSF, 1% lidocaine (up to a total of 5 cc) is usually given.

Complications
Proper technique will reduce the likelihood of pneumothorax and negative aspiration the likelihood of intravascular injection.

Intrapleural Nerve Blocks
Indications
This block can be used for the control of pain after thoracotomy, cancer pain, malignant lesions of the liver and lung, postherpetic neuralgia, and fractures of the ribs. A catheter can be tunneled into the intrapleural space to provide continuous medications to the area. Neurolytic agents can also be administered into the space to relieve intractable pain due to malignancy.

Anatomy

The pleural cavity is the cavity which surrounds the lungs. The region between the pleural sacs is called the mediastinum. The pleura is one of the three serous membranes in the body. From the apex of the lung to the pleura, there are many structures that collectively are described as intrapleural. Pain related to irritation of the lower part of the costal pleura will be referred along its nerve distribution. The visceral pleura, however, is innervated by sensory autonomic nerves. Successful intrapleural blockade most likely involves both intercostal and visceral drug distribution.

Technique

Sympathetic nerves as well as somatic nerves can be blocked by pooling of local anesthetic into the interpleural gutter next to the thoracic spine. The position of the patient determines, to a great extent, the types of nerves that can be blocked. For the treatment of sympathetically mediated pain the affected side should be up, whereas placing the affected side down will block the thoracic somatic nerves, the thoracic sympathetic chain, and the intercostal and the thoracic spinal nerves. The eighth rib is first identified on the affected side. At a point 10 cm from the origin of the rib an 18-gauge 3.5-in. styletted needle is inserted in a sterile fashion until the rib bone is encountered. The needle is then walked off the superior margin of the rib, the stylet is removed, and the needle is connected to a 5-cc syringe with air. The pleural space is identified by the loss of resistance to air technique. A pleural catheter is then advanced 6–8 cm into the cavity, and 20–30 cc of local anesthetic solution is introduced in incremental doses (Fig. 13.11). In the presence of inflammation, 80 mg of methylprednisolone can be added to the local anesthetic with the initial block and 40 mg of methylprednisolone can be added with subsequent blocks.

Complications

Again, pneumothorax, though not typical, can occur.

Trigger Point Injections
Indications

Myofascial trigger points are tender points in muscle thought to originate from tissue trauma. They may cause pain and a resultant decreased range of motion. The trigger points may be located by palpation of a small lump or cord in the muscle by the examiner in concordance with discomfort by the patient. There is a very long list of etiologies of myofascial trigger points.

Anatomy

A myofascial trigger point, also known as a central trigger point, is a hyperirritable foci in skeletal muscle. It is associated with hypersensitive palpable nodule in a taut band. The region is tender and painful to palpation. Widespread, generalized pain and tenderness, as compared with one distinct myofascial trigger point, are often part of a constellation of findings in fibromyalgia. Controversy exists whether this represents a unique syndrome or is a continuum of other pain processes.

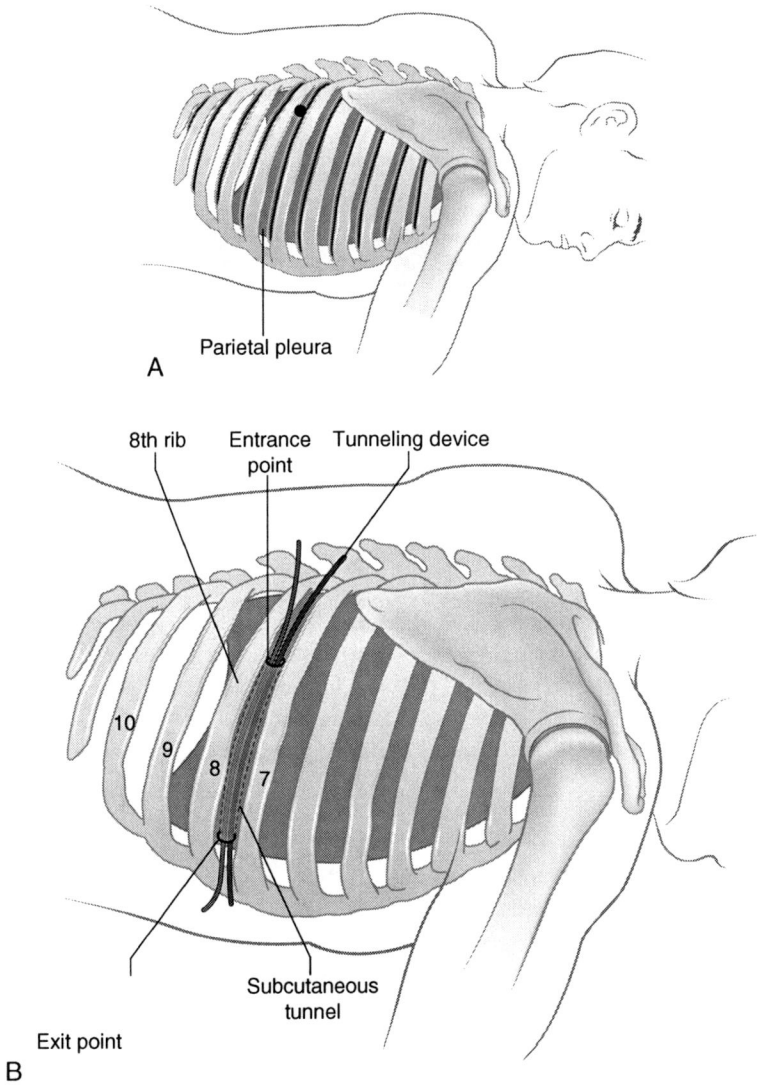

Figure 13.11   Interpleural nerve block: tunneled catheter technique.

Technique

Insertion of a needle into the trigger point may elicit a local twitch response (LTR) which confirms the injection site. Trigger point injections are usually performed in a regular examination room. Patients are positioned in a manner to facilitate access to the trigger points as well as minimize potential patient movement. After marking the injection sites, the area should be prepped with cleansing solution. Local anesthetic with or without steroid is then drawn into a sterile control syringe for injection. Under sterile technique the trigger point is fixed with one hand and the other guides the syringe. Several cubic centimeters of medication may be injected and should elicit discomfort in the patient's usual area of pain.

Complications
Complications include bleeding, infection, pneumothorax, viscus perforation, and vessel or nerve damage (Lavelle et al. 2007).

Sympathetic Ganglion Blockade for Extremities
Stellate Ganglion Block
Indications
The stellate ganglion block is utilized for the diagnosis and treatment of complex regional pain syndromes of the upper extremity. The block may be utilized as well in clinical situations where increased upper extremity blood flow is warranted. The block can be effective for pain in the head and neck, upper extremity, and upper thoracic dermatomes. Clinically, the most common indications in the upper extremity include chronic regional pain syndrome, malignancy, and vascular insufficiency and hyperhydrosis.

Anatomy
The stellate ganglion is the most caudal sympathetic ganglion affecting the head and neck. It is also one of the more cephalad ganglion affecting the upper limb. It is formed by the fusion of the inferior cervical ganglion (C7) and the first thoracic ganglion (T1) and star shaped, yielding its name. It is located in the anterior part of the neck, and the classic block is performed from anterior directed toward the lateral process of C6, "Chassignac's" tubercle, on the affected side.

Technique
Stellate Ganglion Block: Anterior Approach
Although the ganglion is located caudal to the C6, this anterior approach provides a higher level of safety. The important vascular structures are retracted laterally as a 22-gauge 1.5-in. needle is advanced to the tubercle. After contact with bone, it is withdrawn slightly and aspirated and then a test dose of the LA is given. If there are no untoward effects after a minute the remaining LA is injected slowly with frequent aspiration checks. The patient is brought to a 30° head-up position after the injection block to increase caudal migration of the local anesthetic.

Stellate Ganglion Block: Posterior Approach
The posterior approach to the stellate ganglion is performed with the patient in the prone position. The block is approached lateral to the spinous process of the T1–T2 vertebrae. A 22-gauge 10-cm needle is inserted 4 cm lateral to the spinous process of T1–T2. The lamina of the vertebra is contacted after which the needle is slightly withdrawn and redirected laterally and inferiorly to be adjacent to the anterolateral aspect of the vertebral body; then, 5–7 cc of local anesthetic solution is injected. If there is an inflammatory component, then a total of 80 mg of depot steroid can be used for the initial block, followed by 40 mg of depot steroid for successive blocks.

Stellate Ganglion Block: Vertebral Body Approach

With this approach, the patient is placed in the supine position with the cervical spine placed in a neutral position. The point of injection of the local anesthetic is at the junction of the transverse process of C7 and the vertebral body medial to the carotid pulsations. This procedure is done with a 22-gauge 3.5-in. spinal needle. Neurolysis of the stellate ganglion can also be performed with 6.5% phenol or alcohol.

Skin temperature in the blocked extremity should elevate a few degrees due to vasodilatation. Horner's syndrome and recurrent laryngeal nerve paralysis and hoarseness are common side effects. It should be noted that pneumothorax is the most common complication with a stellate ganglion block done with a posterior approach.

Complications

Complications include pneumothorax, and intravascular and subarachnoid injection can be catastrophic complication (Figs. 13.12 and 13.13).

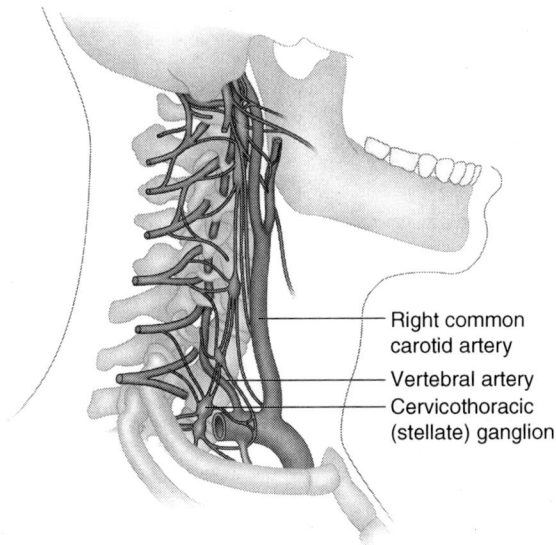

Figure 13.12 Sagittal cervical spine showing sympathetic nerves and ganglia.

RF lesioning of the stellate ganglion block can be performed via the anterior approach. The junction of the C7 transverse process with the vertebral body is identified with fluoroscopic guidance. A 54-cm RF 20-gauge needle with a 4 mm active tip is inserted at this junction. After bony contact is made, the needle is withdrawn slightly and 3–5 cc of the mixture of local anesthetic and contrast medium is injected. First a trial stimulation of 50 Hz and 0.9 V for sensory nerves and a stimulation of 2 Hz and 2 V for motor nerves is done to ensure that the recurrent laryngeal nerves and the phrenic nerves would not be affected by the RF lesioning. The RF lesioning is performed by heating at 80°C for 60 s or by pulsed radiofrequency at 45 or 50°C for a longer period of time. Second lesioning at the medial aspect of the

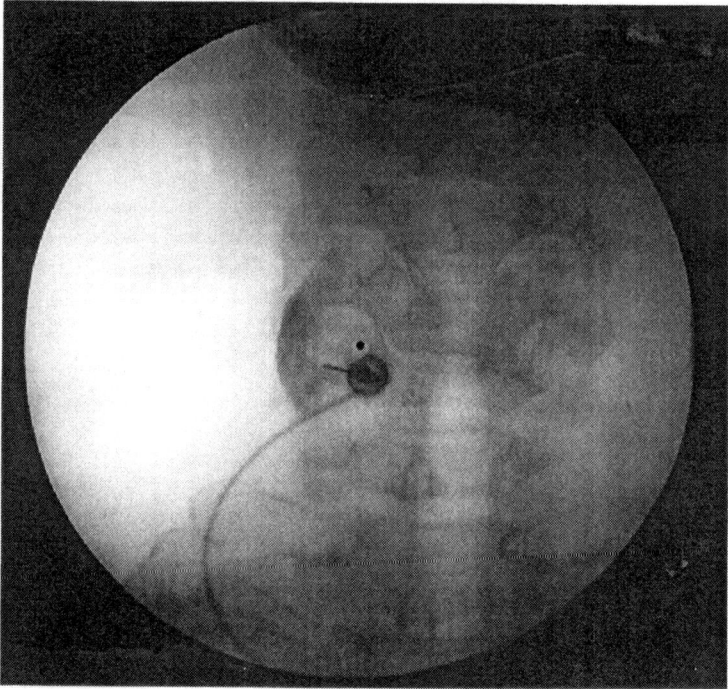

Figure 13.13 AP fluoroscopic image of a right stellate ganglion block with contrast dye.

transverse process and a third lesioning at the uppermost junction of the C7 transverse process and vertebral body may be performed if there is no stimulation of the motor and sensory nerves.

Lumbar Sympathetic Ganglion Block and Radiofrequency
Lumbar Sympathetic Blocks
Indications
The stellate ganglion block is utilized for the diagnosis and treatment of complex regional pain syndromes of the lower extremity. The block may be utilized as well in clinical situations where increased lower extremity blood flow is warranted.

Anatomy
The *lumbar plexus* conducts the sympathetic innervation to the lower extremity. It encompasses the first three lumbar sympathetic ganglia. Fusion of the first and the second lumbar ganglia can be seen in many patients. The sympathetic chains run along the anterior portion of the vertebral bodies and are blocked from a posterior approach at L2 or L3 with diffusion cephalocaudad along the anterior portion of the vertebral bodies and the sympathetic chains.

Technique
A 22-gauge spinal needle is guided almost to the anterior line of the vertebral body, closely approximated to the vertebrae, aspirated, then a test dose given as above. The indications

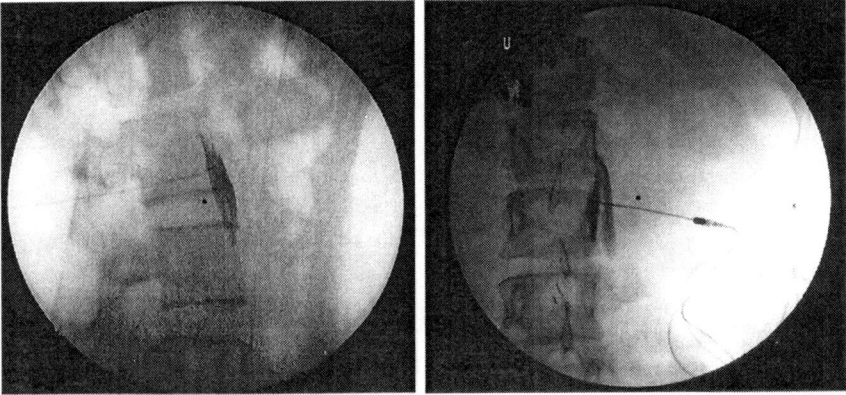

Figure 13.14 Lumbar sympathetic block lateral and AP. Note the two patterns of spread on the AP. The more lateral column of dye is along the psoas muscle. The needle is advanced slightly, and the proper dye spread is observed closer to the vertebral body.

for the lower extremity are similar to those in the upper extremity. Complications include intravascular injection and viscus perforation (Fig. 13.14).

Radiofrequency Lesioning of the Lumbar Sympathetic Ganglion

Radiofrequency lesioning of the lumbar sympathetic ganglion is performed with the patient in the prone position. The spinous process of the vertebra just above the nerve to be blocked is identified, and a 150-mm 20-gauge radiofrequency needle with a 10 mm active tip is inserted in a sterile fashion at this point and advanced at a 35–40° angle to the skin. At a depth of about 2 in., the lateral portion of the L2 vertebral body is usually encountered, after which the needle is walked off the lateral portion of the L2 vertebral body. The needle is then advanced approximately 1/2 in. deeper to the anterior-lateral aspect of the vertebral body. The position of the needle is checked with contrast medium. After negative aspiration of CSF or blood, a trial stimulation at 50 Hz and 1 V is performed. The pain encountered should be localized to the lower back. If the pain is in the groin or in the lower extremity, the needle should be repositioned. Motor stimulation is then performed. If it is negative at 2 Hz and 3 V trial, a lesion is created for 60 s at 80°C.

Visceral Nerve Blockade

Indications

There are a number of blocks that can be performed for visceral pain syndromes of the abdomen. These include the celiac plexus block, the hypogastric plexus block, and the ganglion impair block. There are a number of intraabdominal pain states that can be treated, including malignancy.

Celiac Plexus Block

Anatomy

The celiac plexus is located at T12–L1. It receives sympathetic fibers from the greater, lesser, and least splanchnic nerves. The visceral afferents from the liver, pancreas, gall bladder, stomach, esophagus, spleen, kidneys, intestines, adrenals, and associated vasculature course through this plexus. Indications include pain secondary to malignancy and other chronic processes in one of the above structures.

Technique

There are several commonly used approaches performed in the prone position using fluoroscopy: retrocrural, transcrural, periaortic, and transaortic. Transabdominal approaches directed by computed tomography (CT) as well as a transgastric approach via upper endoscopy are other approaches to deliver analgesic and neurolytic medications to the plexus. The block is performed with the patient in the prone position (Fig. 13.15). Two 20-gauge, 13-cm styletted needles are inserted bilaterally to block both of the celiac ganglia, but on some occasions good spread to both sides is achieved with just using one needle. The needle entry point is just below the tip of the 12th rib, and with the help of fluoroscopic guidance, the needle is advanced until it hits the side of the L1 vertebra. The needle is withdrawn slightly and then redirected forward until it is in the area of the celiac plexus, avoiding the aorta and inferior vena cava. Radio-opaque dye is injected to confirm the correct placement of the needle, and then the appropriate mixture is injected. For a diagnostic block, 10–15 ml of 1% lidocaine or 3% 2-chloroprocaine is used on each side. For a therapeutic block, 10–15 ml of 0.5% bupivacaine is administered on each side and 10–12 ml of either absolute alcohol or 6.0% aqueous phenol is injected on each side for a neurolytic block.

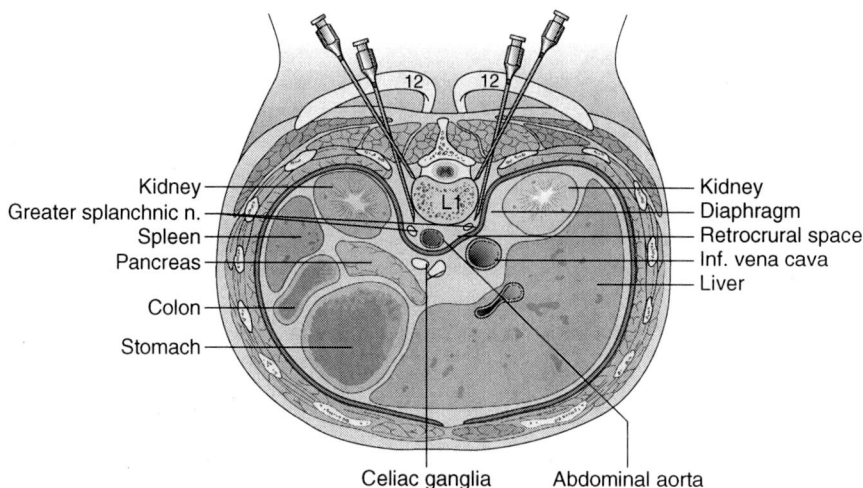

Figure 13.15   Classic two-needle retrocrural technique.

Complications

Since the block causes dilatation of the upper abdominal vessels, venous pooling can occur, leading to hypotension. Since this can be exacerbated by preexisting dehydration, adequate intravenous hydration is needed before performing the block. Diarrhea is another common side effect. Other complications include bleeding due to aorta or inferior vena cava injury by the needle, paraplegia from injecting phenol into the arteries that supply the spinal cord, sexual dysfunction (injected solution spreads to the sympathetic chain bilaterally), and lumbar nerve root irritation (injected solution tracks backward toward the lumbar plexus).

Hypogastric Plexus Block
Indication
The hypogastric plexus block can be utilized for numerous lower abdominal pain states.

Anatomy
Located in the retroperitoneal space between the lower third of the fifth lumbar and the upper third of the first sacral vertebrae. It provides the sympathetic innervation to the pelvic organs such as the bladder, uterus, vagina, prostate, and rectum, as well as conducts nociceptive fibers. Pain arising from malignancy, postsurgical conditions, and chronic pelvic pain secondary to gynecologic or intestinal pathology can be effectively treated by this block (Fig. 13.16).

Technique
The block procedure is very similar in each of the targets mentioned above. A spinal needle is fluoroscopically guided to the desired anatomic location, and the position of the tip is further

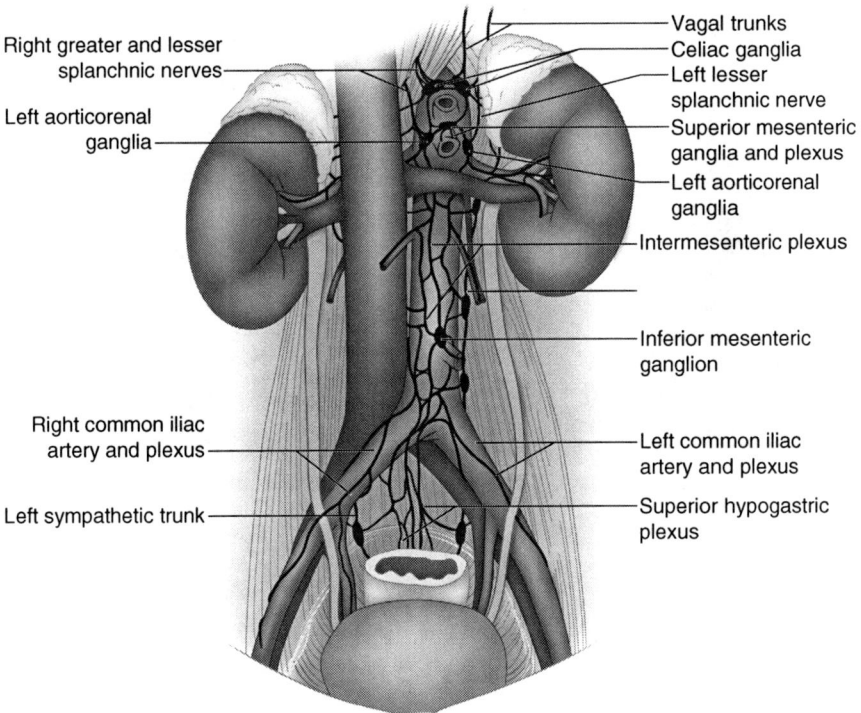

Figure 13.16 Abdominal sympathetic nerves and ganglia.

defined with the use of contrast material. The injectate may consist of local anesthetic for trial procedures or alcohol or phenol for neurolysis (de Leon-Casasola 2000).

Ganglion Impar Block
Indication
The ganglion impar block can be utilized for perineal pain, most likely arising from the vagina and the rectum, including malignancy.

Anatomy
The ganglion impar is a solitary structure at the end of the sympathetic chains in the pelvis. It is just anterior to the sacrococcygeal junction. Visceral afferents from perineum, distal rectum, anus, distal urethra, distal 1/3 of vagina, and the vulva may project to the ganglion. Blocking it can be very effective for perineal pain secondary to pathology in one of the above structures. It is commonly blocked for pain from rectal cancer. It may be approached from beneath the tip of the coccyx, from the side of the sacrococcygeal junction, or transcoccygeal with a spinal needle under fluoroscopy (Fig. 13.17).

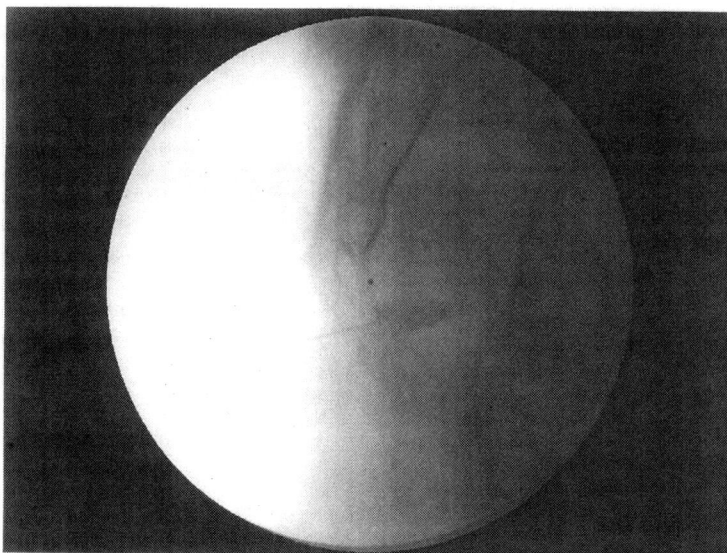

Figure 13.17 Fluoroscopic image of a ganglion impar block from the lateral approach at the sacrococcygeal junction.

Complications
A particular risk of the ganglion impar injection is perforation of the rectum and infection.

Penile Blocks
Penile Block
Indication
This block is usually performed for a circumcision, along with a ring block of the penis.

Anatomy

The penis is innervated by the left and the right dorsal nerves, both of which are derived from the pudendal nerve. The right and the left dorsal nerves are separated by the suspensory ligament of the penis. Each dorsal nerve passes inferior to the inferior ramus of the pubis, after which it penetrates the superficial fascia to supply the skin. After penetrating the superficial fascia, each dorsal nerve gives off a branch to the corpus cavernosus of the penis.

Technique

EMLA cream can be applied to the prepuce and the mucosal surfaces of the penis for a period of 45 min to ease the performance of the penile block. With the patient in the supine position, a 27-gauge needle is inserted at the base of the penis over the middle of the pubic arch, until it touches the pubic symphysis. The needle is then withdrawn and redirected to pass below the symphysis and 3–5 mm deeper depending on the size of the patient. It is preferable to direct it slightly laterally into the pear-shaped space and then to reinsert it on the other side, depositing equal volumes on each side. After negative aspiration, a total of 5–7 cc of a mixture of 0.25% bupivacaine and 1% lidocaine is given on either side.

Complications

Avoiding the midline injection reduces the chance of penetrating the dorsal vessels of the penis and causing hematoma.

Ring Block of the Penis

This block is performed along with the penile block to provide anesthesia for circumcision. The ring block is a subcutaneous injection at the base of the penile shaft usually performed with a 27-gauge needle. A total of 10 cc of a mixture of 0.25% bupivacaine and 1% lidocaine can be given via two injection sites – one dorsally and one ventrally.

Spine Injections

Back pain is one of the most common reasons for patients to seek medical attention.
About two-thirds of adults will experience low back pain at least once in their lifetime (Rubin 2007).
Its etiology is often unclear given that similar complaints and symptoms may result from various pathologic conditions and imaging studies do not always correlate. This makes accurate diagnosis and treatment difficult. Occupational injuries, compensation, and secondary gain issues confound the situation even more. A thorough history and physical examination, as well as development of a cohesive and consistent treatment plan incorporating diagnostic procedures and therapeutic interventions yield the most effective care (Waldman 1996) (Table 13.1).

Back pain can be generalized into two categories, axial and radicular, but patients commonly have components of both. Axial back pain commonly originates with the facet joints but can be secondary to pathology related to the intervertebral disk. Radicular pain usually results from nerve root irritation which may be the end result of many different processes. There are different approaches to diagnosis and treatment of axial and radicular back pain through interventional procedures, but significant overlap exists. Patient responses to the procedures are difficult to predict, and evidence-based outcomes are difficult to interpret.

Table 13.1 Diagnostic tests in patients with back pain.

Diagnostic test	Accuracy (%)	Sensitivity	Specificity
Clinical examination	46–76	0.80	0.82
Radiography	34	–	–
Myelography	72–91	0.67–0.95	0.76–0.96
CT/MRI	70–100	0.80–0.96	0.68–0.95
Discography	30	0.83	0.63–0.78
Electromyography	78	0.66–0.72	–

CT – computed tomography; MRI – magnetic resonance imaging.
Adapted from Rubin (2007).

Epidural Steroid Injections

Interlaminar, Transforaminal, and Caudal Epidural Steroid Injections

Indications

Epidural steroid injections (ESIs) are the most commonly performed injection for back pain. They may be performed in all segments of the spine, but are most commonly done in the lumbar and cervical regions. The usual approach is through the interlaminar window, but this is not always possible. Removal of bone and ligament, hardware implantation, and postsurgical scarring can make the interlaminar approach both difficult and risky. Transforaminal, caudal, and sacral approaches to steroid injections may be necessary due to the anatomic alterations or pathologic changes in the spine. Clinical practice data have shown that cervical interlaminar ESI is safer than cervical transforaminal injection. Lumbar interlaminar ESIs compared with lumbar transforaminal injection are equally safe and efficacious.

Interlaminar ESI

Technique

The interlaminar ESI is usually performed in the prone position under fluoroscopic guidance. The targeted level is identified by counting the lumbar or cervical vertebrae from a known level such as T1 (first rib-bearing vertebrae), T12 (last rib-bearing vertebrae), or the skull or sacrum. Anatomic variants such as a sacralized L5 or a lumbarized S1 may be present, so counting up and down is recommended. After a prep and drape and under standard sterile technique, the skin is anesthetized and a Tuohy needle (18 or 20 gauge) is advanced through the skin and interspinous ligament until the ligamentum flavum is engaged. The loss of resistance technique with saline or air is used to access the epidural space. In the cervical spine the hanging drop technique may also be used. The needle tip location is confirmed with a lateral film and also by injection of radio-opaque contrast, which shows a characteristic pattern (Fig. 3.18). The steroid is then injected, followed by a small amount of preservative-free saline or local anesthetic. The addition of local anesthetic not only provides some immediate pain relief but also increases the risk of post-injection weakness. It requires monitoring after the procedure for prolonged weakness or potential intrathecal injection. The injections are targeted at or below the corresponding level of the symptoms and the pathology shown on imaging. Severe stenosis or disk herniation would suggest injection below the level, as risk of

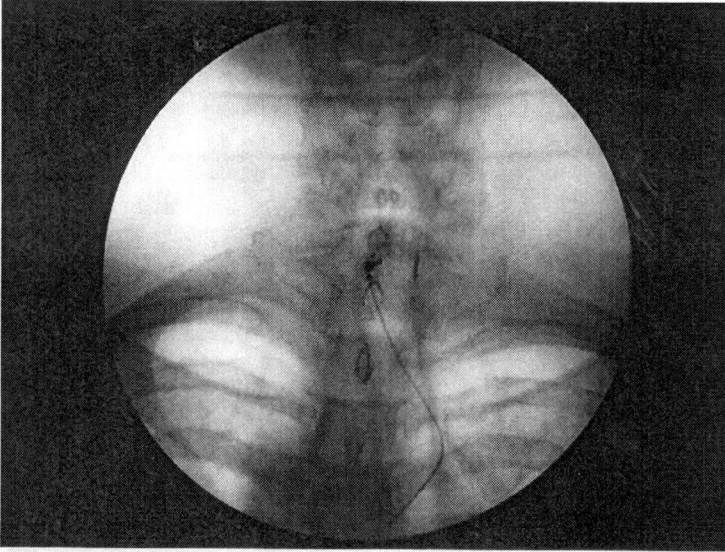

Figure 13.18 Cervical epidural injection at C7–T1 interspace with spread of contrast outlining fat globules in the epidural space.

a wet tap or neurologic injury is increased. The effects of the steroid usually occur within 24–48 h and reach their maximum potential benefit by 7–10 days. They may be repeated monthly up to three times per year without significant systemic side effects from the steroids. Diabetics may experience elevated blood glucose levels for up to several weeks.

Transforaminal Injections

Transforaminal steroid injections target the nerve root laterally as it exits the neural foramen created between two vertebral segments. Depending on practice, they are performed for the same indications of intralaminar injections or after failure of interlaminar injections. Additionally, transforaminal injections are utilized in patients whose anatomy does not allow for safe performance of the interlaminar approach. A 22-gauge spinal needle is used to approach the nerve root in the foramen. A fluoroscopic view about 22° lateral oblique shows the characteristic "scotty dog" appearance of the vertebral body and pedicle. The needle is advanced toward the "neck," or 6 o'clock position just beneath the transverse process. This area above the nerve root is considered safer with respect to risk for intravascular injection and contact with the nerve root itself. This approach is also used for diagnostic nerve root blocks utilized in preoperative planning.

Complications

Intravenous injection is prevented with contrast dye. Intraneural injection can be reduced following present American Society of Interventional Pain Physicians guidelines that require a patient be communicative, such that initiation of an intraneural injection will be met with a scream of discomfort from the patient and cessation of injection at that anatomical point.

Intra-arterial injection of particulate steroids in this approach can cause spinal cord infarction. The use of contrast to assess for vascular runoff and verify spread along the nerve root and even to the epidural space is a must. It should be noted that the risk of intra-arterial injection is even higher when performing transforaminal injections in the cervical spine (Figs. 13.19 and 13.20). Cervical epidural injection with the use of a lateral view can reduce risk of inadvertent improper location of injection and mitigate the risk of catastrophic cord injection.

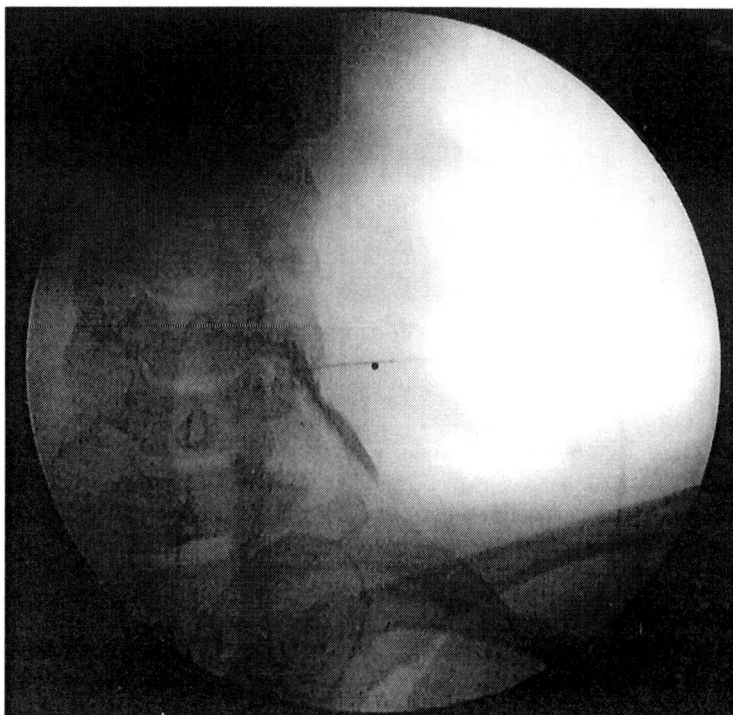

Figure 13.19   Fluoroscopic image of left C6 nerve root injection.

Caudal ESI

The caudal ESI delivers steroid to the epidural space by entry through the sacral hiatus. The external palpable landmarks to this are the sacral cornu and the tip of the coccyx, and a lateral fluoroscopic view is very helpful in directing the Tuohy needle. After a prep, local anesthesia, and fluoroscopic views AP and lateral are obtained, the Tuohy needle is advanced through the skin just below the sacral hiatus and advanced to the sacrococcygeal ligament. The needle approach angle is then flattened almost to the same axis as the patient and advanced through the ligament. The injection may be delivered via the needle at this location or an epidural catheter may be advanced further to a more cephalad location. Dye may be used to confirm the spread, and a flush with 7–10 ml of preservative-free saline also helps to achieve cephalad spread of the medication.

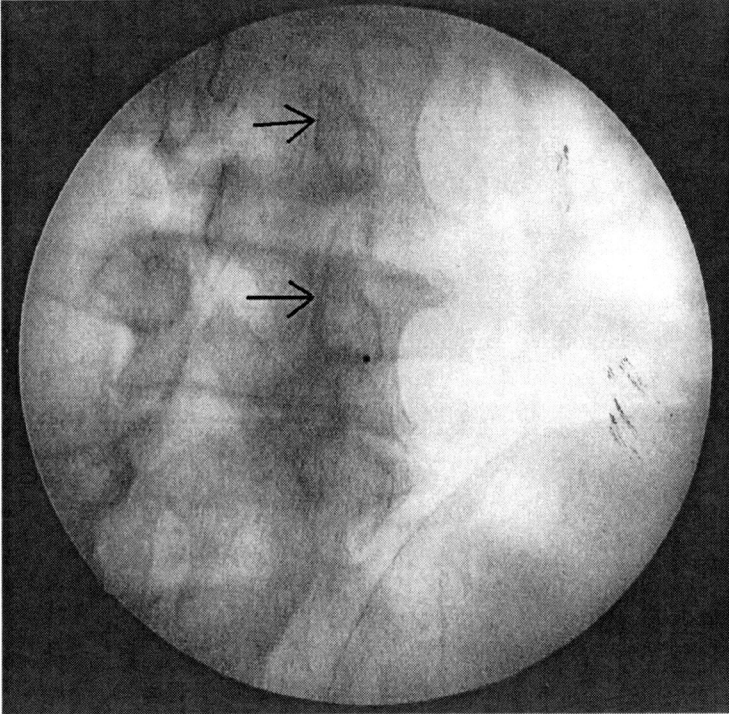

Figure 13.20 The *arrows* are pointing to the left L3–4 and L4–5 facet joints. From this angle a transforaminal or nerve root injection for L4 would be made at the *dot*.

Epidurolysis

Epidural fibrosis or "adhesions" may form spontaneously or after a surgery. They may cause back pain or radicular symptoms in addition to limiting the effectiveness of epidural injections. The adhesions can restrict the flow of medication to the nerve roots thus limiting their spread and absorption. Epidural lysis of adhesions is a percutaneous procedure with parts similar to an epidural steroid injection. It may be performed from the sacral, interlaminar, or transforaminal approaches. With the patient prone under fluoroscopy, a Tuohy needle is used to access the epidural space and a steerable catheter is advanced in the epidural space to the affected area. Injection of contrast shows characteristic filling defects which are the target of the procedure. Repeated passes of the catheter in combination with injection of large volumes of saline are administered in attempts to disrupt the fibrosis tissue. The injectate may be normal or hypertonic saline sometimes in combination with hyaluronidase which softens scar tissue. It may be followed by steroids and or local anesthetic. The catheters may be left in place for repeated treatments over a several-day period (Racz et al. 2008). An additional approach to perform the lysis of adhesions is done under direct visualization called epiduroscopy. A flexible scope is inserted into the epidural space via the caudal approach to the sacral hiatus. Pressure from the scope in combination with infusions of saline is used to break adhesions.

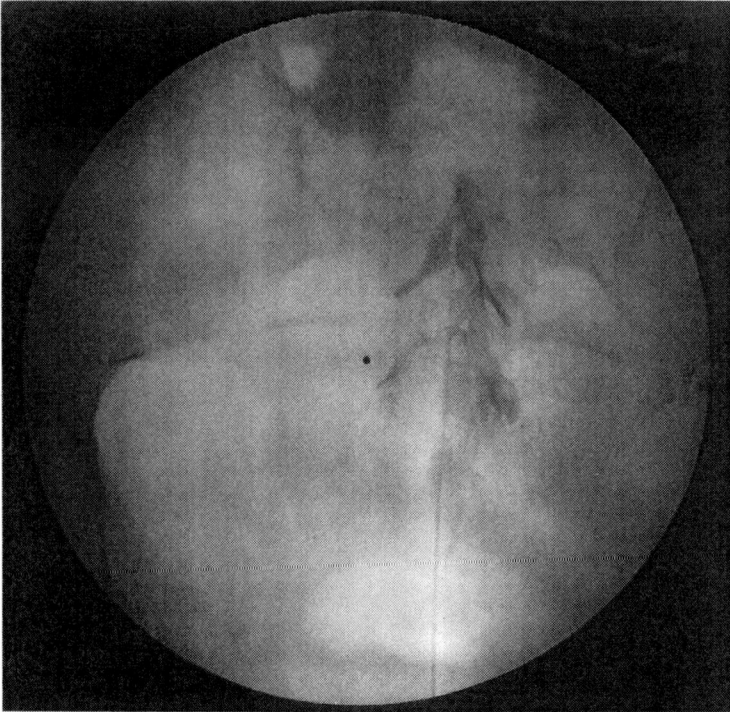

Figure 13.21   Fluoroscopic image of caudal approach to epidural steroid injection. Radio-opaque catheter and contrast display a characteristic "Christmas tree" pattern outlining the sacral roots.

Complications include dural puncture, headache, epidural abscess, bleeding, sensory deficit, and catheter shearing. The procedure may be repeated several times in a year (Geurts et al. 2002) (Fig. 13.21).

Sacral Nerve Blocks
Indications
Sacral injections through the S1 foramen can be used to deliver steroids to the epidural space if other approaches are not technically feasible. A spinal needle is advanced into the superior aspect of the foramen under fluoroscopy, and contrast is injected to verify epidural spread.

Complications
The risks of the above injections vary in degree based on the approach. They include bleeding, infection, dural puncture causing CSF leak and headache, weakness, increased pain, nerve damage, and medication reactions.

Facet Joint Injections
Indications
The facet joints are small synovial joints located between each vertebrae posteriorly and are implicated in axial back pain.

Anatomy

They function in alignment of the spine and allow for forward flexion and extension and smaller amounts of lateral flexion, extension, and rotation. Abnormalities in their structure and alignment may cause substantial discomfort which follows a characteristic referral pattern. After a failure of conservative measures, injections are targeted into the joint itself or to the sensory innervation of the joint (Figs. 13.22 and 13.23).

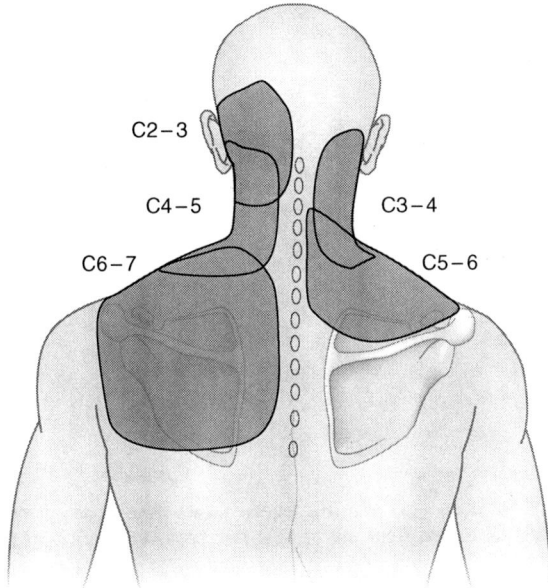

Figure 13.22   Pain referral patterns from cervical facet disease.

Technique

Facet injections are performed in the prone position under fluoroscopy with a spinal needle. It is directed into the joint space which can only support 1–2 ml of fluid. Diagnostic injections would include LA alone, while a mixture of LA and steroid provides longer relief. Each facet receives sensory innervations from the dorsal nerve root above and below it (Raj et al. 2002) (Fig. 13.24). These nerves, the "medial branches," may be anesthetized with local anesthetic diagnostically as well. This block establishes not only the specific contribution of the injected facet joint to the patients overall back pain but also the ability to treat them with radiofrequency neurolysis. The procedure is performed under fluoroscopic guidance in the prone position. A spinal needle is directed to the lamina where the medial branches come off the dorsal roots at levels above and adjacent to each symptomatic level. A small amount of long-acting LA, usually less than 0.5 cc, is injected to anesthetize each medial branch. Pre- and post-injection pain scores and level of function are compared to establish efficacy, and patients also track their pain over the ensuing hours during normally painful activities. Response to the MBB's correlates a response to radiofrequency neurolysis. Because of the potential for false positives, the right and left sides may be blocked separately, and

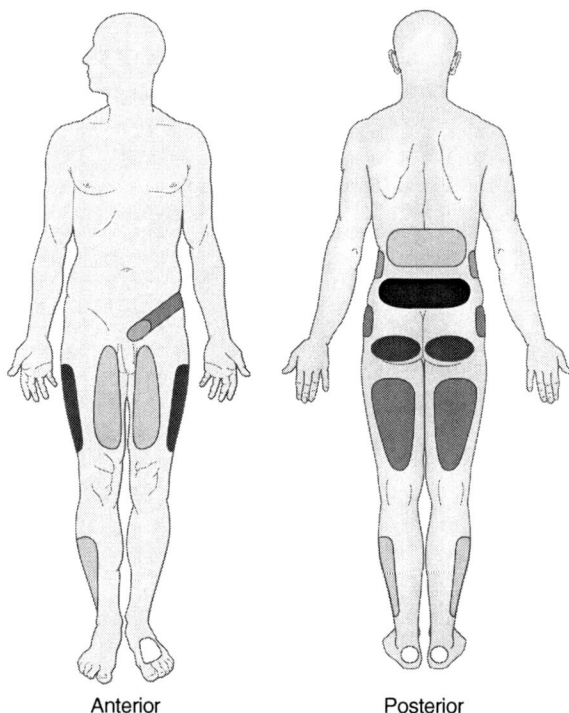

Anterior   Posterior

Figure 13.23   Pain referral patterns from the lumbar facet joints. In descending order, the most common referral patterns extend from the *darkest* (low back) to the *lightest* regions (flank and foot).

it has been suggested that a second diagnostic block be performed to confirm the diagnosis (Schwarzer et al. 1994) (Fig. 13.25).

Due to the anatomic differences between the vertebrae in the different regions of the spine, the approach to the medial branches varies. In the cervical spine there are no distinguishable transverse processes as landmarks. The needle is directed to the groove formed between the superior and the inferior articular processes at each level visualized by a 10° medial oblique angle (Fig. 13.26).

Cervical Facet Injections

All the cervical joints are true joints since they are lined with synovium and have a capsule, except for the Atlanto-occipital and the Atlanto-axial joints. Cervical facet blocks can be done by the intra-articular technique as well. This can be achieved by means of a "blind" technique where the point of entry of the needle is two spinal levels below and 2.5 cm lateral to the facet joint to be blocked. An 18-gauge needle is used as an introducer, and a 25-gauge 3.5-in. styletted spinal needle is inserted to reach the area below the joint to be blocked. As the needle is advanced, a pop is felt when the spinal needle enters the facet joint. Two cubic centimeters of preservative-free local anesthetic is injected into the joint for pain relief. In the presence of inflammation, 80 mg of depot steroid can be added for the first block and 40 mg of depot

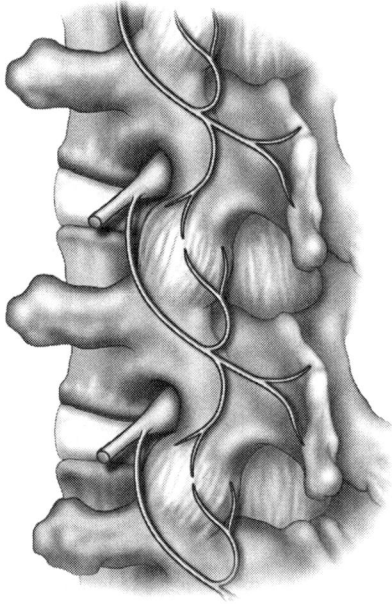

Figure 13.24   The facet joints are innervated by the medial branches of the dorsal ramus from the level above and same level as the joint.

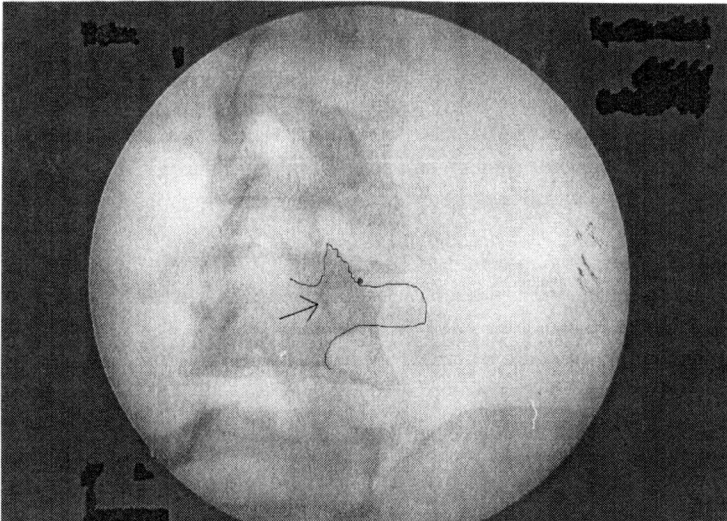

Figure 13.25   The *arrow* indicates the left pedicle on L4, and the *dot* indicates the location for a medial branch block in the lumbar region.

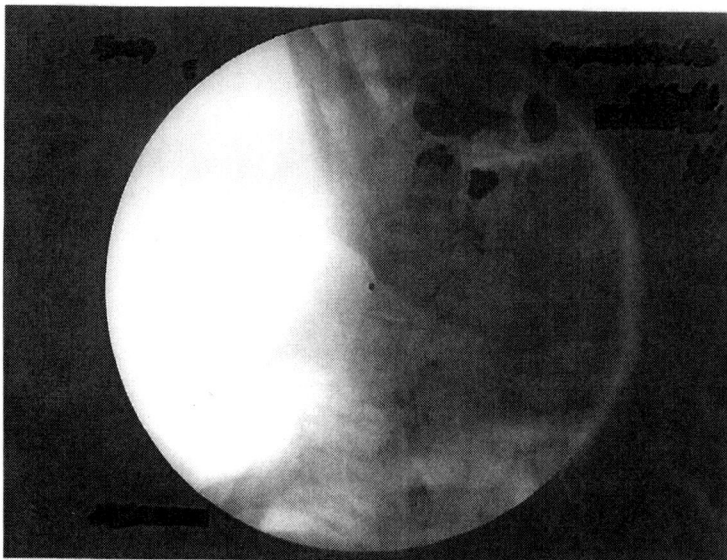

Figure 13.26 Fluoroscopic image of the C-spine from a 10° oblique angle to visualize the MBB target groove between articular processes.

steroid can be added for the consequent block. Many practitioners utilize larger volumes (up to 5 ml) for bathing of associated ligaments, paraspinal muscles, and support structures which can provide additional beneficial affects.

Thoracic Facet Block: Medial Branch Technique

Indications
The medial branch technique is the most common technique for treating thoracic facetogenic pain syndrome. Physical examination with pain on facet loading or a Kemp's test is highly suggestive of a facetogenic mediated pain syndrome.

Technique
The patient is placed in a prone position, and the spinous process at the level to be blocked is identified. After anesthetizing the skin with 1% lidocaine, a 25-gauge 3.5-in. styletted needle is inserted through an 18-gauge introducer needle at a point 5 cm lateral and slightly inferior to the spinous process. The needle is pointed to the junction of the transverse process and the vertebra at the level to be blocked (Fig. 13.27). The needle is then advanced to the most lateral aspect of the border of the articular process. The stylet is removed, and if no blood or CSF fluid is observed after aspiration, about 1.5 cc of local anesthetic solution is injected. If an inflammatory process is suspected then depot steroid can be added with the local anesthetic usually 80 mg for the initial block and 40 mg thereafter. The block can also be done under fluoroscopic guidance with contrast medium injected before injection of the local anesthetic to ensure that the needle is not in the intrathecal space.

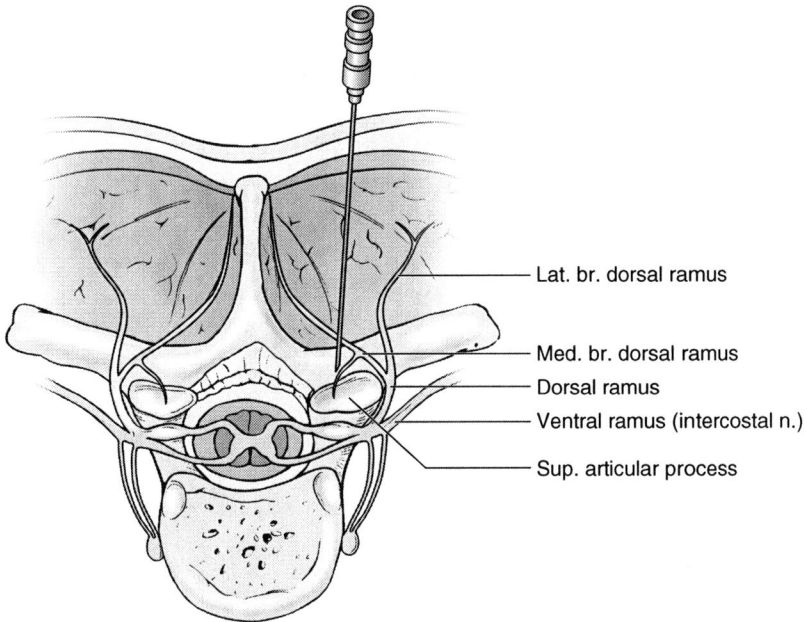

Lat. br. dorsal ramus

Med. br. dorsal ramus

Dorsal ramus

Ventral ramus (intercostal n.)

Sup. articular process

Figure 13.27   Thoracic facet block: medial branch technique.

Thoracic Facet Block: Intra-articular Technique

The thoracic facet block can also be done by an intra-articular technique when the needle is inserted two spinal levels below and 2.5 cm lateral to the spinous process to be blocked. Similar to the medial branch technique, an 18-gauge 1-in. needle is used as an introducer for a 25-gauge 3.5-in. styletted spinal needle that is used for the block. The needle is advanced to impinge on the bone of the articular pillar and is advanced until it slides into the facet joint. After negative aspiration a total of 1 cc of local anesthetic is injected. If there is an inflammatory process then 80 mg of depot steroid can be added to the local anesthetic for the initial block and 40 mg of depot steroid for subsequent blocks. The procedure can also be done with fluoroscopic guidance and the injection of 1 cc of contrast medium before the injection of local anesthetic to ensure correct placement of the needle.

Lumbar Facet Joint Block Technique

The lumbar spine is visualized and approached from a 22° oblique angle. Thoracic facet disease is much less common but may be approached in a similar fashion. Patient participation during needle manipulation aids placement. Sedation can be used but is discouraged since it may alter subjective relief of symptoms (Cohen and Raja 2007).

Radiofrequency neurolysis or ablation (RFN or RFA) of facet joints is a neurodestructive procedure utilizing RF energy delivered through the tip of an insulated needle to a specific location, in this case the medial branch of the dorsal root which gives sensory innervation to the facet. After successful diagnostic medial branch blocks with local anesthetic, RF energy can be applied to the same location, achieving sensory denervation of the facet joint for a much longer duration. Both cervical and lumbar RFA of the medial branches have been

Lumbar Facet Block

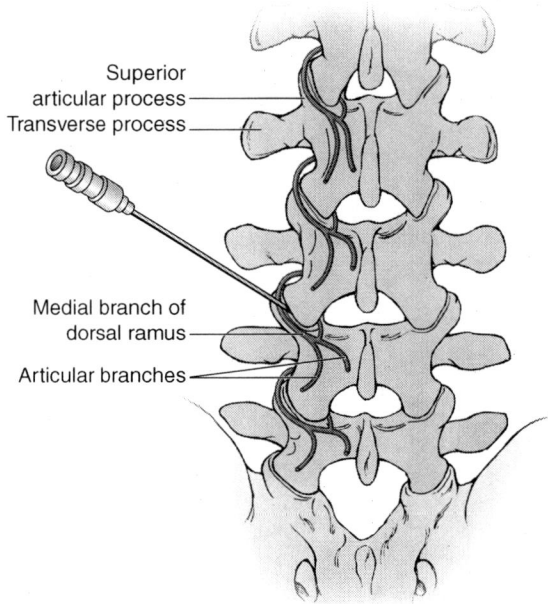

Figure 13.28 Lumbar facet block: radiofrequency lesioning of the medial branch of the primary posterior rami.

shown to be effective in multiple studies after a single successful diagnostic block (Leclaire et al. 2001, Tekin et al. 2007, van Kleef et al. 1999, van Wijk et al. 2005, Dreyfuss et al. 2002, Dreyfuss et al. 2000, Lord et al. 1996) (Fig. 13.28). Needle placement technique and target are the same as the medial branch blocks. After placement of the RF needle, testing is done to confirm a safe distance from both the dorsal and the ventral roots so that they are not damaged while treating the medial branch. Lesions are made by using high-frequency and varying current, maintaining a temperature of 80° C. The procedure is usually effective for 6–12 months or longer. A variation of the technique using pulsed radiofrequency at 2 Hz for 4 min at 42° C has also been shown to be effective (Tekin et al. 2007). Complications include pain, bleeding, infection, and nerve damage.

Genitofemoral Nerve Blocks
Indications
This block is for the treatment of groin pain and genitofemoral neuralgia and also for the provision of surgical anesthesia for groin surgery and inguinal herniorrhaphy when combined with ilioinguinal and iliohypogastric blocks.

Anatomy
The genitofemoral nerve arises out of the L1 nerve root and also occasionally has a contribution from the T12 nerve root. It emerges on the abdominal surface opposite L3 or L4 and

then divides into the genital branch and the femoral branch above the inguinal ligament. In males the genital branch passes through the inguinal canal.

Technique
The block is done in a supine position. In order to block the genital branch it is important to identify the pubic tubercle and the inguinal ligament. A point just lateral to the pubic tubercle below the inguinal ligament is the point of entry. A 1.5–in., 25-gauge needle is used to pierce the skin, and 5 cc of 1.0% preservative-free lidocaine is injected into the subcutaneous tissues after negative aspiration. In the presence of inflammation 80 mg of depot steroid can be used with the initial block and 40 mg of depot steroid with subsequent blocks.

Ilioinguinal Nerve Blocks
Anatomy
The ilioinguinal nerve is a branch of the L1 nerve with occasional contribution from the T12. The ilioinguinal nerve pierces the transverse abdominis muscle at the level of the anterior superior iliac spine. It provides sensory innervation to the skin in the inner side of the upper thigh, the root of the penis, and the upper scrotum in males or the lateral part of the labia and the mons pubis in females.

Technique
To perform the block a point 2 in. medial and 2 in. inferior to the anterior superior iliac spine is identified. The area is prepped and draped in sterile fashion. A 25-gauge 1.5-in. needle is entered at the point identified and advanced obliquely toward the pubic symphysis. A total of 5–7 cc of 1% lidocaine is injected in a fan-like fashion to block the ilioinguinal nerve.

Iliohypogastric Blocks
Anatomy
The L1 nerve root gives fibers to the iliohypogastric nerve. Contribution from the T12 is also seen in some patients. The iliohypogastric nerve perforates the transverse abdominis muscle and lies between this muscle and the external oblique muscle. The nerve divides into a lateral and an anterior branch. The lateral branch gives sensory innervation to the posterior-gluteal region, while the anterior branch provides sensory innervation to the skin above the pubis after piercing the external oblique muscle.

Technique
The block is performed by identifying a point 1 in. medial and 1 in. inferior to the anterior superior iliac spine. A 25-gauge 1.5-in. needle is inserted obliquely toward the pubic symphysis, and about 5–7 cc of 1% lidocaine is injected in a fan-like fashion. Methylprednisolone 40 mg can be injected with the local anesthetic if there is an inflammatory component to the pain.

Sacroiliac Joint Injections
Indications
Sacroiliac (SI) joint dysfunction is a common cause of low back pain and also a frequently missed diagnosis. It occurs independently or in conjunction with facet disease, sometimes

being confused with it. Physical examination with a positive Patrick's test is highly suggestive of sacroiliac joint-mediated pain. A local anesthetic block of the joint can be used to diagnose it, and steroids may be added to the injection for therapy.

Technique

With the patient positioned prone, fluoroscopy is used to visualize the joint space obliquely, medial to lateral. The joint is accessed in the inferior portion with a 22- or 25-gauge spinal needle. Intra-articular placement is verified with contrast. The joint has a large surface area, but not a tremendous capacity, so only a small amount, several cubic centimeters, of local anesthetic or LA/steroid is tolerated. RF treatment of the joint is also possible and has been shown to be effective versus placebo (Ferrante et al. 2001, Vallejo et al. 2006, Maugars et al. 1996). Standard RF lesions are performed at the L5 medial branch and along the medial portions of the S1 and S2 foramen. This covers the innervation of the upper half of the joint. Then two RF probes are used as bipolar leads to create lesions in a stepwise fashion along the SI joint from the mid portion to the bottom to continue the RF lesion for the remainder of the joint. A "railroad track" down the joint is made by successively placing the needles about 5 mm apart along the medial side of the joint from the mid portion to the inferior edge and creating lesions between them. Motor testing should be performed prior to treating the branches as described in RFN. The effects usually last for 6–12 months.

Cryoneurolysis

Cryoneurolysis is a neurodestructive procedure that uses cooling to induce nerve damage. The cryoprobes consist of an inner tube and an outer tube and a cooling chamber at the tip. They come in 12, 14, or 16 gauges. Either nitrous oxide or carbon dioxide is pressurized through the needle and tip which cools causing a 3.5–5.5 mm expansion of ice in the surrounding tissue. Like radiofrequency, there are several steps to the treatment procedure. First, a diagnostic block should be performed to identify the nerve location and contribution. On another occasion just before treatment, both sensory and motor stimulation should be performed. Lesions are made for 90–120 s. As the nerve regenerates the lesion can be repeated.

Discography

Discography is a diagnostic procedure used to identify pain-generating intervertebral disks in preoperative evaluation and planning. Under fluoroscopy with the patient prone, a needle is guided into the vertebral disk. Contrast dye is injected to verify placement of the needle into the disk. The disk is then pressurized via the needle in attempts to reproduce painful symptoms. The procedure is repeated at levels above and below, and pain scores are reported after injections into each level. Comparison is made from symptomatic to non-symptomatic or control discs. Due to the variability in technique and its basis on subjective patient reports, its use is limited (Fig. 13.29).

Intradiscal Electrothermal Therapy

Intradiscal electrothermal therapy (IDET) is a therapeutic technique used to treat discogenic pain. It involves passage of a catheter under fluoroscopy into the pain-generating ruptured intervertebral disk. The catheter is then heated to 80–90° for 5–6 min. This thermal treatment

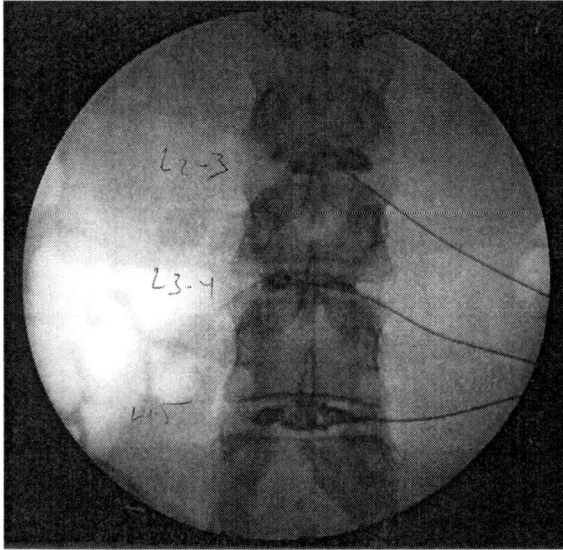

Figure 13.29 Lumbar discogram.

is postulated to stop the disk contents from leaking as well as improve pain. Despite its initial popularity, its efficacy is inconclusive and because of patient discomfort and risk of diskitis its use has been limited (Bogduk et al. 2004).

Spinal Cord Stimulation

Spinal cord stimulation (SCS) is a treatment modality whereby electrical stimulation is applied to the dorsal columns of the spinal cord to treat pain by "covering" it with sensory interference. It is an "augmentation" therapy as compared to the "ablative" therapies previously mentioned performed by neurosurgery, but similar to the neurosurgical procedures in that it is an endpoint therapy. Although the actual mechanisms are not known, the theories initially spawned from Melzack and Wall's "gate control theory." Neuropathic, sympathetic, and nociceptive pain can all be treated with varying efficacy. Different theories exist for each of the different types of pain treated, but "the precise mechanism of action seems to be complex and may vary depending on the clinical condition for which the device was placed. A single, simple, unifying mechanism of action of SCS is not evident at this time (Schmidek and Roberts 2006)."

Refractory neuropathic pain after back surgery, post-laminectomy pain syndrome or failed back surgery syndrome, chronic regional pain syndrome (CRPS) (Kumar et al. 1997), and ischemic pain from peripheral vascular disease and refractory angina (Ansari et al. 2007) are the most common and very effectively treated with SCS (Bala et al. 2008). It is also used successfully in the treatment of diabetic neuropathy, posttherapeutic neuralgia, and limb amputation pain. Implantation of the electrodes outside the CNS has been valuable in the treatment of peripheral nerve injuries and occipital neuralgia (Jasper and Hayek 2008) (Fig. 13.30). Leads can also be placed subcutaneously for "field stimulation" in non-dermatomal pain syndromes.

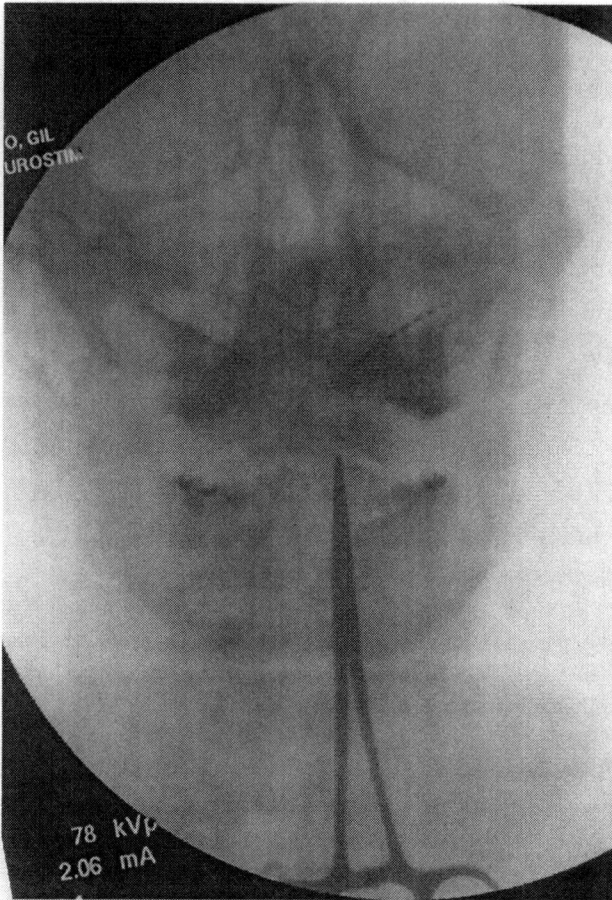

Figure 13.30 Intraoperative film of bilateral occipital nerve stimulator leads, tip of the instrument is at the C1–C2 interspace.

Technique

The procedure involves several phases, but may be condensed depending on the institution. After appropriate patient screening process including a mental health evaluation (Prager and Jacobs 2001), a several-day stimulation trial is performed. Percutaneous implantation is performed in an operating room setting with the patient under a light anesthetic. With the patient prone, a Tuohy needle and the loss-of-resistance technique are used to access the epidural space several vertebral levels below the desired location. A shallow-angled approach minimizes movement at the skin. The lead is then threaded to the desired level and side adjacent to the dorsal columns with the aid of a steerable central wire and fluoroscopy (Figs. 13.31 and 13.32). Coverage is tested with patient participation so that the lead can be maneuvered for optimal pain coverage. The lead is carefully taped to the skin and attached to an external generator.

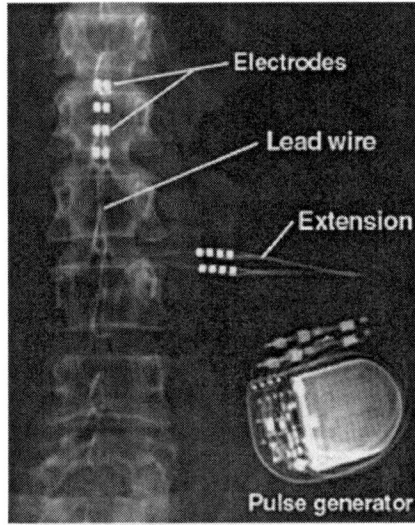

Figure 13.31   Spinal cord stimulation (SCS) system diagram labeled.

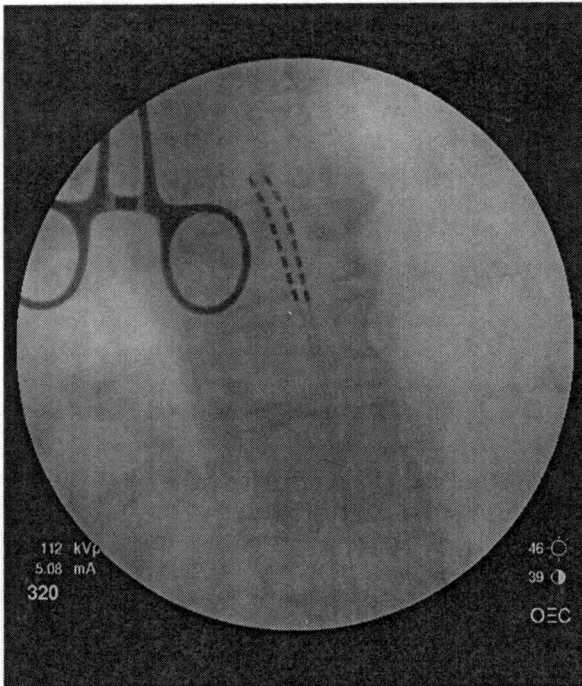

Figure 13.32   Intraoperative fluoroscopic image of dual percutaneous thoracic leads.

Complications

Complications include epidural hematoma and abscess, dural puncture, infection, and lead migration, the last two being the most common.

If greater than 50% pain relief is achieved over the trial period (about a week), the patient is a suitable candidate and they return for removal of the temporary percutaneous lead and scheduled for a permanent device. If a permanent lead has been implanted for the trial, they return for generator implantation. The generator is implanted in a separate pocket created by blunt dissection at a depth of about 1 cm. The small size of the newer generators permits implantation in many locations: lateral to the entry site, in the abdomen, chest wall, or upper buttocks. Both regular and rechargeable batteries are available. It is essential that the pocket fits the generator snugly to minimize movement of the implant. The lead is tunneled from the anchor site to meet the pocket, and any excess length is coiled beneath it. Standard surgical techniques are utilized. Postoperative infection usually mandates explantation of the device. Lead migration, the most common complication, usually requires a revision and placement of a paddle lead in the epidural space via laminotomy (Fig. 13.33).

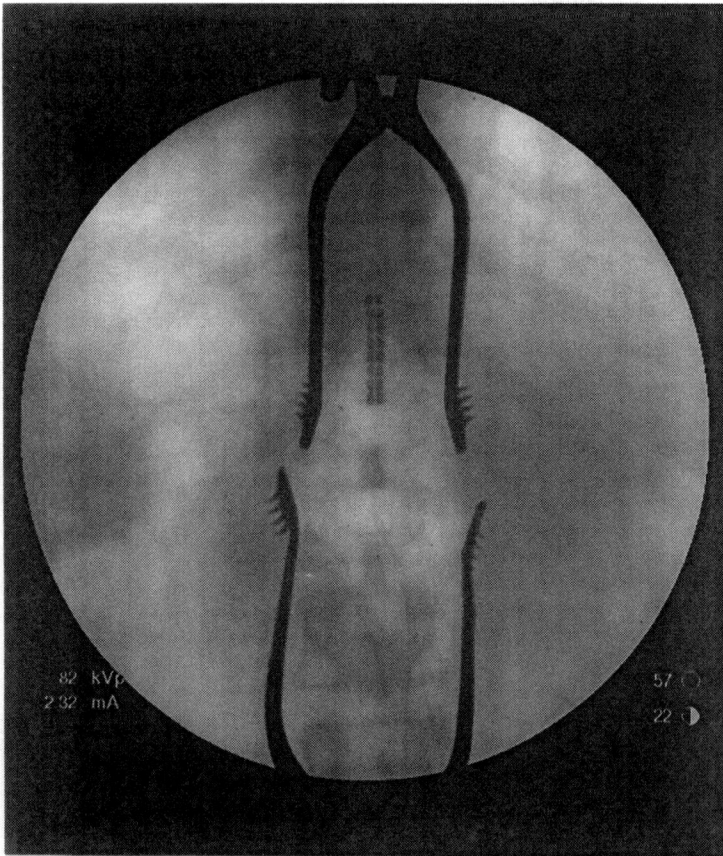

Figure 13.33   Intraoperative film of thoracic paddle lead placement via laminotomy.

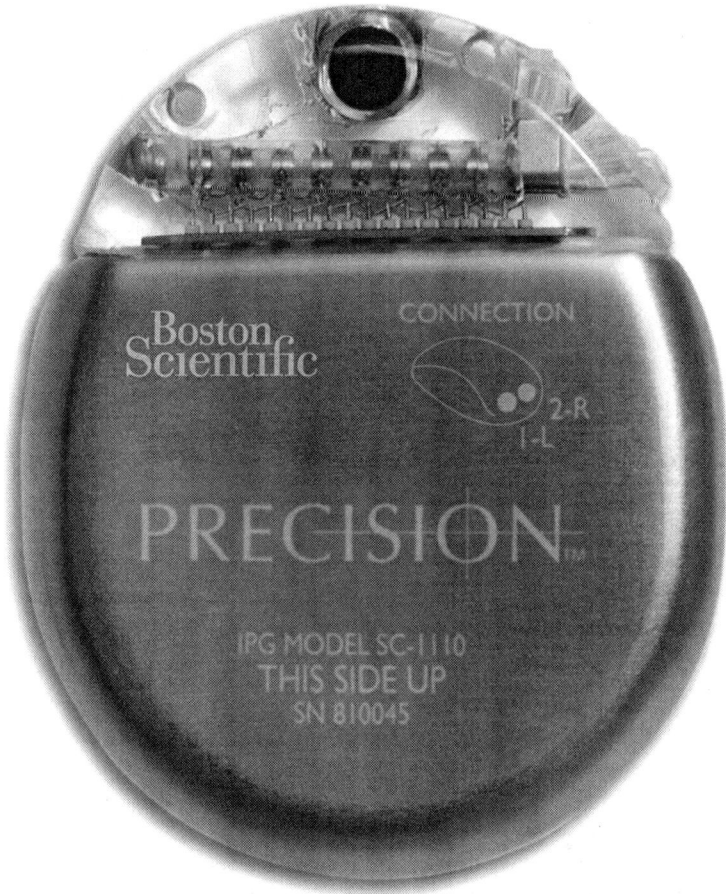

Figure 13.34 Boston Scientific generator and paddle lead. With permission from Boston Scientific, Natick, MA.

Detailed programming of the stimulators takes place in recovery after the procedure. The lead electrode arrays allow for an almost infinite number of stimulation programs varying the amplitude, frequency, pulse width, and contacts used. The programming and charging of the device take place via remote placed next to the skin. There are three main manufacturers of the devices: Medtronic Corporation (Minneapolis, MN; www.medtronic.com), Boston Scientific (Natick, MA; www.bostonscientific.com), and St. Jude Medical – formerly ANS (St. Paul, MN; www.sjm.com). Extensive physician and patient information can be found on the web sites listed (Figs. 13.34 and 13.35).

Intrathecal Drug Delivery
Indications
Intrathecal drug delivery is an invaluable tool for the pain management physician. Oral and even intravenous medication requirements may exceed acceptable side effect profiles in some pain conditions, particularly malignancy. Administration of pain intrathecal medications can

286 · ESSENTIALS OF PAIN MANAGEMENT

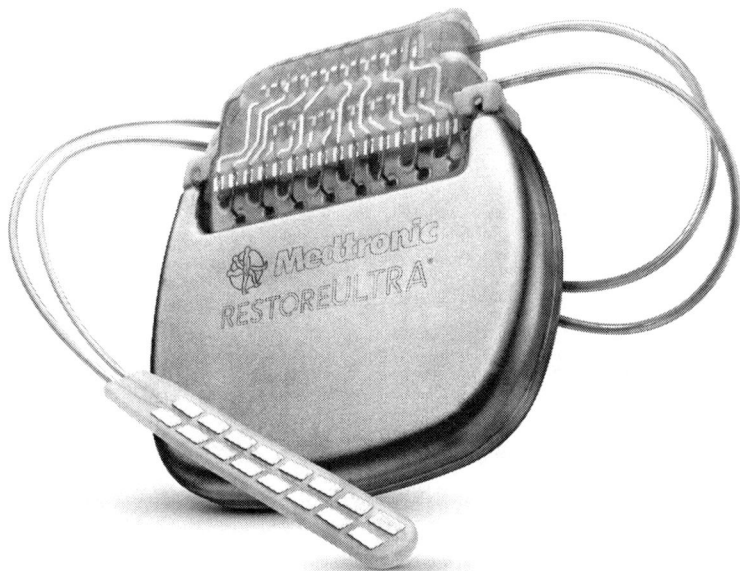

© 2010 Medtronic, Inc.

Figure 13.35 Medtronic rechargeable generator. With permission from Medtronic Corporation, Minneapolis, MN.

provide substantially higher levels of pain control or relief of spasticity without many of the systemic side effects.

General Technique
In the short term, a percutaneous intrathecal catheter may be placed very similarly to an epidural. These are usually done under fluoroscopy with the patient in the lateral decubitus position. Many of these patients will not tolerate prone positioning due to both pain and deconditioning. The catheters are threaded up the intrathecal space to mid thoracic levels. They are usually tunneled from the access point laterally to facilitate dressing application and maintenance and also to reduce infection risk. Patients can be discharged home with indwelling catheters and home nursing maintenance or hospice to maintain the infusion and external pump.

History
Implantable intrathecal systems have been in use since the early 1980s. First morphine in 1982, then baclofen in 1984 was delivered with these systems. In 1991, the Medtronic Corporation released a permanent implantable pump system for cancer-related pain. The system was not much different from pumps implanted today.

Modern Devices
Currently, the pumps are made up of three sealed chambers: an electronic module and battery, a peristaltic pump and drug reservoir, and the last chamber contains an inert (stable)

gas. Medications are injected into the pump through the reservoir fill port and then through a valve to the reservoir. The inert gas inside the device pressurizes the reservoir and forces medication through a bacteria-retentive filter into the peristaltic pump. The pump delivers medication at a very slow rate through the catheter. An externally programmable microprocessor controls the medication delivery rate. It is capable of delivering multiple drugs in a mixture, as well as varying infusion rates and blousing over the course of the day (Medtronic 2008) (Fig. 13.36).

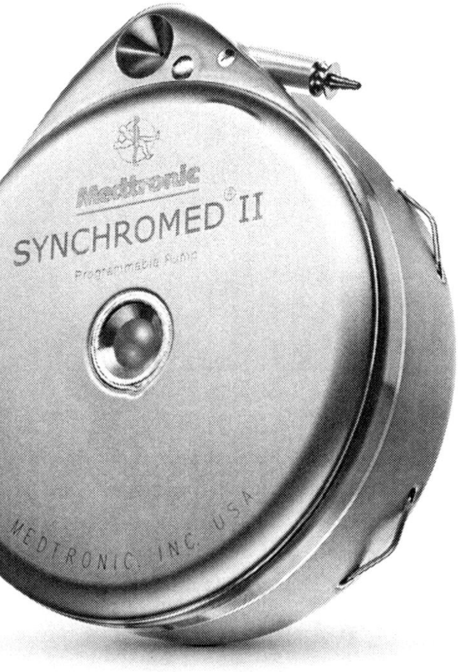

© 2010 Medtronic, Inc.

Figure 13.36   The Medtronic Synchromed II implantable intrathecal delivery system. With permission from Medtronic Corporation, Minneapolis, MN.

Patient Selection

Patient selection in treating non-cancer pain is crucial, since negative variables such as major psychopathology, addiction, and social or economic stressors can significantly affect outcomes (Oakley and Staats 2000) (Table 13.2).

Drug Selection

In drug selection for pain control, continuous intrathecal infusion of morphine is the gold standard. Other opioids used include hydromorphone, fentanyl, sufentanil, and meperidine. Local anesthetics may be combined with the opioid or infused alone. These include bupivacaine, ropivacaine, and tetracaine. Clonidine is an alpha agonist effective at the spinal cord level that may be added to the infusion for improved pain control as well

Table 13.2 Selection criteria for implantable intrathecal pump.

Exclusion criteria
Relative
Emanciated patient
Ongoing anticoagulation therapy
Child before fusion of the epiphyses
Occult infection possible
Recovering drug addict
Lack of social or family support
Socioeconomic problems
Lack of access to medical care
Absolute
Aplastic anemia
Systemic infection
Allergy to implant materials
Allergy to intended medications
Certain psychological–behavioral features
Inclusion criteria
Pain type and generator appropriate
Demonstration of opioid responsiveness
Psychological clearance
Successful completion of screening trial

Adapted from Waldman (1996).

(Anderson 1984, Coombs et al. 1982, Hassenbusch et al. 1990, Krames et al. 1985, Magora et al. 1980, Shetter et al. 1986, Winkelmuller and Winkelmuller 1996, Deer et al. 2007, Fanciullo et al. 1999, Coombs et al. 1985, Hassenbusch and Porteney 2000) (Tables 13.3 and 13.4).

The medication infusate is highly concentrated to allow for a long duration between pump refills. Commercial preparations are available, and doses and mixtures can be tailored by a compounding pharmacy. The older Medtronic system (Synchromed EL) has a reservoir volume of 18 ml, and the updated system (the Synchromed II) is available with a reservoir volume of 20 or 40 ml.

Additional Pearls

Morphine and *hydromorphone* are stable up to 90 days, the maximum refill interval even if a patient is on small doses (Hildebrand et al. 2001, Hildebrand et al. 2003, Classen et al. 2004).

Ziconotide is additional Food and Drug Administration (FDA)-approved medication for intrathecal use. It is a calcium channel blocker which has been shown to be useful in neuropathic pain where other treatments have failed. Psychiatric side effects may limit its use.

Baclofen is a gamma aminobutyric acid (GABA) agonist used for the treatment of spasticity and pain. It is administered both oral and intrathecal routes. If patient symptoms are unresponsive to maximum oral doses, an intrathecal baclofen trial may be performed. After 50–100 mcg of baclofen is injected by spinal, the response, which is variable, is then serially measured and quantified using the Ashworth scale. Significant improvement may be treated with an intrathecal delivery system. Pump malfunction is an emergency, since baclofen withdrawal can be life threatening.

Table 13.3 Recommended algorithm for intrathecal polyanalgesic therapies. Progression begins from first line initial medications through sixth line which are experimental medications.

Line 1	(a) Morphine	◄►	(b)Hydromorphone	◄►	(c)Ziconotide
Line 2	(d) Fentanyl	◄►	(e) Morphine/hydromorphone + ziconotide	◄►	(f) Morphine/ hydromorphone + bupivacaine/clonidine
Line 3	(d) Clonidine	◄►	(h) Morphine/hydromorphone/fentanyl Bupivacaine + clonidine + ziconotide		
Line 4	(i) Sufentanil	◄►	(j)Sufentanil + bupivacaine + clonidine + ziconotide		
Line 5	(k) Ropivacaine, buprenorphine, midazolam Meperidine, ketorolac				
Line 6	Experimental drugs Gabapentin, octreotide Conopeptide, neostigmine, adenosine XEN2174, AM336, XEN, ZGX 160				

Adapted from Racz (2008).

Table 13.4 Percent of physicians using different medications/combinations for intrathecal pumps.

Drug	% of Surgeons (total sample n = 413)	Low managers (n = 199)	High managers (n = 214)	Mean # patients	# of Patients	% Patients
Morphine alone	99	99	98	15.5	6339	48
Morphine + bupivacaine	68	55	80	5.9	1649	12
Hydromorphone alone	58	48	67	4.7	1142	8
Morphine + clonidine	55	44	66	4.8	1099	8
Hydromorphone + bupivacaine	35	26	44	3.9	566	4
Morphine + clonidine + bupivacaine	34	22	48	5	700	5
Morphine + baclofen	34	21	46	2.8	395	3
Fentanyl alone	21	13	29	2.4	212	1
Clonidine alone	21	12	30	1.9	168	1
Sufentanil alone	16	8	23	2.3	153	1
Other	24	19	29	9.2	919	7

Adapted from Geurts (2002).

Implantation

Implantation is performed in the operating room under anesthesia. Abdominal placement lateral to the umbilicus and above the beltline is usually chosen for easy accessibility and implant tolerance. The patient is positioned in lateral decubitus to allow for access to the spine, tunneling area, and implant site (Fig. 13.37). A Tuohy needle is used to access the intrathecal space via the L1–L2 interlaminar window under fluoroscopy. After free flow of CSF is verified, the implantable catheter is threaded into the intrathecal space up to the symptomatic level. An incision is opened above and below the Tuohy needle and catheter, and blunt dissection is used to expose the thoracolumbar fascia. A purse-string suture is made around the needle entry point and tied after the Tuohy needle is removed, making sure to maintain free flow of CSF. An anchor is then sutured to the thoracolumbar fascia and a loop of catheter coiled in the recess before attention is turned to creation of a pocket for the pump. The pocket should be approximately 1.5–2 cm in depth, and the use of a template is helpful. A supplied tunneling device is used to connect the pocket to the back incision. Excess catheter may be removed but is generally coiled beneath the pump for consistency of catheter volume. Patients should be admitted for overnight observation.

Complications from the procedure include bleeding, infection, seroma, cerebrospinal fluid leak or hygroma, and post-dural puncture headache. Opiate infusions can cause granuloma formations at the catheter tip next to the spinal cord and should cause hesitation when placement for nonmalignant pain syndromes is considered. The incidence may be as high as 3% (Medtronic 2008). Spinal cord compression and permanent neurologic injury may result. Some institutions perform yearly monitoring with CT and fine-cut magnetic resonance imaging (MRI) studies to evaluate the catheter tip. If a granuloma is found, the intrathecal infusion must be transitioned to saline and replaced by oral opiates, a daunting task. Device problems include catheter occlusion, disconnection, pump failure, and pump battery depletion. Medication side effects such as nausea, vomiting, urinary retention, weakness, and pruritus may occur with escalating doses. Different medications or combinations can be used to minimize escalation of single drug doses and side effects.

Pump Refills and Reprogramming

Pump refills and reprogramming are performed percutaneously and transcutaneously, respectively. Pumps are interrogated with a remote control and then accessed with a 22-gauge Huber needle under sterile conditions included in the refill kit. Unused medication is removed, and the reservoir is refilled with new medication. Discrepancies between the expected and the actual residual volume can be indicative of a problem with the system. After removal of old medication, 5 cc of the new medication is injected, aspirated back as a confirmatory step, and then the full volume can be slowly instilled. After refill, the pump is reprogrammed to the new reservoir volume and the new refill date is calculated. Errors in medications, concentrations, rates, and boluses as well as pump access and sterility can be life threatening. All reprogramming and drug changes should be confirmed with another experienced provider.

Infusion rates may be adjusted for increases in pain. Panel guidelines suggest dose increases for nonmalignant pain of up to 30% and increases of up to 50% for malignancy pain

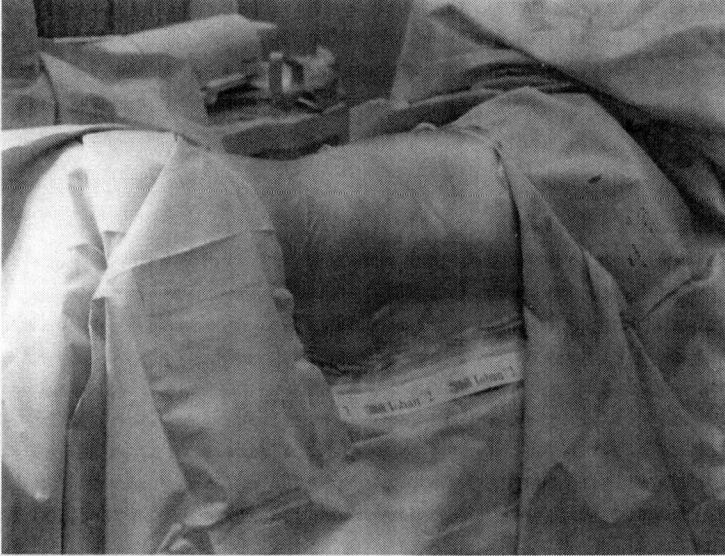

Figure 13.37 Patient positioned and draped in left lateral decubitus in the operating room for pump and intrathecal catheter implantation.

(Deer et al. 2007). Magnetic resonance imaging will cause the pump to stall, and interrogation should be performed after each study. If functioning normally, it will restart within 15 min.

Neurosurgical Procedures for Chronic Pain

Neurosurgical ablative procedures are neurodestructive treatments targeted at the peripheral and central nervous systems that permanently alter the anatomy. They have most commonly been used for cancer pain, but are performed less frequently today because of their poor risk benefit ratio and the development and widespread use of augmentative therapies. These include spinal and peripheral nerve stimulation and implantable intrathecal infusion pumps. Careful patient selection can optimize outcomes: treatment of nociceptive pain not relieved by analgesics, opioid-intolerant patients, or palliation of pain in a patient with a short life expectancy. One of the major concerns with many of the ablative procedures is deafferentation pain. About 6–9 months after the procedure the original pain may return at a heightened level, while the induced deficits may remain. Hence the reservations in utilizing these procedures in patients with a longer life expectancy or until other avenues have been exhausted (Loyd and Fanciullo 2005).

Peripheral Nerves as a Therapeutic Target

Peripheral nerves can be a source of significant pain after trauma or ligation precipitates the formation of a neuroma or abnormal growth of the nervous tissue. The neural tissue may be resected by a procedure called neurectomy, but motor deficit may result since most nerves have both sensory and motor components. This procedure is not highly successful for nerve ligations in amputations, but may be effective for meralgia paresthetica and post-herniorrhaphy pain. Pain signals can also be targeted peripherally at a level closer to the CNS, at the sensory nerve root. A dorsal rhizotomy involves lesioning of the dorsal nerve root. A similar procedure called ganglionectomy targets the dorsal root ganglion and may be more effective since there are additional sensory fibers in the ventral motor root that pass through the DRG. Ablation of the DRG by ganglionectomy ligates these afferents as well and may provide more pain relief. Both of these procedures require a general anesthetic and a multilevel laminectomy.

Doral Root Entry Zone Lesioning

The spinal cord may be targeted for pain reduction by performing dorsal root entry zone lesioning (DREZ) and cordotomy. In a DREZ procedure, lesions are created in the superficial layers of the dorsal horn of the spinal cord called Rexed's laminae. Second-order afferent nociceptive fibers (A-beta) terminate here primarily lamina # 3, but can also be # 1, 2 (C-fibers). Patient selection is important since anatomically well-defined lesions respond best, and the procedure requires a general anesthetic for a multilevel laminectomy. DREZ lesioning is highly effective in treating chronic pain from brachial plexus avulsion injuries, postherpetic neuralgia, and malignancy pain from a pancoast tumor. Spontaneous abnormal activity, hyperactivity, and corticospinal tract damage resulting in motor deficits may result from the procedure (Fig. 13.38).

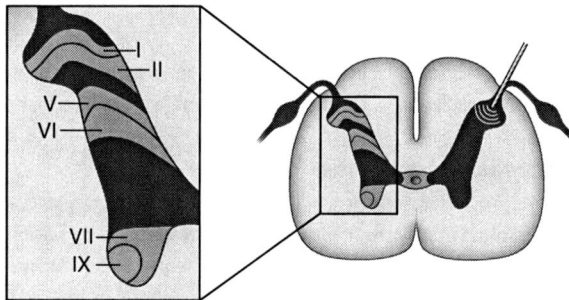

Figure 13.38 T10 spinal cord cross section showing a radiofrequency dorsal root entry zone (RF-DREZ) lesion. Window shows organization of Rexed's lamina in the gray matter.

Cordotomy

Cordotomy is sectioning of the spinothalamic tract located at the anterior-lateral portion of the spinal cord. It carries pain and temperature sensation from the periphery. Since the fibers cross over to the opposite side, or "decussate," two to five levels cephalad to their entry point into the cord, lesions of the tract cause loss of these senses two to five levels below it, on the opposite side (Figs. 13.39 and 13.40).

Brainstem

Brainstem mesencephalotomy is used to treat pain in the head, neck, and upper extremity by targeting the lateral spinothalamic tracts. At this level the spinothalamic tract affects the contralateral side as it has already decussated. Lesioning is performed in the periaqueductal gray

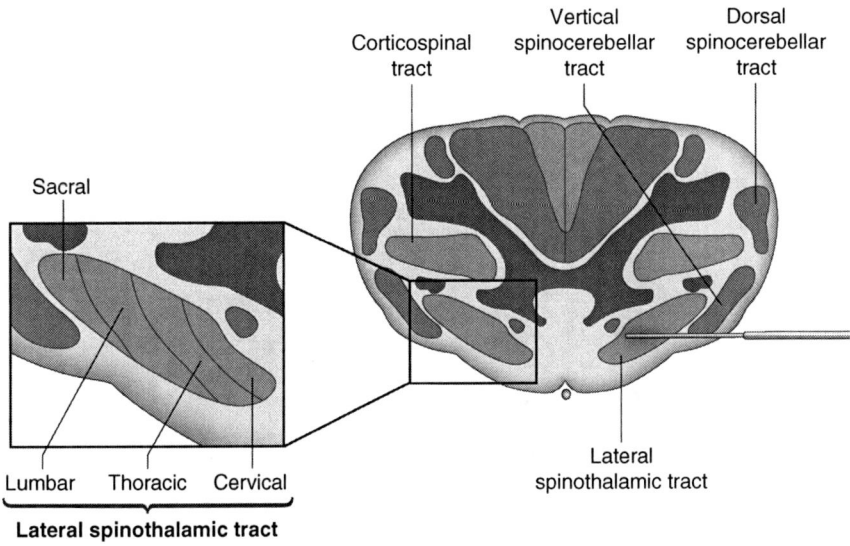

Figure 13.39 Cross section of spinal cord at C1–C2 showing the spinothalamic tract and window detailing the somatotopic organization. Probe on left side for percutaneous radiofrequency.

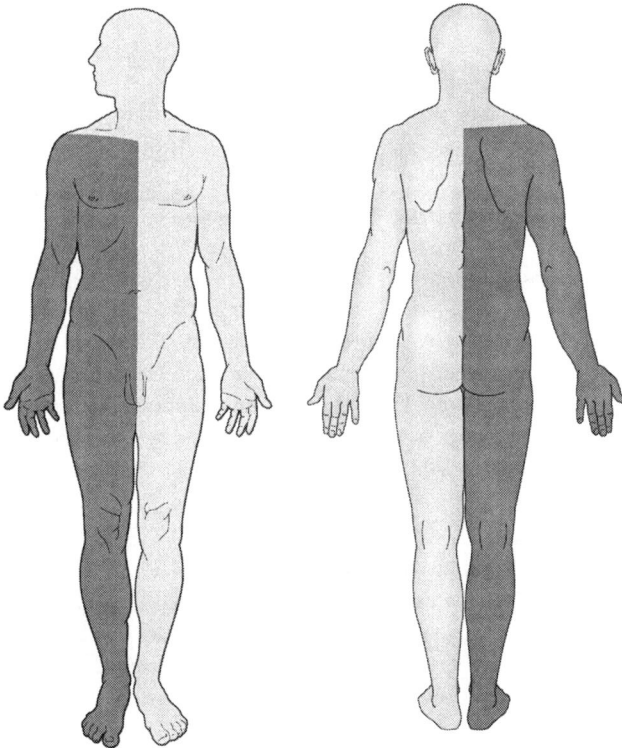

Figure 13.40 Analgesic area after C1–C2 unilateral left cordotomy.

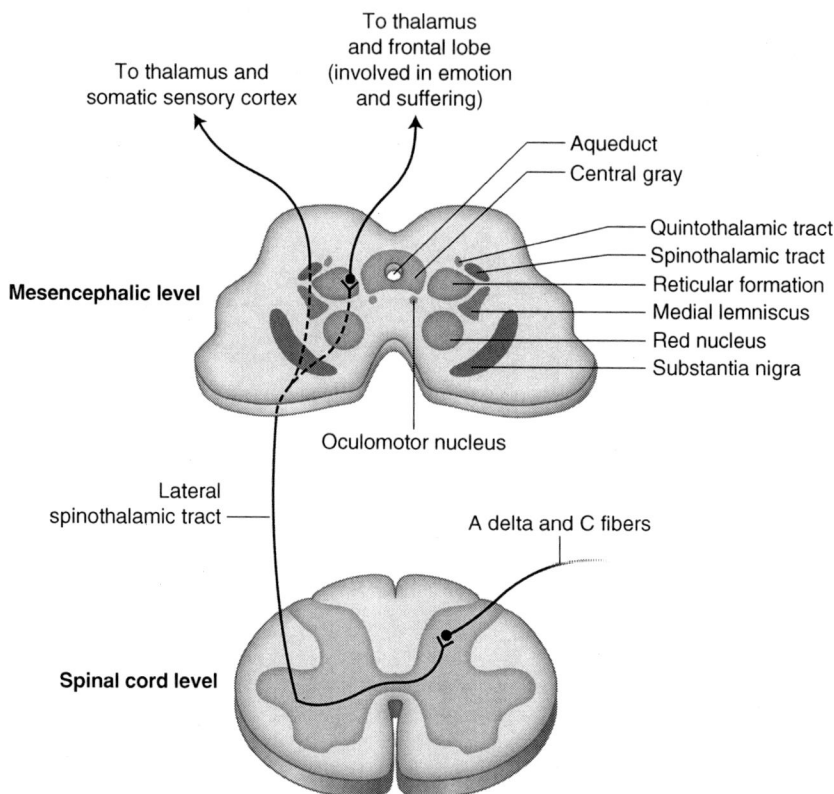

Figure 13.41 A delta and C-fibers decussate in the spinal cord and ascend in the spinothalamic tract to the midbrain where they can be lesioned under sedation guided by magnetic resonance imaging (MRI).

matter or the reticular formation. An additional tract that may be lesioned is the quintothalamic tract. It is located superomedial to the spinothalamic tract. This decreases transmission of extralemniscal emotional suffering. The best results have been using stereotactic approaches for the treatment of nociceptive head and neck pain secondary to malignancy and neuropathy. The main untoward side effects are dysesthesias and oculomotor dysfunction (Fig. 13.41).

Brain-Targeted Surgical Interventions

In the *brain*, a hypophysectomy can be performed for intractable pain in association with hormonally responsive cancers. The transsphenoidal approach is used for resection or ablation with radiofrequency or alcohol. Both metastatic breast and prostate cancer pain have been treated with very good results. Cingulotomy is usually performed for psychiatric illness, particularly obsessive compulsive disorder and depression, but is also used to treat chronic pain syndromes. Lesioning the cingulate gyrus, part of the limbic system, disrupts the perception of pain. The pain is still felt by the patient, but it does not

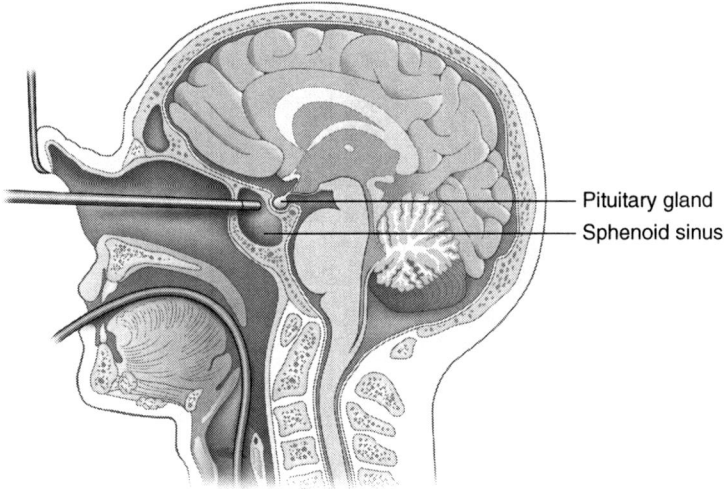

Pituitary gland
Sphenoid sinus

Figure 13.42   Transsphenoidal hypophysectomy.

bother them. Aside from the operative risks, there can be cognitive side effect as well (Fig. 13.42).

Case Scenario

Michael A. Cosgrove, MD, David K. Towns, MD, and Gilbert Fanciullo, MS, MD

You have been asked to see George, a 48-year-old man with a history of metastatic rectal cancer in remission for 5 years with recent recurrence. He had an abdominoperineal resection with adjuvant chemotherapy and radiation on his initial presentation with the malignancy. The recurrence was heralded by increasing pelvic floor and perineum pain due to local recurrent disease that is inadequately controlled with oral opioids and antiseizure medications. Further surgical resection is not an option, and he does not want chemotherapy. He has a poor prognosis and is expected to succumb in several months. His oncologist has referred him for possible interventional techniques to help with his pain.

What are your options for managing his pain?

Neuroaxial, sympathetic, or somatic nerve blocks with neurolytic agents is an option worth considering.

Pain in the lower pelvis, from the rectum and perineum, may be sympathetically mediated via the ganglion impar (ganglion of Walther). Blockade of the ganglion is effective in malignancy-related pain in this area. Normally, a block with local anesthetic would be performed initially to establish efficacy, but his dire circumstances might preclude the additional procedure and a neurolytic block might be the starting point. His post-resection anatomy actually reduces risk, as there is no bowel or anus at risk of perforation.

You perform the block, and he has immediate pain relief and goes home. A week later George is back to see you. He is in severe pain. He would like to try something which will give him long-term pain relief.

What could be done to help George?
Obviously, the pain relief from the block was short-lived. The alternate option now is to consider intrathecal drug delivery after careful evaluation of its feasibility. An MRI should be done to rule out intraspinal metastasis or areas of tumor that could interfere with percutaneous placement into the L1–L2 or L2–L3 interspace. A percutaneous intrathecal catheter would be most likely, but if he were still fairly functional and independent, a permanent implanted device would provide more flexibility and portability in his final months.

Is there a role for epidural analgesia?
The epidural route is commonly selected for delivering pharmacological agents if the patient is unlikely to survive more than 3 months. The intrathecal route is preferred if long-term survival is likely as drugs can be delivered by implanted pumps. The dose requirement of spinal infusion is significantly less, and refill intervals are much longer than epidural infusions. In addition, the intrathecal route provides analgesia that is more predictable.

References

Anderson EF. Epidural and intrathecal narcotics for pain relief. S D J Med. 1984;37(1):7–12.

Ansari,S, Chaudhri K, Moutaery K. Neurostimulation for refractory angina pectoris. Acta Neurochir Suppl. 2007;97(Pt 1):283–8.

Bala MM, et al. Systematic review of the (cost-)effectiveness of spinal cord stimulation for people with failed back surgery syndrome. Clin J Pain 2008;24(9):741–56.

Bogduk N, Dreyfuss P, et al. International spine intervention society practice guidelines for spinal diagnostic and treatment procedures. San Francisco, CA: International Spine Intervention Society; 2004.

Classen AM, Wimbish GH, Kupiec TC. Stability of admixture containing morphine sulfate, bupivacaine hydrochloride, and clonidine hydrochloride in an implantable infusion system. J Pain Symptom Manage 2004;28(6):603–11.

Cohen SP, Raja SN, Pathogenesis, diagnosis, and treatment of lumbar zygapophysial (facet) joint pain. Anesthesiology 2007;106(3):591–614.

Coombs DW, et al. Intrathecal morphine tolerance: use of intrathecal clonidine, DADLE, and intraventricular morphine. Anesthesiology 1985;62(3):358–63.

Coombs DW, et al. Epidural narcotic infusion reservoir: implantation technique and efficacy. Anesthesiology 1982;56(6):469–73.

Deer T, Hassenbusch SJ, et al. Polyanalgesic consensus conference 2007: recommendations for the management of pain by Intrathecal (Intraspinal) drug Delivery: Report of an Inderdisciplinary Expert Panel. Neuromodulation: Technology At The Neural Interface, 2007, p. 10.

de Leon-Casasola OA, Critical evaluation of chemical neurolysis of the sympathetic axis for cancer pain. Cancer Control 2000;7(2):142–8.

Dreyfuss P, et al. Radiofrequency facet joint denervation in the treatment of low back pain: a placebo-controlled clinical trial to assess efficacy. Spine 2002;27(5):556–7.

Dreyfuss P, et al. Efficacy and validity of radiofrequency neurotomy for chronic lumbar zygapophysial joint pain. Spine 2000;25(10):1270–7.

Fanciullo GJ, et al. The state of implantable pain therapies in the United States: a nationwide survey of academic teaching programs. Anesth Analg. 1999;88(6):1311–6.

Ferrante FM, et al. Radiofrequency sacroiliac joint denervation for sacroiliac syndrome. Reg Anesth Pain Med. 2001;26(2):137–42.

Geurts JW, Kallewaard JW, Richardson J, Groen GJ. Targeted methylprednisolone acetate/hyaluronidase/clonidine injection after diagnostic epiduroscopy for chronic sciatica: a prospective, 1-year follow-up study. Reg Anesth Pain Med. 2002;27(4): 343–52.

Hassenbusch SJ, et al. Constant infusion of morphine for intractable cancer pain using an implanted pump. J Neurosurg. 1990;73(3):405–9.

Hassenbusch SJ, Portenoy RK, Current practices in intraspinal therapy – a survey of clinical trends and decision making. J Pain Symptom Manage 2000;20(2):S4–11.

Hildebrand KR, Elsberry DE, Anderson VC, Stability and compatibility of hydromorphone hydrochloride in an implantable infusion system. J Pain Symptom Manage. 2001;22(6): 1042–7.

Hildebrand KR, Elsberry DD, Hassenbusch SJ. Stability and compatibility of morphine-clonidine admixtures in an implantable infusion system. J Pain Symptom Manage. 2003;25(5):464–71.

Jasper JF, Hayek SM. Implanted occipital nerve stimulators. Pain Physician 2008;11(2): 187–200.

Krames ES, et al. Continuous infusion of spinally administered narcotics for the relief of pain due to malignant disorders. Cancer 1985;56(3):696–702.

Kumar K, Nath RK, Toth C. Spinal cord stimulation is effective in the management of reflex sympathetic dystrophy. Neurosurgery 1997;40(3):503–8; discussion 508–9.

Lavelle ED, Lavelle W, Smith HS. Myofascial trigger points. Med Clin North Am. 2007;91(2):229–39.

Leclaire R, et al. Radiofrequency facet joint denervation in the treatment of low back pain: a placebo-controlled clinical trial to assess efficacy. Spine 2001;26(13):1411–6; discussion 1417.

Loyd R, Fanciullo G. Surgical procedures for intractable cancer pain. Palliat Pain Med Improving Care Patients Serious Illn. 2005;9(3):167–76.

Lord SM, et al. Percutaneous radio-frequency neurotomy for chronic cervical zygapophyseal-joint pain. N Engl J Med. 1996;335(23):1721–6.

Magora F, et al. Observations on extradural morphine analgesia in various pain conditions. Br J Anaesth. 1980;52(3):247–52.

Maugars Y, et al. Assessment of the efficacy of sacroiliac corticosteroid injections in spondyloarthropathies: a double-blind study. Br J Rheumatol. 1996;35(8):767–70.

Medtronic. Available from: http://www.medtronic.com/neuro/paintherapies. Accessed December 2008.

Medtronic, Urgent Medical Device Correction: Updated information-Inflammatory Mass (granuloma) At or Near the Distal Tip of Intrathecal Catheters. 2008, January.

Moore DC. Regional block; a handbook for use in the clinical practice of medicine and surgery. 4th ed. Springfield, IL: C. C. Thomas; 1965. p. xvii, 514p.

Oakley J, Staats PS. The use of implanted drug delivery systems. In: Raj PP, editor. The practical management of pain. St. Louis, MO: Mosby; 2000. pp. 768–78.

Ogoke BA, The management of the Atlanto-occipital and Atlanto-axial joint pain. Pain Physician 2000;3(3):289–93.

Prager J, Jacobs M. Evaluation of patients for implantable pain modalities: medical and behavioral assessment. Clin J Pain. 2001;17(3):206–14.

Racz GB, Heavner JE, Trescot A. Percutaneous lysis of epidural adhesions – evidence for safety and efficacy. Pain Pract. 2008;8(4):277–86.

Raj PP, Benzon AB, et al. Facet syndromes and blocks. In: Ross A. editor. Practical management of pain. 3rd ed. St. Louis, MO: Mosby; 2002. p. 746.

Rosenberg M, Phero JC. Regional anesthesia and invasive techniques to manage head and neck pain. Otolaryngol Clin North Am. 2003;36(6):1201–19.

Rubin DI. Epidemiology and risk factors for spine pain. Neurol Clin. 2007;25(2):353–71.

Schmidek HH, Roberts DW. Schmidek & Sweet operative neurosurgical techniques: indications, methods, and results. 5th ed. Philadelphia, PA: Saunders Elsevier; 2006. 2 v. p. xxxix, p. 2337, 67p.

Schwarzer AC, et al. The false-positive rate of uncontrolled diagnostic blocks of the lumbar zygapophysial joints. Pain 1994;58(2):195–200.

Shanahan EM, et al. Suprascapular nerve block (using bupivacaine and methylprednisolone acetate) in chronic shoulder pain. Ann Rheum Dis. 2003;62(5):400–6.

Shetter AG, Hadley MN, Wilkinson E. Administration of intraspinal morphine sulfate for the treatment of intractable cancer pain. Neurosurgery 1986;18(6):740–7.

Simpson BA. Spinal cord stimulation. Br J Neurosurg 1997;11(1):5–11.

Tekin I, et al. A comparison of conventional and pulsed radiofrequency denervation in the treatment of chronic facet joint pain. Clin J Pain. 2007;23(6):524–9.

Vallejo R, et al. Pulsed radiofrequency denervation for the treatment of sacroiliac joint syndrome. Pain Med. 2006;7(5):429–34.

van Kleef M, et al. Randomized trial of radiofrequency lumbar facet denervation for chronic low back pain. Spine 1999;24(18):1937–42.

van Wijk RM, et al. Radiofrequency denervation of lumbar facet joints in the treatment of chronic low back pain: a randomized, double-blind, sham lesion-controlled trial. Clin J Pain. 2005;21(4):335–44.

Waldman HJ. Neurophysiologic testing in the evaluation of the patient in pain. In: Waldman SD, Winnie AP, editors. Interventional pain management. Philadelphia, PA: WB Saunders; 1996;407–411.

Winkelmuller M, Winkelmuller W. Long-term effects of continuous intrathecal opioid treatment in chronic pain of nonmalignant etiology. J Neurosurg. 1996;85(3):458–67.

Chapter 14

Functional Restoration of Patients with Pain

Ali Nemat, MD and Yogi Matharu, DPT, OCS

Introduction

This chapter will introduce a different group of clinicians who treat pain with a primary focus of improvement in functional mobility of the patients. One of these disciplines is physical medicine and rehabililtation, also called *physiatry*. Like any other clinician, a physiatrist follows the established algorithms for the diagnosis and treatment of a variety of medical conditions. The same is true for the evaluation and treatment of pain patients. A physiatrist evaluates the pain patient, orders appropriate diagnostic studies, and then treats the patient with appropriate therapeutic modalities including the medication and interventional procedures. One factor that differentiates the physiatrists from other clinicians is their focus of treating the patient as a whole, looking not only at the area of disability but also the patients' functional capability and the tasks that they are able to accomplish. The ideal model for the treatment of pain is a multidisciplinary approach, meaning that a variety of clinicians from different disciplines address the treatment of complicated pain syndromes. This does not necessarily mean that each individual pain patient will require an elaborate program to receive appropriate care. In fact, many of these patients could and should be able to get adequate treatment at a primary care level. However, when required, a multidisciplinary setting will enable the clinicians to treat pain effectively. This will eventually result in an overall reduction of the number of chronic pain patients in the community. The training curriculum for the physiatrist includes the musculoskeletal system as well as the peripheral nervous system. Combining the findings from a thorough physical examination and appropriate diagnostic studies enables the physiatrist to make the diagnosis and then develop an effective treatment plan. Even though the treatments offered to patients with pain generally follow the similar algorithm, as mentioned earlier the main focus here will be the functional restoration for the patients.

Another group of clinicians who are closely involved in the treatment of patients with pain are physical therapists who are uniquely qualified to provide functional restoration through evaluation, treatment, and disease prevention strategies. Physical therapy intervention by a licensed physical therapist has been shown to be a very effective short- and long-term method of managing pain.

While it is difficult to give a complete listing of the qualifications of physical therapists, it is important to recognize that like many other health-care professionals, not all physical therapists are trained the same or will treat each problem in the same manner. A clinician

N. Vadivelu et al. (eds.), *Essentials of Pain Management*,
DOI 10.1007/978-0-387-87579-8_14, © Springer Science+Business Media, LLC 2011

ought to develop referral relationships with a variety of physical therapists that specialize in treating a wide range of diagnoses and personalities. Physical therapists are educated at the post-baccalaureate level and must pass a state and national licensing examination. Many physical therapists are Doctors of Physical Therapy (DPT) and many have completed specialized residency training. Board certification is available in orthopedics, neurology, pediatrics, geriatrics, sports, cardiopulmonary, and clinical electrophysiology. Physical therapists are licensed by their respective State Board of Physical Therapy. It should be emphasized that treatment by non-licensed persons should not be considered of high quality and should not be billed as physical therapy. Finally, before it is decided whether a patient has failed physical therapy intervention and requires other treatments, it is important to make a thorough assessment of the type and quality of the treatment the patient has received.

In this chapter, we will discuss the evaluation of a patient with musculoskeletal pain, appropriate diagnostic tools, and then available treatment options including physical therapy. It should be emphasized, however, that this is only an introduction to the field of physiatry and physical therapy, and the interested reader is encouraged to refer to other resources for detailed information.

Obtaining History of a Patient with Musculoskeletal Pain

This step follows the same basics taught to students while in training. However, there are several points that will assist the clinician to gather most information in the allocated time.

Listening to the Patient

First and foremost, when obtaining the history from a pain patient, it is essential to listen to the patient. Successful clinicians are the ones who let their patients tell them about their symptoms. For example, when a patient complains of pain in the calves after walking a short distance, this could be a clue toward the diagnosis of peripheral vascular disease or lumbar spinal stenosis. When a patient complains of pain in one or both wrists especially while typing on a keyboard, it could be secondary to the diagnosis of carpal tunnel syndrome. A patient describing a sharp shooting pain starting in the low back area, with radiation to the distal lower extremity, might be suffering from S1 radiculopathy. However, in light of the current health-care environment it is also very important to manage time efficiently. Hence, asking focused questions will guide the process in a productive way.

Functional Mobility

Another important piece of information to inquire from patients is their baseline functional history. This will assist the clinician in overall evaluation of the patient providing invaluable data in regards to the patient's ability to perform activities of daily living (ADLs) and also the extent of their limitations or disability. It will also give clues as to the etiology of the disease process and the amount of time required for rehabilitation. For example, a patient who has been experiencing gradual decline in functional mobility over the course of the past 5 years will require more intensive and lengthy rehabilitation than one with a 3-month history of functional deficits. Included in this section are questions about the patient's use of any assistive devices, such as canes or walkers that not only confirm the disability but also highlight other issues such as decreased balance (O'Dell et al. 2007).

Other Co-Morbidities

When evaluating a patient to find out whether he/she is an appropriate candidate for a functional restoration rehabilitative program, we need to determine if that patient is physically, mentally, and emotionally suited to participate. For example, the patient's cardiopulmonary status will affect the level/intensity of such treatment. If a patient presents with depressed mood or emotional distress, this will adversely affect the outcome of the rehabilitative program. Hence, it is vital in such a case scenario, especially when dealing with chronic pain, to obtain a psychological history. In many instances, this might require a referral to a pain psychologist for appropriate evaluation and treatment. Another example is a patient who presents for his physical therapy following a head on collision with bodily injury. In many such cases the ensuing traumatic brain injury is underdiagnosed but will come to attention when the patient presents with cognitive impairments and/or learning disabilities.

Medication

One of the other important components of the history is the complete list of current medication as well as those the patient has tried in the past. For example, many elderly patients who are undergoing treatment with pain medications with anti-cholinergic side effects might present with loss of balance and, hence, increased incidence of falls (Mintzer and Burns 2000). The list can also provide insight into other medical conditions that the patient may not have revealed in the initial interview.

Evaluation

Thorough evaluation of a patient's mobility warrants a detailed knowledge of the anatomy of the muscles in the affected limb(s). A well-trained clinician is knowledgeable of muscles in the upper and lower limbs, origins, insertions, nerve supply, and finally their function. Many of the pathologies originating from the muscles in the limbs could be diagnosed by recognized diagnostic tests for the particular muscle/tendon. In regards to the nerve supply, it is very important to become familiar with the innervations to the upper and lower limbs (Perotto 2005). Basically, these nerves originate from the brachial plexus for the upper limb and the lumbar plexus to the lower limb. Tables 14.1 and 14.2 summarize sample muscles in the upper and lower limbs, respectively, with the corresponding innervations. Adequate knowledge of these structures anatomically and functionally will enable the clinician to narrow down the list of differential diagnoses after a complete history and physical examination.

Table 14.1 Selected muscles in the upper limb with the corresponding innervation and function.

Muscle	Peripheral nerve	Nerve root	Function
Deltoid	Axillary	C5, C6	Abduction of the arm
Biceps	Musculocutaneous	C5, C6	Flexion of the forearm
Triceps	Radial	C7, C8, T1	Extension of the elbow
Flexor carpi radialis	Median	C6, C7, C8	Flexion of the wrist
Extensor pollicis longus	Posterior interosseous	C7, C8	Extension of the thumb
Abductor pollicis brevis	Median	C8, T1	Abduction of the thumb

Table 14.2 Selected muscles in the lower limb with the corresponding innervation and function.

Muscle	Peripheral nerve	Nerve root	Function
Gluteus maximus	Inferior gluteal	L5, S1, S2	Extension of the hip
Tensor fascia lata	Superior gluteal	L4, L5, S1	Abduction of the thigh
Vastus lateralis	Femoral	L2, L3, L4	Extension of the knee
Extensor hallucis longus	Deep peroneal	L5, S1	Extension of the big toe
Gastrocnemius	Tibial	S1, S2	Flexion of the foot
Abductor hallucis	Medial plantar	S1, S2	Abduction of the big toe

During the initial evaluation, the physical therapist will also perform a physical and environmental evaluation of the factors contributing to the patient's pain problem. The therapist will review the medical history and inquire about the patient's clinical course, limitations, deficits, and aggravating and alleviating factors. The physical therapist will then perform a biomechanically based physical examination which includes evaluation of range of motion, flexibility, strength, sensation, and reflexes; performing special tests; testing functional limitations; and finally observing movement patterns that may be causing or perpetuating injury. Also, in this section they evaluate the patient's gait, posture, and activity-specific patterns. These data are used in conjunction with the subjective evaluation to formulate the prognosis and short- and long-term risk of injury. The patients are then educated about their physical therapy diagnosis, the risks and benefits of treatments involved, and finally what is expected from them throughout and the role they can play in their own recovery. A personalized plan of care is then developed based on the patient's dysfunction, goals, and schedule.

We should now discuss the issue of altered movement patterns in pain patients. If a patient has pain, he/she will try to compensate by using other muscles and modifying movement patterns. Often these compensations lead to the development of myofascial pain (Table 14.3) on top of the original pain source and may even cause injury to other body segments or systems. If the patient is unable to compensate (or as pain of compensation increases), his/her function will decline. As function decreases, the muscles become weaker, joints become stiffer, motor control decreases, and cardiovascular performance suffers. In fact, over time, the patient does less and less. This decline in function might result in emotional distress which could present itself as anxiety, decreased self-esteem, loss of stress management strategies, decreased social interaction, isolation, inactivity, and depression. The dysfunction also causes strain on relationships due to increased workload on the partner and family as well as financial hardship if the person in pain must decrease overall participation in the home, recreational, and employment activities.

Recovery

In some cases, patients are able to identify which movements are causing their pain. They are able to modify their activity and allow healing to occur. However, in other cases, particularly when there is latency (time delay) between their movement and the onset of pain, the patient is not able to modify the activity correctly.

Table 14.3 Original pain source varies depending on location and nature of original injury. Compensatory patterns can cause myofascial pain dependent on the specific patterns the individual patient chooses.

Types of pain	Typical region	Possible reason
Original pain source	Any area	Trauma
		Repetitive use
		Degeneration
		Idiopathic
Myofascial pain from compensatory patterns	Joints —one to two levels proximal or distal to the affected area Other joints specific to the patients chosen compensatory movement pattern	Altered movement patterns and postures

In order to recover completely, the patient must be educated to recognize the current functional status. This is of critical importance. If a patient continues to keep the "best" or "pre-injury" functional level as the baseline, he/she will continue to make errors in judgment leading to increased pain. For example, if a patient has a 5-min walk tolerance, but decides to walk for 25 min, it results in a "flare up." The patient often says that "I used to walk for 60 min so 25 should be no problem." This inability to recognize current compromised level of function and the subsequent failure feed to their psychological dysfunction. In the above example, had the patient attempted to increase the time by small proportions, for example, to 7 min, this might have been a successful attempt with positive emotional/psychologic effect. It is important that the physical therapist and physician determine tolerance for activity. These include walking tolerance on level ground, hills, up/downstairs; standing tolerance; sitting tolerance; and sleep tolerance (including total hours and uninterrupted time). This establishes the intensity of the treatment plan and helps monitor functional progress for the patient, clinician, and third-party payers. It can also be used to determine alternative activities that do not cause pain (i.e., sitting desk activities versus standing activities if walk and stand tolerance is an issue). Detailed examples of activity-specific tolerance and ensuing functional limitation and secondary effect on the patient's life are presented in Table 14.4.

To establish a recovery plan, the patient and clinician must have a clear understanding of aggravating and alleviating factors. Simply stated, to improve, a patient must do more of what alleviates symptoms and less of what aggravates. Generally speaking, a patient continues to aggravate and maintain the symptoms by not only moving in a suboptimal pattern but also with "too much" movement at the injured area. In some cases, the patient is able to move appropriately, but can only do so for a short period of time or when the load is low (endurance and strength deficit). When the patient becomes fatigued, he/she switches to an altered pattern which results in pain. The physical therapist must identify these problems and educate the patient to avoid these movements and activities, adopt appropriate movement strategies (for permanent or temporary use depending on the ability to recover from disease process), rehabilitate their joint (mobility) and muscle (strength and length) deficits, and then retrain appropriate motor control. Depending on the injury, there will be a varying degree of recovery versus compensatory strategies. Ultimately, the patient's goal is to return to their baseline,

Table 14.4   Examples of specific tolerances and functional limitations.

Activity tolerance	Functional limitations	Participation in life
Sit tolerance	Cannot drive, work at desk, sit through movie, meeting	Avoids social events, work duties, family activities
Stand tolerance	Cannot wait in line at grocery store, socialize at parties, go to museum	Avoids social events, stops doing own shopping, has to carry equipment or use wheelchair
Walk tolerance level ground	Cannot walk to activities, attend social functions, visit friends, makes shopping and other activities difficult	Avoids social events, may not be able to work, avoids activities, becomes more isolated
Walk tolerance hills	Cannot access certain environments, cities, ramps, sports such as golf	Avoids uncertain or unusual environments
Walk tolerance stairs up/down	Cannot enter certain buildings, homes	Avoids environments, stays in home, may not be able to leave home
Sleep tolerance -Total time -Uninterrupted time -Position	Cannot obtain restorative sleep and does not heal, may cause other injuries by assuming harmful positions, decreased concentration, increased irritability	Avoids activities, becomes more depressed, avoids travel that may further affect sleep strategies

being able to perform the activities that they want without pain. It is important, however, that the compensatory strategies do not cause injury over time by increasing stress on other body segments. Frequently, to meet this need, physical therapists will teach the patient to move in a way that optimizes body mechanics and shifts forces to stronger, larger muscle groups over multiple body segments. All treatment plans will incorporate preparation for this goal by muscle strengthening and motor control training. It should be emphasized that full recovery requires communication between the physician and the physical therapist about disease processes and treatment plan. If this is not done, the patient may lose confidence, develop fear, and may not participate fully in the program.

Goals

The goals of treatment in physical therapy are ultimately to restore normal function and to prevent disease progression. Goals from the patient's perspective are to

- minimize functional limitation due to pain,
- reduce self-perceived pain frequency, intensity, duration, disability, and depression,
- increase self-perceived functional status, quality of life, and health status, and
- return to work, recreational, and home activities.

Treatment

Physical therapy treatment addresses all aspects of a patient's pain including the impairments, functional limitations, and diminished ADL life. Frequently, clinicians approach a pain problem with a surgery; however, it is often more effective to address the limitations directly while the pain is being addressed medically via pharmacologic and interventional strategies. If this fails, then at least the patient is stronger, more flexible, and better educated. The same patient will also have improved movement patterns and is otherwise better able to recover from surgical intervention. Often, physicians use a sequential algorithm for treatment. For example, they first try pain medication, followed by interventional techniques such as injections, then physical therapy, and finally surgery. Usually, the next treatment is only begun when the previous one has failed. We feel that a complimentary approach is more effective. In other words, physical therapy intervention ought to be started early and in conjunction with the other treatments. In this way, the physical therapist can capitalize on the (possibly temporary) pain reduction achieved with the intervention by implementing treatments for improving function. Typically, patients attend physical therapy one to three times per week for sessions lasting 30–60 min long. This treatment is a combination of active and passive treatments. Many physicians suggest treatment courses lasting 6–12 weeks. In many cases this is appropriate, whereas in other cases a shorter or alternately a longer course is more appropriate.

We feel that the frequency of these treatment sessions should be increased or decreased based on the patient's ability to participate, goals, motivation, and progress during treatment. The reason for this is that often patients are seen —two to three times per week but are not able to tolerate this intensity of treatment and often are not able to implement the behavioral changes that are necessary. In other cases, the treatment is limited by physiology. For example, it takes several weeks to obtain significant muscle strength changes. If a patient's movement pattern is limited by strength but he/she is able to demonstrate the ability to correctly perform a home exercise program, it may be more beneficial (and cost-effective) to see a patient once every few weeks to progress the program and check exercise technique rather than several times per week. On the other hand, seeing a patient once per month to advise on body mechanics and progress program might be the best plan in these other cases. In extremely complex cases, we have followed patients once every 3 months to progress their program and prevent relapse. Many patients report that they are more willing to *self-progress* their function and activities if they know that they have a follow-up visit scheduled. This also allows the patient to use the physical therapist as a resource rather than stalling until they have severely exacerbated symptoms. In some simple cases, few visits with a physical therapist are enough for the patient to learn the tools they need to manage their own condition (Chou and Huffman 2007, Madigan et al. 2009, Assendelft et al. 2004, Deyo and Weinstein 2001).

The following segment includes the treatment interventions that a physical therapist may use as part of their treatment program.

Patient Education

Patients must actively manage their own condition. They must understand what actions they are taking that are causing the pain and also behavioral changes they must make in order to eliminate the pain. In the case of most causes of pain, the condition may not ever resolve completely, so a patient will need to manage the symptoms in perpetuity. Education about their condition decreases the fear associated with the condition, builds confidence in their care provider, and improves compliance with the prescribed program.

Activity Modification and Dosing

Patients must complete certain harmful activities to meet their daily life responsibilities. These activities must be modified into a format that the patient can perform safely. This may mean changing how the activity is performed by using compensatory strategies or by changing the frequency or intensity of the activity. Other activities are not essential but are the patient's choice. These activities, if harmful, ought to be reduced so that the patient's relative activity is reduced to allow healing. Patient education is helpful to effect these behavior changes. If it is possible, the patient may arrange with co-workers or family members to decrease these activities temporarily. For example, a college professor presents with wrist pain. He works on the computer 8 h per day while at work. He is not in the position to reduce this time. However, the interview reveals that when he comes home, he spends an additional 6 h per night on a hobby that involves use of the computer. In this situation, if the patient can reduce his hobby time by 4 h, he will still be able to work and still obtain a relative decrease in repetitive wrist activity level.

Posture Training

Patients often assume maladaptive or non-ideal postures because of pain, prolonged work positions, weakness, and decreased flexibility or because of congenital or developmental deficits. These postures often lead to other problems, limit the ability of the patient to compensate, or perpetuate pain. As the physical therapist works on flexibility, strength, joint mobility, and pain sources, it is important to train the patient to hold themselves in more optimal positions. Good posture improves readiness to move, decreases the need to more muscle activity, and makes activities such as breathing more efficient. This can be a lengthy process and the patient may need to enlist the help of family members and also use outside reminders such as timers.

Body Mechanics Training

Patients often sleep or work in positions that cause pain, increase injury, and contribute to the development of maladaptive movement patterns and postures. Addressing posture issues is very important as the patient may not be aware of these situations and the assumed positions throughout the day. It is of particular use to assist the patient in identifying the best sleep position to protect their injured site and to improve wellness. The key is to first gain the flexibility and strength to move a certain way, then train the patient on how to move in the best pattern, and then repetitively perform the activity in a variety of contexts so that the patient will perform the correct movement automatically. If the patient can perform the movement correctly most of the time, their body will be able to tolerate the few times they perform the movement incorrectly.

Joint Mobilizations/Manipulations (Manual Physical Therapy)

At times, patients might develop movement problems secondary to an acute injury while at other times they develop joint mobility problems over time which is more of a chronic nature and is due to increased stress on a particular area, which might eventually result in an injury. Manual physical therapy in the form of joint mobilization and manipulation has been shown to be effective in providing long-lasting relief of pain and movement dysfunction. Furthermore, it improves the mobility of a joint allowing for movement re-education and/or compensatory movement patterns. The physical therapist provides joint mobilization by gliding or tractioning (separating) the joint using a variety of specialized techniques. In some cases, the decreased mobility in a non-painful area may be causing the problem in another area. For example, a patient presents with shoulder pain. It appears that the joint is being strained at the end of range for overhead movement. The therapist determines that this is the result of decreased spinal extension and performs joint mobilizations to the thoracic spine restoring normal extension. This then results in an increase of functional overhead range of motion and decreases the amount that the shoulder has to move thereby reducing the stress and allowing it to heal (Kulig et al. 2004, Cleland et al. 2007, Brosseau et al. 2008a).

Soft Tissue Mobilization (Manual Physical Therapy)

Frequently, pain results in muscle tightness and decreased mobility. In other instances, the patient may develop decreased mobility because of compensatory muscle activation or may develop this over time. As a person ages, there is a loss of tissue extensibility and resiliency. Soft tissue mobilization appears to the layperson to be a type of massage. However, unlike generalized massage that causes muscle relaxation, soft tissue mobilization is utilized in a specific location with the intent of improving mobility and improving blood flow to the region. This is often used in conjunction with joint mobilization techniques. After mobility is restored, the patient is taught how to move within the new range of motion and perform exercises to utilize and maintain the acquired mobility (Kulig et al. 2004, Cleland et al. 2007, Brosseau et al. 2008a).

Neuromuscular/Movement Re-education

Often patients move in suboptimal patterns. This might be compensatory due to pain or it is just because they have originally learned the movement incorrectly. Frequently, they lack the strength or mobility to move correctly. Movement re-education involves retraining correct movement and muscle activation by using verbal and physical cues. This is usually done in a variety of positions, speeds, and loads. Frequently this is performed after manual therapy to maintain and utilize improvements in mobility.

Gait Training

This is specific to conditions where the patient has an altered walking movement pattern. The alterations in gait may be idiopathic or may be the result of injury or surgery. The physical therapist uses verbal and physical cues to retrain walking in a manner that protects painful areas and allows optimal muscle reactivation. This is frequently performed after gaining increased mobility and/or after strength improvements.

Balance Training

Balance is the key ingredient of any safe movement. Good balance allows efficient muscle activation and allows the patient to use multiple body segments and large muscle groups. The lack of balance often results in overuse of certain muscles and injury. There is evidence that injury can lead to balance deficits. Balance training includes proprioceptive, visual, and vestibular systems.

Taping/Bracing

Taping and bracing can support deficient structures permanently or temporarily. These techniques can also decrease mobility to prevent injury and allow healing or can be utilized to teach modified movement patterns. Tape generally provides proprioceptive effect rather than structural effect. Bracing is also used temporarily after certain surgeries to prevent movement or to ease pain.

Adaptive Equipment

In many cases, a patient may not be able to perform an activity safely. Adaptive equipment can be used on a permanent or temporary basis to allow a movement, to decrease stress on an injured area, or to transfer stress to another region. Examples of equipment are reachers, canes, walkers, crutches, large handled utensils and ergonomic equipment such as modified chairs, keyboards, or other similar devices.

Therapeutic Exercise

Exercise is an important part of all physical therapy treatment. Exercise has the ability to aggravate symptoms if chosen incorrectly or dosed too high (too many repetitions) or to improve symptoms by improving mobility, motor control, or increasing strength and endurance. Exercise under the prescription of a physical therapist is different than just physical activity. The therapist has the ability to choose appropriate exercise based on the dysfunction, the patient's other medical issues, and the desired functional improvement. Generalized exercise has not been shown to be effective in all conditions. Specific exercises have been shown to have efficacy. Often, treatment may include transferring forces to proximal or distal segments. Specific strengthening is utilized to prepare target muscles for the movement re-education that is to follow. Strengthening in these non-painful areas also serves to improve general function and decrease a patient's fear of pain as the treatment does not initially focus on the painful region. Exercise serves to improve motor control and coordination, decreases stress, improves mood, and improves cardiovascular performance. Physical therapists dose exercise based on frequency, intensity (load, number of repetitions, rest time), and speed that the exercise is performed (Brosseau et al. 2008b, Kulig et al. 2009, Hayden et al. 2005, French et al. 2006).

Home Program

The home program is an integral part of long-term symptom control. This may include an exercise program consisting of stretching and strengthening movements, behavior changes to control symptoms, movements or techniques to alleviate symptoms, and strategies for setting up their environment (including use of adaptive equipment). The home program empowers the patient to control their own symptoms and is advanced over time until the patient is independent. It is important that the size of the program fits into the time that the patient is available. Otherwise, the patient will not be compliant, and the resulting failure can fuel further psychological dysfunction. We recommend using a written home program that includes diagrams or pictures so that the patient does not forget what is expected. The clinician should check the program at each visit to make sure that the patient is following it and to address any difficulty that the patient might encounter.

Modalities

Modalities have been used for symptom control for many decades. Some have better effect than others. Some of these are believed to work via the gate theory of pain control or by improving circulation to the injured body part. Often times, physical therapy treatment and consultation are confused with physical therapy modalities or physical agents such as ultrasound, ice, heat, electrical stimulation, and light therapy. Physical therapists do sometimes use these modalities as part of their treatment. However, to say that the practice of physical therapy is applying modalities is similar to saying that the practice of medicine is only prescribing pain killers and giving shots.

Some examples include

Moist Hot Packs

Hot packs are placed on the area of symptoms. The heat helps relax the patient and causes vasodilation of the surrounding blood vessels thereby increasing circulation to the region. This decreases muscle tension and can be used to increase compliance with suggestions such as lying down to decrease pain in the low back. Hot packs can also be used as a way of preparing a tissue for manual physical therapy, stretching, or exercises. The physiologic effect is only approximately 1 mm deep. The alternative could be immersion in a warm water bath which can result in a more significant effect as the core body temperature is raised (Santamato et al. 2009).

Cold Packs/Ice

Cold packs are made using ice or gel material. The packs are placed on the area of pain to transfer cold to the patient's skin. Alternatively, ice is massaged on the area of symptoms, or the limb is immersed in an ice water bath. This application of cold causes vasoconstriction of the blood vessels in the area resulting in decreased pain and inflammation. After the cold pack is removed, hyperemia is noted as blood returns to the area in order to restore normal temperature. The physiologic effect can be up to several centimeters deep depending on the technique utilized. Cold packs can be used to manage symptoms or can be utilized to control inflammation after injections, exercise, or manual physical therapy intervention (Santamato et al. 2009).

Ultrasound

Therapeutic ultrasound is a modality that involves the use of a transducer to transmit sound waves into the patient's tissue. This causes warming in the deep tissues and into the muscles. This also results in increased blood flow to the region temporarily, which may improve the healing process. The sound waves may also improve the permeability of the tissue to topical medications. Most physical therapists use this as an adjunct to treatment rather than as an independent treatment modality (Alexender et al. 2010, Leaver et al. 2010).

Transcutaneous Electrical Nerve Stimulation (TENS)

TENS is applied to selected tissues (specifically sensory nerves) using a machine that transmits electricity into the skin via electrodes. The current is adjustable in a variety of ways depending on the patient's needs. The patient feels a tingling sensation that disrupts the transmission of pain signal to the brain. The pain relief could last for several hours after application or may cease when the machine is shut off. Patients are able to use small pocket-sized battery-operated devices so that they can move about while using TENS. Based on our experience, when a good quality professional model is used, the pain relief can be dramatic.

Neuromuscular Electrical Stimulation (NMES)

Electrical stimulation uses similar electrodes to deliver a current into muscles causing them to contract. This enables the physical therapist to teach the patient how to contract specific muscles. This process can assist in improving muscle strength and overcoming muscle inhibition resulting from pain.

Other Electrical Stimulation

There are several other types of electrical current including interferential, H-wave, and microcurrent. These can be utilized to improve wound healing, increase blood flow, decrease pain, and decrease muscle spasm. They are effective in certain patient population depending on the pathology.

Laser

The use of light for the treatment of pain is many centuries old. The use of laser has the promise for the future treatment of pain and healing of damaged tissue. However, at this time, its use is considered experimental (Alexander et al. 2010, Leaver et al. 2010, Chow et al. 2009).

Summary

The treatment of a patient with pain requires a thorough subjective and objective evaluation consisting of patient interview, clinical tests, and diagnostic studies. We have presented how both physiatrists and physical therapists utilize the information obtained to develop a treatment plan resulting in functional restoration of the patients with pain. On many occasions, especially when treating chronic pain patients, an optimal outcome will be very unlikely unless a variety of resources including psychological, interventional, pharmacologic, behavioral, physical agents, and movement-based treatments are implemented under the umbrella of a multidisciplinary approach.

Case Scenario

Imrat Sohanpal, MbChB, FRCA, FFPM

Eva, a 53-year-old woman presents to your clinic with a 2-year history of persistent left arm pain. The pain was initially thought to be due to ulnar neuropathy for which she had an ulnar decompression at the elbow. The pain is classically neuropathic in description. Since the operation, the pain actually became worse and has resulted in significant loss of function. As a result, she has endured repeated interventions to help ease her suffering, none of which have been successful. Eva is known to suffer from chronic obstructive pulmonary disease, she smokes 10 cigarettes a day and drinks occasionally.

How would you assess this patient's pain?

The assessment of pain is crucial in establishing the etiology and impact it has on function, quality of life, and psychological well-being. Therefore, a biopsychosocial multidimensional assessment should be utilized, including musculoskeletal examination and assessment of baseline dysfunction.

This patient describes severe allodynia in the region of her elbow down to her hand, including the scar site from surgery over the medial epicondyle. She has hyperhidrosis of the palm and sporadic shooting electrical pains up her arm. She also complains of neck and shoulder pain on the same side where she has arm pain. Musculoskeletal assessment shows contracted flexion of the left little and ring fingers, swelling of the hand, and weakness of the long flexors. There is also wasting of the hypothenar eminence and decreased pinprick sensation over C6, C7, and C8 sensory dermatomes of the hand. There is also evidence of myofascial pain of the posterior neck and trapezius muscles.

She has been taking slow-release preparation of morphine. Unfortunately, the benefit was limited due to side effects at higher doses. In the past she has tried several anti-neuropathic agents with little effect or stopped them due to anti-cholinergic and over-sedating side effects.

Impact of pain: Eva is unable to work as a cleaner as a result of the disability. She is unable to do simple tasks such as hold a cup of tea or cook. Fear avoidance behaviors are evident. For example, she is very reluctant to the leave home for fear of her arm being bumped, potentially causing severe pain. As a result, she has become socially isolated, leading to a downward spiral in overall function and mood.

Psychological history: Recently Eva has been feeling suicidal and actually visualiszed amputating the arm to ease the pain. She blames the pain as the reason for her separation from her partner of 10 years. In the past Eva received counselling for posttraumatic stress due to an abusive husband.

What is your first impression regarding the diagnosis?
Her symptoms are suggestive of chronic regional pain syndrome following trauma to the nerve, likely a result of surgery.

What is the cause of her myofascial pain?
This is most certainly related to the compensatory mechanism implemented to reduce load and movement of the affected arm by putting extra strain on the shoulder and neck muscles.

To what types of specialists would you consider referring this patient to help manage her pain?
When treating biopsychosocial disorders, the interventions required must also have biological, psychological, and social dimensions. The psychological information adds a new dimension to the condition and alters the clinical picture significantly. Depression with suicidal urges is a potentially life-threatening condition; therefore an immediate referral to a **psychiatrist** is warranted.

Functional restoration is key to reducing disability and improving quality of life. In this case a referral to a **hand therapist** and to nerve injury unit may help achieve this. Regarding her overall pain, a **musculoskeletal physiotherapy** team may be of benefit.

Cognitive behavioral therapy is another avenue to pursue once the acute depressive phase has been dealt with, to help educate about pain behaviors and pacing.

What intervention could be done to help treat the CRPS?
Repeated stellate ganglion blocks and intravenous regional block with guanethidine or a brachial plexus block can all be tried to bring about pain relief and facilitate active exercise and rehabilitation.
Eva underwent a series of stellate ganglion blocks in conjunction with hand therapy sessions. This combination produced excellent results by reducing disability and achieving the goals set out in the treatment plan.

After successful pain reduction and eradication of the CRPS, Eva was left with ulnar neuropathy that was manageable. However, her main problem was poor mobility of the effective limb and abnormal posture secondary to her myofascial pain.

The above biomechanical issues were reconditioned in an intensive physiotherapy program as well as being entered into a pain management program. Eva was able to integrate the coping skills learnt into her everyday life after the sessions had finished. During this period she was able to stop her morphine and was treated for her depression. Depression was a major factor affecting her compliance and motivation and was preventing her from achieving a reasonable level of function and quality of life.

This case is an example of a situation where without a multidisciplinary approach, a successful outcome would have not been achieved.

References

Alexander LD, Gilman DR, Brown DR, Brown JL, Houghton PE. Exposure to low amounts of ultrasound energy does not improve soft tissue shoulder pathology: a systematic review. Phys Ther. 2010 Jan;90(1):14–25.

Assendelft WJ, Morton SC, Yu EI, Suttorp MJ, Shekelle PG. Spinal manipulative therapy for low back pain. Cochrane Database Syst Rev. 2004;1.

Brosseau L, Wells GA, Tugwell P, Egan M, Wilson KG, Dubouloz C-J, Casimiro L, Robinson VA, McGowan J, Busch A, Poitras S, Moldofsky H, Harth M, Finestone HM, Nielson W, Haines-Wangda A, Russell-Doreleyers M, Lambert K, Marshall AD, Veilleux L. Ottawa panel evidence-based clinical practice guidelines for Aerobic fitness exercises in the management of fibromyalgia: part 1. Phys Ther. 2008a;88:857–71.

Brosseau L, Wells GA, Tugwell P, Egan M, Wilson KG, Dubouloz C-J, Casimiro L, Robinson VA, McGowan J, Busch A, Poitras S, Moldofsky H, Harth M, Finestone HM, Nielson W, Haines-Wangda A, Russell-Doreleyers M, Lambert K, Marshall AD, Veilleux. Ottawa panel evidence-based clinical practice guidelines for strengthening exercises in the management of fibromyalgia: part 2; Phys Ther. 2008b;88:873–86.

Chou R, Huffman LH. Non pharmacologic therapies for acute and chronic low back pain: a review of the evidence for an American Pain Society/American College of Physicians clinical practice guideline.; American Pain Society; American College of Physicians. Ann Intern Med. 2007;147(7):492–504.

Chow RT, Johnson MI, Lopes-Martins RA, Bjordal JM. Efficacy of low-level laser therapy in the management of neck pain: a systematic review and meta-analysis of randomised placebo or active-treatment controlled trials. Lancet. 2009 Dec 5;374(9705):1897–908.

Cleland JA, Glynn P, Whitman JM, Eberhart SL, MacDonald C, Childs JD. Short-term response of thoracic spine thrust versus non-thrust manipulation in patients with mechanical neck pain: a randomized clinical trial. Phys Ther. 2007;87:431–40.

Deyo RA, et al. Low back pain. N Engl J Med. 2001;344(5):363–70.

French SD, Cameron M, Walker BF, Reggars JW, Esterman AJ. A cochrane review of superficial heat or cold for low back pain. Spine. 2006;31(9):998–1006.

Hayden JA, van Tulder MW, Malmivaara A, Koes BW. Exercise therapy for the treatment of non-specific low back pain. Cochrane Database Syst Rev. 2005;(3).

Kulig K, et al. Segmental lumbar mobility in individuals with low back pain: in vivo assessment during manual and self-imposed motion using dynamic MRI. J Orthop Sports Phys Ther. 2004;34(2):57–64.

Kulig K, Beneck GJ, Selkowitz DM, Popovich JM Jr, Ge TT, Flanagan SP, Poppert EM, Yamada KA, Powers CM, Azen S, Winstein CJ, Gordon J, Samudrala S, Chen TC, Shamie AN, Khoo LT, Spoonamore MJ, Wang JC. Physical therapy clinical research network; an intensive, progressive exercise program reduces disability and improves functional performance in patients after single-level lumbar microdiskectomy. Phys Ther. 2009;89:1145–57.

Leaver AM, Refshauge KM, Maher CG, McAuley JH. Conservative interventions provide short-term relief for non-specific neck pain: a systematic review. J Physiother. 2010;56(2):73–85.

Madigan L, Vaccaro AR, Spector LR, Milam RA. Management of symptomatic lumbar degenerative disk disease. J Am Acad Orthop Surg. 2009 Feb;17(2):102–11.

Mintzer J, Burns A. Anticholinergic side effects of drugs in elderly people. J R Soc Med. 2000;93:457–62.

O'Dell MW, Lin D, Panagos A, Fung NQ. The physiatric history and physical examination. In: Braddom RL, editor. Physical medicine & rehabilitation. 3rd ed. Philadelphia, PA: Saunders Elsevier; 2007. pp. 1–35.

Perotto AO, editor. Anatomical guide for the electromyographer: the limbs and trunk. 4th ed. Springfield, IL: Charles C Thomas; 2005.

Santamato A, Solfrizzi V, Panza F, Tondi G, Frisardi V, Leggin BG, Ranieri M, Fiore P. Short-term effects of high-intensity laser therapy versus ultrasound therapy in the treatment of people with subacromial impingement syndrome: a randomized clinical trial. Phys Ther. 2009 Jul;89(7):643–52.

Chapter 15

Occupational Therapy in Client-Centered Pain Management

Janet S. Jedlicka, PhD, OTR/L, Anne M. Haskins, PhD, OTR/L, and Jan E. Stube, PhD, OTR/L

Introduction

Occupation has been defined as, "activity in which one engages that is meaningful and central to one's identity (Hussey et al. 2008)." The role of an occupational therapist in assessing, treating, and collaborating with clients who experience pain of a psychological or physical origin has a primary focus on the client's ability to function in his/her everyday life in those activities or "occupations" that hold meaning for the client.

Regardless of etiology, the presence of acute or chronic pain has significant ramifications for a person's experience of quality of life, productivity, independence, and psychosocial well-being. It is the aim of occupational therapy to facilitate a person's return to engaging in a more fulfilling quality of life as an *occupational being* through physical and psychosocial client-centered interventions.

Treatment Settings

Occupational therapists (OT) practice in a variety of treatment settings including hospitals, outpatient centers, burn units, pain management clinics, rehabilitation centers, school systems, skilled nursing facilities, community settings, home health, and work settings. Subsequently, persons with acute or chronic pain may be referred to OT at various points in their recovery. Table 15.1 provides a summary of diagnoses associated with pain that OT commonly treat. Ideally, clients are referred to OT during early stages of acute pain or upon initial diagnosis of a chronic pain-related syndrome to provide early intervention or prevent increased dysfunction.

Occupational Therapy Evaluation and Intervention Overview

Occupational therapy evaluation and intervention is a complex procedure that begins with a physician's referral. An overview of the occupational therapy evaluation and intervention process is in the subsequent sections followed by more specific descriptions of treatment methods.

N. Vadivelu et al. (eds.), *Essentials of Pain Management,*
DOI 10.1007/978-0-387-87579-8_15, © Springer Science+Business Media, LLC 2011

Table 15.1 Common client diagnoses and examples of occupational therapy interventions.

Diagnostic category	Examples of common diagnoses	Intervention examples
Pain related to non-traumatic diagnoses	Lateral/medial epicondylitis DeQuervain's tendonitis Rotator cuff tendonitis Shoulder impingement syndrome Osteoarthritis Rheumatoid arthritis Fibromyalgia Multiple sclerosis Peripheral nerve compression	Physical agent modalities Therapeutic exercise Nerve gliding exercises Manual techniques • Trigger point release • Deep tissue massage • Transverse friction massage Functional splinting • Elbow/wrist/hand orthotics • Kinesiotaping Work/activity modification and education Body mechanics education Relaxation techniques
Pain related to traumatic injuries or post-surgical care	Upper and lower extremity fractures Joint dislocations Tendon lacerations Crush injuries Injection injuries Reflex sympathetic dystrophy Amputations Peripheral nerve lacerations Rotator cuff tear	Wound care/scar management/ stump shaping Edema management Manual techniques Physical agent modalities Splinting Therapeutic exercise Sensory re-education/desensitization Client education/relaxation techniques Functional activity

Physician Referrals

Occupational therapy is not a stand-alone service in most states, and treatment provision that will be submitted to third-party payers can be initiated only with a referral from a physician. A physician's referral is always required with patients who have Medicare coverage (The American Occupational Therapy Association 2008a). Physicians may choose to provide a referral with detailed instructions or provide a less detailed referral to allow for a more dynamic and adjustable treatment planning (Groth 2008) (Fig. 15.1). Referrals for clients must be updated every 30 days or when there is a significant change in a client's status.

The relationship between a physician and an occupational therapist is a critical aspect of promoting client recovery, and open communication is an important component of that relationship. Physicians and occupational therapists should seek to build professional, collaborative relationships conducive to a client's recovery (Groth 2008).

Occupational Therapy Evaluation Considerations

Following a physician referral, an occupational therapist will evaluate first the client's ability to perform in a variety of areas. These *areas of occupation* include *activities of daily living* (ADLS) (such as dressing, bathing, sexual activity), *instrumental activities of daily living* (IADLS) (such as caring for others, health management, meal preparation), *sleep and rest, education, work, leisure, play,* and *social participation* (The American Occupational Therapy Association 2008b). As the occupational therapist assesses the client's functional

Physician Referral for Occupational Therapy

Department of Occupational Therapy

Physician Referral for Treatment

Client Name: _____

Diagnosis: _____

Date of Injury/Date of Surgery: _____

Precautions: _____

> If you prefer the therapist to exercise greater clinical reasoning in treating your client, you may select only 'Evaluate & Treat'. The therapist will then choose the intervention options most suitable for the client.

❐ Evaluate & Treat	❐ Evaluation Only	❐ Continue OT Treatment

Prescribed Treatment

❐ Therapeutic Activity	❐ Work Simplification	❐ Job Analysis
❐ Therapeutic Exercise	❐ Ergonomic Evaluation	❐ Relaxation Education
❐ Neuromuscular Re-education	❐ Functional Capacity Evaluation	❐ Deep Tissue Massage
❐ AROM	❐ Work Conditioning	❐ Stress Management/
❐ AAROM	❐ Myofascial Release	Coping
❐ PROM	❐ Home Safety Evaluation	❐ Energy Conservation
❐ Wound/Scar Management		❐ Joint Protection
		Education

Splinting

❐ Physical Agent Modalities PRN

❐ Resting Hand Splint	❐ Physical Agent Modalities as Directed
❐ Wrist Cock-Up Splint	
❐ Thumb Spica Splint	❐ Ultrasound
❐ CMC Splint	❐ Fluidotherapy
❐ Long Arm Splint	❐ Light Therapy
❐ Zipper Splint	❐ Transcutaneous Electrical Stimulation
❐ Elbow Splint	❐ Thermotherapy
❐ Finger Splint	❐ Iontophoresis w/ Dexamethasone
	❐ Neuromuscular Electrical
Other: _____	Stimulation
	❐ Laser Therapy
	❐ Phonophoresis
	❐ Cryotherapy

> If you choose an intervention that includes a medication, also include a prescription for that medication.

Additional Instructions:_____

_____

_____   _____

Physician Signature   Date

Figure 15.1 Physician referral for occupational therapy.

ability, he/she further evaluates a multitude of factors including the client's *neuromuscu-loskeletal, movement, sensory–perceptual, emotional regulation, communication and social, pain, cognitive, cardiovascular, respiratory, skin,* and *related structures function* using objective and subjective assessments (The American Occupational Therapy Association 2008b). Table 15.2 provides a summary of assessment tools commonly used by occupational therapists. Throughout the assessment process, the occupational therapist seeks to understand the client's values, beliefs, culture, home and work environment, roles, habits, and routines to

Table 15.2 Examples of standardized and non-standardized assessments of pain and function used in occupational therapy.

Assessment category	Assessment tool	Purpose
ADL and IADL	• Barthel Index of ADL[a] • Canadian Occupational Performance Measure[b] • Disability of the Arm, Shoulder, and Hand (DASH)[c] • Functional Independence Measure[d,e] • Occupational Profile[f]	Measure clients' functional abilities; a number assessments also include pain assessment subtests; occupational profile provides a summary of the clients occupational history
Pain	• Numeric or visual analogue scales • McGill Pain Questionnaire[g] • Pain Drawing Instrument[h] • Pain Patient Profile (P-3®)[i]	Describe the uni- or multidimensional subjective and emotional experience of pain and provides a description of the quality and intensity of pain; also provides localization of pain experience
Ergonomic, work and/or functional capacity evaluations	• Ergo Science Physical Work Performance Evaluation (PWPE)[j] • Isernhagen Work Systems Functional Capacity Evaluation[k,l] • Joule 3.0 FCE System by Valpar[m]	Provide work performance and ergonomic assessments of the clients' work, home, and/or leisure environments to ascertain areas of needed modification for symptom reduction and/or prevention
Coping/psychosocial areas	• Stress Profile[n] • Perceived Stress Questionnaire[o] • Rhode Island Stress and Coping Inventory (RISCI)[p]	Assess clients' coping behaviors as related to stress management and coping

[a]Collin and Wade (1988), [b]Carswell et al. (2004), [c]Hudak et al. (1996), [d]Hamilton et al. (1987), [e]Gosman-Hedstrom and Svensson (2000), [f]The American Occupational Therapy Association (2008), [g]Melzack (1975), [h]Margolis et al. (1986), [i]Pearson Education, Inc. (2009), [j]Lechner et al. (1994), [k]Isernhagen et al. (1999), [l]Reneman et al. (2004), [m]Valpar International Corporation (2009), [n]Nowack (2009), [o]Fliege et al. (2005), [p]Fava et al. (1998).

design a client-centered treatment plan (The American Occupational Therapy Association 2008b).

Occupational Therapy Interventions

Occupational therapy treatment interventions may be classified into three broad categories: *preparatory methods, purposeful activity,* and *occupation-based interventions* (The American Occupational Therapy Association 2008b) (Table 15.3). Preparatory methods include interventions intended to prepare the client for engaging in activity and may include splinting, edema management, physical agent modality application, and therapeutic exercise (The American Occupational Therapy Association 2008b). Purposeful activity includes interventions designed to remediate specific mental or physical skills to allow the client to engage in his/her occupation (The American Occupational Therapy Association 2008b). For example, a client may have a goal of independently caring for his grandchildren with controlled pain. To reach this goal, the client may engage in specific education, cooking, or dressing activities designed to increase range of motion and strength; provide an opportunity for feedback regarding pacing or ergonomics; and provide a platform for client–therapist discussion focused on educating and empowering the client as an agent of change. Occupation-based interventions are treatment methods that include the client's participation in occupations that he/she finds meaningful, preferably in the environment in which the client would normally

Table 15.3 Common occupational therapy intervention strategies addressing physical, psychosocial, and environmental aspects of pain.

	Preparatory techniques	Purposeful activity	Occupation-based activity
Physical management	Physical agent modalities Therapeutic exercise Joint mobilization Nerve gliding exercises Wound care Trigger point release	Functional activities designed to address the client's physical dysfunction. For example, client may wipe off a table to address shoulder range of motion Work conditioning includes work-simulated tasks	Occupations such as gardening may address balance, proprioception, range of motion, strength but are intended to accomplish a client-centered goal (i.e., the client needs to wash laundry at home) Perform work hardening in the client's actual environment
Psychosocial management	Ideally, psychosocial management techniques (cognitive behavioral interventions, assertiveness training, relaxation, guided imagery, yoga, tai chi, etc.) should be used in all activity categories. As the activities progress from preparatory to occupation-based activity, the occupational therapist must encourage the client to integrate those interventions into his/her lifestyle to establish a habit or routine		
Environmental/contextual adaptations	Ergonomic modification Work simplification education Energy conservation education Adaptive technology education	Work simplification principle application in a simulated work environment	Work simplification principle application in a client's actual work environment

complete the occupation (The American Occupational Therapy Association 2008b). For instance, a client with chronic pain who engages in work conditioning tasks at his/her place of employment with an occupational therapist would be engaging in an occupation-based intervention (Fig. 15.2). The intervention occurs not only as the client is completing tasks required for his/her position but also as the therapist provides feedback and direction, analyzes the client's posture, implements workstation modifications, and provides educational experiences. During the process of occupational therapy pain management intervention, the client's occupational performance is a central focus.

Acute and Chronic Pain Management with a Focus on Occupation

Occupational therapy treatment of clients with pain is dependent on the client's personal experience, occupational background and functional status, diagnosis, symptoms, and duration of pain. Broadly, an occupational therapist seeks to understand the client's pain experience from its onset. Typically, acute pain can occur instantaneously and its duration can be from momentary to days, while chronic pain duration is much longer (Bracciano 2008). Acute pain is associated with inflammation, damage to surrounding tissue, and normal injury or disease process while chronic pain persists beyond usual healing time and can become a separate diagnosis (Bracciano 2008, National Institute of Neurological Disorders

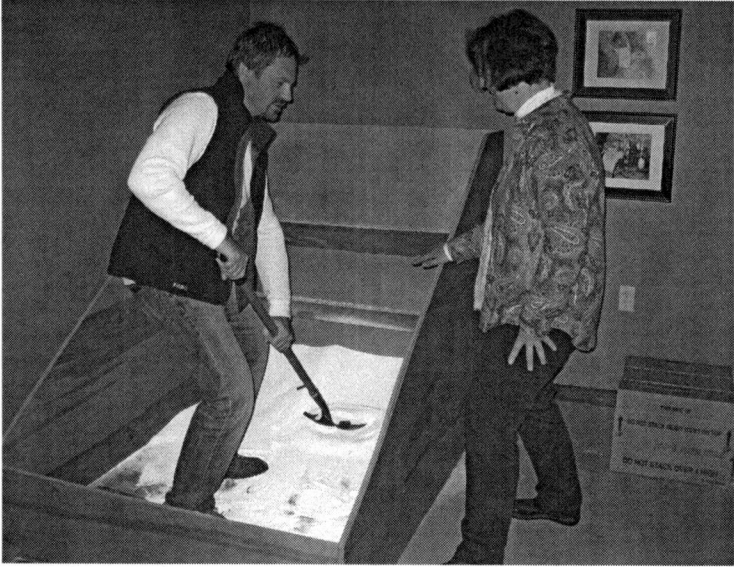

Figure 15.2   Work simulation task during occupational therapy session.

and Stroke 2009, Rochman and Kennedy-Spaien 2007). Occupational therapists differentiate pain further into the categories of persistent, abnormal, and referred pain (Fedorczyk
and Barbe 2002). The determination of the duration of the client's experience of pain has
significant ramifications for treatment planning.

Management of Acute Pain

The foci of occupational therapy treatment of persons experiencing acute pain include symptoms reduction, facilitation of a healthy inflammatory process, and short-term adaptation
of occupational functioning. While occupational therapists may seek to educate clients on
adaptive techniques to complete functional tasks to maximize independence during the acute
stage of their injury or disease process, the primary objective of treatment is on clients' healing
process to achieve independence.

Management of Chronic Pain

Persons who experience chronic pain have reported the "life changing" (Fisher et al. 2007)
characteristic of its presence and changes in their relationships (Fisher et al. 2007), quality
of life (Fisher et al. 2007, Neville-Jan 2003), ability to function (Fisher et al. 2007, Neville-
Jan 2003), and psychological well-being (Fisher et al. 2007, Neville-Jan 2003). Within the
context of chronic pain, occupational therapy offers treatment interventions intended to
facilitate clients' adaptation to pain and enhancement in functional engagement, physically
and psychologically. To address this, many occupational therapists implement a biopsychosocial foundation that also includes "behavioral, cognitive–affective, and environmental
factors (Bracciano 2008)." Due to the holistic nature of treatment, occupational therapy is an
important partner on the multidisciplinary pain management team.

Occupational therapy intervention approaches the individual client from a holistic perspective, focusing on the overall functioning and adaptability of the client to be able to manage those daily tasks and occupations that they find valuable and meaningful. Following a comprehensive evaluation, occupational therapy works with the client to identify areas of difficulty and the occupations and routines that are the most meaningful to the client. Based on the findings of the evaluation and the collaboration process, a comprehensive intervention plan is developed. Occupational therapy interventions focus on providing the client with the resources and skills to be able to effectively manage his/her pain and engage in the activities/occupations that are meaningful and productive. Research supports using a multidisciplinary approach and the biopsychosocial model in pain management (Guzman et al. 2007, Turk 2002). Supporting the biopsychosocial model, occupational therapy interventions can be grouped into areas that impact an individual's ability to successfully engage; these include physical management, psychosocial management, and environment/contextual adaptations (Table 15.3).

Physical Management of Pain

Approaches for the physical management of pain include client education and training in methods to protect joints, prevention of pain and inflammation, work simplification, proper body mechanics, therapeutic exercise, work hardening programs, and physical agent modalities. The goal is to control pain and educate the client on strategies that can be used to more effectively manage the pain and allow engagement in enjoyable and meaningful occupations. Joint protection, work simplification, proper body mechanics, and positioning are used in both acute and chronic pain management intervention programs. The intent is to provide education and resources to minimize pain levels and prevent further complication or exacerbation of symptoms.

Joint protection principles include respecting pain by not overdoing activity, maintenance of range of motion and muscle strength, stabilization of joints to reduce the force and effort required to complete an activity, and use of correct patterns of movement (Deshaies 2006). In addition, individuals are encouraged to use the strongest joints available. For example, carrying a purse on the shoulder rather than on the wrist, using a rolling cart to transport home or work items, using the palm of the hand to open jars (Yasuda 2008).

Work simplification and energy conservation strategies focus on promoting independence and safety and preventing additional stress or trauma to the individual while engaging in purposeful activity/occupations. Key principles include using both hands to complete a task whenever possible, working within normal reach (not over extending or reaching), gathering supplies needed for the task prior to beginning, sliding heavy objects rather than carrying, and using gravity to decrease energy expenditure. Work simplification also addresses the storage and organization of work spaces, placing commonly used items in a place where they are easy to reach and use, sitting whenever possible, and determining the appropriate height of the work surface for the individual and the actual tasks being performed (Grangaard 2006, Sabata et al. 2008).

Proper body mechanics principles include maintaining a straight back, maintaining a good posture bending from the hip, avoiding positions in which twisting might be required to lift and hold objects, carrying objects close to the body, and lifting with one's legs using a wide base of support (Grangaard 2006). The goal is to reduce back stress and prevent any additional trauma that might result in increased pain levels. In addition to body mechanics, occupational therapists also work with clients in the area of proper positioning for activities of daily living including intimacy and sexual activity.

Therapeutic exercise and neuromuscular interventions are other important occupational therapy interventions for persons experiencing acute or chronic pain. Reasons for these interventions include reduction of edema and prevention of joint stiffness, restoration or maintenance of joint motion and muscle strength, effective muscle use patterns, as well as improvement in task participation without discomfort (Rochman and Kennedy-Spaien 2007, Fedorczyk and Barbe 2002, Hand Rehabilitation Center of Indiana 2001). Common techniques taught to clients include gentle stretch and individualized strengthening programs involving combinations of passive, active-assisted, to active or resistive exercises. Gentle stretch programs often involve client education to perform self-stretches. Clients who exhibit low neurogenetic pain irritability can participate in "nerve gliding" or gentle neural tension exercises as a method of pain modulation (Fedorczyk and Barbe 2002). Joint weight-bearing exercise, often referred to as "stress loading," facilitates graded sensory stimuli to the extremity and is recommended for such painful conditions as complex regional pain syndrome (Li et al. 2005, Walsh and Muntzer 2002). Although therapeutic exercise is a recommended intervention, occupational therapists help clients learn a healthy balance of active participation with stress-free, pain-limited motion.

Work hardening and work conditioning are interventions often implemented with injured workers who are preparing to return to work. While often used interchangeably, there are significant differences. Work hardening is interdisciplinary and composed of a combination of job tasks the client would perform within his/her job capacity with consideration for strength, endurance, pacing, range of motion, and differential movements specific to the client's job (Keegan and Kahlert 2006, King and Olson 2009). Ideally, a job analysis (during which the occupational therapist evaluates physical, mental, and psychological demands of the job) would be completed prior to the development of the client's work conditioning treatment plan. This would allow the occupational therapist to tailor the work hardening treatment plan to the client's work-related needs. Additionally, work hardening is unique as it includes intervention targeting the client's psychosocial factors such as self-esteem, confidence, and anxiety related to his/her job performance (King and Olson 2009); a critical component as psychological adjustment has been found vital to successfully returning injured workers to employment (Adams and de C Williams 2003). Conversely, work conditioning is less intensive than work hardening, involves fewer disciplines, and has a primary focus on physical functioning (King and Olson 2009). Additionally, injured employees may benefit from the inclusion of self-directed, occupational therapist-facilitated wellness program in which the client engages outside of the occupational therapy clinic. Occupational therapists are qualified to develop wellness programs to promote health and prevent disease with consideration for the individual client's lifestyle, exercise regimen, nutrition, and psychosocial and mental well-being (Jaegers 2008).

Manual techniques are preparatory occupational therapy interventions and useful measures in controlling acute and chronic pain. These techniques include passive range of motion, joint mobilization, myofascial release, deep tissue massage including trigger point release, and manual edema mobilization. Passive range of motion may be used to elongate tissues. Joint mobilization is used to enhance the integrity of the joint capsule and to control pain (Lundon 2007). Myofascial release may be implemented to decrease the tension of the body's soft tissue structures and inhibit active trigger points that may be limiting range of motion and causing pain (Dávila 2002). Deep tissue massage, including trigger point release, is used to inhibit the presence of point tenderness and taut muscular bands that often cause referred and myofascial pain (Kasch 2002, Simons et al. 1999). Manual edema mobilization is used to stimulate the lymphatic system and facilitate drainage of localized and generalized edema to promote tissue health and reduce pain (Priganc 2008). There are multitudes of additional manual techniques that may be employed to reduce a client's pain. Each should be applied in conjunction with other therapeutic interventions.

Physical agent modalities (PAMS) are composed of the application of light, water, temperature, sound, and/or electricity to produce a soft tissue response (Bracciano 2008). In occupational therapy, these are most commonly used as a precursor to working with the client in purposeful or occupation-based interventions (McPhee et al. 2003) or following a client's occupational therapy session as means of controlling for a resultant inflammatory response. Common PAMS include cryotherapy such as ice massage and cold packs, thermotherapy such as hot packs, fluidotherapy and paraffin wax, thermal or non-thermal ultrasound, electrical stimulation, iontophoresis, infrared, neuromuscular stimulation (NMES), and transcutaneous electrical nerve stimulation (TENS). An occupational therapist's selection of PAMS is dependent on the acute or chronic nature of the client's pain. Often, therapists will employ a combination of PAMS. For example, a client who is 2-month status post a distal radius open reduction internal fixation surgery may benefit from thermotherapy to increase muscular extensibility prior to occupational therapy activity and cryotherapy following therapy to control any minor edema incurred during treatment. PAMS are not intended to be the sole treatment modality and should always be applied in conjunction with other methods of therapeutic intervention (Bracciano 2008). In occupational therapy, PAMS are used to prepare the client's tissue for movement and/or provide the individual with relief of pain prior to or following the client's engagement in functional activity or occupations. Primary objectives of PAMS implementation are to provide the client with limited pain, enhance the client's willingness to engage in movement and activity, and, ultimately, decrease the fear avoidance response when the client is able to engage in activity without increasing the pain. When appropriate, and depending on the nature of the PAM, clients may be educated in self-application of PAMS to implement as preventative or post-activity pain control method (Fig. 15.3). This is applicable particularly with clients who have chronic pain conditions as a measure to build responsibility for symptom management (Rochman and Kennedy-Spaien 2007, Moscony 2002).

Splinting and bracing may be needed to provide pain relief for the client. Occupational therapists may fabricate customized dynamic or static splints for clients, or they may fit clients with prefabricated splints. The purposes of splints are to provide rest, maintain joint alignment, and support the client's anatomy in functional positions. The goals are to increase function, prevent or correct deformities, protect healing structures, and restrict painful or harmful motion (Fess 2005). Splints are provided commonly to treat acute pain, but they may also be used to provide support and proper alignment with individuals experiencing chronic pain.

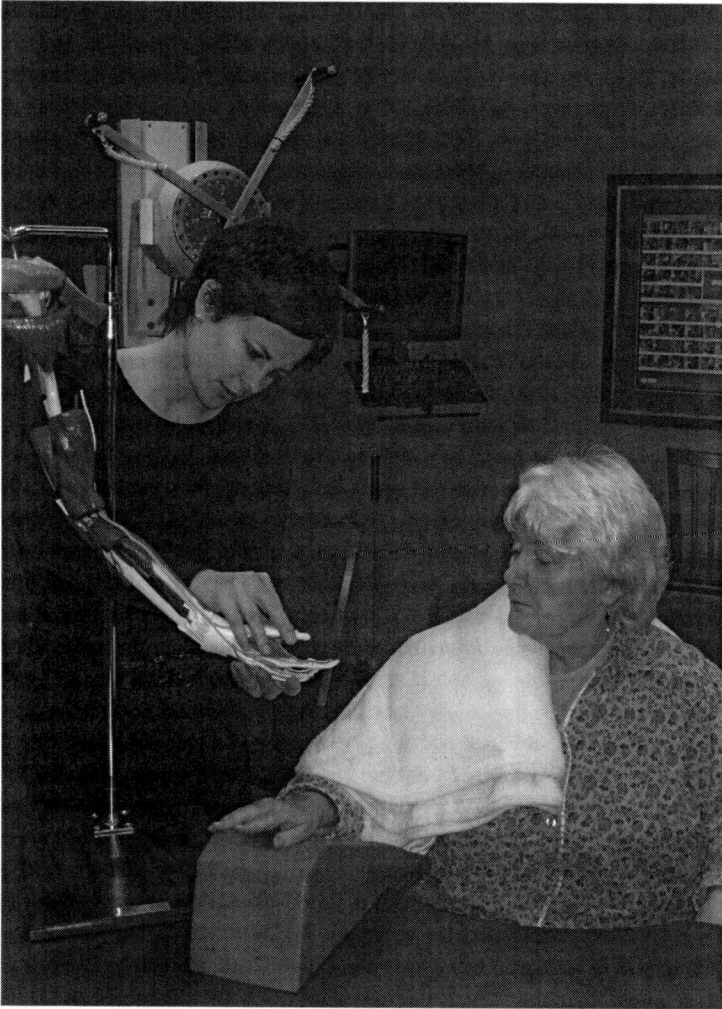

Figure 15.3. Client education during thermotherapy intervention.

Another approach commonly used by occupational therapists in the treatment of clients with pain is kinesiotaping. Kinesiotaping can be used to control inflammation through the enhancement of lymphatic drainage (DeBono 2007) to reduce pressure on pain receptions. It is also used as an external support as it provides proprioceptive feedback to clients, a quality that can assist clients in remediating dysfunctional movements (DeBono 2007, Kase 2000).

Occupational therapy plays an important role in the provision of physical pain management intervention. In addition, essential to a client's return to function is the area of psychosocial management.

Psychosocial Management of Pain

There is a strong psychological overlay to pain. Pain experiences have the potential to limit an individual's engagement in functional activities and social interaction. This affects the meaning and quality of life and needs to be addressed systematically in providing intervention. Pain can have a significant impact on the client's engagement of activities and involvement in social participation and resuming productive roles. Strategies used to manage the acute phase of pain become detrimental in managing chronic pain. These include guarding the body part, decreased activity, and rest. Cognitive behavioral approaches have been found to be effective in helping individuals become aware of the connections between thoughts, feelings, and behaviors and how these three combine to influence the effective management of pain (Kavanagh 1995, Strong 1998, Wiskin 1998). Occupational therapists are concerned with helping clients become active participants in their care and promoting increased self-efficacy and learning new coping strategies. Coping strategies include goal setting, activity pacing, time management strategies, stress management, relaxation training, and assertiveness training.

The process of goal setting and attainment can be an outcome measure of the multidisciplinary treatment team (Fisher and Hardie 2002). It can also be a way to develop realistic client expectations and engage clients in more effectively managing their pain and engaging in activities (Rochman and Kennedy-Spaien 2007).

Activity pacing is defined as the process of breaking down activities/tasks into smaller more manageable time frames while incorporating regular periods of rest (Gatchel and Turk 1996). It involves the processes of slowing down, changing positions according to time, delegating tasks, incorporating frequent rest periods, increasing activity levels, prioritizing activity, and planning ahead (Birkholtz et al. 2004).

Pain affects how individuals use time and engage in productive activities. Occupational therapists use activity configurations to provide a visual display of how an individual is currently spending time throughout the day and then to begin to identify changes the client would like to make in his/her routines. The focus is on developing strategies to prioritize tasks, developing reasonable to-do lists, balancing the activity demands of the week rather than the day, and building in rest time.

Many individuals experiencing pain also experience high levels of stress. This can be associated with decreased engagement in valuable occupations, managing multiple medical demands and regimes. With a comprehensive stress management program, the first step is to work with the individual to identify current stressors and the impact they are making on the daily routine. The occupational therapist can then work with the client to address his/her perceived level of stress and develop strategies to more effectively handle situations that are within his/her control. Areas to consider include socially connecting with others, participating in support groups, planning regular exercise, eating balanced nutritious meals, and addressing the spirituality needs of the clients as indicated (Roth and McCune 2005).

Relaxation training includes diaphragmatic breathing, guided imagery, progressive muscle relaxation, and biofeedback. Diaphragmatic breathing is described as one of the most basic relaxation techniques; it involves the process of deep breathing using the diaphragm or lower stomach muscles to increase an individual's state of relaxation (Seaward 2006). Guided imagery includes the use of the imagination and pleasant visual descriptions, such as lying on a warm sunny beach with the wind gently blowing across your body to promote relaxation and provide a setting where additional techniques can be learned (Seaward 2006, Cole 2005). Progressive muscle relaxation uses tensing and then relaxing muscle groups throughout the body; it is done in a systematic manner to decrease muscle tension that may be associated with pain symptoms (Seaward 2006, Stein and Cutler 1998). Biofeedback focuses on the monitoring of physiological body functions including measuring pulse, heart, and respiration rates as well as body temperatures (Cole 2005, Stein and Cutler 1998). The purposes of these aforementioned interventions are to help clients increase awareness of muscle tension, anxiety, and stress associated with the physiological response to pain. The ultimate goals would be to provide tools to self-manage more effectively the symptoms associated with pain and increase the client's functional ability and engagement in meaningful occupations.

Occupational therapists work with clients to address their confidence and assertiveness. An assertive individual is able to express directly his/her feelings, wants, and needs. This individual is able to set limits and balance his/her stress levels by saying no. This is an important skill in managing both acute and chronic pain. Assertiveness training allows the individual to appropriately ask for assistance, say no to requests that would be over tiring or increase pain levels, and to communicate directly how he/she is feeling to loved ones and health-care providers.

Tai chi and yoga are two non-pharmacologic interventions for total body activity endurance and pain management accompanying a variety of medical conditions. Both interventions have been shown to provide short-term benefits and/or stress reduction for chronic pain management in older adults who have osteoarthritis or rheumatoid arthritis (Reid et al. 2008, Yocum et al. 2000). Studies of tai chi among the elderly resulted in improved lower extremity muscular strength and endurance (Lan et al. 2000). For adults with chronic low back pain, superior benefits of a yoga group in comparison to exercise alone were reported in a randomized controlled trial (RCT) (Sherman et al. 2005). Authors of a systematic review found "fair evidence" for the use of yoga for chronic low back pain (Chou and Huffman 2007). For persons with carpal tunnel syndrome, a Cochrane Intervention Review reported short-term benefits from participation in yoga (O'Connor et al. 2003); additionally, one RCT reported a significant improvement in grip strength and pain reduction (Garfinkel et al. 1998). Yet other studies indicated limited or conflicting evidence to support yoga for pain management of carpal tunnel syndrome (Gerritsen et al. 2002, Goodyear Smith and Arroll 2004, Piazzini et al. 2007). To date, the evidence supporting the use of yoga over tai chi is more promising for pain management; yet both can be considered as low-risk interventions with beneficial effects (Bauer 2007).

Psychosocial management of pain encompasses education and training for the development of more effective coping skills. In providing holistic care, occupational therapists also need to consider the environmental/contextual adaptations for pain management.

Environment/Contextual Adaptations for Management of Pain

Occupational therapists not only have the skills to effectively analyze activities but also evaluate environments and contexts to support engagement in occupations. Occupational therapists recognize that occupation takes place in a physical and social environment within a larger context of personal, temporal, and cultural expectations (The American Occupational Therapy Association 2009). Analyzing the environment provides opportunities to make simple changes such as placing commonly used items on the countertop to avoid painful reaches, adjusting the height of a computer workstation for upper extremity/neck/back comfort, or encouraging social activity choices such as smoke-free environments that enhance rather than discourage a healthy lifestyle. Contextual adaptations include such recommendations as balancing activity or exercise with rest throughout the day to promote endurance and limit painful participation, limiting face-to-face meeting or travel in lieu of phone or e-mail interaction, or using assertive social communication to avoid painful greetings via handshake. Often, the client's use of cognitive behavioral strategies and assertive communication are paramount to promoting a better quality of life. At other times the environment can be changed to promote a more comfortable and effective routine. For some clients, more specialized environmental adaptation approaches can be found through the process of home evaluations, ergonomic evaluations, and worksite job analyses conducted by occupational therapists. These consultative activities allow individuals with family members and/or employers to find the best work routines, schedules, or practices to allow the client to return to productive activity. In the case of home modification, installation of grab bars within the bathroom facilitates safety and prevents painful jarring of joints or muscles; lever-style door handles prevent increased external force on painful joints or smaller muscles of the wrist and hand. Other personal adaptive devices may be recommended, such as dressing aids, particularly during the acute pain management phase.

The client is educated by occupational therapists to use personal strategies to facilitate his/her own comfort and participation in social, home, and/or work lives. In addition, occupational therapists can be instrumental in adapting the environment and contexts to promote engagement in activities valued by each individual.

Summary

Occupational therapy is an integral member of a multidisciplinary team of health-care practitioners who provide evaluation and intervention for clients learning to manage symptoms of pain. The effectiveness of occupational therapy has been documented in number of studies including those involving clients with reflex sympathetic dystrophy (Oerlemans et al. 2000) and complex regional pain syndrome (Singh et al. 2004). Similarly, clients with diagnoses of fibromyalgia, whiplash disorders, low back pain disorders, myalgia, and chronic pain disorders have demonstrated improvements in occupational performance and satisfaction with their functional ability following occupational therapy as part of inter-professional pain management treatment (Persson et al. 2004, Stark Schier and Chan 2007).

Unique aspects of occupational therapy in the realm of pain management include such services as evaluating each client as an individual with a unique set of symptoms, reactions, and circumstances affecting his/her occupational performance. Occupational therapists focus on providing a variety of interventions such as physical management of pain, psychological coping techniques, ways to adapt environments, and consultation with others (such as employers) for necessary modifications. Each entry-level occupational therapy practitioner will possess the necessary background knowledge and skills to evaluate and provide intervention for clients who are experiencing acute or chronic pain conditions. Ultimately occupational therapists strive to promote full participation in valued occupations, thereby enhancing each client's quality of life.

Case Scenario

Janet S. Jedlicka, PhD, OTR/L, Anne M. Haskins, PhD, OTR/L and Jan E. Stube, PhD, OTR/L

Ryan, a 25-year-old construction worker, fell from a 2-story scaffolding structure onto the construction site. He suffered a left upper extremity brachial plexus injury with left shoulder dislocation and a tibia–fibula fracture of the left lower extremity. He was medically stabilized and had reasonable control of his pain with IV ketorolac. Now he is concerned that he might not regain the full functions of his limbs and runs the risk of losing his livelihood.

How could you help Ryan?
Early intervention and liaison between the treating physician and the occupational therapist can help in restoration of functional ability of the patient and also play a significant role in controlling pain.
During an initial evaluation, on day 3, conducted by the occupational therapist (OT), a medical record review and an occupational profile interview established that the client had been previously healthy and living independently. He is single, living with two male roommates, and interests include frequenting nightclubs, skiing, and all terrain vehicle racing. His physical and cognitive/psychosocial skills by OT evaluation concludes the following. Ryan's left upper extremity (UE) has minimal passive range of motion (PROM) at the shoulder, all planes, with pain self-rated at 8 on a scale of 0–10. Distally, Ryan has full active range of motion (AROM) and functional strength from the elbow distally, including the hand. He has some mild loss of tactile pain discrimination and touch awareness sensation at the left shoulder region only; otherwise, he has intact sensation of his left UE. He self-limits use of his left UE presently due to pain and expresses frustration that he "can't do anything" using only one hand. He wears a shoulder stabilization soft brace, which limits passive and active motion at the shoulder only. The OT notes that Ryan is visually sensitive to sunlight in his hospital room and loses his concentration easily. The OT plans and discusses intervention with Ryan, then documents the findings and agreed-upon goals.

Enumerate the possible occupational therapy interventions?
OT interventions fall broadly into three major types: physical management, psychosocial management, and environment/contextual adaptations. All these can be used in the case of Ryan. After OT consultation with the attending orthopedic surgeon's physician assistant, safe parameters have been set regarding OT intervention (1) for left UE range of motion, actively and passively, to within pain tolerance and (2) to promote use of the UE in activity, as client tolerates. The soft shoulder brace may be removed for bathing and left UE activity.
By day 5, the occupational therapist has been seeing Ryan once daily for UE passive to active-assisted exercise, teaching Ryan to perform specified exercises on his own once to twice daily. Breathing techniques, visual imagery, and goal-focused strategies have been used to assist Ryan in making gains in motion at his left shoulder. Ryan's occupational

therapy has also included transfers to his bedside chair. In sitting, Ryan has been engaged in practice and problem-solving OT sessions to promote use of his left arm and hand as an "assist" for two-handed activities of daily living (ADLs) such as cutting meat, spreading jam on toast, holding paper as he writes, fastening his clothing. Further, Ryan has been encouraged by practice with his OT to assertively ask for controlling the lighting in his room, to request rest breaks, and to communicate his other needs to his health-care providers, family members, and friends.

By day 7, Ryan has been prepared by his occupational therapist, other health-care professionals, and discharge-planning professional for return to his family's home. From an OT perspective, Ryan will require minimal assistance for bathing at home (provided by his family), will be independent with adaptive strategies for dressing, and will require maximal assistance for heavy home management tasks over the next month. Driving and return-to-sedentary work have been postponed for 4 weeks. Outpatient occupational therapy has been ordered by the orthopedic surgeon for fortnightly sessions over the upcoming month for continuation of left UE ROM and strength improvements, increasing ADL independence, and evaluation for safe return to driving and work.

References

Adams JH, de C Williams AC. What affects return to work for graduates of a pain management program with chronic upper limb pain? J Occup Rehabil. 2003;13:91–106.

Bauer B, ed. Mayo clinic guide to alternative medicine. New York, NY: Time Incorporated; 2007.

Birkholtz M, Aylwin L, Harman RM. Activity pacing in chronic pain management: one aim, but which method? Part one: introduction and literature review. Br J Occup Ther. 2004;67:447–452.

Bracciano AG. Physical agent modalities – theory and application for the occupational therapist. 2nd ed. Thorofare, NJ: Slack, Incorporated; 2008.

Carswell A, McColl MA, Baptiste S, Law, M, Polatajko H, Pollock N. The Canadian occupational performance measure: a research and clinical review. Can J Occup Ther. 2004;71:210–222.

Chou R, Huffman LH. Nonpharmacologic therapies for acute and chronic low back pain: a review of the evidence for an American Pain Society/American College of Physicians clinical practice guideline. Ann of Int Med. 2007;147:492–504.

Cole MB. Group dynamics in occupational therapy: the theoretical basis and practice application of group intervention. 3rd ed. Thorofare, NJ: Slack, Incorporated; 2005.

Collin C, Wade DT. The Barthel ADL Index: a reliability study. Intl Disabil Stud. 1988;10: 64–67.

Dávila SA. Therapist's management of fractures and dislocations of the elbow. In: Mackin EJ, Callahan AD, Skirven TM, Schneider, LH, Osterman AL, Hunter JM, editors. Rehabilitation of the hand and upper extremity. 5th ed. St. Louis, MO: Mosby, Incorporated; 2002. pp. 1230–1244.

DeBono V. Integration of taping techniques with myofascial therapy. In: Hammer WI, editor. Functional soft-tissue examination and treatment by manual methods. Sudbury, MA: Jones and Barlett Publishers; 2007. pp. 675–688.

Deshaies L. Arthritis. In: Pendleton HM, Schultz-Krohn W, editors. Pedretti's occupational therapy: practice skills for physical dysfunction. St. Louis, MO: Mosby Elsevier; 2006. pp. 950–82.

Fava J, Ruggiero L, Grimely D. The development and structural confirmation of the Rhode Island stress and coping inventory. J Behav Med. 1998;21:601–11.

Fedorczyk JM, Barbe MF. Pain management: principles of therapists' intervention. In: Mackin EJ, Callahan AD, Skirven TM, Schneider, LH, Osterman AL, Hunter JM, editors. Rehabilitation of the hand and upper extremity. 5th ed. St. Louis, MO: Mosby, Incorporated; 2002. pp. 1725–41.

Fess EE. A history of splinting. In: Fess EE, Gettle KS, Philips CA, Janson JR, editors. Hand and upper extremity splinting: principles & methods. 3rd ed. St. Louis, MO: Mosby Elsevier; 2005. pp. 3–43.

Fisher GS, Emerson L, Firpo C, Ptak J, Wonn J, Bartolacci G. Chronic pain and occupation: an exploration of the lived experience. Am J Occup Ther. 2007;61:290–302.

Fisher K, Hardie RJ. Goal attainment scaling in evaluating a multidisciplinary pain management programme. Clin Rehabil. 2002;16;871–7.

Fliege H, Rose M, Arck P, Walter OB, Kocalevent RD, Weber C, Flapp, BF. The Perceived Stress Questionnaire (PSQ) reconsidered: validation and reference values from different clinical and health adult samples. Psychosom Med. 2005;67:78.

Garfinkel M, Singhal A, Katz W, Allan D, Reshetar R, Schumacher Jr H. Yoga-base intervention for carpal tunnel syndrome: a randomized trial. JAMA. 1998;280;1601–3.

Gatchel RJ, Turk DC. Activity-rest cycling. In: Gatchel RJ, Turk DC, editors. Psychological approaches to pain management – a practitioner's handbook. New York, NY: Guilford; 1996. pp. 272–4.

Gerritsen AA, de Krom MC, Struijs MA, Scholten RJ, de Vet HC, Bouter LM. Conservative treatment options for carpal tunnel syndrome: a systematic review of randomized controlled trials. J Neurol. 2002;249:272–80.

Goodyear Smith F, Arroll B. What can family physicians offer patients with carpal tunnel syndrome other than surgery? A systematic review of nonsurgical management. Ann Fam Med. 2004;2:267–73.

Gosman-Hedström G, Svensson E. Parallel reliability of the functional independence measure and the Barthel ADL Index. Disabil Rehabil. November 2000;22:702–15.

Grangaard L. Low back pain. In: Pendleton HM, Schultz-Krohn W, editors. Pedretti's occupational therapy: practice skills for physical dysfunction. St. Louis, MO: Mosby Elsevier; 2006. pp. 1036–55.

Groth GN. Clinical decision making and therapists' autonomy in the context of flexor tendon rehabilitation. J Hand Ther. 2008;21:254–9.

Guzman J, Esmail R, Karjalainen KA, Malmivaara A, Irvin E, Bombardier C. Multidisciplinary bio-psycho-social rehabilitation for chronic low-back pain. Cochrane Database Syst Rev. 2007 Jul;18(2):CD 000963.

Hamilton BB, Granger CV, Sherwin FS, Zielezny M, Tashman JS. A uniform national data system for medical rehabilitation. In: Fuhrer MJ, editor. Rehabilitation outcomes: analysis and measurements. Baltimore, MD: Brookes; 1987. pp. 137–47.

Hand Rehabilitation Center of Indiana. Diagnosis and treatment manual for physicians and therapists. 4th ed. Indianapolis, IN: Author; 2001.

Hudak PL, Amadio PC, Bombardier C, and The Upper Extremity Collaborate Group (UECG). Development of an upper extremity outcome measure: The DASH (Disabilities of the Arm, Shoulder and Hand) [corrected]. Am J Ind Med. September 1996;3:372.

Hussey SM, Sabonis-Chafee B, O'Brien JC. Introduction to occupational therapy. 3rd ed. St. Louis, MO: Mosby Elsevier; 2008.

Isernhagen SJ, Hart DL, Matheson LM. Reliability of independent observer judgment levels of lift effort in a kinesiophysical functional capacity evaluation. Work 1999;12:145–50.

Jaegers LA. Ergonomics, health, and wellness in industry: a holistic approach. Am Occup Ther Assoc Work Ind Spec Int Sec Q. 2008;22:1–4.

Kasch MC. Therapist's evaluation and treatment of upper extremity cumulative trauma disorders. In: Mackin EJ, Callahan AD, Skirven TM, Schneider, LH, Osterman AL, Hunter JM, editors. Rehabilitation of the hand and upper extremity. 5th ed. St. Louis, MO: Mosby, Incorporated; 2002:1005–17.

Kase K. Illustrated kinesiotaping. 3rd ed. Albuquerque, NM: Ken'i Kai; 2000.

Kavanagh J. Management of chronic pain using the cognitive-behavioral approach. Brit J Ther Rehabil. 1995;2:413–8.

Keegan DM, Kahlert RC. Industrial rehabilitation services. In: Burke SL, Higgins JP, McClinton MA, Saunders RJ, Valdata L, editors. Hand and upper extremity rehabilitation – a practical guide. 3rd ed. St. Louis, MO: Elsevier; 2006:727–38.

King PM, Olson DL. Work. In: Blesedell Crepeau E, Cohn ES, Boyt Schell BA, editors. Williard & Spackman's occupational therapy. 11th ed. Philadelphia, PA: Wolters Kluwer/Lippincott Williams & Wilkins; 2009. pp. 615-31.

Lan C, Lai J-S, Chen S-Y, Wong M-K. Tai Chi Chuan to improve muscular strength and endurance in elderly individuals: a pilot study. Arch Phys Med Rehabil. 2000;81:604-7.

Lechner, DE, Jackson, JR, Roth D, Straaton KV. Reliability and validity of a newly developed test of physical work performance. J Occup Med. 1994;36:997-1004.

Li Z, Paterson Smith B, Smith TL, Koman LA. Diagnosis and management of complex regional pain syndrome complicating upper extremity recovery. J Hand Ther. 2005;18:270-6.

Lundon K. The effect of mechanical load on soft connective tissues. In: Hammer WI, editor. Functional soft-tissue examination and treatment by manual methods. Sudbury, MA: Jones and Bartlett Publishers; 2007. pp. 15-30.

Margolis RB., Tait RC, Krause SJ. A rating system for use with patient pain drawings. Pain 1986;24:57-65.

McPhee SD, Bracciano AG, Rose BW. Physical agent modalities: a position paper. Am J Occup Ther. 2003;57:650-1.

Melzack R. The McGill pain questionnaire: major properties and scoring methods. Pain 1975;1:277-99.

Moscony AM. Enabling occupational competence: evaluation and treatment for the painful extremity: part II. Am Occup Ther Assoc Phy Dis SIS Q. 2002;25:1-4.

National Institute of Neurological Disorders and Stroke – National Institutes of Health. NINDS chronic pain information page. February 23, 2009. Available at: http://www.ninds.nih.gov/disorders/chronic_pain/chronic_pain.htm. Accessed 2 Apr 2009.

Neville-Jan A. Encounters in a world of pain: an autoethnography. Am J Occup Ther. 2003;57:88-98.

Nowack KM. Stress Profile. Western Psychological Services. 1999. Available at: http://portal.wpspublish.com/pdf/sp.pdf. Accessed 20 Oct 2009.

O'Connor D, Marshall S, Massy-Westropp N. Non-surgical treatment (other than steroid injection) for carpal tunnel syndrome. Cochrane Database Syst Rev. 2003;1:CD003219.

Oerlemans HM, Oostendorp RA, de Boo T, van der Laan L, Severens JL, Goris JA. Adjuvant physical therapy versus occupational therapy in patients with reflex sympathetic dystrophy/complex regional pain syndrome Type I. Arch Phys Med Rehabil. 2000;81:49-56.

Pearson Education, Inc. Pain Patient Profile by Tollison CD & Langley JC. Available at: http://psychcorp.pearsonassessments.com/HAIWEB/Cultures/en-us/Productdetail.htm?Pid=PAg509. Accessed 20 Oct 2009.

Persson E, Rivano-Fischer M, Eklund M. Evaluation of changes in occupational performance among patients in a pain management program. J Rehabil Med. 2004;36:85–91.

Piazzini DB, Aprile I, Ferrara PE, et al. A systematic review of conservative treatment of carpal tunnel syndrome. Clin Rehabil. 2007;21:299–314.

Priganc VW, Ito MA. Changes in edema, pain, or range of motion following manual edema mobilization: a single-case design study. J Hand Ther. 2008;21:326–35.

Reid MC, Papaleontiou M, Ong A, Breckman R, Wethington E, Pillemer K. Self-management strategies to reduce pain and improve function among older adults in community settings: a review of the evidence. Pain Med. 2008;9:409–24.

Reneman MF, Brouwer S, Speelman Meinema A, Dijkstra PU, Geertzen, JHB, Groothoff JW. Test-retest reliability of the Isernhagen work systems functional capacity evaluation in health adults. J Occup Rehabil. 2004;14:295–305.

Rochman DL, Kennedy-Spaien E. Chronic pain management – approaches and tools for occupational therapy. OT Pract. 2007;12:9–15.

Roth S, McCune CC. The client and family experience of mental illness. In: Cara E, MacRae A, editors. Psychosocial occupational therapy: a clinical practice. 2nd ed. Clifton Park, NY: Thomson Delmar Learning; 2005. pp. 3–25.

Sabata DR, Shamberg S, Williams M. Optimizing access to home, community, and work environments. In: Radomski MV, Trombly Latham CA, editors. Occupational therapy for physical dysfunction. 6th ed. Baltimore, MD: Lippincott Williams & Wilkins; 2008. pp. 951–73.

Seaward BL. Managing stress: principles and strategies for health and well-being. 5th ed. Sudbury, MA: Jones and Bartlett; 2006.

Sherman K.J, Cherkin DC, Erro J, Miglioretti DL, Deyo RA. Comparing yoga, exercise, and a self-care book for chronic low back pain: a randomized, controlled trial. Ann Int Med. 2005;143:849–856.

Simons DG, Travell JG, Simons LS. Travell & Simons' Myofascial pain and dysfunction – the trigger point manual. Vol. 1. The upper half of the body. 2nd ed. Baltimore, MD: Williams & Wilkins; 1999.

Singh G, Willen SN, Boswell MV, Janata JW, Chelimsky T. The value of interdisciplinary pain management in complex regional pain syndrome Type I: a prospective outcome study. Pain Physician. 2004;7:203–209.

Stark Schier J, Chan J. Changes in life roles after hand injury. J Hand Ther. 007;20;57–69.

Stein F, Cutler SK. Psychosocial occupational therapy: a holistic approach. San Diego, CA: Singular; 1998.

Strong J. Incorporating cognitive-behavioral therapy with occupational therapy: a comparative study with patients with low back pain. J Occup Rehabil. 1998;8:61–71.

The American Occupational Therapy Association. Occupational therapy practice framework: domain & process. 2nd ed. Am J Occup Ther. 2008b;62:625–83.

The American Occupational Therapy Association: Reimbursement and Regulatory Policy Department. Fact sheet: Medicare basics. 2008a. Available at: http://www.aota.org/Practitioners/Reimb/Pay/Medicare/FactSheets/37788.aspx. Accessed 14 May 2009.

Turk DC. Clinical effectiveness and cost-effectiveness of treatments for patients with chronic pain. Clin J Pain. 2002;18:355–65.

Valpar International Corporation. Interrater reliability of Joule, an FCE System. 1999. Available at: http://www.valparint.com/JOULSTD2.htm. Accessed 20 Oct 2009.

Walsh JT, Muntzer E. Therapist's management of complex regional pain syndrome (reflex sympathetic dystrophy). In: Mackin EJ, Callahan AD, Skirven TM, Schneider, LH, Osterman AL, Hunter JM, editors. Rehabilitation of the hand and upper extremity. 5th ed. St. Louis, MO: Mosby, Incorporated; 2002:1707–1724.

Wiskin LF. Cognitive-behavioral therapy: a psychoeducational treatment approach for the American worker with rheumatoid arthritis. Work 1998;10:41–48.

Yasuda YL. Rheumatoid arthritis, osteoarthritis, and fibromyalgia. In: Radomski MV, Trombly Latham CA, editors. Occupational therapy for physical dysfunction. 6th ed. Baltimore, MD: Lippincott Williams & Wilkins; 2008. pp. 1214–43.

Yocum DE, Castro WL, Cornett M. Exercise, education, and behavioral modification as alternative therapy for pain and stress in rheumatic disease. Rheum Dis Clin N Am. 2000;26:145–59.

Chapter 16

Acupuncture

Shu-Ming Wang, MSci, MD

Introduction

The word acupuncture is derived from Latin *acus* "with a needle" and *pungere* "puncture through the skin (Kaptchuk 2000)." Acupuncture has been used in China for more than 3000 years as a therapeutic procedure for pain relief, but only recently (1970s) a greater understanding of the underlying mechanism of acupuncture analgesia developed (NIH consensus developmental panel on acupuncture 1998). Similar to many ancient healing traditions, acupuncture has accumulated a wealth of anecdotal experiences documenting its clinical effectiveness in a variety of pain conditions. In 1997, a National Institutes of Health (NIH) conference released the consensus statement that acupuncture is effective in treating migraine headache, back pain, and dysmenorrhea (NIH consensus developmental panel on acupuncture 1998, Patel et al. 1989, Ter Riet and Keipachild 1990, Ezzo et al. 2000). The main focus of this chapter is to review the philosophy and history of acupuncture, to uncover the physiology of pain perception, to understand the underlying physiologic mechanisms of acupuncture analgesia, and to review current use of acupuncture in pain management for selected acute and chronic pain conditions.

History of Acupuncture

Acupuncture is one of many therapeutic interventions utilized in traditional Chinese medicine (TCM). The seminal TCM textbook, Huang Di Nei Jing (Inner Canon of the Yellow Emperor or The Inner Canon of Huangdi), was compiled around 305–204 BCE (Fig. 16.1). This textbook covered the theoretical foundation of Chinese medicine (Unschuld 1985). It is composed of two volumes: Shu Wen and Ling Shu. Each volume has 81 chapters and is written in a question and answer format between the mythical Huangdi and his ministers. The first volume, Shu Wen, also known as "Simple Questions" basically covers the theoretical foundation of Chinese medicine and its association with diagnosis and treatment methods. The second volume, Ling Shu, also known as "Spiritual Pivot" mainly describes meridians, acupuncture points, and acupuncture techniques and has laid a solid foundation for clinical acupuncture theory. Due to the complexity and the depth of the original "Ling Shu," there were great discrepancies among the interpretations from generations to generations (DeWoskin 1983, Epler 1980, Farquhar 1994). Despite the differences in interpretation, there is agreement that acupuncture is not an ideological belief. It is a system of thoughts and

N. Vadivelu et al. (eds.), *Essentials of Pain Management*,
DOI 10.1007/978-0-387-87579-8_16, © Springer Science+Business Media, LLC 2011

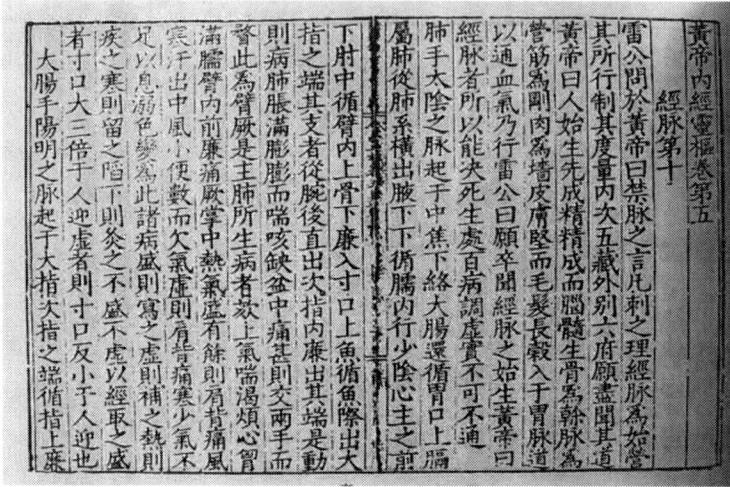

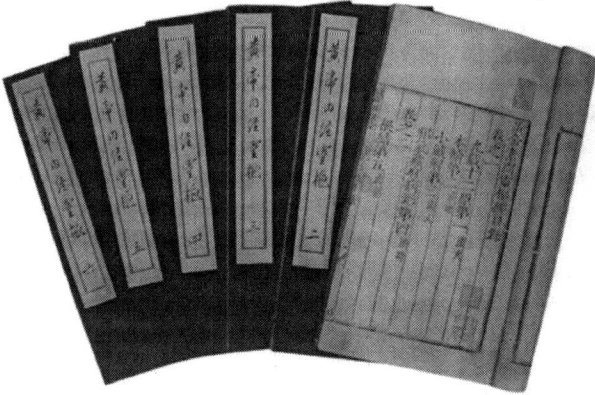

Figure 16.1   The ancient Chinese textbook.

practices that are based on investigating the natural phenomenon, understanding the principles of realism, and applying them to the prevention and treatment of human ailments. The instruments used for acupuncture in the ancient time are as illustrated in Fig. 16.2.

The first known European account of the use of acupuncture came from a 16th century Roman Catholic Church in Canton, China, and was reported by Portuguese, Dutch, Danish, and French missionaries. "A Treatise on Acupuncturation" was the first English text known to describe the practice of acupuncture that was published in 1823 by a surgeon named James Morss Churchill (Churchill 1821). It described the practice as having the most success in the treatment of rheumatic conditions, sciatica, and back pain. In 1972, Mr. James Reston describing his experience in acupuncture analgesia in a front-page article in *The New York Times* is credited with sparking an increased interest in acupuncture in the United States. This was followed by stories told by the physicians, who accompanied President Nixon on a

da	chang	hao	yuanli	pi	feng	ti	yuan	chan
大	長	毫	圓利	鈹	鋒	鍉	圓	鑱

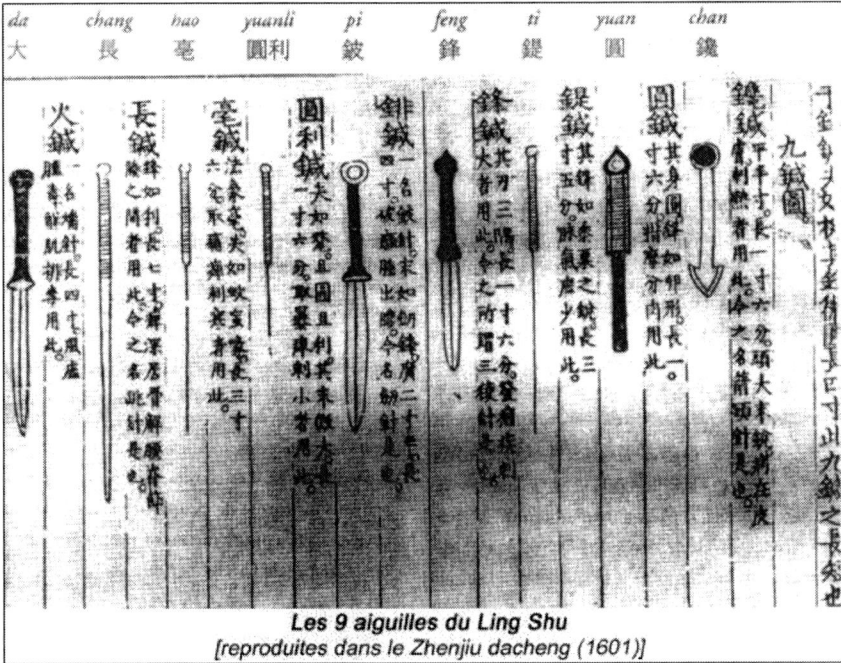

Les 9 aiguilles du Ling Shu
[reproduites dans le Zhenjiu dacheng (1601)]

Figure 16.2   The instruments used in ancient time to perform acupuncture.

visit to China, where he witnessed open-heart surgery performed under acupuncture analgesia. This overwhelming press release soon led to scientific efforts designed to test the clinical effectiveness and elucidate the underlying mechanism of acupuncture for analgesia. In 1974, California became the first state to designate acupuncture as a legal experimental procedure (McRae 1982). In 1996, the Food and Drug Administration (FDA) changed the status of acupuncture needles from Class III to Class II medical devices, i.e., acupuncture needles are regarded as safe and effective instrument by licensed practitioners. In 1997, the NIH gathered all available documentations published and a group of experts around the world to attest the clinical efficacy of acupuncture in various pain conditions (NIH consensus developmental panel on acupuncture 1998). Subsequently, the release of a consensus statement has enhanced the popularity and acceptance of acupuncture in the United States. Soon after, the establishment of the National Center for Complementary Alternative Medicine (NCCAM) has further supported the research endeavors aimed at exploring the scientific validity of using acupuncture for various pain problems and the underlying mechanism of acupuncture analgesia (www.nih.gov/about/almanac/organization/NCCAM.htm).

Traditional Principle of Acupuncture

Traditionally acupuncture is embedded in a complex theoretical framework that provides conceptual and therapeutic directions. Acupuncture relies on ordinary human sensory awareness, and its fundamental assertion is similar to the kindred philosophical systems of Confucianism and Taoism (Hahn 1982). The contemplation and reflection on sensory perceptions and ordinary appearances are sufficient to understand the human condition, including both health and illness. The foreign-sounding key words of acupuncture "language" such as Yin, Yang, dampness, wind, fire, dryness, cold, and earth as well as strange concepts have acted as a formidable barrier for acceptance by many Westerners. In reality, these key words represent human "meteorologic" conditions, which are sometimes pathologic and disruptive, but sometimes necessary and healthy (Kaptchuk). The following examples are to illustrate the Chinese prospective of Yin–Yang and Qi and how acupuncture works (Liu and Akira 1994).

Yin–Yang

Yin and Yang are two conditions that are complementary and opposite to each other. Yin and Yang have been successfully intertwined for additional descriptive refinement (Fig. 16.3). Yin is associated with cold, darkness, feminine, stagnation, and passiveness. In contrast, Yang is associated with heat, brightness, masculine, hyperdynamic, and aggressiveness. In a healthy

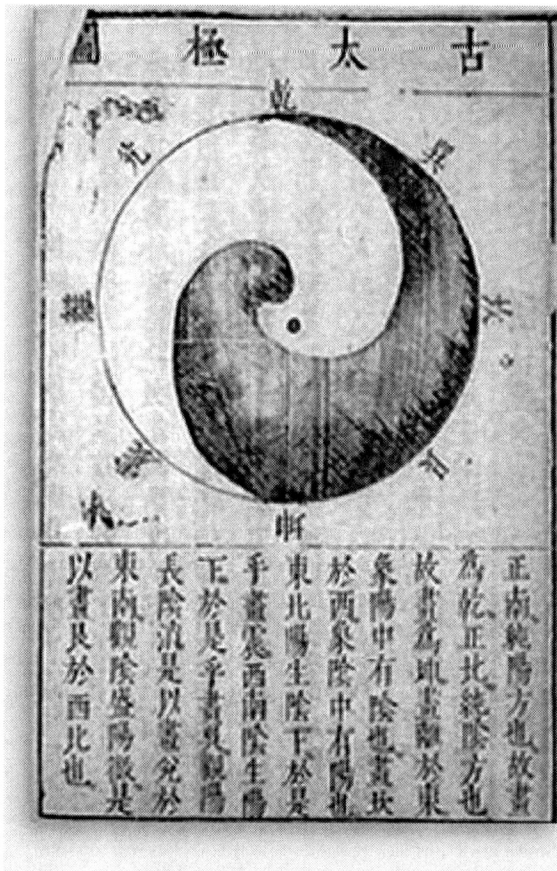

Figure 16.3   Yin-Yang.

condition, Yin and Yang are balance complements to each other; however, when Yin and Yang are imbalance manifesting, specific symptoms are manifested which affect the well-being of a person. The Ancient Chinese believed that the changing of climate actually affects the balance between Yin and Yang. Through their observation that certain diseases or illnesses commonly manifest themselves at the certain seasons, there is a special focus on prevention of imbalance of Yin and Yang at the time of season changes.

Qi and Meridians

Qi is considered as the essence of life (i.e., "vital energy") that cycles around the body and maintains all organs' functions (Fig. 16.4). Qi flows through a hypothetical network of channels called meridians that interconnect the various organs. Figures 16.5a and b are illustrations of Conception Vessel Meridian and Heart Meridians listed in the TCM textbook. Along the meridians, there are acupuncture points where Qi travels immediately below the skin surface. Qi appears to not only provide the linkage between internal organs but also carry vital information from internal organs to the skin surface. In the normal healthy condition, Qi flows in regular rhyme. However, any state of disharmony or any imbalance in Yin–Yang will also cause disturbances in Qi flow. The disturbances of Qi lead to manifestation of symptoms of illnesses.

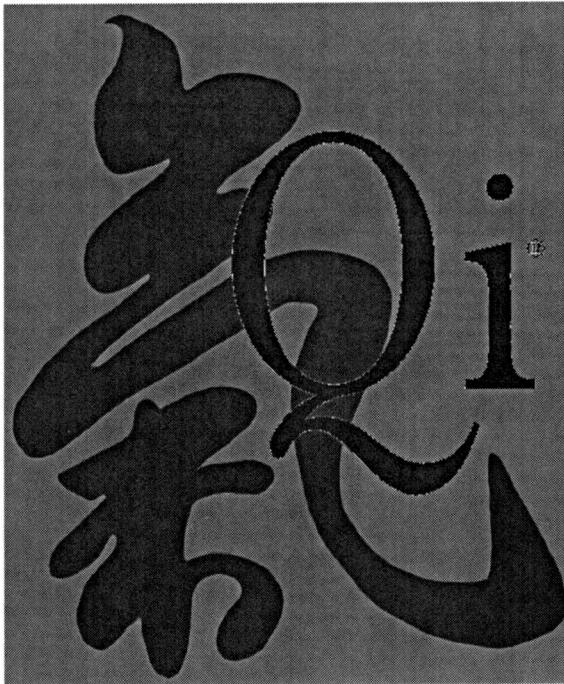

Figure 16.4   Chinese character for Qi.

Acupuncture Therapy

Any imbalance in Yin–Yang and Qi has to be dynamically harmonized in order to restore the body back to a healthy condition. By applying acupuncture therapy onto specific points of the body, one can shift a person's illnesses into a healthy condition. It appears that acupuncture has the capacity to dry, cool, warm, augment, deplete, redirect, reorganize, unblock, restore, and stabilize based on the specific needs of a particular illness. Several interventional techniques are commonly described to perform traditional acupuncture (Fig. 16.6a–f; Table 16.1). The most common technique is one that inserts hair-thin needles into specific acupuncture points on the body to correct disruptions in harmony. Heat stimulation is a technique also known as *moxibustion*, which burns the herb *Artemisia vulgaris* either onto acupuncture points through needles or indirectly near the acupuncture point. The whole purpose of applying moxibustion is to warm or move the Qi. Vacuum stimulation is also

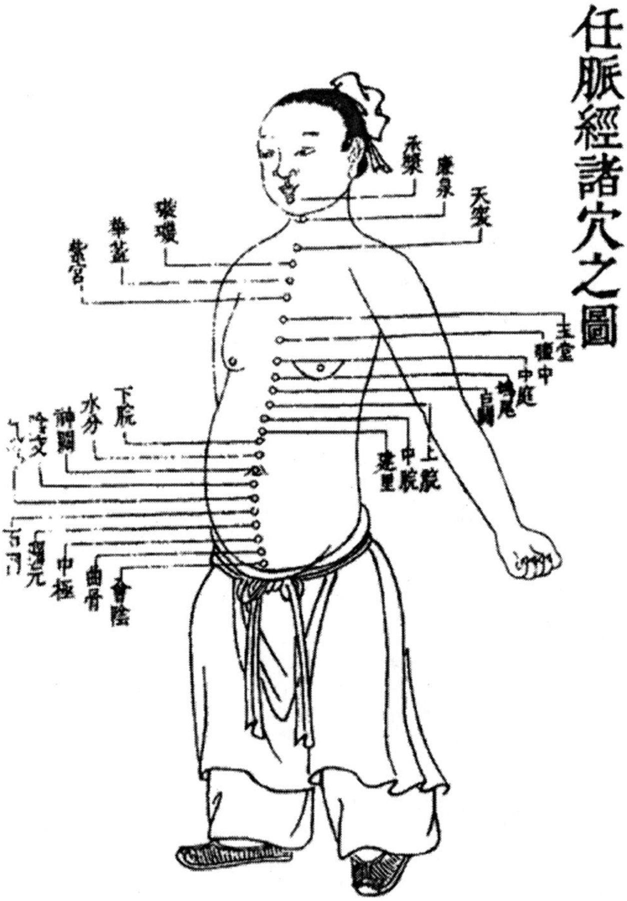

Figure 16.5 (a) Conception Vessel Meridian. (b) Heart Meridian.

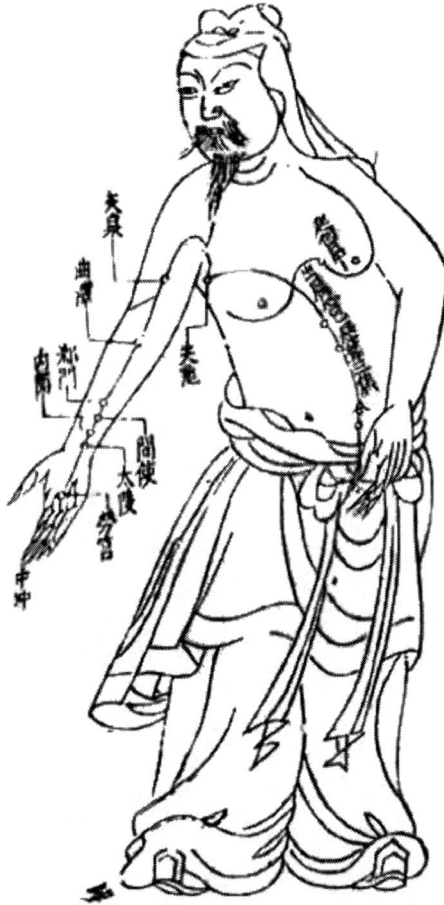

Figure 16.5 (Continued)

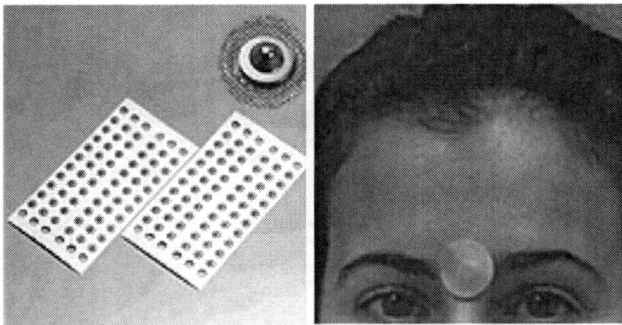

Figure 16.6 (a) Acupressure bead and practice. (b) Acupuncture needles and practice. (c) Moxa and Moxibustion. (d) Cups and cupping. (e) Laser and practice. (f) Electrical stimulator and practice.

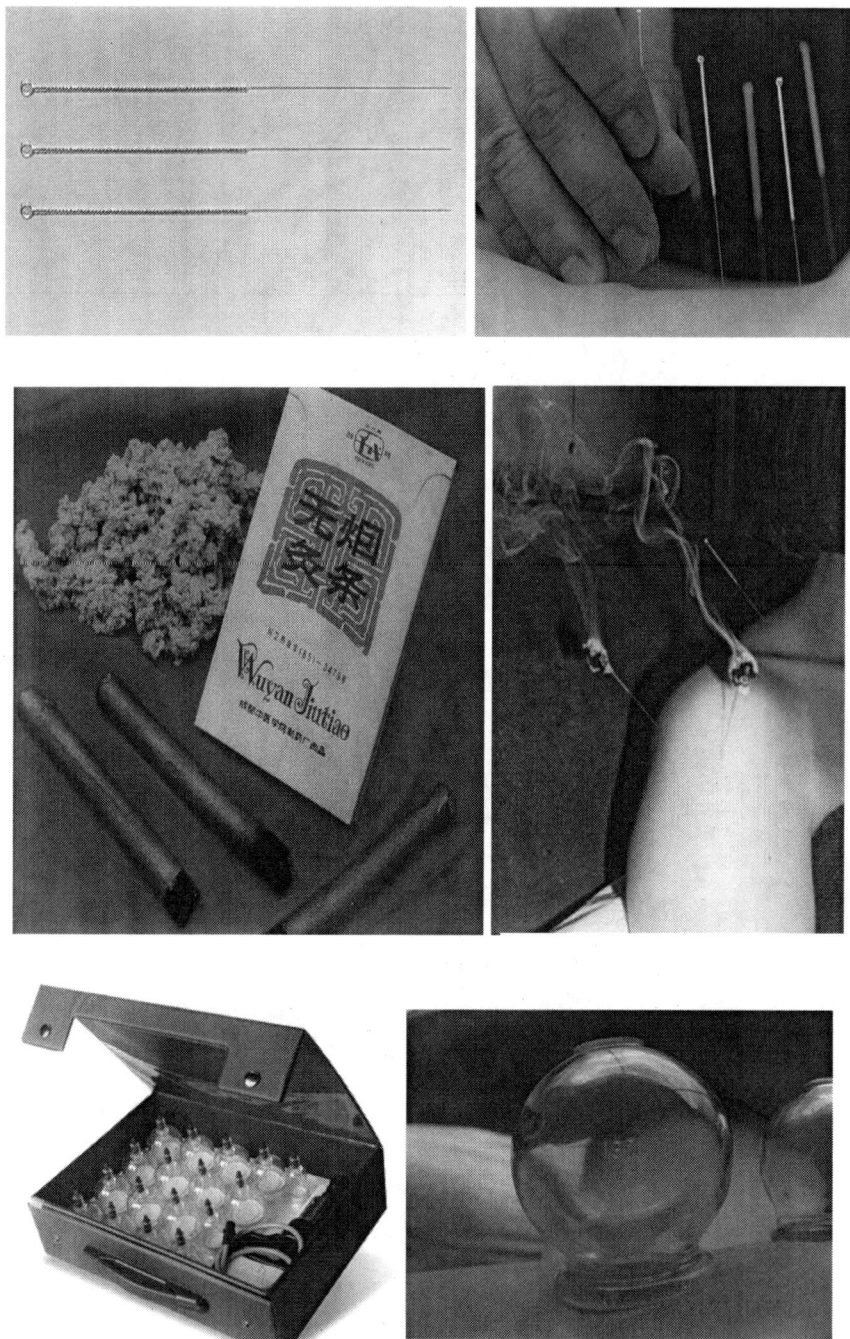

Figure 16.6   (Continued)

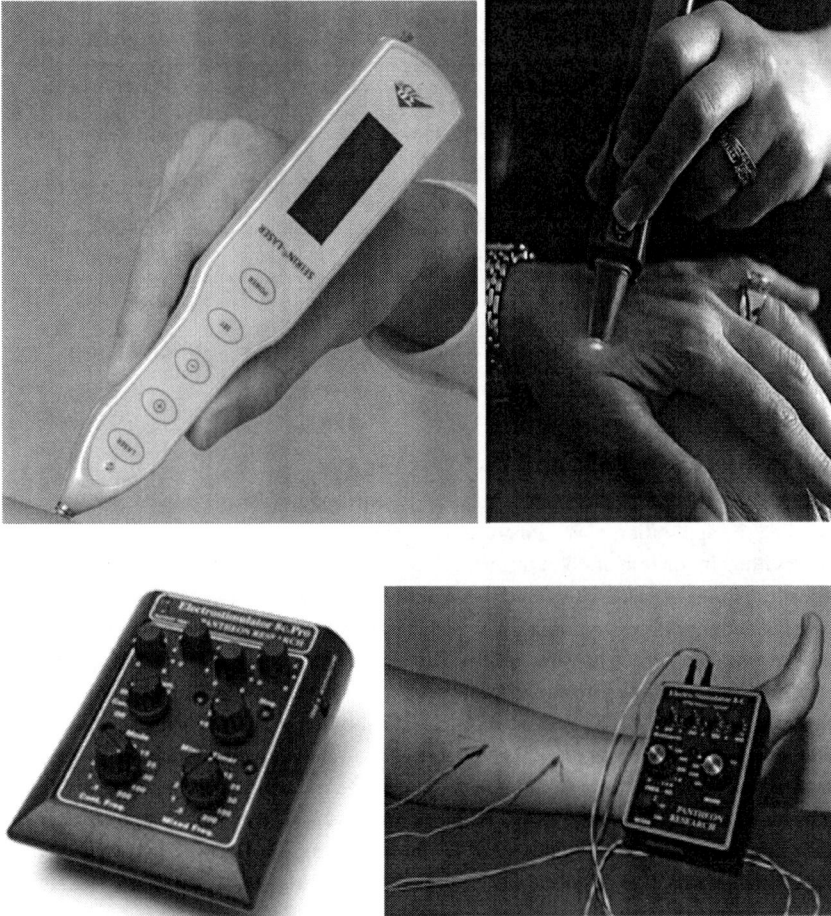

Figure 16.6 (Continued)

known as cupping, which applies the suction cup onto the acupuncture point with or without the needles. Cupping is used to remove excessive energy or soothing the turbulence of Qi. Hand pressure is sometimes applied to relieve mild symptoms. All these physical stimuli are applied to one acupuncture point to restore harmony and health. Electroacupuncture, laser, and hydroinjection are recent developments in acupuncture stimulation techniques (Wang et al. 2008).

The premise of acupuncture is that internal pathology can be diagnosed and treated using surface evaluation and stimulation by taking advantage of somatovisceral and viscerosomatic reflexes, which occurs via stimulation at one site of the body resulting in a "harmonizing" effect on the body. In other words, the stimulation does not have to be applied directly to the affective area to achieve the optimal therapeutic effect (Biella et al. 2001).

Table 16.1 The family of techniques utilized as acupuncture stimulation.

Pressure: Application of fingers pressure, pressure pellet available commercially to the acupuncture point also known as acupressure
Needle: Usually application of hair-thin needle into the acupuncture point also known as traditional body acupuncture, manual acupuncture, etc
Moxibustion: Application of dried mugwort to the acupuncture point by attaching the dried herb to the handle of acupuncture needle place into the acupuncture point or above the acupuncture point
Cupping: Application of suction cups onto the acupuncture point with or without the acupuncture needle already in place
Laser: Application of laser to the acupuncture point
Electrical stimulation: Application of electrical stimulation through surface electrodes (transcutaneous electrical acupoint stimulation – TEAS) or through needle placed into the acupuncture point (electroacupuncture or electrical acupoint stimulation – EA)
Hydroinjection: Injection of fluid of medication into the acupuncture point also known as acupoint injection

The Principle of Pain and Its Physiology

Chinese theory indicates that pain is frequently associated with stagnation or obstruction of "Qi," and the application of acupuncture stimulation unblocks this obstruction and stagnation resulting in the resolution of this pain (Liu and Akira 1994). The Western physiology of pain perception and modulation describes a multilevel system that is activated once an injury occurs under normal circumstances. The peripheral activation leads to a series of events processing toward the central nervous system. This leads to a sequence of events including signal processing along neural pathways, immunologic, hormonal release, and psychobehavioral responses (Wang et al. 2008). Pain perception and inhibition accept a dynamic, malleable, and complex set of interacting neurons with gene regulation and expression producing a variety of neuropeptides and cytokines at both the peripheral and the central nervous systems (Besson 1999, Melzack and Wall 1965, Bolay and Moskowitz 2002). The recognition of the plasticity of the nervous system has revolutionized the understanding of pain, especially chronic pain. The neuroanatomy of nociception can be organized into three major domains. The periphery is composed of small-fiber sensory axons that respond to various types of noxious input called nociceptors. At the spinal cord level, the interneurons, which receive nociceptive and non-nociceptive afferent information, act on the side of dynamic neurons and others ascend the order neuron to alter the retrograde processing of "pain" signals from the periphery. In the brain, these signals are mediated further by norepinephrine, serotonin, and acetylcholine and endogenous opioids. The well-identified opioid receptor sites of the brain and spinal cord include the hypothalamus, limbic system, basal ganglia and periaqueductal gray area, nucleus raphe magnus, reticular activating system, and dorsal horn of the spinal cord (Besson 1999).

Mechanism of Acupuncture Analgesia
The Action of Acupuncture at the Peripheral Acupuncture Point

De Qi sensation has been described in the TCM as the therapeutic signal for acupuncture treatment. This "De Qi" sensation has been characterized by the patient as a sensation of heaviness, numbness, and soreness and aching (Wang et al. 1985). In the meantime, the acupuncturist experienced the sensation of needles being caught. It is now believed that "De Qi" sensation is caused by the activation of $A\beta$ and C fibers in the skeletal muscle (Wang et al. 1985, Pomeraez 1998), and recent studies have also demonstrated the insertion and rotation of acupuncture needles resulting in the reorganization of the local connective tissue fibers and illicit difference type of mechanical signals-post-stimulation being processed (Langevin et al. 2001a, Langevin et al. 2001b).

The Action of Acupuncture at the Central Nervous System

The central pathways of acupuncture were mapped by the use of functional magnetic resonance imaging (fMRI) techniques. Interestingly, scientists discovered that the areas of brain affected by acupuncture stimulations include the hypothalamus, nucleus accumbens, rostral part of the anterior cingulate cortex, the amygdale formation, and the hippocampal complex. Most of the activated areas are shared with areas activated in acute and chronic pain states (Besson 1999, Anderson et al. 1997, Casey et al. 1996, Parienet et al. 2005). This indicates that acupuncture could relieve pain by unbalancing the equilibrium of distributed pain-related central networks.

At present, acupuncture stimulation may affect peripheral tissue organization and interfere with pain signal processing along the central nervous system, either through direct signal interference or by the release of chemical substrates.

Acupuncture in the Clinical Setting – The United States Experience

In the early 1990s, by an act of congress, the NIH formed an Office of Alternative Medicine, which subsequently became the National Center for Complementary and Alternative Medicine (NCCAM). The main objective of the center was to fund basic and clinical research in various complementary alternative medicine (CAM) therapies with the ultimate goal of proving clinician's evidence-based approaches. With the support from NIH, the first consensus guidelines for clinicians summarized the evidence on the use and effectiveness of acupuncture in a variety of medical conditions. Although the consensus statement did not strongly recommend the use of acupuncture for all the pain syndromes, acupuncture has been accepted as a technique for peripheral sensory stimulation in the therapy of painful syndromes. Similar to other CAM researches, the validity of clinical acupuncture studies and their outcomes are significantly affected by the methodological approach employed. Important study variables include study design, sample size, proper placebo or sham, treatment duration, post-treatment follow-up, and outcome measurements.

Over the last three decades, more than 500 randomized, controlled trials have evaluated the efficacy of acupuncture (Greenwood 2002). A growing number of systemic reviews and meta-analysis that use stringent inclusion criteria have begun to synthesize this research. The reviews most often report that trials of acupuncture efficacy are equivocal or contradictory. This chapter will discuss the efficacy of acupuncture for both acute and chronic pain symptoms. Table 16.2 outlines common acupuncture points used for pain in various clinical acupuncture trials.

Chronic Pain Conditions

Chronic Lower Back Pain

In the United States, chronic low back pain (LBP) is the most common cause of activity limitation in people younger than 45 years and the second most frequent reason for physician office visits. It also ranks as the fifth common cause of hospital admission

Table 16.2 Acupuncture points commonly used in clinical acupuncture studies.

- **LR3 Taichong**: On the dorsum of the foot, in the fossa distal to the junction of the first and second metatarsal bones, 2 in. proximal to the margin of the web of the toe; this acupuncture point has been used in migraine and adjunct for lithotripsy studies
- **SP6 Sanyinjiao**: 3 in. directly above the tip of the medial malleolus, in the fossa posterior to the medial margin of the tibia; this acupuncture point has been used in migraine headache, colonoscopy, and labor analgesia studies
- **ST36 Zusanli**: In the fossa 1 fingerbreadth lateral to the anterior margin of the tibia and 3 in. inferior to the acupoint Dubi (ST 35), which is located at the lower border of the patella, in the depression lateral to the patellar ligament; this acupuncture point has been used in osteoarthritis, migraine, colonoscopy, and postoperative pain studies
- **LI4 Hegu**: On the dorsum of the hand, between the first and the second metacarpals, at the midpoint of the radial margin of the second metacarpal bone; this acupuncture point has been used in adjunct for lithotripsy labor pain, colonoscopy, migraine, neck, and shoulder pain
- **PC6 Neiguan**: On the palmar side of the forearm, 2 in. above the transverse crease of the wrist and between the tendons of the flexor carpi radialis and palmaris longus muscles; this acupuncture point has been used in migraine, angina, nausea, and vomiting studies
- **GB20 Fengchi**: At the posterior lateral aspect of the neck, in the fossa between the superior margins of the trapezius and sternocleidomastoid muscles; this acupuncture point has been used in migraine, neck, and shoulder studies
- **GV20 Baihui**: At the middle of the vertex, on the line connecting the apexes of the two ears. This acupuncture point has been used in labor analgesia and migraine studies
- **SP6** (San Yin Jiao, the sixth point on the spleen channel): On the medial side of the lower leg, three-finger breadth superior to the prominence of the medial malleolus, in a depression close to the medial crest of the tibia. This acupuncture point has been used in colonoscopy, labor analgesia, and migraine studies
- **LR3 Taichong**: On the dorsum of the foot in a depression distal to the junctions of the first and second metatarsal bones; this acupuncture point has been used in adjunct for lithotripsy, migraine, and labor analgesia studies

(www.ninds.nih.gov/disorders/backpain/detail_backpain.htm). Most importantly, LBP is the third most common indication for surgical procedures. In average, about 2% of the US workforces are compensated for back injuries each year. Both surgical and pharmacologic interventions have been prescribed as a treatment for patients suffering from LBP. There are a growing number of clinical data supporting that acupuncture and related intervention may serve as a treatment for LBP as well. Carlsson and colleagues (Carlsson and Sjolund 2001) conducted a sham randomized controlled trial (RCT) study of patients suffering from chronic LBP and found that both manual and electrical acupuncture were superior to sham electrical stimulation in reducing pain, improving sleep patterns, and analgesic consumption. These effects were sustained 4–6 months post-intervention. However, they could only demonstrate these positive responses in women. As a result these investigators suggest that gender may have an effect on the therapeutic effect of acupuncture and related techniques. Leibing et al. (2002) found that LBP patients who received a series of 26 sessions of interventions, consisting of a combination of ear and body manual acupuncture and physical therapy, was superior to those of patients who received 26 sessions of standard physical therapy alone for the reduction of pain, disability, and psychological distress for 3 months. However, the beneficial effects of combined ear and body manual acupuncture were present, and at 9 months post-intervention there were no differences between the two study groups. The results of this study suggest that in order for a sustained clinical effect, "maintenance" acupuncture therapy may be indicated to sustain the prolonged benefit in patients with LBP. A similar observation was also noted in a more recent RCT that found that the combination of true acupuncture and conservative orthopedic treatment was superior to sham acupuncture combined with conservative orthopedic treatment or conservative orthopedic treatment alone. However, the beneficial effects lasted only 3 months (Molsberger et al. 2002). Sator-Katzenschlager et al. (2004) compared different acupuncture-related techniques and found that electrical auricular acupuncture is superior to semi-permanent press needle acupuncture in decreasing the severity of LBP and improving the psychological well-being, activity, and sleep for 3 months after treatment. Similarly, Meng et al. (2003) found that electrical acupuncture is superior to standard therapy such as non-steroidal anti-inflammatory drugs (NSAIDs), muscle relaxants, paracetamol, and back exercises in elderly patients who suffer from low blood pressure (LBP). In summary, acupuncture and related interventions can serve as a short-term adjunct treatment for LBP management. This lack of long-term benefit may be related to quick degradation of acupuncture-induced endogenous endorphins and duration of treatment protocol and may require follow-up and additional treatment.

Chronic Neck and Shoulder Pain

In the United States, more than 10% of the population has experienced pain in the neck and shoulder at some point in their life (Côté et al. 1998). Chronic neck and shoulder pain is another clinical entity that is commonly seen in women more than men. This clinical entity is frequently associated with certain adverse working condition such as repetitive working under time restraints (awkward and repetitive work), and the aging of the workforce appears to contribute to the widespread concern about chronic neck and shoulder pain (Cassou et al. 2002). Acupuncture and related interventions are frequently considered as treatment for this clinical entity (He et al. 2004). Irnich and colleagues (2001) found that although acupuncture was superior to massage therapy, it was not superior to "sham" acupuncture (i.e., the intervention mimicking acupuncture but can be different from the true acupuncture in the depth of needle insertion or in the locations where needles are placed). Interestingly the study data were reanalyzed by Vickers (2001) and found that acupuncture was superior to massage and to sham therapies as short-term treatments for chronic neck pain. Vickers and Irnich (Nabeta and Kawakita 2002) conducted another study and found that manual needle stimulations at specific acupuncture points are superior to both direct needling of local trigger points and laser sham acupuncture in improving motion-related pain and range of movement in chronic neck pain patients. Nabeta et al. (Irnich et al. 2002) conducted a similar study as did Vicker and Irnich, and the investigators found that acupuncture indeed provided a greater immediate relief for the neck and shoulder pain than other interventions, but the therapeutic effect did not last and there was no long-term benefits. Thus, the readers can speculate that in order to have a sustained long-term benefit, a repeated acupuncture intervention is required. Sator-Katzenschlager and colleagues (2003) compared the efficacy of 6-weekly treatments of manual and electrical auricular acupuncture for the treatment of chronic neck and shoulder pain. The investigators found that electrical auricular acupuncture is superior to manual auricular acupuncture in reducing the severity of pain, analgesic consumption, and return to full-time employment. This study again illustrated that in order to achieve long-term therapeutic effects, acupuncture should be administered continuously or with a maintenance schedule. In addition, the stimulating techniques applied to the acupuncture needles once they are in place can affect the magnitude of pain relief. In a large-scale trial that was conducted in the United Kingdom, patients were randomized to receive either transcutaneous electrical acupoint stimulation (TEAS) or sham-TEAS (White et al. 2004). In this study, a total of eight treatments were administered over a 4-week period and outcome assessments included neck pain, the neck disability index, the Short Form (SF)-36, and analgesics consumption. Patients in the TEAS group reported significantly less pain as compared to patients in the sham-TEAS group. However, the neck disability index and SF-36 scores did not differ significantly between the two groups. Finally, a small-scale sham-RCT was conducted with 24 subjects who suffered from chronic neck and shoulder pain (He et al. 2004). In this study, subjects were randomized to receive a series of 10 acupuncture or sham acupuncture treatments combined with daily acupressure at acupuncture points or at sham points over a 3–4-week period. Following this very intensive regimen, the investigators found that the patients in the acupuncture group had better sleep quality, less anxiety and pain, less depression, and a higher satisfaction with life as compared to patients in the sham acupuncture group. This difference was seen both at the 6-month and at the 3-year follow-up evaluations (He et al. 2004). Similar to the studies of acupuncture in patients with chronic LBP, the clinical data indicate that acupuncture and related interventions have decreased the pain and disability effectively in patients suffering from chronic neck and shoulder pain. Preliminary data also suggest that these interventions may have long-term benefit for chronic neck and shoulder pain, if the treatment period is sustained over a month. Lastly, the additional electrical stimulation applied to the needles may enhance the analgesic effect.

Osteoarthritis of the Knee

More than 20 million Americans have osteoarthritis (OA) of the knee. This clinical entity is one of the most frequent causes of physical disability among adults (www.nih.gov/news/pr/dec2004/nccam-20.htm). A recent study conducted at the University of North Carolina at Chapel Hill suggested that nearly 50% of US adults and nearly two-thirds of obese adults will develop painful knee OA by age 85 (uncnews.unc.edu September 2, 2008). According to the Forbes.com, OA of the knee is listed among the top 10 most expensive medical condition, costing 34 billion dollars. Berman et al. (1999) investigated the efficacy of acupuncture as an adjunctive therapy in elderly patients suffering from OA of the knee using a randomized crossover study design. These investigators found that patients randomized to acupuncture treatments had improvement on both McMaster University's OA index and Lequesne's indices at 4 and 8 weeks. The same research team then conducted a large-scale sham-controlled RCT that included 570 patients randomized to receive acupuncture treatment, sham treatment, or an educational intervention over a 6-month period (Berman et al. 2004). The research team found that patients in the acupuncture group experienced significantly greater improvement than the sham group in both McMaster University's OA index function and pain scores. A recent sham-controlled RCT published in *Lancet* randomized patients with OA of the knee to receive 8 weeks of acupuncture, sham, or waiting list control (Witt et al. 2005). The study found that patients in the acupuncture group experienced improved joint movement and significantly less pain. However, a follow-up at 1 year revealed no differences between the various study groups (Witt et al. 2005). At present, the available clinical data support the efficacy acupuncture as a short-term treatment of OA of the knee. Unfortunately, long-term benefits from acupuncture treatment have not been demonstrated to date.

Migraine Headache

Migraine is a very common disorder being characterized by enhanced sensitivity of the nervous system. The attack is associated with activation of the trigeminal vascular system. In 1989, a self-administered questionnaire was sent to a sample of 15,000 households (Srewart et al. 1992). A designated member of each household initially responded to the questionnaire. Each household member with severe headache was asked to respond to detailed questions about symptoms, frequency, and severity of headaches. After a single mailing, 20,468 subjects (63.4% response rate) between 12 and 80 years of age responded to the survey (Srewart et al. 1992). Migraine headache cases were identified on the basis of reported symptoms using established diagnostic criteria. An estimated 17.8% of women and 5.7% of men, i.e., about 8.7 million females and 2.6 million males, experiencing migraine found to have one or more migraine headaches per year in the United States (Srewart et al. 1992). Of these, 3.4 million females and 1.1 million males experience one or more attacks per month. Similar results were also obtained by a subsequent epidemiological study. In this subsequent study (Liptom et al. 2001), the investigators reported that many respondents reported the severity of their headaches resulted in substantial impairment of activities or required bed rest (Liptom et al. 2001). Approximately 31% missed at least 1 day of work or school in the previous 3 months because of migraine; 51% reported that work or school productivity was reduced by at least 50% (Liptom et al. 2001). When comparing the data collected in 1989, the researchers found that the prevalence and distribution of migraine remained stable over a 10-year period. The study concluded that migraine-associated disability remains substantial and pervasive. The number of those suffering from migraine has increased from 23.6 million in 1989 to 27.9 million in 1999 commensurate owing to the growth of the population. Migraine is an important target for public health interventions because of its highly prevalent and associated disabilities. The etiology of migraine remains unclear. However, the mechanism of this central pain may be related to a dysfunction in the endogenous opioid antinociceptive system (Baischer 1995). Acupuncture may be beneficial in migraine treatment as an ample number of studies in the acupuncture analgesia indicate that acupuncture modulates the pain perception through activating the release of endogenous opioids (Wang et al. 2008).

Baischer (1995) conducted a clinical study to evaluate the long-term stability of treatment effects on 26 patients (19 women, 7 men) suffering from chronic migraines. These patients documented frequency, duration, and intensity of attacks as well as analgesic intake in a migraine diary, for 5-week periods prior to acupuncture treatment, immediately after treatment, and 3 years later. Data showed improvement greater than 33% for 18 patients (69%) at post-treatment and 15 patients (58%) at 3-year follow-up. Drug intake was reduced by 50%. Treatment outcome was associated with personality traits, but not depending on demographic data or severity of migraine Baischer (1995). In a randomized controlled trial conducted by Allais evaluating the effectiveness of acupuncture versus flunarizine in preventing migraine attack over a 6-month period, we evaluated the effectiveness of acupuncture versus flunarizine in the prophylactic treatment of migraine without aura (Allais et al. 2002). A total of 160 women with migraines were randomly assigned to acupuncture treatment (the treatment regime is one session per week of acupuncture and then once per month for 4 months) or to an oral therapy with flunarizine (10 mg flunarizine was given daily for the first 2 months and then for 20 days per month for the next 4 months). The investigators found that the frequency of attacks and use of symptomatic drugs significantly decreased during treatment in both groups. The number of attacks after 2 and 4 months of therapy was significantly lower in patients who received acupuncture treatment than those who took flunarizine. The analgesic consumption was significantly lower in patients in the acupuncture group at 2 months of treatment. However, there was no difference in the analgesic consumption at 6 months between the groups. Pain intensity was significantly reduced only by acupuncture treatment, and fewer side effects were reported in patients who received acupuncture treatment than those received flunarizine.

In 2002, a systemic review was conducted to assess whether there is evidence that acupuncture is effective in the treatment of recurrent headaches. Among the 22 trials, 15 trials were performed in migraine patients. The majority of the trials, comparing true and sham acupuncture, showed at least a trend toward true acupuncture. A large-scale randomized trial was conducted in Germany to investigate the effectiveness of acupuncture compared with sham acupuncture and with no acupuncture in patients with migraine. A total of 302 patients were enrolled in the study from April 2002 to January 2003; patients were treated at 18 outpatient centers in Germany (Linde et al. 2005). These patients were randomized into acupuncture, sham acupuncture, or waiting list control. Acupuncture and sham acupuncture were administered by specialized physicians and consisted of 12 sessions per patient over 8 weeks. All the patients completed headache diaries from 4 weeks before to 12 weeks after randomization and from week 21 to week 24 after randomization. The investigators found that the number of dates with headache of moderate or serve intensity decreased in both acupuncture and sham acupuncture groups during weeks 9–12 as compared to 4 weeks before the interventions. The improvement of headache in either acupuncture or sham acupuncture group patients is superior to that of waiting list control. The investigators concluded that any acupuncture intervention, regardless of the locations or depth of needle insertion, can decrease the severity of migraine. Thus whether any needle interventions can improve of the migraine or bias of the operator and patients contributed to the "positive" outcome of this study remain to be determined (Streitberger and Kleinhenz 1998).

In the pediatric population, acupuncture has also been used as a treatment for migraine. Pintov and colleagues (1997) conducted a RCT to test the effectiveness of acupuncture in childhood migraine. The investigators found that children who received acupuncture treatments had significant clinical reduction in both migraine frequency and intensity. At the same time, the investigators also discovered that panopioid activity showed a gradual increase in plasma, which correlated with the clinical improvement. In addition, a significant increase in β-endorphin levels was observed in the migraine patients who were treated in the true acupuncture group as compared with the values before treatment or with the values of the placebo acupuncture group. The results suggest that acupuncture may be an effective treatment in children with migraine headaches and that it leads to an increase in activity of the opioidergic system. A prospective, randomized, double-blinded, placebo-controlled trial of low-level laser acupuncture was performed in 43 children with chronic headache (Meichart et al. 2002). Again, children who received laser acupuncture had significant reduction in the severity and frequency of headache. Overall, the existing evidence suggests that acupuncture has a role in the treatment of recurrent headaches. However, the quality and amount of evidence are not fully convincing. There is urgent need for well-planned, large-scale studies to assess effectiveness and efficiency of acupuncture under real-life conditions.

Dysmenorrhea

Dysmenorrhea refers to the occurrence of painful menstrual cramps of uterine origin and is a common gynecological complaint. Based on epidemiologic studies, at least 72.7% of female adolescents reported "pain or discomfort" during their period and almost 58.9% of them reported decreased activity and 45.6% reported school or work absenteeism (Taylor et al. 2002). A survey conducted on a group of female adolescents indicated that the majority of the respondents identified dysmenorrhea as one of the problems interfering with their academic performance and school absenteeism. Thus dysmenorrhea and premenstrual symptoms are common pediatric pain problems (Helms 1987). Common treatment for dysmenorrhea includes medical therapy such as NSAIDs or oral contraceptive pills (OCPs). Both modalities work by reducing myometrial activity (contractions of the uterus). The efficacy of conventional treatments such as NSAIDs is considerable. However, the failure rate can be as high as 20–25%. It is not surprising, therefore, that acupuncture and related interventions have been considered as treatments or adjunct treatments for dysmenorrhea. A RCT indicates that an acupressure garment (the Relief Brief®; Underworks, Miami, FL) decreases pain and symptoms associated with dysmenorrhea (Taylor et al. 2002). Sixty-one young women with moderately severe primary dysmenorrhea were randomized and assigned to the standard treatment control group or the Relief Brief® acupressure device group. The researchers found that patients who received Relief Brief® had less pain and used less pain medication ($P < 0.05$). The use of Relief Brief® was associated with at least a 50% decline in menstrual pain intensity in more than two-thirds of the women (Taylor et al. 2002). The researchers recommended that this acupressure device might serve as an adjuvant therapy to medication in more severe cases of dysmenorrhea.

Helm (1987) conducted a RCT to study the effectiveness of acupuncture in managing the pain of primary dysmenorrhea. Forty participants were randomized into one of the four groups: the real acupuncture group was given appropriate acupuncture and the placebo acupuncture group was given random point acupuncture on a weekly basis for three menstrual cycles; the standard control group was followed without medical or acupuncture intervention; the visitation control group had monthly non-acupuncture visits with the project physician for three cycles (Helm 1987). The investigator found that 10 of 11 (90.9%) participants in real acupuncture group, 4 of 11 (36.4%) in the placebo acupuncture group, 2 of 11 in the standard control group, and 1 of 11 in the visitation control group showed improvement. There was a 41% reduction in analgesic medication usage by the women in the real acupuncture group after their treatment series than those of other intervention groups (Helm 1987). Similarly, transcutaneous electrical nerve stimulation (TENS) and acupuncture have been used as adjunctive treatment for primary dysmenorrhea. Lastly, intramuscular injection of vitamin K_3 into the acupuncture point was evaluated as a treatment for primary dysmenorrhea (Wang et al. 2004). One hundred and eighty patients with history of dysmenorrhea or pelvic inflammatory diseases were enrolled in the study. All these patients had been previously treated without relief using Chinese herbal or Western medicine. They were divided into three groups according to the history of their illness, pelvic examination, and ultrasonography: group A consisted of 60 patients with primary dysmenorrhea, group B of 60 patients with chronic pelvic inflammation, and group C of 60 patients with endometriosis. Patients with primary dysmenorrhea were subdivided into three subgroups according to the pain-relieving efficacy of analgesics and the influence of the illness on the patients' daily life. Pain that was relieved by the analgesics and where daily life was not impacted was considered as mild symptoms; pain which was partly relieved by analgesic and constrained daily activity was considered moderate symptoms, and when the pain could not be relieved by analgesic at all and daily life was arrested, it was considered as severe. Patients in this study received intramuscular injection of a total 8 mg of vitamin K_3 (4 mg in each acupoint) into the spleen 6 acupuncture points. These patients were followed for three menstrual cycles. The researchers found that 95% of patients in the mild dysmenorrhea group had significant improvement in their pain and daily activities ($P < 0.05$). Sixty-three and 65% of patients in moderate and severe groups, respectively, also had reduction in their pelvic pain. The researchers concluded that bilateral intramuscular injection of vitamin K_3 into spleen 6 is effective in decreasing the pain and dysfunction associated with primary dysmenorrhea. Thus at present, acupuncture and related intervention may be considered as an effective adjunctive treatment for primary dysmenorrhea (Wang et al. 1997). However, there is a lack of clinical data supporting the long-term benefit of acupuncture and related treatments in patients with primary dysmenorrhea owing to the study design and follow-up.

Acute Pain Conditions
Procedural Analgesia
Acupuncture and related techniques have been used to alleviate pain and discomfort during many medical procedures such as colonoscopy, lithotripsy, and oocyte aspiration. Wang and colleagues (1997) demonstrated that pain and serum beta-endorphins, epinephrine, norepinephrine, and dopamine levels were similar between patients who received electroacupuncture (EA) and patients who received meperidine during colonoscopy procedures. These investigators also found that patients receiving EA had fewer side effects such as dizziness. Since these investigators did not include a sham control group, their findings should be interpreted cautiously. Fanti et al. (2003) conducted a sham-RCT to evaluate the analgesic effects of EA in a group of patients who were undergoing colonoscopy procedures. Patients in both the acupuncture and the sham acupuncture groups received the same frequency (100 Hz) of stimulation for 20 min prior to the procedure and throughout the duration of the procedure. The investigators found that patients in the acupuncture group reported non-significantly reduced pain during the procedures as compared to those of the sham acupuncture group. Therefore, currently available data do not support the use of acupuncture as an analgesic adjuvant during colonoscopy (Quatan et al. 2003).

Rogenhofer and colleagues (2004) conducted a non-randomized cohort study and also indicated that acupuncture might be beneficial for patients undergoing shock wave lithotripsy procedure. A recent randomized sham control study conducted by Wang and colleagues (2007) indicated that the combination of auricular acupuncture and electroacupuncture (EA) stimulations decreased the amount of alfentanil usage in patients undergoing lithotripsy procedures who also received midazolam as a sedative. Based on the available clinical data in the literature, acupuncture and related interventions may be considered as adjunct analgesics for procedures such as lithotripsy. In addition, infertility specialists have used EA as a means of analgesia for women undergoing oocyte retrieval as a method to reduce or alleviate the need for narcotics. Sterner-Victorin and colleagues (1999) conducted a series of studies using EA stimulation for oocyte aspiration and in vitro fertilization. The investigators found that although women in the EA group indicated higher stress and experienced greater discomfort than women who received alfentanil, the implantation rate, pregnancy rate, and take-home baby rate were significant higher than those women who received alfentanil for oocyte aspiration procedure. As a result, the investigators suggested that EA may be a good alternative to alfentanil during oocyte aspiration. In contrast, Gejervall and colleagues (2005) randomized a total of 160 women undergoing oocyte aspiration. The investigators found that the level of pain was significantly higher during and immediately following oocyte aspiration. However, the participants who received acupuncture were less tired and confused as compared to those who received conventional analgesia. Based on the study, the investigators suggested that EA cannot be generally recommended as a sole method for pain relief during oocyte aspiration but may be an alternative for women desiring a non-pharmacological method. Overall, despite a preoperative difference in pain rating, experts in infertility and reproductive medicine still recommend that EA, given a few minutes prior to oocyte aspiration procedure, is a good alternative to conventional analgesia because the procedure is well tolerated, the duration of hospitalization is much shorter, and the cost is much (Humaidan and Sterner-Victorin 2004).

Surgical Analgesic

Anecdotal reports from China indicate that acupuncture can be used successfully as a sole analgesia method for a variety of surgical procedures such as open-heart surgery (Cheng 2000). However, there are limited data from the Western world to support the claim and experience demonstrated in the Chinese experience. The data available in the literature are inconsistent. In early 1970, Schaer (1979) conducted a study using EA as surgical analgesia in a group of women undergoing gynecological procedures. Based on the hemodynamic changes during the surgery, a small dose of fentanyl would be administered. The investigator found that EA was as effective as 0.27 µg/kg of fentanyl given intravenously every 10 min. Grief and colleagues (Greif et al. 2002) performed electrical stimulation at the lateralization control point near the ear tragus and reported that this intervention significantly decreased the desflurane anesthetic requirements (~25%). Similarly, Taguchi and colleagues (2002) who applied auricular acupuncture stimulation at Shen Men, thalamus, tranquilizer, and master cerebral points also observed a similar anesthetic-sparing effect.

In contrast, Sim et al. (2002) conducted a sham-controlled RCT study of EA in a group of women scheduled for lower abdominal surgery. The investigators found no difference in morphine consumption between preoperative EA and sham EA groups. Additionally, postoperative patient-controlled analgesia (PCA) morphine consumption was not different between the groups. Similarly, Morioka and colleagues (2002) found that EA failed to decrease desflurane anesthetic requirements, and Kvorning et al. (2003) found that EA actually increased sevoflurane anesthetic requirements. Thus there are no conclusive data to support or deny the effectiveness of the use of intraoperative acupuncture or the analgesia modality. Wang et al. (2007) indicated that the type of anesthesia can have a significant damping effect on the acupuncture-induced central activities. Additional studies need to be conducted to verify whether the level of consciousness or depth of anesthesia affects the therapeutic effects of acupuncture. At the current time, there is inconsistency in the literature suggesting that more studies are needed to determine whether acupuncture can be used as a sole surgical analgesic or as an adjunct to local and general anesthesia for surgery.

Acute Postoperative Pain

Since July 26, 1971, the landmark event documenting that Mr. James Reston received acupuncture for acute post appendectomy pain, the Western medical society has been fascinated by the acupuncture analgesia (www.eastwestacupuncture.net/reston.htm). There are numerous acupuncture techniques that can be used for the management of acute postoperative pain. Kotani et al. (2001) conducted a RCT that applied intradermal needles to "Back Shu" acupoints in a group of patients who were scheduled to undergo major abdominal procedures. These acupuncture needles were inserted 2 h before induction of anesthesia and retained in place for 48 h postoperatively. The investigators found that patients in the acupuncture group reported a significant reduction in postoperative pain and analgesic requirements and postoperative nausea and vomiting when compared to the sham group. Usichenko et al. (2005) conducted a RCT to determine the analgesic effect of auricular acupuncture in a group of patients undergoing a total hip arthroplasty. Sixty-one patients, who were scheduled to have total hip arthroplasty, were randomized to receive either auricular acupuncture or sham (auricular) acupuncture perioperatively. The acupuncture semi-permanent press needles were placed the evening before surgery and retained for 36 h postoperatively. The investigators found that analgesic consumption during the first 36 h postoperatively was lower in the auricular acupuncture as compared to the sham auricular acupuncture group. In contrast to the above "positive" studies, Gupta et al. (1999) conducted a sham-controlled RCT to evaluate the effect of intraoperative acupuncture intervention on the analgesic requirement following knee arthroscopy. However, the investigators were unable to demonstrate any reduction in postoperative analgesic effect in the acupuncture treatment group. Based on these clinical studies, it appears that acupuncture is effective in decreasing the severity of postoperative pain, only *when* the acupuncture stimulation is performed prior to induction of anesthesia and/or during the postoperative period. In contrast, acupuncture administered while the patient is under general anesthesia was found to be ineffective in decreasing postoperative analgesic requirement. Also, these studies suggested that the timing at which manual acupuncture stimulation is administered in relation to the delivery of general anesthesia has significant effect on the acupuncture analgesia for postoperative pain.

Electroacupuncture has been used as part of postoperative analgesia for many years. In 1989, Christensen et al. (1989) conducted a RCT involving 20 healthy women who underwent gynecological surgery and received either EA or no treatment. The intervention was administrated while these women were emerging from anesthesia but still receiving 70% nitrous oxide. Postoperatively, the investigators found that patients who received EA consumed significantly less (40%) pethidine use in the postoperative acute unit (PACU) as compared to the control group. The same research team did a follow-up study to determine whether a longer duration of the EA may be even more beneficial for postoperative analgesia than the previous study (Christensen et al. 1981). The investigators administered continuous EA from the preoperative period throughout the intraoperative and postoperative period. To their surprise they found no differences in postoperative analgesic consumption between the acupuncture and the control groups. The potential reasons for this may be twofold: there are animal experimental data indicating that prolonged acupuncture stimulation leads to a reversal of acupuncture analgesia (Han and Tang 1981), and acupuncture administered under general anesthesia may not be as effective as has been shown in an adult volunteer study (Wang et al. 2007).

In 1997, Wang et al. (1997) conducted a sham-controlled RCT evaluating the analgesic effects of postoperative TEAS in patients undergoing lower abdominal surgery. Following a standardized anesthetic protocol, TEAS was applied either to acupuncture points or to the para-incisional dermatomes, and the intensity of the electrical stimulation delivered was high (9–12 mA) or low (4–5 mA) level. The investigators found that the TEAS treatment of these locations demonstrated a 30–35% reduction in postoperative opioid analgesic requirements. They also found that high-intensity TEAS was more effective in decreasing postoperative analgesic requirement than low-intensity TEAS. Chen and colleagues (1998) conducted a similar study with surgical patients randomized to receive either transcutaneous electrical stimulation at one of the three locations: an acupuncture point, a non-acupuncture point, or at the dermatome corresponding to the surgical incision. The authors found that both TEAS and TENS at para-incisional dermatomes were effective in producing a similar analgesic-sparing effect after surgery. Importantly, simultaneous stimulation at both acupoints and dermatomes resulted in additive opioid-sparing effects. Lin et al. (2002) performed a large-scale RCT to examine effects of various frequencies of preoperative EA on postoperative pain and opioid-related side effects. They found that the postoperative analgesic effect is positively correlated to the frequency of the electrical stimulation. That is, 100 Hz of EA resulted in less analgesic consumption in the first 24 h postoperatively (Lin et al. 2002).

In conclusion, acupuncture is effective as an adjunctive treatment for the treatment of acute postoperative analgesia if administered to surgical patients in the postoperative period. Future studies should examine whether the efficacy of EA and related techniques is affected by the depth of anesthesia, types of anesthetics (i.e., intravenous versus volatile), and different states of anesthesia or types of anesthetics. It also seems that the analgesic effect of electroanalgesia is affected by the duration, amplitude, and frequencies of stimulation. Location of electrode placement plays a less significant role in the analgesic effect, and the placement of electrodes should be either an appropriate acupuncture points or at the peripheral nerves corresponding to the surgical incision.

Labor Analgesia

Acupuncture and related interventions have been considered as alternatives for pain relief for epidural labor analgesia. Acupuncture and related interventions were compared with meperidine consumption for labor analgesia. A randomized, non-blinded, controlled study found a decrease in the requirement for meperidine in the acupuncture group as compared to a control group with the same parity (Ramnero et al. 2002). Chung and colleagues applied acupressure as the analgesic for the first stage of labor (Chung et al. 2003). These investigators found that during the first stage of labor the patients who received acupressure reported significantly less labor pain compared to patients who received sham or no treatment. A recent study by Lee et al. (2004) performed a sham-controlled RCT to evaluate the analgesic effects of acupressure on the intensity of labor pain and duration of labor. These investigators reported that labor pain score during the first hour following the intervention was lower and the total labor time (i.e., delivery time) was significantly shorter in the acupressure versus sham control group. Therefore, available data indicate that acupuncture and related techniques may be effective for pain relief in the early stages of labor. However, more data are needed to establish the effectiveness of acustimulation techniques during the entire labor process.

Summary

To date, acupuncture and related interventions appear to serve as alternative and adjunctive treatment for various acute and chronic pain conditions. Since the release of NIH consensus, many high-quality scientifically valid clinical studies have been conducted examining this technique for a variety of pain syndromes. However, due to variations in the study designs and the duration of treatment and follow-up periods, available data do not support the long-term use or efficacy of acupuncture analgesia. The use of acupuncture and its timing in relation to anesthesia, duration of treatment, and frequency of acupuncture-related stimulation also play a significant role in the effectiveness of this modality. With the development of placebo needle techniques and the advancement of study design combined with imagining techniques, the effectiveness and the optimal timing for acupuncture in the perioperative period will be elucidated.

Case Scenario

Shu-Ming Wang, MSci, MD, Janet S. Jedlicka, PhD, OTR/L, Anne M. Haskins, PhD, OTR/L, and Jan E. Stube, PhD, OTR/L

Harris is a 45-year-old, otherwise healthy man suffering from lower back pain. He over exerted himself lifting a heavy box from the floor. He did not experience immediate pain until the following morning. He complained that his pain was very severe and had significantly affected his movement. He stated that he experienced sharp pain associated with every movement. The pain radiated downward over the buttocks and both legs. He had no other symptoms, and an MRI of his back was normal. The patient received several sessions of massage, but his symptoms and pain did not subside. As a result, he is here to receive acupuncture treatment.

Compare the pathological interpretation of low back pain in Chinese medicine to modern medicine?

Chinese medicine and modern medicine have radically different concepts regarding the etiology of back pain: Chinese concept of pathological changes is as follows. **The local muscles of the lower back were injured followed by overexertion. Consequently, the circulation of blood was retarded, which led to blood stasis. The development of blood stasis intensifies the pain and restriction of movement. On the other hand, modern medicine interprets the pain in terms of damage to anatomical structures.** Following the local muscle injury, inflammation occurred causing local release of lactic acid and substance P, which worsens the inflammation. Owing to pain and fear of pain, abnormal posturing is adopted to guard against pain and limited movement develops. The abnormal posture causes further inflammation that initiates the development of chronic low back pain.

Describe your treatment as an acupuncturist?
Manual acupuncture is administered include at the UB 63, and patient experiences instant relief of his low back pain. Other points considered include UB 57 and GB 34. UB 63 is an acupoint located on the lateral side of the foot, directly below the anterior border of the external malleolus, on the lower border of the cuboid bone. This particular point is called Jin Men, the Xi Cleft point in Chinese acupuncture and the intersection point of the bladder and Yang Wei meridians.

Harris responds to acupuncture therapy and he returns to normalcy. He is very grateful for your expertise.

Two years later, he develops a headache. It is an episodic and right-sided headache distributed along the temporal region. The headache is frequently triggered by stress and anxiety. The headache is fixed in the right temporal region, and the pain becomes worse when the patient feels sad or upset. In addition to headache, he suffers from occasional left-sided chest pain, which is not severe. His right upper arm feels uncomfortable, but there is no actual pain or limitation of movement. He sees a pain specialist, and acupuncture is his first choice. Therefore, he is back to consult you. You make the following diagnosis: right-sided headache represents obstruction in the channel, association of the pain with emotional changeless Yang dysfunction. Left-sided chest pain is associated with poor circulation of Qi in the chest.

According to the Chinese theory of headache, the right-sided headache is considered the lesser Yang channel and gallbladder Qi obstruction.

Briefly describe how modern medicine would interpret Harris' condition?
There is no single cause for stress headache (tension headache). In some people, this tension headache is caused by tightened muscle in the back of the neck and scalp or permanent structural change. In others, it is not the cause.

Describe your acupuncture treatment?
Manual acupuncture at the GB 20, GB 21, Li 3, and GV20 is one of the master analgesic points for any pain related to head and neck. GV20 is considered to have a calming, sedative effect. Other acupuncture points to be considered are GB20 – a local point for the neck muscle. Please refer to www.yinyanghouse.com for the locations of acupuncture points.

References

Allais G, De Lorenzo C, Quirico PE, Airola G, Tolardo G, Mana O, Benedetto C. Acupuncture in prophylactic treatment of migraine comparison with flunarizine. Headache 2002;42: 855–61.

Anderson JL, Lilja A, Hartvig P, Langstrom B, Gordh T, Handwerker H, Torebjork E. Somatotopic organization along the central sulcus, for pain localization in human as revealed by positron emission tomography. Exp Brain Res. 1997;117:192–9.

Baischer W. Acupuncture in Migraine: Long-term outcome and predicting factors. Headache 1995, 35:472–4.

Berman BM, Lao L, Langenberg P, Lee WL. Ilpin AM, Hochberg MC. Effectiveness of the knee: a randomized controlled trial. Ann Intern Med. 2004;21:902–20.

Berman BM, Singh BB, Lao L, Langengerg P, Lee H, Hadhazy V, Bareta J, Hochberg M. A randomized trial of acupuncture as an adjunctive therapy in osteoarthritis of the knee. Rheumatology 1999;38:346–54.

Besson JM, The neurobiology of pain. Lancet 1999;353:1610–5.

Biella G, Sotgiu ML, Pellegata G, Pauleus E, Castiglioni I, Fazio F. Acupuncture Procedures central activations in pain regions. Neuroimage 2001;14:60–6.

Bolay H, Moskowitz MA. Mechanism of pain modulation in chronic syndromes. Neurology 2002;59(Suppl 2):S2–7.

Carlsson C, Sjolund B. Acupuncture for chronic low back pain: a randomized placebo-controlled study with long-term follow-up. Clin J Pain. 2001;17:296–305.

Casey K, Minoshima S, Morrow T, Koeppe R. Comparison of human cerebral activation pattern during cutaneous warmth, heat pain and deep cold pain. J Neurophysiol. 1996;76:571–81.

Cassou B, Derriennic F, Monfort C, Norton J, Touranchet A. Chronic neck and shoulder pain, age, and working condition: longitudinal results from a large random sample in France. Occup Environ Med. 2002;59:537–44.

Chen L, Tang J, White PF. The effect of location of transcutaneous electrical nerve stimulation on postoperative opioid analgesic requirement: acupoint versus non-acupoint stimulation. Anesth Analg. 1998;87:1129–34.

Cheng T. Acupuncture anaesthesia for open-heart surgery. Heart 2000;83:256

Christensen PA, Noreng M, Andersen PE, Nielsen JW. Electroacupuncture and postoperative pain. Br J Anaesth. 1989;62:258–62.

Christensen PA, Rotne M, Vedelsdal R, Jensen RH, Jacobson K, Husted C. Electro-acupuncture in anaesthesia for hysterectomy. Br J Anaesth. 1993;71:835–8.

Chung U, Hung L, Kuo S, Huang C. Effects of LI4 and BL 67 acupressure on labor pain and uterine contractions in the first stage of labor. JNR. 2003;11:251–60.

Churchill JM. A Trestise on Acupuncturation being a description of a surgical operation peculiar to the Japanese and Chinese and by them demonstrated zin-king, now introduced into European practice, with directions for it's performance and cases illustrating its success. London: Simpkin and Marshall; 1821.

Côté P, Cassidy JD, Carroll L. The Saskatchewan health and back pain survey. The prevalence neck pain and related disability in Saskatchewan adults. Spine 1998;23:1689–98.

DeWoskin KJ. Doctors, diviners, and magicians of ancient China: biographies of Fang-Shih. New York, NY: Columbia University Press; 1983.

Epler DC Jr. Bloodletting in early Chinese medicine and its relation to the origin of acupuncture. Bull Hist Med. 1980;54:337–67.

Ezzo J, Berman B, Hadhazy VA, Jadad AR, Lao I, Singh BB. Is acupuncture effective for the treatment of chronic pain ? A systemic review. Pain 2000;86:217–25.

Fanti L, Gemma M, Passaretti S, Testoni P, Casati A. Electroacupuncture analgesia for colonoscopy, a prospective, randomized placebo-controlled study. Am J Gastroenterol. 2003;98:312–6.

Farquhar J. Knowing practice: the clinical encounter of Chinese medicine. Boulder, CO: Westview Press; 1994.

Gejervall A, Sterner-Victorin E, Möller A, Janson PO, Werner C, Bergh C. Elecrtoacupuncture versus conventional analgesia: a comparison of pain levels during oocyte aspiration and patients' experiences of well-being after surgery Hum Reprod. 2005;20(3):728–35.

Greenwood MT. Acupuncture and evidence-based medicine: a philosophical critique. Med Acupunct J. 2002;13:2.

Greif R, Laciny S, Mokhtarani M, Doufas AG, Bakhshandeh M, Dorfer L, Sessler DI. Transcutaneous electrical stimulation of an auricular acupuncture point decreases anesthetic requirement. Anesthesiology 2002;96:306–12.

Gupta S, Francis JD, Tillu AB, Sattirajah I, Sizer J. The effect of pre-emptive acupuncture treatment on analgesic requirements after day-case knee arthroscopy. Anaesthesia 1999;54:1204–19.

Hahn RA. 'Treat the patient, not the lab': internal medicine and the concept of 'person'. Cult Med Psychiatry. 1982;6:219–36.

Han JS, Tang J. Tolerance to electroacupuncture and its cross tolerance to morphine. Neuropharmacology 1981;20:593–6.

He D, Bo Veiersted K, Høstmark A, Ingulf Medbø J. Effect of acupuncture treatment on chronic neck and shoulder pain in sedentary female workers: a 6 month and 3 year follow up study. Pain 2004;109;299–307.

Helms JM. Acupuncture for the management of primary dysmenorrhea. Obstet Gynecol. 1987;69:51–6.

Humaidan P, Sterner-Victorin E. Pain relief during oocyte retrieval with a new short duration electro-acupuncture techniques-an alternative to conventional analgesic methods. Hum Reprod. 2004, 19(6):1367–72.

Irnich D, Behrens N, Gleditsch J, Stor W, Schreiber M, Schops P, Vickers A, Beyer A. Immediate effects of dry needling and acupuncture at distant points in chronic neck pain: results of a randomized, double-blind, sham-controlled crossover trial. Pain 2002;99: 83–9.

Irnich D, Behrens N, Molzen H, Konig A, Gleditsch J, Krauss M, Natalis M, Senn E, Beyer A, Schops P. Randomised trial of acupuncture compared with conventional massage and "sham" laser acupuncture for treatment of chronic neck pain. Br Med J. 2001;322:1574–77.

Kaptchuk TJ, The web that has no weaver: understanding Chinese medicine. 2nd ed. Lincolnwood, IL: Contemporary Books (McGraw-Hill); 2000.

Kaptchuk TJ. Acupuncture: theory, efficacy, and practice. Complementary and alternative medicine series, Series Editor. Eisenberg DM and Academia and Clinic.

Klein JR, Litt IF. Epidemiology of adolescent dysmenorrhea. Pediatrics 1981;68:661–4.

Kotani N, Hashimoto H, Sato Y, Sessler DI, Yoshioka H, Kitayama M, Yasuda T, Matsuki A. Preoperative intradermal acupuncture reduces postoperative pain, nausea and vomiting, analgesic requirement, and sympathoadrenal responses. Anesthesiology 2001; 95:349–56.

Kvorning N, Christiansson C, Beskow A, Bratt O, Akeson J. Acupuncture fails to reduce but increases anaesthetic gas required to prevent movement in response to surgical incision. Acta Anaesth Scand. 2003;47:818–22.

Langevin HM, Churchill DL, Cipolla MJ. Mechanical signaling through connective tissue: A mechanism for the therapeutic effect of acupuncture FASEB J. 2001b;91:2275–82.

Langevin HM, Churchill DL, Fox JR, Badger GJ, Garra BS, Krag MH. Biomechanical response to acupuncture needling in humans. J Appl Physiol. 2001a;91:2471–8.

Lee M, Chang S, Kang D. Effects of SP6 acupressure on labor pain and length of delivery time in women during labor. J Alt Complem Med. 2004;10:959–65.

Leibing E, Leonhardt U, Koster G, Goerlitz A, Rosenfeldt J, Hilgers R, Ramadori G. Acupuncture treatment of chronic low-back pain – a randomized, blinded, placebo-controlled trial with 9-month follow-up. Pain 2002;96:189–96.

Lin J, Lo M, Wen Y, Hsieh C, Tsai S, Sun W. The effect of high and low frequency electroacupuncture in pain after abdominal surgery. Pain 2002;99:509–14.

Linde K, Streng A, Jügens S, Hopps A, Brinkhaus B, Witt C, Wagenpfell S, Pfaffenrah V, Hammes G, Weldenhammer W, Willich S, Mechart D. Acupuncture for patient with migraine JAMA. 2005;293:2118–25.

Liptom RB, Stewart WF, Diamons S, Diamond ML, Reed M. Prevalence and burden of migraine in the United States: data from the American migraine study II. Headache 2001;41:646–57.

Liu G, Akira H. Basic Principle of TCM. In Liu G, Akira H; Eds. Fundamentals of acupuncture and moxibustion. Tianjin, China: Tianjin Science and Technology Translation and Publishing Corporation; 1994. pp. 9–32.

McRae G. A critical overview of U.S. Acupuncture regulation. J Health Policy Law. 1982;7:163–96.

Meichart D, Linde K, Fischer P, White A, Vicker A, Berman B. Acupuncture for recurrent headache: A systematic review of randomized controlled trials. Cephalalgia 2002; 19:779–86.

Melzack R, Wall PD. Pain Mechanism: a new theory. Science 1965;150:971–9.

Meng C, Wang D, Ngeow J, Lao L, Peterson M, Paget S. Acupuncture for chronic low back pain in older patients: a randomized, controlled trial. Rheumatology 2003;42:1508–17.

Molsberger A, Mau J, Pawelec D, Winkler J. Does acupuncture improve the orthopedic management of chronic low back pain – a randomized, blinded, controlled trial with 3 months follow up. Pain 2002;99:579–87.

Morioka N, Akca O, Doufas A, Chernyak G, Sessler DI. Electro-acupuncture at the Zusanli, Yanglingquan, and Kunlan points does not reduce anesthetic requirement. Anesth Analg. 2002;95:98–102.

Nabeta T, Kawakita K. Relief of chronic neck and shoulder pain by manual acupuncture to tender points – a sham-controlled randomized trial. Complem Ther Med. 2002;10:217–22.

NIH consensus developmental panel on acupuncture. JAMA. 1998;280:1518–24.

Parienet J, White P, Frackowiak RSJ, Lewith G. Expectancy and brief modulate the neural substrates of pain treated by acupuncture. Neuroimage 2005;25:1161–7.

Patel M, Gutawillwe F, Paccaud F, Marazzi A. A meta-analysis of acupuncture for chronic pain. Int J Epidemiol. 1989;18:900–6.

Pintov S, Lahat E, Alstein M, Vogel Z, Barg J. Acupuncture and the opioid system: implications in management of migraine. Pediatr Neurol. Sep 1997;17(2):129–33.

Pomeraez B. Scientific basis of acupuncture. In: Stux G, Pomweanz B, editors. Basis of acupuncture. 4th ed. Heidelberg: Springer; 1998:7–9.

Quatan N, Bailey C, Larking A, Boyd PJ, Watkin N. Stick and stones: use of acupuncture in extracorporeal shockwave lithotripsy. J Endourol. 2003;17:867–70.

Ramnero A, Hanson U, Kihlgren M. Acupuncture treatment during labour – a randomised controlled trial. Br J Obstet Gyn. 2002;109:637–44.

Rogenhofer S, Wimmer K, Blana A, et al. Acupuncture for pain in extracorporeal shockwave lithotripsy. J Endourol. 2004;18:634–7.

Sator-Katzenschlager S, Scharbert G, Kozek-Langenecker S, Szeles J, Finster G, Schiesser A, Heinze G, Kress H. The short- and long-term benefit in chronic low back pain through adjuvant electrical versus manual auricular acupuncture. Anesth Analg. 2004;98:1359–64.

Sator-Katzenschlager S, Szeles J, Scharbert G, Michalek-Sauberer A, Kober A, Heinze G, Kozek-Langenecker S. Electrical stimulation of auricular acupuncture points is more effective than conventional manual auricular acupuncture in chronic cervical pain: a pilot study. Anesth Analg. 2003;97:1469–73.

Schaer H. Zur Quantifizierung der analgetisch. Anaesthesist 1979;28:52–5.

Sim CK, Xu PC, Pua HL, Zhang G, Lee TL. Effects of electroacupuncture on intraoperative and postoperative analgesic requirement. Acupunct Med. 2002;20:56–65.

Stewart WF, Lipton RB, Celentano DD, Reed ML. Prevalence of migraine headache in the United States. Relation to age, income, race and other sociodemographic factors. JAMA. 1992;267:64–69.

Sterner-Victorin E, Waldenström, Nilsson L, Wikland M, Janson O. A prospective randomized study of electroacupuncture versus alfentanil as anaesthesia during oocyte aspiration in in-vitro fertilization. Hum Reprod. 1999;14:2480–4.

Streitberger K, Kleinhenz J. Introduction a placebo needle into acupuncture research. Lancet 1998;352:364–5.

Taguchi A, Sharma N, Ali SZ, Dave B, Sessler DI, Kurz A. The effect of auricular acupuncture on anaesthesia with desflurane. Anaesthesia 2002;57:1159–63.

Taylor D, Miaskowski C, Kohn J. A randomized clinical trial of the effectiveness of an acupressure device (Relief Brief®) for managing symptom of Dysmenorrhea. J Complem Altern Med. 2002;8:357–70.

Ter Riet G, Keipachild P. Acupuncture and chronic pain: a criteria-based meta-analysis J Clin Epidemiol. 1990;43:1191–9.

Thomas M, Lundeberg T, Björk G, Lundström-Lindstedy V. Pain and discomfort in primary dysmenorrhea is reduced by preemptive acupuncture or low frequency TENS. Eur J Phys Med Rehabil. 1995;5:71–6.

Unschuld PU. Medicine in China: history of idea. Berkeley, CA: University California Press; 1985.

Usichenko T, Dinse M, Hermsen M, Witstruck T, Pavlovic D, Lehmann C. Auricular acupuncture for pain relief after total hip arthroplasty – a randomized controlled study. Pain 2005;114:320–7.

Vickers A. Acupuncture for treatment of chronic neck pain: reanalysis of data suggests that effect is not a placebo effect. Br Med J. 2001;323:1306–7.

Wang B, Tang J, White PF, Naruse R, Sloninsky A, Kariger R, Gold J, Wender RH. Effect of the intensity of transcutaneous acupoint electrical stimulation on the postoperative analgesic requirement. Anesth Analg. 1997;85:406–13.

Wang H, Chang Y, Liu D, Ho Y. A clinical study on physiological response in electroacupuncture analgesia and meperidine analgesia for colonoscopy. Am J Chin Med. 1997;25:13–20.

Wang K, Yao S, Xian Y, Hou Z. A study on the receptor field on acupoints and the relationship between characteristics of needling sensation and groups of afferent fibres. Sci Sin. 1985;28:963–71.

Wang L, Zhao W, Yu J. Cardini F, Forcella E, Regalia AL, Wade C. Vitamin K Acupuncture point injection for severe primary dysmenorrhea: an international pilot study. MedGenMed 2004;6:45–54.

Wang SM, Constable RT, Tokoglu FS, Weiss DA, Freyle D, Kain ZN. Acupuncture-induced blood oxygenation level dependent signals in awake and anesthetized volunteers: a pilot study. Anesth Analg. 2007;105:499–506.

Wang SM, Punjala M, Weiss D, Anderson K, Kain ZN. Acupuncture as an adjunct for sedation during lithotripsy. J Alternat Complem Med. 2007;13;241–6.

Wang SM. Kain ZN. White PF. Acupuncture analgesia (I): the scientific basis (I). Anesth Analg. 2008;106:602–10.

White P, Lewith G, Prescott P, Conway J. Acupuncture versus placebo for the treatment of chronic mechanical neck pain: a randomized, controlled trial. Ann Int Med. 2004;141:911–9.

Wilson CA, Keye WR Jr. A survey of adolescent dysmenorrhea and premenstrual symptom frequency. A model program for prevention, detection, and treatment. J Adolesc Health Care. 1989;10:317–22.

Witt C, Brinkhaus B, Jena S, Linde K, Streng A, Wagenpfeil S, Hummelsberger J, Walther H, Melchart D, Willich S. Acupuncture in patients with osteoarthritis of the knee: a randomised trial. Lancet 2005;366:136–43.

www.eastwestacupuncture.net/reston.htm

www.nih.gov/about/almanac/organization/NCCAM.htm

www.nih.gov/news/pr/dec2004/nccam-20.htm

www.ninds.nih.gov/disorders/backpain/detail_backpain.htm

Chapter 17

Nursing Perspective on Pain Management

Ena Williams, MBA, MSM, RN

Introduction

Clinicians who care for patients have an ethical obligation to relieve pain and suffering using a combination of approaches including medical, pharmacological, and psychological. According to the Agency of Healthcare Research and Quality (AHRQ), the most reliable indicator of the existence and intensity of pain is the patient's self-report (Potter and Perry 2009).

The AHRQ developed clinical practice guidelines on acute pain management and contends that all patients should be assessed and reassessed for severity of pain using a rating scale or a visual analogue scale. Pain is now classified as the fifth vital sign which then requires that pain should be assessed and reassessed at a minimum when vital signs are obtained (Smeltzer et al. 2008). It is important to remember that not all patients respond to pain in the same manner. Basic measures of pain intensity should be prioritized with the patient's self-report as the most important measure. Other measures of pain intensity include exposure to a painful procedure; behavioral signs, such as crying or restlessness; a proxy pain rating by someone who knows the patient well; and the psychological indicators such as elevated vital signs.

The clinician must accept and respect the patient's report of pain and proceed with an appropriate assessment and treatment. The clinician is entitled to a personal opinion but should not allow it to guide practice. Patients of differing cultures respond to pain and express pain differently, and the clinician needs to be aware of this (Smeltzer et al. 2008).

Symptomatic relief of pain should be provided while the investigation of cause proceeds. Unrelieved pain may be dangerous and is unacceptable. Postoperative pain can delay healing and contribute to complications that can be life threatening. Acute pain warns of actual or potential tissue damage and resolves when healing has occurred. Unrelieved postoperative pain is a complication or risk, not an acceptable consequence of surgery (2). Good pain management promotes healing and can result in shorter hospital stays and reduce admissions and readmissions.

The Joint Commission which accredits health-care institution provides guidelines for how facilities should educate, assess, and manage pain. The standard states that "the hospital must assess and manage pain." The Joint Commission also encourages patients to speak up and provides tools for clinician to use in informing patients (Fig. 17.1) (JC.org 2010).

N. Vadivelu et al. (eds.), *Essentials of Pain Management*,
DOI 10.1007/978-0-387-87579-8_17, © Springer Science+Business Media, LLC 2011

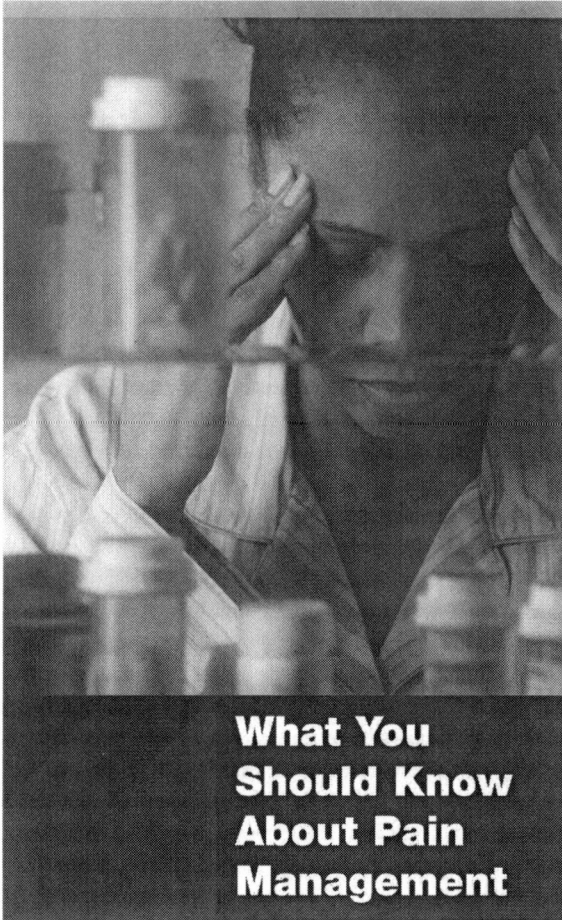

Figure 17.1   JC speak up brochure for pain management. With permission from Joint Commission Resources, Oakbrook Terrace, IL.

What Is Pain?

The International Society of Pain (IASP), defined pain as an uncomfortable feeling and/or an unpleasant subjective, sensory and emotional experience associated with the actual or potential tissue damage or described in terms of such damage. The presence of pain often is an indication that something is wrong. Pain can appear suddenly or can come about slowly. It is also described as whatever the experiencing person says it is, existing whenever the person says it does. The guiding principle in pain care is that pain is whatever the patient says it is (Potter and Perry 2009).

Each individual is the best judge of his or her own pain. Feelings of pain can range from mild and occasional to severe and constant. Pain can be classified as acute pain or chronic pain.

Acute Pain

Acute pain begins suddenly and is usually sharp in quality. It serves as a warning of disease or a threat to the body. Acute pain might be caused by many events or circumstances, including

- surgery,
- broken bones,
- dental work,
- burns or cuts, and
- labor and childbirth.

Acute pain might be mild and last just a moment, or it might be severe and last for weeks or months. In most cases, acute pain does not last longer than 6 months, and it disappears when the underlying cause of pain has been treated or has healed. Unrelieved acute pain, however, might lead to chronic pain.

Chronic Pain

Chronic pain persists despite the fact that the injury has healed. Pain signals remain active in the nervous system for weeks, months, or years. Physical effects include tense muscles, limited mobility, a lack of energy, and changes in appetite. Emotional effects include depression, anger, anxiety, and fear of reinjury. Such a fear might hinder a person's ability to return to normal work or leisure activities. Common chronic pain complaints include

- headache,
- low back pain,
- cancer pain,
- arthritis pain,
- neurogenic pain (pain resulting from damage to nerves), and
- psychogenic pain (pain not due to past disease or injury or any visible sign of damage inside).

Chronic pain might have originated with an initial trauma/injury or infection, or there might be an ongoing cause of pain. However, some people suffer chronic pain in the absence of any past injury or evidence of body damage (www.myclevelandclinic.org).

How Is Pain Treated?

Depending upon its severity, pain might be treated in a number of ways. Symptomatic options for the treatment of pain might include one or more of the following:

- Non-steroidal anti-inflammatory drugs (NSAIDs), a specific type of painkiller such as Motrin® (Pfizer, New York, NY) or Aleve® (Bayer Pharmaceuticals, Morristown, NJ)
- Acetaminophen (such as Tylenol®; Ortho-McNeil-Janssen, New Brunswick, NJ)

- Opioids (such as morphine or codeine)
- Localized anesthetic (a shot of a painkiller medicine into the area of the pain)
- Nerve blocks (the blocking of a group of nerves with local anesthetics)
- Acupuncture
- Electrical stimulation
- Physical therapy
- Surgery
- Psychotherapy (talk therapy)
- Relaxation techniques such as deep breathing
- Biofeedback (treatment technique in which people are trained to improve their health by using signals from their own bodies)
- Behavior modification

Some pain medicines are more effective in fighting pain when they are combined with other methods of treatment. Patients might need to try various methods to maintain maximum pain relief (Donofrio and Labus 2007).

The role of the nurse is critical in the management of pain. It is primarily the nurse that will be assessing, treating, and reassessing pain status. It is therefore critical for the patient to have a plan of care which includes pain management. Several pain intensity and distress scales are available for assisting the patient and health-care giver with pain management. The following information offers important information about the role of the nurse in assessment and reassessment of pain. There are some basic guiding principles to be aware of when managing pain especially related to surgical intervention.

Principles

- Patients who may have difficulty communicating their pain require particular attention. This includes patients who are cognitively impaired, psychotic, or severely emotionally disturbed; children; the elderly; patients who do not speak English; and patients whose level of education or cultural background differs significantly from that of the health-care team.
- Unexpected intense pain, particularly if sudden and associated with altered vital signs, such as hypotension, tachycardia, or fever, should be evaluated immediately, and new diagnosis such as wound dehiscence, infection, or deep vein thrombosis, should be considered.
- Family members should be involved when appropriate.

The preoperative preparation of the patient cannot be overemphasized. This will enhance the recovery period and prepare the patient in understanding their role and the clinician's role in managing their pain. Inform patients that it is easier to prevent pain than to chase it and reduce it after it has become established, and that communication of unrelieved pain is essential to its relief. Emphasize the importance of factual report of pain.

The following things should be considered in the preoperative preparation of the patient. It is important to discuss the patient's previous experiences with pain and beliefs about the preferences for pain assessment and management. Provide the patient information about pain management therapies that are available and the rationale underlying their use. Develop with the patient a plan for pain assessment and management, select a pain assessment tool and teach the patient to use it, and provide the patient with education and information about pain control, distraction, imagery, and massage.

Management of pain can be so varied that various types of pain assessment tools have been developed. It should be remembered that the most reliable indicator of the existence and intensity of pain and any resultant distress is the patient's self-report. Self-report measurement scales include numeric or adjective ratings and visual analogue scales (see Chapter 5). The tools should be reliable, valid, and easy for the patient and the nurse and physician to use. One may use these tools by showing a diagram to the patient to indicate the appropriate rating. One may also use tools by simply asking the patient for a verbal response: "on a scale of 0–10 with 0 being as no pain and 10 being as the worst pain possible, how would you rate your pain?" Tools must be appropriate for the patient's developmental, physical, emotional, and cognitive status.

Postoperatively the patient's perception along with behavioral and psychological response should be carefully assessed. Observations of behavior and vital signs should not be used instead of self-reporting, unless the patient is unable to communicate.

Pain should be assessed and reassessed frequently during the immediate postoperative period. The frequency of assessment should be based on the operation performed and the severity of the pain. Pain should be assessed every 2 h during the first postoperative day of the major surgery. If necessary, increase the frequency of assessment and reassessment if the pain is poorly controlled or if interventions are changing. Pain intensity and response to intervention should be recorded in an easily visible and accessible place, such as a bedside flow sheet. Observations of behavior and vital signs should not be used instead of self-reporting, unless the patient is unable to communicate.

Review with the patient before discharge the interventions used and their effectiveness and provide specific discharge instructions regarding pain and its management (Rothrock 2011).

Pain Assessment

Once a patient answers yes to whether they have pain or not, a licensed health-care provider should perform a comprehensive pain assessment and an appropriate pain assessment scale selected. The assessment should include a comprehensive evaluation of

- pain history (acute, chronic, or both),
- location,
- characteristics,
- onset/duration,
- frequency,
- quality,
- intensity/severity,
- precipitating factors, and
- alleviating factors.

Additional factors to include are conditions affecting pain response and who is providing the information:

- Cultural/spiritual
- Presence of chronic/persistent pain
- Gender
- Extent of tissue damage
- Psychosocial
- Behavioral/physiologic signs of discomfort (especially in those who have difficulty or are unable to communicate)
- Information provider
  - Patient
  - Family
  - Other primary caregiver (Potter and Perry 2009)

Pain Assessment Scales

These are tools clinicians such as nurses use to assist in assessment of the patient's pain. It is always important to remember that the single most important and reliable indicator of pain is the patient self-reporting. Some patients, however, may be unable to communicate, and in these cases, objective pain assessment scales are needed. The nurse is guided by the recommendations of the Joint Commission that the "hospital uses methods to assess pain that are consistent with the patient's age, conditions, and ability to understand (www.JC.org)."

0 – 10 Numeric Rating Scale (page 1 of 1)

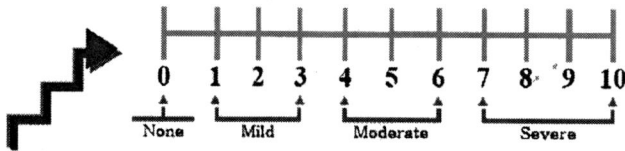

Indications Adults and children (> 9 years old) in all patient care settings who are able to use numbers to rate the intensity of their pain

Instructions:

1 The patient is asked any one of the following questions
   - What number would you give your pain right now?
   - What number on a 0 to 10 scale would you give your pain when it is the worst that it gets and when it is the best that it gets?
   - At what number is the pain at an acceptable level for you?
2. When the explanation suggested in #1 above is not sufficient for the patient, it is sometimes helpful to further explain or conceptualize the Numeric Rating Scale in the following manner
   - 0 = No Pain
   - 1-3 = Mild Pain (nagging, annoying, interfering little with ADLs)
   - 4–6 = Moderate Pain (interferes significantly with ADLs)
   - 7-10 = Severe Pain (disabling, unable to perform ADLs)
3 The interdisciplinary team in collaboration with the patient/family (if appropriate), can determine appropriate interventions in response to Numeric Pain Ratings

Figure 17.2 Example of a pain intensity instrument/scale – numeric rating scale. National Institutes of Health, Warren Grant Magnuson Clinical Center. Pain Intensity Instruments, July 2003.

Once the nurse has made a plan of care for the patient, pain assessments are to be completed using the Assessment, Intervention, and Reassessment (AIR) cycle of the patient's pain. This is used with the chosen pain assessment scale and is performed according to the institution's guideline.

The nurse must be knowledgeable of the different pain scales and how they are to be applied and included in the pain plan of care (Figs. 17.2 and 17.3; Table 17.1; also see Chapter 5). Pain scores should be assessed and documented at a minimum as follows:

- prior to any pain-relieving intervention (pharmacological or non-pharmacological),
- with any new report of pain, and
- with complete set of vital signs (temperature, pulse, blood pressure, respiratory rate, and oxygen saturation).

Checklist of Non-Verbal Indicators (CNVI) (page 1 of 1)

	With Movement	At Rest
Vocal Complaints – nonverbal expression of pain demonstrated by moans, groans, grunts, cries, gasps, sighs)		
Facial Grimaces and Winces – furrowed brow, narrowed eyes, tightened lips, dropped jaw, clenched teeth, distorted expression		
Bracing – clutching or holding onto siderails, bed, tray table, or affected area during movement		
Restlessness – constant or intermittent shifting of position, rocking, intermittent or constant hand motions, inability to keep still		
Rubbing – massaging affected area		
Vocal complaints – verbal expression of pain using words, e.g., "ouch" or "that hurts;" cursing during movement, or exclamations of protest, e.g., "stop" or "that's enough "		
TOTAL SCORE		

Indications: Behavioral Health adults who are unable to validate the presence of or quantify the severity of pain using either the Numerical Rating Scale or the Wong-Baker Faces Pain Rating Scale.

Instructions:
1. Write a 0 if the behavior was not observed
2. Write a 1 if the behavior even briefly during activity or rest
3. Results in a total score between 0 and 5.
4. The interdisciplinary team in collaboration with the patient (if appropriate), can determine appropriate interventions in response to CNVI scores.

Figure 17.3 Non-verbal indicators. National Institutes of Health, Warren Grant Magnuson Clinical Center. Pain Intensity Instruments, July 2003.

Table 17.1 Face, Legs, Activity, Cry, Consolability (FLACC) Scale.

Category	Scoring		
	1	2	3
Face	No particular expression or smile	Occasional grimace or frown, withdrawn, disinterested	Frequent to constant quivering chin, clenched jaw
Legs	Normal position or relaxed	Uneasy, restless, tense	Kicking or legs drawn up
Activity	Lying quietly, normal position, moves easily	Squirming, shifting back and forth, tense	Arched, rigid, or jerking
Cry	No cry (awake or asleep)	Moans or whispers, occasional complaint	Crying steadily, screams, or sobs, frequent complaints
Consolability	Content, relaxed	Reassured by occasional touching, hugging, or being talk to, distractable	Difficult to console or comfort

Each of the five categories (F) Face, (L) Legs, (A) Activity, (C) Cry, (C) Consolability is scored from 0 to 2, which results in a total score between 0 and 10. Adapted from Merkel et al. (1997).

Pain Interventions

Pain interventions can be pharmacological and non-pharmacological. A combination of both is often the best intervention. The nurse collaborates with the LIP to communicate the effectiveness of the pain management so that appropriate medications can be ordered and administered as needed or as prescribed. The nurse must check the orders and ensure that all specific elements are included especially in titrated and range orders. The nurse must closely monitor the effect of the titration, any negative and positive effects, and documents in the patient's medical record. The nurse also administers the site of intramuscular medications for redness and hematoma and the patient for respiratory depression, nausea, and vomiting and mental status changes. The nurse frequently collaborates with the physician/LIP to implement the appropriate medications for achieving the patient's pain goal.

Non-pharmacological approach may include massage, meditation, counseling, relaxation, music, distraction, heat/cold, and deep breathing (Smeltzer et al. 2008).

Patient and Family Education

The nurse must constantly teach the patient and family about pain control methods. They should be encouraged to participate in effective pain management and educated about the pain tools and how management of the pain will improve their quality of life. Also, it is important to teach the patient about pain medications and side effects.

Summary

The nurse plays a critical role in assisting the patient with effective management of their pain. The nurse should be knowledgeable and sensitive in his/her interaction with all patients, with an understanding that patients vary in their experience, response, and treatment modalities for pain.

Case Scenario

Ellie Sutton, MBBS

Kumar is an 85-year-old man who fell in his garden and fractured right neck of his femur. His co-morbidities include hypertension (treated with thiazides), ischemic heart disease (he had a myocardial infarction 3 years ago and had a CABG on the same admission), benign prostatic hypertrophy, and asthma (for which he uses inhalers as needed). He is admitted to the hospital with a femur traction and you are the nurse taking care of Kumar. He is awaiting surgery that afternoon. He has had hydromorphone in the emergency department and has been prescribed oral hydromorphone and acetaminophen PRN.

Describe your preoperative preparation for this patient with respect to pain management?
Kumar is an elderly gentleman and it is essential to develop a rapport with him and to have a comprehensive assessment with regard to his background, communication abilities, and emotional needs – in addition to his medical and surgical problems. You need to discuss with Kumar his previous experiences with pain and explain pain treatment options available. You will also require selecting an appropriate pain assessment tool that is understood by the patient.

Kumar appears to be stoic with well-preserved mental capacity. He understands and agrees to use the verbal scoring system for pain assessment. He tells you that at present the pain score is about 3 on a maximum scale of 10 at rest and it is about 5 with movement. Fifteen minutes later he calls you and says he is "in agony."

How would you assess the pain?
You have to follow the AIR cycle (see chapter). Use the verbal scoring system to assess pain. The next step would be to find out the cause for the abrupt increase in pain. Kumar points to his hip and says the pain score is now 9 out of 10. He is now tachycardic and hypertensive. He mentions that the pain shot up when he tried to lift his right leg. You lift up the blanket **and you suddenly notice that the femoral traction has slipped out of the pulley!** You get help and set the traction right; the pain score settles back to 3 within minutes.

Soon he is transferred to the OT and later returns to your ward after undergoing a hemiarthroplasty of the hip under general anesthesia combined with fascia iliaca compartment block. His postoperative analgesia included a hydromorphone PCA. He has stable vital signs and is sleepy but easily aroused. Once he is settled, you assess the pain, and Kumar mumbles a score of 2.

What is a PCA and how does it work? How is it beneficial to patients and nursing staff?
PCA stands for patient-controlled analgesia, and it is an electronically controlled infusion pump that delivers a prescribed amount of intravenous analgesia (in this case hydromorphone) to the patient when he/she activates a button. This form of analgesia gives the patient more control over their pain: they can receive analgesia when they need it, and greater patient satisfaction has been reported compared to

IV PRN administration by the nurse. From the nursing perspective, PCA reduces the workload because it is preloaded with multiple doses and it can also help reduce medication errors and opioid-related oversedation.

You set up the monitor, PCA, make sure that the nasal prongs are delivering oxygen, and leave to attend to another patient. When you recheck on Kumar you find him restless, agitated, and attempting to pull out all his IV lines and nasal prongs.

Describe your management?
You have to execute the AIR cycle. You check his respirations and other vital signs and then undertake a review of all medications recently administered. A review of PCA pump shows that he has made several successful attempts at pressing the PCA button and has received 2 mg of hydromorphone within the last hour. However, Kumar is unable to comply with your assessment of pain score. He is hypertensive and tachycardic. He is attempting to touch his lower abdomen, and he is trying to tug on the urinary catheter. You notice that there is suprapubic swelling and the urine bag is empty. The urine output since he came to the ward has been minimal. On palpation you notice that he has a distended urinary bladder.

What would you do next?
The most likely cause of Kumar's distress appears to be a distended bladder. The first step is to evaluate the Foley catheter. You flush the catheter with 50 ml sterile water using a bladder syringe. You notice that when you do this the water is leaking from around the catheter. You then notice that the catheter tip is outside the bladder. You decide to insert a new, sterile catheter, which consequently drains about 600 ml of urine. Kumar settles down and appears to be very much relieved. You assess the pain score now and he states it is a "2."

References

American Society of Peri-Anesthesia Nurses. ASPAN pain and comfort guideline. http://www.aspan.org/Portals/6/docs/ClinicalPractice/Guidelines/ASPAN_ClinicalGuideline_PainComfort.pdf. Accessed 29 Oct 2009.

American Society of Peri-Anesthesia Nurses. Standards of peri-anesthesia nursing practice. Cherry Hill, NJ: The Society; 2008–2010.

Barash PG, Cullen BF, Stoelting RK, Cahalan MK, Stock, MC. Clinical anesthesia. Philadelphia, PA: Lippincott Williams & Wilkins; 2009.

Cancer Pain Management in Children. http://www.childcancerpain.org/content.cfm?content=assess08. Accessed 29 Oct 2009.

Doe JB. Conceptual planning: a guide to a better planet, 3rd ed. Reading, MA: Smith Jones; 1996.

Donofrio J, Labus D. Fundamentals of Nursing Made Incredibly Easy. 1st ed. PA: Lippincott Williams & Wilkins; 2007.

Fishman SM, Ballantyne JC, Rathmell JP. Bonica's management of pain. 4th ed. Philadelphia, PA: Lippincott Williams & Wilkins; 2010.

McCaffery M, Beebe A. Pain management for nursing practice. Baltimore, MD: Mosby Company; 1993.

Merkel S, et al. The FLACC: a behavioral scale for scoring postoperative pain in young children. Pediatr Nurse. 1997;23(3):293–7.

Partners Against Pain. http://www.partnersagainstpain.com. Accessed 29 Oct 2009.

Potter PA, Perry AG. Fundamentals of nursing. 7th ed. Mosby Elsevier; 2009.

Smeltzer SC, Bare BG, Janice HL, Kerry CH. Brunner and Suddarth's textbook of medical-surgical nursing. 11th ed. Philadelphia, PA: Lippincott Williams & Wilkins; 2008.

Rothrock JC. Alexander's care of the patient in surgery. 13th ed. St. Louis, MO: Mosby; 2007.

The Cleveland Clinic Website: Pain Management. http://my.clevelandclinic.org/services/pain_management/hic_acute_vs_chronic_pain.aspx. Accessed 29 Oct 2009.

The Joint Commission Website. http://www.jointcommission.org/NR/rdonlyre. Accessed 29 Oct 2010.

Chapter 18

Post-surgical Pain Management

Darin J. Correll, MD

Introduction

Why should we care about controlling pain in the postoperative period? Better pain control, depending on the agent(s) and modalities used, leads to benefits in terms of cardiovascular and respiratory complications as well as endocrine, immunologic, gastrointestinal, and hematological outcomes (Liu 2007). Another reason is that patients are often more concerned about being in pain than they are about the primary reason for being in the hospital. In addition, the quality of recovery is improved, and acute pain may become chronic/persistent if not treated properly (Carr 1999).

Pain Assessment and Mechanism of Pain

Listen to and believe the patient; pain is always subjective and one must accept the patient's report of pain. It is important to ask the patient what analgesic therapies have either worked or not worked in the past, as well as if they were taking any analgesic agents prior to admission, and if so the exact doses. Ask about all the *locations* where the patient is experiencing pain and any *radiation* from the primary location(s). Have the patient rate the *intensity* of the pain on a regular basis using scales appropriate for the patient (see Chapter 5).

The most commonly used measurement tools for intensity of pain in the postoperative setting are the single dimension scales. A frequently used variation of this scale is the verbal numeric scale where patients are asked to verbally state a number between 0 and 10, where 0 is "no pain at all" and 10 is "the worst pain imaginable," to correspond to their present pain intensity (see Chapter 5).

In order to choose the correct therapy for treating pain, the underlying mechanism or generator of the pain needs to be determined (Table 18.1). One of the best ways to determine this is to have the patient use adjectives to describe the *character* of the pain (e.g., aching, burning, dull, electric-like, sharp, shooting, stabbing, tender, throbbing). In the postoperative period it is still important to determine the *impact* of the pain on the patient's functional ability; specifically does the pain affect the patient's ability to cough, get out of bed, and ambulate while in the hospital.

Analgesic Modalities

There is no one correct way to treat a patient in pain, but a multimodal approach is always better than using a single modality to its "limit"; this can include both pharmacologic and

N. Vadivelu et al. (eds.), *Essentials of Pain Management*,
DOI 10.1007/978-0-387-87579-8_18, © Springer Science+Business Media, LLC 2011

Table 18.1 Mechanisms of pain.

Pain mechanism	Character	Examples	Treatment options
Somatic	• Usually well localized • Constant • Aching, sharp, stabbing	• Laceration • Fracture • Burn • Abrasion • Localized infection or inflammation	• Heat/cold • Acetaminophen • NSAIDs • Opioids • Local anesthetics (topical or infiltrate)
Visceral	• Not well localized • Constant or intermittent • Ache, pressure, cramping, sharp	• Muscle spasm • Colic or obstruction (GI or renal) • Sickle cell crisis • Internal organ infection or inflammation	• NSAIDs • Opioids • Muscle relaxants Local anesthetics (nerve blocks)
Neuropathic	• Localized (i.e., dermatomal) or radiating, can also be diffuse • Burning, tingling, electric shock, lancinating	• Trigeminal • Post-herpetic • Post-amputation • Peripheral neuropathy • Nerve infiltration	• Anticonvulsants • Antidepressants • NMDA antagonists • Neural/neuraxial blockade

NSAIDs, non-steroidal anti-inflammatory drugs; GI,gastrointestinal; NMDA, N-methyl-D-aspartate.

non-pharmacologic measures. It is best to individualize therapy for each patient with the addition or alteration of agents when pain control is inadequate and an adjustment or diminishing of agents as the pain resolves. In terms of pharmacologic measures, there are many different agents available that can be divided into three basic categories: non-opioid analgesics, opioids, and adjuvant analgesics (American Pain Society 2008). Most of these agents can be administered through a variety of routes including enteral, parenteral, and neuraxial. The neuraxial, specifically epidural, route will be discussed specifically in the sections on patient-controlled epidural analgesia below. Always discuss the analgesic plan with the patient and family, understand the patient's expectations for pain management, and offer reasonable goals for the therapy. If pain is present most of the time or expected to last for an extended period of time (e.g., greater than a few weeks), order standing analgesics or use long-acting agents. As needed (prn) dosing of immediate release agents is also needed for breakthrough pain. If pain is intermittent or expected to last a short time (e.g., less than a couple weeks) then prn dosing of immediate release agents can be used.

Non-pharmacologic Measures

Applications of cold (to reduce inflammation) or heat (to reduce spasms) to muscles or joints are commonly employed techniques but evidence for an analgesic benefit is mixed. Hypnosis has been shown to reduce pain associated with medical procedures; however, it requires specific training and time to administer. Transcutaneous electrical nerve stimulation (TENS) has shown conflicting results in terms of an analgesic benefit in the acute setting, but it has been shown to reduce the need for pharmacologic analgesics. There is limited evidence of benefit in the acute setting from relaxation and guided imagery. Acupuncture and electro-acupuncture have been shown to be of benefit in the acute setting both to improve pain and to reduce common opioid side effects; however, they require specific training and time to administer.

Non-opioid Analgesics

Table 18.2 lists some of the available non-opioid analgesics. Acetaminophen has opioid-sparing and mild–moderate analgesic effects. Because it has no peripheral effects on prostaglandins, it not only has no incidence of gastrointestinal disturbance or anti-platelet effects but also does not have anti-inflammatory effects; thus, if inflammation is the sole generator of the pain, it will be less effective. Around-the-clock acetaminophen is beneficial for most patients in the postoperative period, except when contraindicated.

The other agents in this class have analgesic effects, opioid-sparing effects leading to decreased side effects and possibly anti-hyperalgesic effects. They are primary analgesics for low-intensity pain associated with headache or musculoskeletal disorders and are used as adjuncts for moderate-to-severe postoperative pain when inflammation is present, which is frequently the case. There is a "plateau effect" such that dosages beyond the recommended range increase the incidence of side effects but do not improve analgesia. No one nonsteroidal anti-inflammatory drugs (NSAIDs) appears to be more effective as an analgesic than any other, but there is great inter-patient variability in response, therefore changing agents may be of benefit if one is not effective. The cyclooxygenase (COX)-2-selective NSAID, celecoxib, has no affect on platelet aggregation, less effect on the gastrointestinal mucosa, but an equal incidence of renal toxicity compared to nonselective NSAIDs. It should not be considered as first-line agent given its high cost and should not be used long term, especially at high doses, given the data that it increases the risk of major cardiovascular events.

Table 18.2 Select Non-opioid analgesics.

Agent	Adult dosing	Maximum daily dose	Comments
Acetaminophen	650–1,000 mg po/pr q 6 h	4,000 mg	Doses above 1,000 mg do not improve analgesia, caution in liver disease
Choline magnesium trisalicylate	1,000–1,500 mg po BID	3,000 mg	Low GI effect incidence, avoid in severe liver disease
Diclofenac	50 mg po BID-QID	200 mg	Low GI effect incidence, but possible increased renal effects, data suggest increased negative CV effects
Etodalac	200–400 mg po q 6–8 h	1,000 mg	Low GI and renal effect incidence, safest NSAID in liver disease
Ibuprofen	400–600 mg po q 4–6 h	3,000 mg	<1,500 mg QD has low risk of GI effects, possible increased renal effects, inhibits CV benefits of aspirin when given concomitantly
Ketorolac	30 mg IV q 6 h	120 mg	High risk of renal and GI complications; use for no more than 5 days; 15 mg q 6 h in renal impairment, age >65 years, weight <50 kg
Nabumetone	750–1,500 mg po QD or BID	1,500 mg	Low GI effect incidence
Naproxen	250–500 mg po q 6–12 h	1,500 mg	Possible increased liver and renal effects, probably least negative CV effects
Celecoxib	100–200 mg po QD	200 mg	Use 100 mg dose if possible; long-term use has increased incidence of negative CV effects

CV = cardiovascular, GI = gastrointestinal, IV = intravenous, po = oral, pr = rectal.

Opioid Basics

Other than asking the patient if a particular agent has worked or not worked in the past, it is not possible to determine which opioid may work best for a given patient. There are, however, some agents which should not be used, at least first line, in the postoperative setting. Codeine is not a good first choice due to the fact that possibly around 10–15% of the population does not have an active form of the enzyme (i.e., cytochrome P450 2D6) necessary to convert codeine into the active drug, morphine. Morphine is relatively contraindicated in patients with severe renal insufficiency due to the accumulation of the metabolite, morphine-6-glucuronide, which can lead to sedation and respiratory depression. Meperidine is not recommended as its active metabolite, normeperidine, can accumulate in a day or two to levels that cause nervous system excitation (tremors, muscle twitching, convulsions). In addition it causes a strong euphoric feeling especially when given intravenous (IV) push and it usually causes more nausea than other agents. Propoxyphene is not recommended because its active metabolite, norpropoxyphene, can accumulate when high doses are used, if renal or hepatic insufficiency exists or in the elderly, leading to nervous system toxicity. Hydrocodone use needs to be monitored closely because of the acetaminophen component in the available preparations which can lead to acetaminophen toxicity. Also, the most frequent non-medical use of a pharmaceutical agent leading to emergency department visits is hydrocodone combination preparations (Weinger 2007).

Opioid Administration

Whenever possible, the enteral route of administration is best as it is the easiest route and offers the most stable pharmacokinetics. If the enteral route is not able to be used or if adequate analgesia is not able to be obtained in a timely manner then intravenous administration should be used. Intramuscular administration is not recommended because it hurts and has unpredictable pharmacokinetics. With a competent patient, the use of an intravenous patient-controlled analgesia (PCA) has been demonstrated to offer the best overall pain management option (see sections on PCA below).

Opioid Dosing

The pronounced individual variability in opioid response, combined with changes in responsiveness over time, mandates individualization of opioid doses based on a continuing process of assessment (analgesia and adverse effects) and dose titration. Table 18.3 lists the recommended starting doses for moderate-to-severe pain in the postoperative period for opioid-naïve patients. If a patient is not receiving enough pain relief at a given dose, increase the dose by 25–50%. If a patient is having pain before the next dose is due, reduce the interval and/or increase the dose.

Rotation from one opioid to another may be necessary in several circumstances. One situation is if a few attempts have been made at increasing the dose of an opioid, such that a patient is on a "reasonable" dose and they are still not receiving *any* pain relief, rotation to a different opioid may provide better analgesia. A second situation is if a patient is having intolerable side effects not treated with appropriate agents, again rotation to a different opioid may provide a better side effect profile. A third situation is if a particular opioid is not available by the route of administration required in a given patient. A fourth situation would be if a patient has been on an opioid for an extended period of time and is

Table 18.3   Recommended starting doses of opioids for adults over 50 kg.

Agonist	Oral	Intravenous (IV)
Codeine	15–60 mg q 3–4 h	n/a
Hydrocodone	5–10 mg q 3–6 h[a]	n/a
Tramadol	50–100 mg q 4–6 h[b]	n/a
Oxycodone	5–10 mg q 3–4 h	n/a
Morphine	10–30 mg q 3–4 h	5–10 mg q 2–4 h
Hydromorphone	2–6 mg q 3–4 h	1–1.5 mg q 3–4 h
Oxymorphone	10–20 mg q 4–6 h	1 mg q 3–4 h

n/a = not applicable.
[a]Daily dose limited by acetaminophen component in available preparations
[b]Maximum recommended 24-h dose: 400 mg in adults <75 years old; 300 mg in adults >75 years old.

demonstrating signs of tolerance to the analgesic effects, again rotation to a different opioid may provide better analgesia, usually at less than the expected equianalgesic dose due to incomplete cross-tolerance. This means that patients will not be "as tolerant" to the new opioid agonist as they were to the one they were on previously. Thus, when converting between opioids, for any of the reasons mentioned, the calculated equianalgesic dose of the new agent must be reduced by 25–75% in order to prevent over-sedation and/or respiratory depression.

Sustained Release or Long-Acting Opioids

Sustained release formulations should generally only be initiated in the acute setting if pain is present most of the time and it is assumed that the pain generator will last for an extended period of time (e.g., >2 weeks). If the pain is more incident related or expected to be of a brief duration, then immediate release agents should be employed. If initiating or increasing a sustained release opioid (e.g., if greater than four rescue doses are needed in 24 h while on a sustained release agent); start or go up on the sustained release agent by 50–100% of the total 24-h breakthrough dose used. When using a sustained release opioid, also provide doses of an immediate release opioid equivalent to 10–15% of the 24 h total, to be used every few hours for breakthrough pain.

Transdermal fentanyl is not appropriate for acute pain, especially in the opioid naïve. There is a black box warning against its use in the acute setting due to the risk of severe respiratory depression from the delayed peak effect of the drug as the pain level decreases. It is intended for use in patients who are already tolerant to opioids of comparable potency.

Methadone is not appropriate as the first-line agent in the acute setting, especially in the opioid naïve. Its use requires an understanding of the unique pharmacology of the drug, especially its extended duration of action and its dose-dependent potency. Also, as it takes a few days to reach a stable plasma concentration, patients will need to be followed closely to monitor for effectiveness and side effects. It must also be realized that methadone is a racemic mixture of a μ agonist and an NMDA antagonist (see the section "Adjuvant Analgesics") which causes patients to have a lesser degree of tolerance development.

Adjuvant Analgesics

Adjunctive agents are needed because pain is not always well controlled with just "standard" therapies, especially in the opioid tolerant, and analgesia can be improved by using a number of different agents together (i.e., multimodal analgesia). Adjuncts can also provide opioid sparing effects to help reduce side effects and reverse or prevent opioid tolerance. They are also used to treat or prevent neuropathic symptoms (e.g., hyperalgesia or allodynia) and potentially the development of chronic pain. Finally, not all pain is well treated with opioids (e.g., muscle spasm), and other agents are needed. Some examples of adjuvant analgesics along with dosing guidelines and common side effects are listed in Table 18.4.

Table 18.4   Select adjuvant analgesics.

Class	Agent	Adult dosing	Side effects/comments
Antiepileptics	Gabapentin	Start with 300 mg po q 8 h, increase by 300 mg QD after a few days as needed to a max of 3,600 mg/day in divided doses	Dizziness and somnolence; do not stop abruptly
	Pregabalin	Start with 50 mg po q 8 h or 75 mg po q 12 h; in 1 week increase to max of 300 mg/day in divided doses if needed	
Antidepressants	Amitriptyline	25 mg po qhs; if needed, increase to max of 150 mg/day in single or divided dose	Anticholinergic symptoms (e.g., dry mouth, confusion), sedation, and hypotension
	Duloxetine	30 mg po QD, increase by 30 mg q week as needed to max of 120 mg/day; usual dose is 60 mg	
Skeletal muscle relaxants	Cyclobenzaprine	5–10 mg po q 8 h	Long-term use can lead to the development of dependence
	Tizanidine	4–8 mg po q 6–24 h	
	Orphenadrine	100 mg po q 12 h 60 mg IV q 12 h	
Antispasmodic	Baclofen	10 mg po q 8 h, titrate slowly to max of 80 mg/day in divided doses as needed	Drowsiness; may impair renal function; abrupt D/C may cause seizures
NMDA antagonists	Ketamine	0.1–0.3 mg/kg/h IV	Sedation, dreams, and hallucinations possible but infrequent at analgesic (low) dose, treat with the addition of benzodiazepine or dose reduction
Alpha-2 agonist	Clonidine	0.2 mg/day via a transdermal patch, left for up to 1 week	Hypotension and sedation; monitor for rebound hypertension on D/C if used for greater than 1 week

NMDA = N-methyl-D-aspartate; IV = intravenous; QD = daily; D/C = discontinuation.

Antiepileptics

The most commonly used agents in this class are gabapentin and pregabalin. They are effective for the treatment of neuropathic pain symptoms and may have analgesic effects in the acute setting as well.

Antidepressants

Doses used for analgesia are lower than those for depression treatment, and the onset of analgesia is faster (i.e., days) than the antidepressant effects (i.e., weeks). They are effective for the treatment of neuropathic pain symptoms.

Skeletal Muscle Relaxants

These agents are useful for relief of muscle injury or spasms.

Antispasmodics

Baclofen is useful for the treatment of pain with a spastic component or in certain neuropathic pain states.

N-Methyl-D-Aspartate (NMDA) Antagonists

Antagonism of the NMDA receptor has no primary analgesic effect but rather it has opioid-sparing, opioid tolerance-reversing, and anti-hyperalgesic/neuropathic effects. Ketamine, in addition to being an NMDA antagonist, interacts with opioid, noradrenergic, and muscarinic receptors and voltage-sensitive calcium channels, thus it has true analgesic properties in addition to the NMDA class effects. Ketamine use improves pain scores and has an opioid sparing effect of up to 50% though there are equivocal benefits in terms of a reduction of opioid-induced side effects.

Alpha-2 Agonists

Clonidine has analgesic and opioid sparing effects when given neuraxially, peripherally (transdermal), or systemically (oral, IV). Dexmedetomidine has documented opioid sparing effect when given as an IV infusion and it may have analgesic effects as well, though this effect may only occur at sedating doses. Thus, it is not a useful agent outside of the sedated intensive care unit (ICU) patient.

Benzodiazepines

These agents may be useful to help with insomnia, making it easier to "deal" with pain or to treat anxiety which can play a role in pain states especially acute pain. However, it must always be remembered that these agents do *not* have any analgesic properties. Therefore they must be used with caution in acute pain, especially when high doses of opioids are required, as significant sedation and respiratory depression can occur in the benzodiazepine-naïve patient. In an anxious patient with pain, adequate titration with analgesics should occur before the addition of a benzodiazepine.

Postoperative Pain in the Opioid Tolerant Patient

Since the patient has had surgery that likely has increased or added to their pain, opioid use can be expected to be higher than just replacement of what they were on before coming in to the hospital and it can be *significantly* higher than in opioid-naïve patients. More pain complaints and higher pain scores should be expected. Discussion of reasonable goals and expectations of analgesic therapy with the patient is crucial. These patients usually know what agents have either worked or not worked for them in the past. The use of multimodal therapy in this patient population is especially important.

Patient-Controlled Intravenous Analgesia

PCA is an excellent therapy for the maintenance of already established analgesia (Grass 2005). If a patient is in moderate-to-severe pain, health-care provider delivered boluses of an opioid must be used to reach an acceptable level of analgesia first because the incremental dosing of a PCA will not allow patients to achieve comfort in a reasonable period of time (Hudcova 2007). PCA may be used in any patient requiring intravenous opioids provided they are alert, oriented, and able to understand how to use the equipment appropriately.

PCA Parameters

All PCA machines allow for the setting of the following parameters: demand (bolus) dose, lockout interval, hourly limit, continuous (basal) infusion, and rescue (loading) dose.

Demand (Bolus) Dose

The demand dose is the amount of opioid the patient receives each time they activate the machine. The amount of the demand dose should be small enough so that side effects are minimized yet large enough to provide effective analgesia.

Lockout Interval

The lockout interval is the amount of time following a successfully delivered demand dose during which the patient can administer no further opioid even if the system is activated. Lockout intervals between 5 and 10 min are commonly used. There does not appear to be any data suggesting that any specific time is more or less effective or safe regardless of the opioid chosen (Macintyre 2001).

Hourly Limit

An hourly limit sets the maximum amount of opioid that can be administered in the given time period. The suggested purpose for this setting is to add a level of safety to the system; however, there is no data to support this claim. An hourly limit is automatically determined by the setting of a demand dose and lockout interval. The use of an hourly limit less than this predetermined limit does not make sense as the patient would be able to get a dose of opioid on schedule for only a part of every given time period and then not be able to receive anything for the remainder of the time.

Continuous (Basal) Infusion

A continuous infusion delivers a set amount of opioid every hour without the need for the patient to activate the system. Continuous infusions are not commonly used, as no documented benefits have been shown for most patients. Continuous infusions are not recommended in the opioid-naïve or high-risk patient populations such as the elderly, concomitant use of other sedatives, those with obstructive sleep apnea, or morbid obesity. The use of continuous infusions increases the overall opioid consumption and has been identified as an independent risk factor for respiratory depression. Continuous infusions have not been shown to improve patient satisfaction or pain rating scores and they do not decrease the frequency of demand dose use.

It may appear to make sense to use a continuous infusion at night when the patient is theoretically sleeping and therefore unable to activate the PCA; however, studies have shown that nighttime basal infusions do not improve sleep or analgesia.

Continuous infusions may be needed in opioid-tolerant patients. If the patient cannot take their usual doses of opioid enterally, then a continuous infusion should be used. One way to achieve this is to determine an intravenous equivalent for the amount of opioid the patient takes in a day (taking into account incomplete cross-tolerance if switching to a different agent) and divide this amount by 24 h and administer this as the hourly continuous infusion rate.

Rescue (Loading) Dose

Rescue doses are a specific amount of opioid delivered by a health-care provider that is generally in excess of the patient's demand dose given when the level of analgesia from the PCA is inadequate. Patients may require a rescue dose for a variety of reasons. There may be brief periods of increased nociceptive input beyond the ability of the demand dose to be effective (e.g., dressing changes). If patients forget to or cannot use the PCA for a period of time (e.g., long period of sleep) they may "get behind" on their analgesia and require an extra or larger amount of opioid to "catch up."

PCA Opioid Choices

There does not appear to be a clearly superior opioid for use in PCA devices. Because morphine has an active metabolite, there can be an accumulation of effects especially in patients with renal failure and/or the elderly, so it is generally best to avoid in these patients. Fentanyl has a shorter duration of action than morphine, which is good if one is concerned about accumulating effects, but "bad" in that patients must frequently activate the PCA. The pharmacology of hydromorphone makes it an excellent choice for postoperative PCA use. Meperidine should only be used in the very, very rare case where a patient has documented intolerance to all other opioid choices and then it is recommended to limit the total dose to 600 mg in a 24-h period for no more than 3 days. Methadone is especially useful in patients who take methadone chronically whereas it is not appropriate as a first-line agent in others given the accumulation of effects over time and since the conversion from methadone to another agent when the patient is taking oral analgesics is difficult given the dose-dependent potency of methadone.

Table 18.5 lists the recommended starting demand doses to be used in opioid-naïve patients. In the opioid-tolerant patient these doses will need to be individualized based on the amount of opioid the patient takes per day leading to higher initial demand doses and possibly the initial use of continuous infusions (see above). High-risk patients, identified as elderly, morbidly obese, or those with a history of obstructive sleep apnea should have lower initial demand doses (e.g., one-half the usual demand dose).

Table 18.5 Initial patient-controlled analgesia demand doses in opioid-naïve patients.

Opioid agonist	Demand dose
Morphine	1–2 mg
Hydromorphone	0.2–0.3 mg
Fentanyl	20–30 mcg
Methadone	1–2 mg
Meperidine	10–20 mg

PCA Management

If the patient does not receive adequate pain relief with a given demand dose, increase the dose per activation using the parameters suggested in Table 18.6.

Table 18.6 Usual patient-controlled analgesia demand dose changes for inadequate analgesia.

Opioid agonist	Demand dose increase
Morphine	0.5–1 mg
Hydromorphone	0.1 mg
Fentanyl	5–10 mcg
Methadone	0.5–1 mg
Meperidine	5–10 mg

A small subset of opioid-naïve patients may "prove" that they need and can be safe with a continuous infusion. For example, if following several demand dose increases over several hours a patient continues to need to use the PCA frequently to maintain analgesia without evidence of side effects (i.e., sedation or respiratory depression) and they repeatedly "get behind," because they fall asleep, and then awaken in severe pain not adequately treated with the demand doses or easily treated with rescue doses, then a low-dose continuous infusion may be appropriate. The starting continuous infusion for the opioid-naïve patient should generally not be more than a single demand dose per hour (e.g., 1–2 mg/h for morphine).

If a continuous infusion is being used in any patient, one must be cautious if the amount of pain is assumed to be decreasing with time (e.g., continued healing following surgery). If a patient has a continuous infusion and they do not need to activate the PCA or if side effects (i.e., pruritus, nausea, sedation) begin to increase, then the basal rate should be decreased or discontinued. This allows for the maintenance of the inherent safety of the PCA device in that the patient controls the amount of opioid received to help reduce the chance of severe side effects (i.e., respiratory depression).

PCA Efficacy

One of the major benefits of PCA is that it helps overcome the wide inter-patient variation in opioid requirements by allowing each individual patient to titrate the amount of opioid they receive based on the response they experience. In addition there is some degree of a placebo effect imparted by the use of a PCA enhancing the overall pain control. The patient-controlled aspect is also one of the major safety features of the PCA in that it is assumed that if a patient is getting sedated they will not activate the PCA thereby limiting the possibility of respiratory depression.

Based on the results of several meta-analyses, when PCA is compared to conventional nurse-administered opioids on an as-needed basis, it has been shown to provide slightly better pain control, improved patient satisfaction, and is preferred by patients. Patients with a PCA use slightly more opioid and experience a higher incidence of pruritus but have similar rates of other opioid-related side effects (e.g., nausea, vomiting, sedation, and respiratory depression). There is also a slight (non-significant) reduction in the length of hospital stay in patients using PCA. Finally there appears to be a lower incidence of pulmonary complications in patients using PCA.

PCA Monitoring

While there are no guidelines for how to monitor patients on a PCA there are recommendations from the Anesthesia Patient Safety Foundation (APSF). The APSF advocates the use of continuous monitoring of oxygenation (i.e., pulse oximetry) and ventilation in patients receiving PCA. The reason for monitoring both oxygenation and ventilation is that pulse oximetry has reduced sensitivity as a monitor of hypoventilation when supplemental oxygen is administered. Therefore, especially when supplemental oxygen is used, monitoring of ventilation should be undertaken with a technology designed to assess breathing or estimate arterial carbon dioxide concentrations. Some type of continuous monitoring is most important for high-risk patients (i.e., elderly, obstructive sleep apnea, morbidly obese) but likely should be applied to all patients.

Patient-Controlled Epidural Analgesia

Patient-controlled epidural analgesia (PCEA) may be used in any patient in whom epidural analgesia is appropriate provided they are alert, oriented, and able to understand how to use the equipment appropriately (Block 2003).

PCEA Parameters

All PCEA machines allow for the setting of the same parameters as described above for a PCA.

Demand (Bolus) Dose

The optimal demand dose for PCEA is not known but is usually set at 2–4 ml. There is no information that a particular demand dose works best with a certain analgesic regimen.

Lockout Interval

Lockout intervals between 10 and 20 min are commonly used. These times are more in line with the peak effect of the analgesics than the lockout intervals used for PCA.

Hourly Limit

If an hourly limit is used it should be the amount mathematically determined by the choice of demand dose, lockout interval, and continuous infusion rate. This will ensure that the patient receives analgesics continuously.

Continuous (Basal) Infusion

Continuous infusions are commonly used for PCEA management. Continuous infusions are usually started at 4–6 ml/h with a usual upper limit of 14 ml/h. The height of the patient does not appear to be a determinant of the correct infusion rate. There is some data to suggest that weight is positively correlated and age is negatively correlated with PCEA requirements. However, it is the location of the surgery that appears to have the strongest correlation with PCEA requirements in that thoracoabdominal operations need higher rates than lower extremity surgery when using the same local anesthetic concentrations. This is likely a function of the number of dermatomes that need to be covered.

Rescue (Loading) Dose

The amount of a rescue dose to be used will be determined by a number of factors including the specific analgesics being used, the number of dermatomes that need to be covered and potentially the hemodynamic status of the patient (see the section "PCEA Management").

PCEA Analgesic Agents

There does not appear to be a clearly superior regimen for use in PCEA devices. Local anesthetics are the most commonly used agents. Typically, bupivacaine is used due to its relative resistance to tachyphylaxis. The cardiotoxicity of bupivacaine has led some to use levo-bupivacaine or ropivacaine instead. The usual ranges of concentration for the various local anesthetics are listed in Table 18.7. Often the higher range of concentrations is used for lower extremity orthopedic procedures and the less concentrated solutions used for thoracic surgery; however, there is not any conclusive data to support this practice.

The next most common agents used for PCEA therapy are the opioids. They are usually used in combination with a local anesthetic. There seems to be no benefit of administering lipophilic opioids (i.e., fentanyl or sufentanil) as the sole agent via the epidural route. The site of action of lipophilic opioids when given epidurally is not clear. Studies looking at the efficacy of fentanyl and sufentanil given epidurally versus intravenously are contradictory. Most studies measuring the plasma concentrations of these opioids when given via an epidural or

Table 18.7 Local anesthetic choices for patient-controlled epidural analgesia.

Local anesthetic	Concentration range (%)
Bupivacaine	0.0625–0.2
Levo-bupivacaine	0.0625–0.2
Ropivacaine	0.1–0.2

IV have shown no difference in levels thus suggesting that the major site of action is not at the spinal cord but rather due to systemic absorption.

Hydrophilic opioids (i.e., morphine or hydromorphone), on the other hand, maintain high cerebrospinal fluid levels for an extended period of time and therefore can act at the opioid receptors in the spinal cord. Table 18.8 lists concentrations documented in the literature for the various opioids when administered via the epidural route; the "correct" dose is not known. When used in combination with local anesthetics the lower end of the concentration ranges are suggested. The total 24-h dose of opioid must be kept in mind if high continuous infusion rates or large frequent demand doses are used. It is best to avoid using opioids in epidural infusions for high-risk patients (i.e., elderly, obstructive sleep apnea, morbidly obese) and if systemic opioids are necessary as well for any reason (e.g., pain outside the area the epidural can be expected to cover).

Table 18.8 Opioid choices for patient-controlled epidural analgesia.

Opioid	Concentration range (mcg/ml)
Fentanyl	1–4
Hydromorphone	10–50
Morphine	20–100
Sufentanil	0.5–1

Other adjunctive agents have been studied for addition to local anesthetics and/or opioids for epidural use; however, they are not used extensively, likely because studies are limited and show equivocal results. The major proposed benefits are improved analgesia and the ability to use a lower concentration of local anesthetics and opioids. Table 18.9 lists the adjuvant agents and offers suggested concentrations from the literature; the "correct" doses have not been determined.

Table 18.9 Other agents for patient-controlled epidural analgesia.

Analgesic	Concentration range (mcg/ml)
Clonidine	1–3
Epinephrine	2–5
Neostigmine	1–7

The major concern with clonidine is an increased incidence of hypotension and sedation. Use of epinephrine has shown improved analgesia with activity though it may lead to an increased incidence of motor block. Epinephrine use also has been shown to reduce plasma concentrations of lipophilic opioids by allowing them to remain in the neuraxis for long enough to actually bind to the opioid receptors in the spinal cord. The concern with neostigmine is that when used for intrathecal administration a dose-dependent incidence of nausea and vomiting occurs as well as sedation; however, epidural use does not seem to have the same incidence of nausea and vomiting and only minimal sedation occurs.

PCEA Complications/Side Effects

The incidence of serious, permanent neurological complications is exceedingly rare and data comprises a handful of case reports. The incidence of spinal hematoma has classically been thought to be 1:150,000 in the presence of normal coagulation, though recent studies have suggested it may be more common. The incidence of epidural hematoma formation in a patient who is anticoagulated is not known, but it is estimated at 1:3,000 in patients receiving therapeutic low molecular weight heparin. A full discussion of epidurals and anticoagulation is beyond the scope of this chapter; the most recent guidelines can be found on the American Society of Regional Anesthesia web site (www.asra.com). Epidural abscess incidence is not known but considered rare (at most 0.05%). Risk factors for abscess formation may be longer times of having the epidural in place (possibly >6 days) as well as use in immunocompromised patients. Intrathecal or intravascular migration of an epidural catheter is estimated at approximately 0.2%, though it is likely much less frequent than this. The incidence of premature catheter dislodgement is estimated at about 6%.

The major side effects due to local anesthetics in epidurals are hypotension, CNS toxicity, and motor block. The probability of hypotension from an epidural does not rise above 1–2% until the "spread" of the epidural is beyond 14 sympathetic dermatomes. Remember that the sympathetic blockade may be another possible six dermatomes beyond the amount of sensory block. The major mechanism by which an epidural might cause hypotension is through decreased venous return (pre-load) from reduced venous capacitance, therefore the most appropriate treatment is increasing pre-load with volume. Hence, hypotension is rarely seen in the supine normovolemic patient. Thus it is often the fluid status of the patient that is more of a causative factor than the epidural itself. This is evidenced by the fact that stopping the epidural infusion in a patient often does not improve blood pressure unless the pain becomes so great that a large sympathetic response occurs.

CNS toxicity (seizures) from systemic accumulation of local anesthetics is obviously based on the total amount of the drug used over time and has an estimated incidence of 0.01–0.1%. Motor block of the lower extremities is estimated at less than 3% when lower concentrations of local anesthetic are used and upward of 25% with higher concentrations. In addition, the level of epidural insertion has much to do with the actual incidence in that lumbar epidurals are more likely to cause motor block than thoracic.

The incidence of nausea/vomiting with opioid-containing PCEA therapy is estimated at between 4 and 15%, though higher incidences have also been reported. The incidence of severe pruritus is between 2 and 17% with the incidence of any degree of pruritus likely being well over 50%. Sedation is reported to occur in about 15% of patients. Respiratory depression is estimated to occur in 0.1–0.4% of patients. However, a higher incidence (approaching 1.5%) of respiratory depression is seen in some studies using morphine.

The respiratory depression seen with epidural opioids is biphasic. Early respiratory depression (within an hour of epidural initiation) is thought to be due to systemic absorption of the opioids via epidural veins and is thus more likely with the lipophilic opioids. Delayed respiratory depression (occurring 4–8 h after epidural initiation) is seen especially when using the hydrophilic opioids and is thought to be due to the cephalad spread of the opioids in the cerebrospinal fluid (Wheatley 2001).

PCEA Management

Inadequate pain relief with an epidural can be due to a number of reasons, and an evaluation of the patient needs to be done in order to determine the best course of action. When a local anesthetic is part of the epidural solution, this evaluation should entail a determination of where the band of analgesia is located, either by testing for pinprick sensation or by temperature differentiation. If the level of analgesia is more or completely one sided the epidural catheter can be pulled out of the epidural space in 0.5–1 cm increments in an attempt to make the block bilateral. The optimal depth of multi-orifice catheters is 3–5 cm in the epidural space. If the level of analgesia is not adequate to cover the entire extent of the surgical incision, then the rate of the continuous infusion can be increased, usually in 2 ml/h increments or the concentration of the local anesthetic can be increased. Either change will increase the number of dermatomes covered, as the total quantity of local anesthetic, in milligrams, is one important factor in the amount of spread. If the patient has an adequate number of dermatomes covered but is still having pain, then the block is likely not dense enough. In this case changing the epidural solution to a more concentrated local anesthetic and/or addition of other agents (i.e., opioid and/or adjunct) should be done. If at any point the patient is in severe pain, a rescue dose of either the epidural infusion (4–8 ml) or a more concentrated local anesthetic bolus (e.g., 3–5 ml of 0.25% bupivacaine) can be used to achieve comfort faster.

Lower extremity motor block can be of any degree from mild to complete. If the level of analgesia does not need to cover the lumbar nerves and it more than adequately covers the surgical incision then the rate of the continuous infusion can be decreased (usually in 2 ml/h increments). If the level of analgesia needs to cover the lumbar nerves or if the level of analgesia is just covering the extent of the surgical incision then the local anesthetic concentration should be decreased to attempt to make the motor block less pronounced. If the patient is not going to be getting out of bed, for reasons other than the motor block from the epidural, then no change in therapy is really necessary especially if the motor block is not bilateral and complete.

The concern with a bilateral, complete motor block, especially one that occurs after the epidural has been running for some time with normal motor function previously, is that it may be a sign of the development of an epidural hematoma. Motor block is the most common presenting symptom of epidural hematomas seen in 46% of cases, followed by back pain in 38% of cases. If an epidural hematoma is suspected the epidural should be stopped and motor function evaluated over the next 2 h. If no resolution of the motor block occurs in this time the patient should be sent for a magnetic resonance imaging (MRI) to rule out hematoma formation. The best chance for recovery of neurological function from an epidural hematoma is to undergo a decompression laminectomy within 8 h from the onset of symptoms.

As stated above if hypotension is seen it is usually best to treat with intravascular volume expansion. If this is not possible then the analgesic level should be established to ensure that the spread is not too excessive for the surgical incision; if it is then a reduction in the continuous infusion rate can be made. If the hypotension is so severe that the epidural infusion needs to be turned off one should ensure that the patient has another means of analgesia (e.g., IV

PCA). In addition, if the blood pressure does not increase significantly after about 2 h then it is not likely that the epidural was at all contributory and the infusion can be restarted.

If the patient is having the opioid-related side effects of nausea/vomiting or pruritus, the options are to treat the particular side effect with a specific therapy or remove the opioid from the epidural solution. To treat nausea/vomiting, any of the available antiemetics can be tried as none has been proven to be more effective than another. The pruritus caused by epidural opioids is generally not due to histamine release, instead being a central μ receptor-related phenomenon. Thus it is best treated with a medication that has μ receptor antagonist properties (e.g., nalbuphine 5 mg IV every 4 h as needed), and not an antihistamine.

Sedation or respiratory depression from epidural opioids definitely requires at least the removal of the opioid from the solution. If either is severe, especially respiratory depression, then naloxone administration may be necessary. Careful titration of naloxone (40 mcg intravenously every couple minutes) is necessary in order to minimize the chance of complete reversal of analgesia and the possible development of hypertension, tachycardia, and pulmonary edema. Naloxone has a relatively short duration of action (about 1 h) and therefore patients should be monitored for return of respiratory depression as opioid agonist effects can last as long as 12 h after discontinuation. Therefore repeat doses of naloxone may need to be given or a naloxone infusion can be used.

PCEA Efficacy Versus Parenteral Opioids

Based on the results of several studies and meta-analyses, epidural analgesia is better than PCA with opioids in a number of ways. Pain control is improved for general surgery, orthopedic, and gynecologic patients. All epidural regimens (except hydrophilic opioids alone) when compared to PCA provide improved analgesia. There is statistically better analgesia at rest and during activity for all types of surgery (through postoperative day four), as well as clinically appreciable differences in pain with activity through postoperative day one. Greater improvements in analgesia are seen when epidurals contain a local anesthetic and when the insertion level is matched to the surgery (i.e., epidural insertion site around the mid-dermatome of the incision).

There is a reduction in pulmonary and cardiac complications (including postoperative myocardial infarction) in major vascular surgery and high-risk patient populations with the use of thoracic epidurals. In addition there is a reduction in the time of postoperative ileus (by 1–1.5 days) following abdominal surgery with the use of local anesthetic containing epidural regimens. There has also been the suggestion that epidurals decrease the time to mobilization, duration of intensive care unit stay, and time to discharge. In lower extremity revascularization, epidurals have been shown to improve the incidence of graft survival. Historically, epidurals have been shown to reduce the incidence of deep vein thrombosis (DVT) and pulmonary embolism (PE); however, no studies have been done with comparison to newer pharmacologic thromboprophylaxis. One negative is that epidural therapy is more expensive than PCA therapy. In terms of side effects, PCA therapy has a higher incidence of nausea and sedation whereas epidurals have a higher incidence of pruritus, urinary retention, and motor block (though this will vary with the agents and concentrations chosen).

PCEA Efficacy Versus Continuous Epidural Infusions

It has been suggested that PCEA compared with continuous epidural infusions (CEIs) optimizes pain control by allowing the patient to "top up" themselves when there is an increase in their pain or in anticipation of a painful event (e.g., prior to getting out of bed or physical therapy) as opposed to having to wait for a health-care provider. Some studies have shown that PCEA compared to CEI provides improved analgesia, whereas others have only shown a decreased requirement for provider-administered boluses. Data is contradictory in terms of which, PCEA or CEI, provides improved analgesia, but PCEA has been suggested to improve patient satisfaction, and PCEA does reduce the total amount of analgesics required. Additionally, PCEA has a decreased risk of motor block and nausea but an increased incidence of pruritus when compared to CEI.

PCEA Safety/Monitoring

Tubing that is clearly marked and differentiated from IV tubing (e.g., different color) is essential to prevent medications other than the intended epidural solution from being injected into the epidural space. While there are no guidelines for how to monitor patients on a PCEA, if the infusion contains an opioid the APSF offers some recommendations as described above for a PCA.

Case Scenario

Darin J. Correll, MD

A 50-year-old man with lung cancer has just undergone a left thoracotomy for left upper lobectomy. He had no contraindication for an epidural, which was placed preoperatively. PCEA has been initiated which contains bupivacaine 0.0625% plus hydromorphone 20 mcg/ml at a rate of 8 ml/h. You get a call from the floor nurse because he is in 8 out of 10 pain an hour after arriving from the recovery room. You have yet to meet the patient.

What questions do you need to ask the patient when you arrive in his room?
You must determine where exactly he is having pain and what it exactly feels like. He tells you that the pain in his chest is "manageable" (3 out of 10 on a verbal rating scale) but his left shoulder is aching (pain 8/10), which is the most disturbing thing for him right now.

You can also take this opportunity to get some background analgesic history from the patient by asking him if he has pain chronically, takes any analgesics on a regular basis (and if so, what and how much) and if he has used any analgesics (e.g., opioids) in the past that have either worked or not worked well for him. The patient relates that he does have some mild osteoarthritis and takes 200 mg of ibuprofen once every few days at most. He is otherwise healthy, and this is the first time he has been in the hospital and therefore has no experience with other analgesics.

What changes are you going to make to his regimen?
The shoulder pain could have several etiologies. It may be from positioning of the arm above his head during surgery, but it could simply be referred pain from "irritation" of his diaphragm either during the operation or from the chest tube. So you ask the

surgeon if it is all right to start the patient on IV ketorolac to help reduce the inflammatory process. The surgeon would rather not use an NSAID at this point because there were several areas of "oozing" during the operation and the output from the chest tube is a bit more blood tinged than usual.

Given that the epidural will not be able to control the shoulder pain regardless of what changes you make to it, you decide to start the patient on an IV PCA of hydromorphone to help control the shoulder pain. You also start the patient on around-the-clock acetaminophen. Even though it is not an anti-inflammatory agent it will still have opioid-sparing effects and offer some added analgesia.

Since you will be starting a parenteral opioid you will need to remove the hydromorphone from the epidural solution so as not to have two different modes of opioid administration and a higher chance for opioid-induced side effects (worst being respiratory depression), especially since the patient is opioid-naïve. You change the order to bupivacaine 0.0625% at a rate of 8 ml/h.

You are called back a few hours later to see the patient because of continued severe pain. Now he relates that his shoulder is feeling better (he thanks you for that) but now he realizes that he cannot take a deep breath or cough because a sharp pain is limiting him from doing this (up to a 10/10 pain).

What would you be looking for in examining the patient?
You need to determine if the epidural is working at all and if it is offering sufficient coverage of the incision on the chest given that the patient cannot perform the activities necessary for recovery from thoracic surgery, specifically taking deep breaths and coughing. You test for the level of anesthesia by using a glove filled with ice water to determine where the difference in temperature sensation is present. The band of anesthesia is from T2 to T8, which is sufficient to cover the entire extent of the surgical incision.

What changes are you going to make to his regimen now?
Since the spread of sensory block from the local anesthetic in the epidural infusion seems to be adequate, increasing the rate will be unlikely to add any additional benefit. Therefore, you decide to change the concentration to make the block "denser" in the given area. You change the epidural infusion to bupivacaine 0.125% at 8 ml/h.

A few hours later the nurse calls again regarding the patient to relate that his pain is now much better controlled while coughing, but he is now complaining of numbness on the medial aspect of his upper extremities extending to his ring and middle fingers.

What is likely happening and what will you do about it?
By going up on the concentration of local anesthetic in the epidural, the total amount (in milligrams) of medication was increased and the spread increased. On testing the level, it now extends from C8 to T9.

You reduce the rate on the epidural to 6 ml/h. You get no further calls on the patient for the rest of the evening, so you and he sleep well.

References

American Pain Society. Principles of analgesic use in the treatment of acute pain and cancer pain. 6th ed. Glenview, IL: American Pain Society; 2008.

Block BM, Liu SS, Rowlingson AJ, Cowan AR, Cowan JA, Wu CL. Efficacy of postoperative epidural analgesia. A meta-analysis. JAMA 2003;290:2455–63.

Carr DB, Goudas LC. Acute pain. Lancet 1999;353:2051.

Grass JA. Patient-controlled analgesia. Anesth Analg. 2005;101:S44–61.

Hudcova J, McNicol E, Quah C, Carr DB. Patient controlled opioid analgesia versus conventional opioid analgesia for postoperative pain. Cochrane Database Syst Rev 2007;4.

Liu SS, Wu CL. Effect of postoperative analgesia on major postoperative complications: a systemic update of the evidence. Anesth Analg. 2007;104:689–702.

Macintyre PE. Safety and efficacy of patient-controlled analgesia. Br J Anaesth. 2001;87:36–46.

Weinger MB. Dangers of postoperative opioids. APSF Newsl. 2007;21:61–3.

Wheatley RG, Schug SA, Watson D. Safety and efficacy of postoperative epidural analgesia. Br J Anaesth. 2001;87:4–61.

Section VI

Acute Pain Management

Chapter 19

Pain Management for Trauma

Neil Sinha, MD and Steven P. Cohen, MD

Introduction

Trauma remains a major cause of morbidity and mortality throughout the world. Medical advances have significantly reduced the mortality associated with trauma, which has led to an increased emphasis on secondary outcome measures, such as psychological well-being, functional improvement, and vocational and social reintegration. Pain has a profound impact on all of these variables. The stress response after multi-trauma exceeds that following elective surgery and includes cytokine and acute phase reactant release, altered immune response, and elevated levels of catecholamines, cortisol, growth hormone, and adrenocorticotropic hormone. Studies have shown that inadequately treated acute pain increases this response, which can result in higher morbidity (Yeager et al. 1987). Poorly controlled inflammatory pain also results in myriad anatomical and physiological changes in the nervous system (i.e., neuroplasticity), which can manifest as chronic neuropathic pain. Trauma patients with high levels of persistent pain are less likely to return to work, more likely to suffer from depression, posttraumatic stress disorder, and other psychological comorbidities, and report greater disability than trauma victims who report less pain (Jenewein et al. 2009, Yang et al. 2009). Even among survivors of severe trauma, the long-term mortality rate is significantly higher compared with matched controls, an effect that may be partly attributable to the sequelae of chronic pain (Naschitz and Lenger 2008).

Burns

Burn injuries are one of the most devastating forms of trauma, and burn pain is one of most debilitating types of pain. Burns may result from a variety of insults including thermal, chemical, light, radiation, friction, and electrical origins. This can cause damage to epidermis, nerve tissue, blood vessels, muscle, and bone, resulting in nociceptive and neuropathic pain (Lee and Astumian 1996). In addition, burn victims may suffer from a number of related, adverse events including shock, infection, respiratory distress, and electrolyte imbalance (Church et al. 2006). More than other types of trauma, negative emotional suffering often develops subsequent to burns as a result of physical scarring and/or deformity (Ward et al. 1987). Consequently, the treatment of burn pain should be a collaborative, multidisciplinary effort that takes into account the physical and emotional sequelae of such an event.

The traditional system classifies burns by degree (Table 19.1). A first-degree burn (e.g., sunburn) involves damage to the epidermis and inflammation of the papillary dermis and

N. Vadivelu et al. (eds.), *Essentials of Pain Management*,
DOI 10.1007/978-0-387-87579-8_19, © Springer Science+Business Media, LLC 2011

Table 19.1 Burn designations.

	Site of injury	Physical exam	Example(s)	Treatment
First degree (superficial thickness)	Damage to epidermis, inflamed papillary dermis	Pain, erythema, +capillary refill	Sunburn	Self-limited, spontaneous healing in 3–4 days
Superficial second degree (superficial partial thickness)	Damage to epidermis, papillary dermis	Pain, erythema, blisters +capillary refill	Scald burn	Self-limited, spontaneous healing in 7–10 days
Deep second degree (deep partial thickness)	Damage to epidermis, papillary and reticular dermis	Mottled skin ± capillary refill ± pain	Scald/grease burn	Spontaneous healing versus surgical excision/grafting
Third degree (full thickness)	Damage to epidermis, dermis, subcutaneous far	White/black, leathery skin –capillary refill –pain	Flame, contact burn	Surgical excision/grafting
Fourth degree (full thickness)	Damage to muscles, tendons, ligaments ± hypodermis	Black, charred –capillary refill –pain	Flame, contact burn	Surgical excision/grafting

presents with erythema and an intact epidermal layer. A second-degree burn invades the dermis (either the papillary or the reticular layers) and is associated with blisters as well as erythema. A third-degree burn involves injury to all cutaneous and subcutaneous tissues and may manifest as a hard, purple eschar. Lastly, a fourth degree burn results in damage to muscles, tendons, and ligaments and may invade the hypodermis. The newer classification of burns distinguishes them by the required surgical intervention and is used to predict outcome. Categories of burns according to this classification are superficial thickness, superficial partial thickness, deep partial thickness, and full thickness (Sharar et al. 2007, Marx et al. 2009).

The treatment of pain in burn victims involves a careful survey of the type and characteristics of the lesion. The depth of the burn, nature of the insult, state of healing, and the patient's demographics including age, gender, and comorbid conditions all influence the type and severity of the pain. Nevertheless, the severity and duration of burn pain is difficult to predict, and careful and frequent analysis of the patient's pain scores in conjunction with monitoring of hemodynamic parameters is necessary in developing a treatment plan (Perry et al. 1981).

Acute burn pain can be broken down into four subtypes. Background pain results from thermal injury and presents as a low–moderate constant pain that resolves with the healing of the wound. Procedural pain occurs during procedures such as wound debridement, dressing changes, and physical therapy. This pain is greater in intensity but shorter in duration and hence may be extremely challenging to treat. Modalities such as regional and preemptive analgesia are often effective in mitigating this. Breakthrough pain can occur at rest or with activity (i.e., incident pain) and is characterized by unexpected intense pain sensations of short duration. One form of breakthrough pain that may be easily remediable is "end-of-dose failure," which is generally experienced as worsening pain before administration of a scheduled opioid. Two strategies to treat this pain include increasing the dose or frequency

Table 19.2 Sample treatment protocols for burn pain.

	Intensive care unit/acute care setting		
	Nil per os (NPO)	Per os (PO)	Hospital floor/discharge anticipated
Background pain	Continuous intravenous opioids (morphine, fentanyl, hydromorphone); methadone, scheduled benzodiazepines when anxiety is suspected	Scheduled sustained release (MSContin, OxyContin), methadone NSAIDs, adjuvants if neuropathic pain is suspected	Acetaminophen, NSAIDs, scheduled sustained release or long-acting oral opioids (if necessary), adjuvants
Procedural pain	Rapidly or short-acting IV or PCA opioids, parenteral ketamine, regional anesthesia, Entonox (50% oxygen and nitrous oxide), benzodiazepines	Preemptive short-acting opioids (oxycodone, hydrocodone) with or without acetaminophen, transmucosal, or buccal fentanyl	Short-acting opioids
Breakthrough pain	Opioids via PCA or prn	PRN oral or transmucosal opioids	PRN short-acting oral or transmucosal or buccal opioids, NSAIDS, acetaminophen
Postoperative pain	Opioids via PCA or prn, regional anesthesia	Opioids via PCA, regional anesthesia	Short-acting opioids

NSAIDS = non-steroid anti-inflammatory drugs; IV = intravenous; PCA = patient-controlled analgesia.

of the "around-the-clock" long-acting opioid. Lastly, postoperative pain manifests as a predictable increase in pain scores after surgical interventions such as skin grafting and burn excision. Recognizing the type of pain is an important step in managing burn pain. Table 19.2 summarizes different pharmacologic approaches to managing each type of pain.

In the acute setting, the initial treatment of burn pain should be based upon the depth of injury. Pain from first-degree burns can often be treated effectively with topical agents (creams, lotions, sprays, etc.) containing local anesthetics such as lidocaine or benzocaine, including eutectic mixture of local anesthetic (EMLA) cream. Non-steroidal anti-inflammatory drugs (NSAIDs) or acetaminophen may also be helpful in these cases. Second-degree burns result in injury to the sensory receptors in the dermis leading to marked hyperalgesia and severe pain. Frequent, controlled, and carefully titrated doses of intravenous opioids are often necessary in the acute setting. Fentanyl, hydromorphone, and morphine are all acceptable choices. Previously, third-degree burns (because of the complete destruction of sensory structures) were thought to cause no pain in the acute setting. However, the transition zones between burned and unburned skin may have inflamed sensory receptors, resulting in pain complaints that need to be addressed.

Burn injuries are associated with a high co-prevalence rate of psychopathology which exceeds 50% in some studies (Davydow et al. 2009). The most common of these are depression, posttraumatic stress disorder, anxiety disorder, and substance abuse (Dyster-Aas et al. 2008). In many cases, pre-existing psychological disorders precede the injury. Burn injuries can also act as psychological stressors that worsen pain, especially in the immediate setting. Not surprisingly, cognitive-behavioral therapy, relaxation techniques, and anxiolytics have all been shown to effectively attenuate pain (Latarjet and Choinere 1995). Other beneficial treatments include psychotherapy, reintegration training, and establishing an adequate social support network.

After the initial presentation, burn pain management should be tailored to the specific type of pain being experienced. Background pain should be treated with pharmacologic agents that achieve a relative steady state in plasma drug concentrations. A continuous intravenous opioid infusion or transdermal fentanyl may be an appropriate option in patients who are nil per os (NPO); those that tolerate enteral medications may do well with sustained release formulations or opioids with long elimination half-lives such as methadone. NSAIDs, ketamine, and adjuvants such as α-2 agonists (e.g., clonidine), tricyclic antidepressants, and membrane stabilizers can be used as pharmacologic adjuvant therapies to decrease opioid requirements. Non-pharmacologic agents such as hypnosis and acupuncture may also be helpful (Pal et al. 1997).

Breakthrough pain in burns victims may occur secondary to changes in opioid requirements (development of tolerance and/or opioid-induced hyperalgesia, changes in plasma protein concentration), inadequate dosing or end-of-dose failure, new or worsening psychosocial matters, specific activities (i.e., incident pain), or from the natural healing process of the wound (i.e., the development of epidermal skin buds). Whenever possible, the underlying cause of breakthrough pain should be identified and addressed (e.g., opioid rotation for tolerance). For breakthrough pain, shorter acting opioids, delivered via intravenous patient-controlled analgesia (IV-PCA) or on a PRN schedule, or oral ketamine (25–50 mg po q3–4 h) may be of benefit. In patients who are NPO, alternatives to parenteral delivery include rectal and other transmucosal formulations.

In contrast to background pain, procedural pain tends to be more intense, but of shorter duration. Studies evaluating the efficacy of analgesic regimens in burn patients have found that nearly half of all patients report undertreatment of procedure-related pain (Choiniere et al. 1990). Procedure-related pain is associated with high levels of anticipatory anxiety that may develop with repeated procedures; inadequate analgesia in prior procedures increases anxiety and arousal, resulting in decreased analgesic effectiveness in subsequent procedures. Consequently, treating procedural pain effectively requires treating the first and all subsequent interventions. The pharmacologic goal is to obtain adequate analgesia without prolonged post-procedure side effects, particularly sedation. This can often be achieved with short-acting agents. In patients without intravenous access, short-acting oral opioids (such as oxycodone or hydrocodone) or transmucosal/buccal fentanyl can be used. These latter two formulations have a rapid onset (<15 min) by virtue of their transmucosal absorption and a short (90–120 min) duration of action, which make them ideal for short procedures. Often, benzodiazepines such as lorazepam or diazepam are incorporated into the regimen to decrease anticipatory anxiety and enhance the effects of opioids (Patterson et al. 2004, Miller et al. 2009).

Ketamine, a dissociative anesthetic which possesses antagonistic effects at the NMDA receptor, is a first-line agent for short procedures such as dressing changes. The major drawback to ketamine is the psychomimetic effects, which may be less common in children and can be reduced with the coadministration of benzodiazepines. In an observational study by MacPherson et al., the authors reported a 98% success rate for burn dressing changes in 44 patients treated with ketamine–midazolam in a 10:0.5 mg ratio delivered by PCA. Among the 13 patients who experienced adverse effects, hallucinations were the most common. A larger study by Owens et al. evaluated the safety and effectiveness of ketamine use by non-anesthesiologists in 347 bedside procedures done in pediatric burn patients, most of which were dressing changes (Owens et al. 2006). The procedure was successfully completed without complications in all but 10 cases for a "success rate" of 97%. Among these 10 sentinel events, eight required airway intervention. In a randomized, double-blind comparative effectiveness study, Tosun et al. (2008) compared the efficacy of propofol–ketamine to propofol–fentanyl for burn dressing changes in 32 pediatric patients. Although both treatments were effective, the lower incidence of restlessness in the propofol-ketamine group prompted the authors to conclude that it was superior to propofol–fentanyl.

Lidocaine can be used topically and systemically to relieve burn pain (Brofeldt et al. 1989, Jonsson et al. 1991). Systemic lidocaine may exert its analgesic properties by depressing conduction of painful afferent stimuli, inhibition of dorsal horn transmission, and reduction of inflammation (Cohen et al. 2004). The main concern with local anesthetics, especially systemic, is neurological and cardiovascular toxicity.

As the intense pain following an acute burn begins to resolve, pruritis is often experienced. Similar to neuropathic pain, some forms of itch may result from damage to small unmyelinated C fibers (i.e., neuropathic itch). Not surprisingly, the pharmacological treatment of neuropathic itch is similar to that of neuropathic pain and includes membrane stabilizers (e.g., gabapentin), capsaicin, and antidepressants. Conventional anti-pruritic drugs such as promethazine and diphenhydramine not only attenuate itch but also enhance the antinociceptive properties of opioids.

In addition to the original injury site, pain may also stem from newly created wounds at the site of skin graft harvesting. Regional techniques may be employed to treat this pain if no contraindications exist and the operative region is well localized. Increasing baseline opioids preemptively may also help to reduce the postoperative pain, but should be done with caution since failure to reduce the dose following pain diminution can result in untoward effects. Although it is frequently overlooked, an informative preoperative conversation with the patient regarding what to expect after the operation can go a long way toward decreasing anxiety and postoperative opioid requirements.

In summary, burns are one of the most devastating forms of trauma, with both profound physical and psychological effects. Treating burn pain effectively requires a careful assessment of the wound characteristics as well as an understanding of the victim and his comorbid conditions. After the initial stage of pain management, analgesia for burn pain should be tailored to the specific type of pain the patient is experiencing. In addition, the presence of a strong emotional support system may decrease anxiety and result in more effective analgesia.

Pain Management for Other Forms of Trauma

Providing analgesia to the trauma patient is a unique and challenging objective for healthcare professionals. The trauma victim often presents with multiple sites of injury resulting in respiratory, cardiovascular, and hemodynamic instability that require immediate attention (Table 19.3). These patients range from young healthy athletes to the debilitated elderly who may have a host of comorbid conditions. Whereas young males represent a disproportionate percentage of trauma victims, it is the elderly who are at highest risk for mortality. Lastly, the trauma itself may serve as a strong emotional stressor that may contribute to pain. These factors must be accounted for when developing an appropriate analgesic strategy.

Pain that arises from trauma often results in a vicious cycle. Increased pain stimuli result in increased firing in primary and secondary afferent neurons, which can lead to central

Table 19.3 Epidemiology, concerns, and analgesic strategies for various types of trauma.

Trauma	Frequency	Causes	Immediate concerns	Analgesic strategies	Long-term sequelae
Blunt chest trauma	8% of trauma admissions	MVC, falls	Pneumothorax, hemothorax, pulmonary/cardiac contusion, cardiac tamponade	Thoracic epidural, lumbar epidural, interpleural catheter, IV-PCA, intercostal nerve blocks, or cryoanalgesia	High incidence of postthoracotomy pain if surgery required
Traumatic brain injury	1.5 million per year in US	MVC, firearms, falls	Intracranial bleed, spinal cord injury, cerebral edema, and hypoxia	Short term: analgesic care plan that minimizes effects on cerebral hemodynamics; long term: it may include prophylactic and/or abortive therapy for headaches, nerve blocks for neck pain, and cervicogenic headaches	Chronic headaches, neck pain, back pain, cognitive impairment, psychological disorders
Traumatic amputation	Trauma accounts for >16% of the >133,000 amputations per year in US. The last sentence should be Most involve digits in the upper extremities	MVC, power tools, lawn mowers, crush injuries, knives, and saws	Blood loss, limb preservation, which can significantly improve long-term function	Mixed evidence for preemptive effect of epidural analgesia to prevent postamputation pain in planned amputations. Treatment of stump pain should focus on underlying cause (e.g., neuroma, heterotopic ossification, adhesive scar tissue, ill-fitting prosthesis). Strongest evidence for short-term benefit for phantom pain is for opioids	Traumatic lower limb amputees have increased morbidity and mortality from cardiovascular disease. High prevalence rates of back pain (>50%), hip pain, bursitis, and other musculoskeletal conditions in lower extremity amputees. Heterotopic ossification is much more common (>50%) in major limb traumatic amputations
Spinal cord injury	100,000 per year in the USA	MVC, falls, sports injuries	Spinal stability, aspiration, hypoventilation	Treatment should be aimed at the different types of pain: central (deafferentation), peripheral neuropathic (radiculopathy, complex regional pain syndrome), spasticity, visceral (e.g., organ distension)	Psychological disorders, pressure ulcers, impaired coping skills

MVC = motor vehicle collision; IV = intravenous; PCA = patient-controlled analgesia.

Table 19.4 Pharmacologic agents used in trauma.

Analgesic agents
Non-steroidal anti-inflammatory drugs (NSAIDs)/acetaminophen
Tramadol
Opioids
Adjuvant agents
Local anesthetics
Ketamine
Tricyclic antidepressants and serotonin–norepinephrine reuptake inhibitors
Anticonvulsants
Clonidine
Benzodiazepines
Antihistamines
Entonox (50:50% nitrous oxide:oxygen mixture)
Corticosteroids

sensitization. A successful analgesic strategy should aim to interrupt this cycle as soon as possible after the injury and provide maintenance relief thereafter. Early and aggressive use of analgesic interventions has been shown to reduce analgesic requirements and improve long-term outcomes for traumatic injuries (Hedderich and Ness 1999). In blunt chest trauma, inadequate analgesia may result in hypoventilation and the inability to clear secretions, leading to the development of atelectasis and pneumonia (Miller et al. 2009). In a study by Gaillard et al. (1990) published in 1990 in over 400 patients with multiple trauma including chest injuries, the authors reported mortality rates of 69, 56, 42, and 38% for flail chest, pulmonary contusion, hemothorax, and pneumothorax, respectively. A larger study by Ziegler and Agarwal reported a mortality rate of 12% in 711 patients with rib fractures secondary to trauma (Ziegler and Agarwal 1994). Table 19.4 summarizes analgesic and other adjuvant agents useful in the trauma setting.

Opioids and Adjuvants

In the acute setting, frequent small doses of intravenous opioids may be used. Hydromorphone, morphine, and fentanyl are all acceptable choices, while meperidine should be avoided because of the potential accumulation of active metabolites and reduction in seizure threshold. Individual patients will have different opioid requirements so doses must be carefully titrated to effect in order to achieve analgesia. Trauma is more likely to occur in young males, individuals with psychiatric disorders, and those with substance abuse problems. Although these patients often require high doses of opioids, and are at increased risk for addiction and aberrant behaviors, there is a clear consensus that these concerns should not affect the short-term goal of adequate pain control (Bourne et al. 2008). In patients who receive parenteral opioids, there is strong evidence that the use of PCA is associated with better pain relief and less side effects than PRN administration. Specific issues that may need to be addressed depending on the circumstances include opioid-hyperalgesia, pain intolerance, poor coping skills, and withdrawal in those with opioid or other drug dependencies. In these cases, the use of multimodal analgesic regimens that include adjuvants, non-steroid anti-inflammatory drugs, ketamine, and regional anesthesia should be implemented whenever possible (Table 19.5).

Table 19.5 Sample pain regiments for the trauma patient.

Initial presentation			
Morphine 1–4 mg q1 h Hydromorphone 0.5–1 mg q1 h Fentanyl 25–50 mcg q20–30 min			

	Intensive care unit (intubated or sedated)	Hospital floor	
		NPO	Tolerating PO
Background pain	Fentanyl 1–2 mcg/kg/h infusion	Opioids via PCA Methadone Continous ketamine infusion	Scheduled long-acting oral opioids (MsContin, OxyContin), Methadone NSAIDs
Breakthrough pain	Morphine 2–10 mg q2 h prn Fentanyl 25–100 mcg q1 h prn Hydromorphone 0.5–2 mg q2 h prn	Hydromorphone PCA 0/0.2/6 Morphine PCA 0/1/6	PRN oral opioids

NPO = nil per os; PCA = patient-controlled analgesia; NSAIDs = non-steroidal anti-inflammatory drugs.

Regional Anesthesia and Other Interventions

The type of trauma influences the pain management plan. Patients with blunt chest trauma have a high mortality rate associated with injury to the heart and lungs and are especially vulnerable to the adverse effects on the respiratory system imposed by pain and opioids. It is therefore generally accepted that regional analgesia should be instituted whenever possible in patients at high risk (e.g., elderly, multiple rib fractures, heart and lung injuries) (Karmakar and Ho 2003, Cohen et al. 2004). This is supported by studies demonstrating the superiority of epidural analgesia compared to parenteral opioids and intercostal nerve blocks after thoracotomy (Moon et al. 1999, Yildirim et al. 2000, Behera et al. 2008) and more recent studies showing that continuous paravertebral blocks provide comparable analgesia to epidurals (Casati et al. 2009, Szebla and Machala 2008). For interpleural analgesia, the results of clinical studies have been mixed at best (Schneider et al. 1993, Miguel and Hubbell 1993). In view of the high systemic blood levels when lipid-soluble opioids are administered epidurally, insertion close to the area of trauma is recommended.

Trauma-related amputations comprise over 15% of all amputations and a majority of upper extremity amputations. Whereas most of these involve digits, many involve full or partial limbs. Trauma-related amputations require frequent revisions, which makes epidural analgesia (lower extremity) and peripheral nerve blocks (upper extremity) ideal techniques. Heterotopic ossification is also more common in trauma-related than planned amputations and can be very painful. Epidemiological studies have found no difference in the prevalence rates of postamputation pain between traumatic and planned amputations (Sherman and Sherman 1985).

There are several factors that may affect the incidence of postamputation residual limb and phantom pain, including pre-morbid psychopathology, location, and preoperative and postoperative pain intensity. The evidence supporting preemptive analgesia to reduce the incidence of phantom pain is mixed and largely irrelevant for traumatic amputations.

However, the strong correlation between postoperative pain intensity and chronic postsurgical pain, the frequent need for multiple procedures, and the other benefits afforded by regional anesthesia strongly augur for the use of epidural and continuous peripheral nerve blocks for traumatic amputations.

Vertebral compression fractures represent a significant cause of morbidity and mortality, especially in the elderly. The prevalence of neurological deficits varies widely in the literature and is contingent on the type, number, location, and extent of injury. However, the incidence of neurological deficits is often reported to exceed 25% (Gertzbein 1992). Along with spinal cord injury and radicular pain, patients with vertebral fractures are at increased risk for facetogenic and discogenic pain.

In addition to NSAIDs and opioids, which are first-line treatments for acute nociceptive bone pain, several other treatment options exist. Vertebroplasty and kyphoplasty may be useful in patients with vertebral fractures secondary to osteoporosis and malignancy, but are generally less beneficial in young patients with traumatic fractures. Contraindications to both techniques include bleeding disorders, unstable fractures with posterior element involvement, and definitive neurological symptoms. Whereas multiple uncontrolled studies have demonstrated efficacy for both vertebroplasty and kyphoplasty, a recent double-blind, placebo-controlled study failed to show benefit for vertebroplasty (Kallmes et al. 2009).

In patients with radicular or other neuropathic symptoms secondary to traumatic vertebral fractures, epidural steroid injections and neuropathic agents may provide pain relief and functional improvement. For bone pain, bisphosphonates and calcitonin have been shown to alleviate pain in addition to preventing future fractures.

Traumatic brain injury (TBI) is another common cause of chronic pain and disability, affecting nearly 1.5 million Americans per year. The prevalence of pain following TBI varies dramatically, ranging from 18% to over 90% depending on the surveillance method, severity, and associated trauma (Cohen et al. 2004). The most common pain complaints in patients with mild TBI (Glasgow Coma Scale 13–15, loss of consciousness <1 h) are headache (69%), neck pain (40%), and back pain (32%). First-line treatments for headache prophylaxis include tricyclic antidepressants, topiramate, and gabapentin. The most frequent cause of neck pain after trauma is facet arthropathy, which may be treated with radiofrequency denervation (Lord et al. 1996, Cohen et al. 2007). Other causes of chronic neck pain after trauma include occipital neuralgia, which may respond to nerve blocks and pulsed radiofrequency, cervical discogenic pain, and myofascial pain.

In patients with moderate to severe TBI, the development of spasticity (especially extensor hypertonia of the lower limbs) can contribute to chronic pain. Tizanidine, cutaneous electrical stimulation, and cryotherapy have been beneficial in relieving spasticity; in refractory cases, intrathecal baclofen and injections of botulinum toxin or alcohol neurolysis have been shown to be effective (Lahz and Bryant 1996, Branca et al. 2004).

Extremity trauma represents the leading cause of survivable war injuries (>67%), sports injuries, and work-related trauma. In patients with orthopedic extremity injuries, peripheral nerve blocks may improve acute pain control, reduce opioid consumption, and facilitate discharge as either stand-alone therapy or an adjunct to systemic opioids. Brachial plexus blocks can be useful in upper extremity trauma, whereas lumbar plexus and sciatic blocks are indicated in patients with lower extremity injuries. When multiple operations or prolonged hospitalization is anticipated, a catheter can be placed to provide continuous analgesia.

Regional techniques, however, may be less useful in patients with multiple injuries and open wounds and contraindicated in patients with untreated infection. Furthermore, the risks of a regional technique may outweigh its benefits in patients who are sedated (i.e., for ventilatory-dependent respiratory failure) or those with acute changes in mental status, as a practitioner may not readily recognize nerve injury during placement or local anesthetic toxicity.

Adjuvants

Trauma victims may develop central or peripheral neuropathic pain, especially following traumatic amputations (>50% after major limb amputation), spinal cord injury (>50%), vertebral fractures (>25%), and crush or burn injuries. Neuropathic pain is initiated or caused by a primary lesion or dysfunction in the nervous system and is often described as shooting, burning, or electrical like. Not infrequently, hyperalgesia, allodynia, or signs of autonomic dysfunction, such as sudomotor and vasomotor changes, are present. The identification of neuropathic pain as the primary cause or a contributor to trauma-related pain is essential in the formulation of an analgesic plan. First-line agents for neuropathic pain include tricyclic antidepressants (and serotonin–norepinephrine reuptake inhibitors in the elderly) and gabapentinoid membrane stabilizers. Second, third, and fourth line agents include NMDA receptor antagonists (e.g., ketamine and dextromethorphan), which may act synergistically with opioids, topical lidocaine (for tactile allodynia), mexiletine, capsaicin cream, clonidine (for sympathetically maintained pain), and cannabinoids, which may be particularly effective for central pain (i.e., spinal cord injury). Finally, corticosteroids have been used to treat trauma-associated pain resulting from spinal cord injury, peripheral nerve injuries (i.e., complex regional pain syndrome type II), and soft tissue damage.

Non-pharmacological Options

Non-pharmacologic options for trauma patients include transcutaneous electrical nerve stimulation (TENS), acupuncture, and relaxation techniques. In general, these therapies tend to be most useful as adjuncts to either nerve blocks or pharmacotherapy or in patients with mild pain. Relaxation techniques such as guided imagery, self-hypnosis, and biofeedback are most beneficial in patients with high anxiety levels, whereas the best candidates for eye movement desensitization and reprocessing (EMDR) and cognitive-behavioral therapies are cognitively intact patients willing to take an active role in treatment. The treatment of coexisting psychopathology is critical to optimizing pain treatment outcomes and should not be underestimated. In fact, long-standing anxiety from poorly managed pain has been associated with depression and posttraumatic stress disorder.

Hemodynamics

Hemodynamics should be carefully monitored, as trauma may cause large-scale fluid shifts and impair the body's ability to respond to stress. For example, patients with spinal cord injury may present in shock or respond poorly to blood loss, and those with chest trauma may have impaired cardiac and lung function. Burn patients require enormous amounts of fluid administration immediately after a burn, which must be monitored and tapered judiciously. Hemodynamic changes can also accompany traumatic limb amputation and head trauma. Hypotension in response to opioid administration may indicate hypovolemia and necessitate further aggressive fluid resuscitation. Sedation and respiratory depression as a consequence of overly aggressive opioid administration must be avoided, as this may interfere with the primary, secondary, and tertiary trauma surveys, as well as recognition of life-threatening conditions such as an occult intracranial hemorrhage (Hedderich and Ness 1998).

Psychological Sequelae

Because of its unexpected and often catastrophic nature, trauma is usually associated with coexisting psychopathology. This may affect how the sensorium of pain is perceived by the victim and limit the effectiveness of pharmacologic analgesia. There are numerous studies conducted in a multitude of pain conditions that show coexisting psychological disorders can adversely affect pain treatment (Kuch et al. 2001, Cohen et al. 2008). As a result, immediate emotional support, in the form of family, religious or spiritual counselors, and psychiatrists, can be beneficial. Financial, legal, and medical issues should be addressed with the patient in an effort to allay the anxiety associated with the trauma. Small doses of anxiolytics may also prove beneficial once the underlying issues have been resolved, but this potential benefit must be weighed against the increased risk for aberrant drug-seeking behavior in young patients with concomitant psychological issues.

Summary

Pain management in trauma patients poses a significant challenge to the health-care provider, as these patients present with a wide range of injuries and comorbid conditions. These injuries exert myriad effects on multiple body systems, all of which can contribute to morbidity and mortality. In recent years, as mortality rates have declined and our understanding of the mechanisms and consequences of pain have improved, it has become increasingly apparent that the early and aggressive treatment of pain can have both short-term and long-term beneficial consequences. In view of the dynamic nature of trauma, frequent assessments of the patient's physical and psychological status and their response to treatment must be undertaken.

Case Scenario

Sreekumar Kunnumpurath, MBBS, MD, FCARCSI, FRCA, FFPMRCA

Meena, a 40-year-old woman is brought to the emergency department with burns affecting her chest, abdomen, and upper limbs. She sustained burns when the bed she was sleeping on caught fire from a cigarette that she had been smoking. As the physician covering emergency calls, you have been requested to attend to her urgently. When you see her, she is anxious, agitated, and screaming from pain.

How would you prioritize your management?
Your initial assessment should follow ATLS guidelines. If this has not already been done, then you have to assess airway, breathing, circulation, and disability (ABCDs). Burn injury could be associated with smoke inhalation, airway burns, both upper and lower, both posing immediate threat to life. There could be coexistence of trauma which should be ruled out during a secondary survey conducted once the patient is stable enough. Then the next step is controlling pain, anxiety, and emotional distress.

On evaluation, you notice that Meena has sustained about 30% burns of varying degree, ranging from first to deep second degree. Luckily, her airway does not appear compromised, and her neck and face are free from burns.

What are the options for pain management during the initial phase?
In this situation, aggressive fluid resuscitation should be initiated along with management of acute pain. For the immediate acute pain management strong opioids are given in frequent, controlled, and carefully titrated doses. Fentanyl, hydromorphone, and morphine are all acceptable. NSAIDs or acetaminophen may also be helpful and these can reduce the opioid requirement. Topical agents (creams, lotions, sprays, etc.) containing local anesthetics such as lidocaine or benzocaine (i.e., EMLA cream) can be applied over areas with first-degree burns. Emotional support and small doses of anxiolytics may also be beneficial.

Meena's pain is under control and she has responded very well to your management. She is then transferred to the burn unit.

Describe your pain management during her stay in the burn unit.
Burn patients can experience various types of pain during recovery such as background pain, procedural pain, postoperative pain, and breakthrough pain. Management should be directed to the specific type of pain being experienced. Various opioids delivered as infusions, PCA, or through enteral route can produce effective analgesia. In the absence of any specific contraindication, these can be combined with acetaminophen and NSAIDs (see chapter 19). Other useful agents include clonidine, tricyclic antidepressants, and ketamine. Ketamine is also useful as a sole anesthetic for minor procedures such as dressing changes.

References

Behera BK, Puri GD, Ghai B. Patient-controlled epidural analgesia with fentanyl and bupivacaine provides better analgesia than intravenous morphine patient-controlled analgesia for early thoracotomy pain. J Postgrad Med. 2008;54(2):86.

Bourne N, et al. Managing acute pain in opioid tolerant patients. J Perioper Pract. 2008;18(11):498–503.

Branca B, et al. Psychological and Neuropsychological Integration in Multidisciplinary Pain Management After TBI. J Head Trauma Rehabil. 2004;19(1):47–50.

Brofeldt BT, Cornwell P, Doherty D, et al. Topical lidocaine in the treatment of partial thickness burns. J Burn Care Rehabil. 1989;10(1):63.

Casati A, Alessandrini P, et al. A prospective, randomized, blinded comparison between continuous thoracic paravertebral and epidural infusion of 0.2% ropivacaine after lung resection surgery. Eur J Anaesthesiol. 2006;23(12):999–1004.

Choiniere M, Melzack R, Girard N, Rondeau J, Paquin M. Comparisons between patients' and nurses' assessment of pain and medication efficacy in severe burn injuries. Pain 1990;40(2):143–52.

Church D, Elsayed S, Reid O, Winston B, Lindsay R. Burn wound infections. Clin Microbiol Rev. 2006;19:403–34.

Cohen SP, Christo PJ, Moroz L, et al. Pain management in trauma patients. Am J Phys Med Rehabil. 2004;83(2):142–61.

Cohen SP, Argoff CE, et al. Management of low back pain. Br Med J. 2008;338(10):100–6.

Cohen SP, Bajwa ZH, et al. Factors predicting success and failure for cervical facet radiofrequency denervation: a multi-center analysis. Reg Anesth Pain Med. 2007;32(6):495–503.

Davydow DS, Katon WJ, Zatzick DF. Psychiatric morbidity and functional impairments in survivors of burns, traumatic injuries, and ICU stays for other critical illnesses: A review of the literature. Int Rev Psychiatry 2009;21(6):531–8.

Dyster-Aas M, Johan D, et al. Major depression and posttraumatic stress disorder symptoms following severe burn injury in relation to lifetime psychiatric morbidity. J Trauma Inj Infect Crit Care. 2008;64(5):1349–56.

Gaillard M, Herve C, et al. Mortality prognostic factors in chest injury. J Trauma 1990;30(1):93.

Gertzbein SD. Multicenter spine fracture study. Spine 1992;17(5):528–40.

Hedderich R, Ness T. Analgesia for Trauma and Burns. Crit Care Clin. 1998;15(1):167–84.

Hedderich R, Ness TJ. Analgesia for Trauma and Burns. Crit Care Clin. 1999;15(1):167–84.

Jenewein J, Moergeli H, Wittmann L, Buchi S, Kraemer B, Schnyder U. Development of chronic pain following severe accidental injury. Results of a 3-year follow-up study. J Psychosom Res. 2009;66(2):119–26.

Jonsson A, Cassuto J, Hanson B. Inhibition of burn pain by intravenous lignocaine infusion. Lancet 1991;338(8760):151–2.

Kallmes DF, Comstock BA, et al. A randomized trial of vertebroplasty for osteoporotic spinal fractures. N Engl J Med. 2009;361(6):569–79.

Karmakar MK, Ho AMH. Acute pain management of patients with multiple fractured ribs. J Trauma Inj Inf Crit Care 2003;54(3):615–25.

Kuch K, et al. Psychological factors and the development of chronic pain. Clin J Pain. 2001;b(4 suppl):S33–8.

Lahz S, Bryant R. Incidence of chronic pain following traumatic brain injury. Arch Phys Med Rehabil. 1996;77(9):889–8.

Latarjet J, Choinere M. Pain in burns patients. Burns 1995;21(5):344–8.

Lee RC, Astumian RD. The physicochemical basis for thermal and non-thermal `burn' injuries. Burns 1996;22(7):509–19.

Lord SM, Barnsley L, et al. Chronic cervical zygapophysial joint pain after whiplash: a placebo-controlled prevalence study. Spine 1996;21(15):1737–44.

Marx JA, et al. Rosen's emergency medicine: concepts and clinical practice. 7th ed. Chapter 60. Thermal Burns: Mosby; 2009.

Miguel R, Hubbell D. Pain management and spirometry following thoracotomy: a prospective, randomized study of four techniques. J Cardiothorac Vasc Anesth. 1993;7(5):529–34.

Miller R, et al. Miller's anesthesia. 7th ed. Chapter 54 Churchill Livingstone: Acutely Burned Patient; 2009.

Miller R, et al. Miller's anesthesia. 7th ed. Chapter 72 Churchill Livingstone: Anesthesia for Trauma and Burns; 2009.

Moon MR, Luchette FA, et al. Prospective, randomized comparison of epidural versus parenteral opioid analgesia in thoracic. Trauma Ann Surg. 1999;229(5):684.

Naschitz JE, Lenger R. Why traumatic leg amputees are at increased risk for cardiovascular diseases. QJM 2008;101(4):251–9.

Owens V, Palmieri T, Comroe C, Convoy J, Scavone J, Greenhalgh D. Ketamine: a safe and effective agent for painful procedures in the pediatric burn patient. J Burn Care Res. 2006;27(2):211–6.

Pal S, Cortiella J, Herdon D. Adjunctive methods of pain control in burns. Burns 1997;23(6):404–12.

Patterson D, Hoflund H, Espey K, Sharar S. Pain management. Burns 2004;30(8):A10–15.

Perry S, Heidrich G, Ramos E. Assessment of pain by burns patients. J Burn Care Res. 1981;2(6):322.

Schneider RF, Villamena PC et al. Lack of efficacy of intrapleural bupivacaine for postoperative analgesia following thoracotomy. Chest 1993;103(2):414–6.

Sharar S, Patterson D, Askay S. Pain Management. Vol. 1. Waldman SD, editor. Chapter 21 Burn Pain Saunders-Elsevier, Philadelphia, PA; 2007. pp. 241–56.

Sherman RA, Sherman CJ. A comparison of phantom sensations among amputees whose amputations were of civilian and military origins. Pain 1985;21(1):91-7.

Szebla R, Machala W. Continuous epidural anaesthesia vs paravertebral block for lung surgery – a comparative study. Anestezjol Intens Ter. 2008;40(3):152-5.

Tosun Z, Esmaoglu A, Coruh A. Propofol-ketamine vs propofol-fentanyl combinations for deep sedation and analgesia in pediatric patients undergoing burn dressing changes. Paediatr Anaesth. 2008;18(1):43-7.

Ward HC, et al. Prevalence of postburn depression following burn injury. J Burn Care Rehabil 1987;8(4):322.

Yang Z, Lowe AJ, de la Harpe DE, Richardson MD. Factors that predict poor outcomes in patients with traumatic vertebral fractures. Injury 2010;41(2):226-30.

Yeager MP, Glass DD, et al. Epidural anesthesia and analgesia in high-risk surgical patients. Anesthesiology 1987;66(6):729-36.

Yildirim V, Akay HT, et al. Interpleural versus epidural analgesia with ropivacaine for postthoracotomy pain and respiratory function. J Clin Anesth. 2000;19(7):506.

Ziegler DW, Agarwal NN. The morbidity and mortality of rib fractures. J Trauma. 1994;37(6):975-9.

Chapter 20

Regional Anesthesia Techniques

Thomas Halaszynski, DMD, MD, MBA, Richa Wardhan, MBBS, and Elizabeth Freck, MD

Introduction

Regional anesthesia (RA) techniques, especially peripheral nerve blocks (PNBs) and central neuraxial anesthesia/analgesia, are more difficult to learn than the basic skills to conduct general anesthesia (GA). RA has not been conducted as a structured rotation for the promotion of consistency as the other subspecialty rotations within anesthesia, but the goals of RA are to develop and cultivate proficiency in motor skills aligned with quality and safe patient care. RA training and practice must impart knowledge, judgment, motor skill proficiency, didactic training, and continued assessment of learned knowledge and skills.

Perioperative use of RA and analgesia (both neuraxial and peripheral) may attenuate adverse perioperative pathophysiology and improve patient outcomes (Liu et al. 2004, Ballantyne et al. 1998, Rigg et al. 2003, Block et al. 2003, Wu et al. 2005). Available data indicates that the perioperative use of RA and analgesia may improve both conventional, rehabilitation, and patient-centered outcomes; however, the benefits on other outcomes (e.g., cognitive dysfunction, immune function) are not as certain (Joshi et al. 2008, Liu and Wu 2007, Jorgensen et al. 2000, Richman et al. 2006, Wu et al. 2004). Although the majority of available data has examined the effect of GA along with epidural anesthesia and analgesia on patient outcomes, an increasing number of recent studies have investigated the effect of peripheral regional techniques on outcomes. Table 20.1 summarizes risks and benefits of different anesthetic techniques, using simple terms and explanations to make it easy for the patient to understand different options available so that he/she can make an intelligent decision. RA provides the anesthesiologist with an alternative to GA for surgery of the abdomen, pelvis, and upper and lower extremities. Many of the RA techniques described may be utilized for anesthesia of the planned surgery, but can also be implemented for the purposes of postoperative analgesia and for reducing the depth of anesthesia during the surgical intervention.

PNBs are gaining widespread popularity for perioperative pain management. PNBs have been identified with many distinct advantages over GA and central neuraxial anesthesia (Table 20.2). Despite the numerous advantages of PNB, the techniques are often underutilized for a variety of reasons, and there are also some documented limitations to PNB. Yet, since the many benefits of PNB are becoming more clinically relevant, some ways to overcome limitations of PNB are suggested in Table 20.3.

N. Vadivelu et al. (eds.), *Essentials of Pain Management*,
DOI 10.1007/978-0-387-87579-8_20, © Springer Science+Business Media, LLC 2011

Table 20.1 Discussing anesthetic options with the patient: Summation of anesthesia, analgesia, and pain relief.

General anesthesia (with or without a breathing tube)	Technique	Medicines put in an IV will result in unconsciousness. A breathing tube or another device may be put into your windpipe or throat after unconsciousness. Medicine breathed through this device will maintain unconsciousness while a machine will breathe for you. Anesthesia gas and/or medications given through the IV will keep you asleep. On the other hand, if numbing medicines are used and a nerve block is performed, you may not need general anesthesia (depends on type of surgery and
	Expected result	patient characteristics)
	Specific risks	You will not be aware during surgery
		Nausea and vomiting, mouth or throat pain, hoarseness, injury to mouth, teeth, or eyes, breathing stomach contents into the lungs, pneumonia, or pain from a nerve injury. A very small risk of becoming aware of what is going on during surgery
Epidural, spinal, or caudal anesthesia	Technique	Medicine put through a needle or tube between the bones of the back resulting in a level of anesthesia (numb body)
	Expected result	Temporarily lose feeling and movement to the lower part of the body or to the chest and belly. Pain relief for a period of time after surgery
	Specific risks	Nausea and vomiting, headache, backache, a seizure, permanent weakness, numbness, or pain from a nerve injury
Peripheral nerve block	Technique	Medicine put through a needle or tube near nerves of the arm, leg, chest, back, or belly will numb a particular portion of the body
	Expected result	Temporarily lose feeling and movement of all or part of a limb, chest, or belly. Pain relief for a period of time after surgery
	Specific risks	Soreness or bruising, injury to a blood vessel, a seizure, permanent weakness, numbness, or pain from a nerve injury. Lung collapse possible with specific types of nerve blocks

Table 20.2 Potential advantages of peripheral nerve blocks.

1. Pain relief with PNB is devoid of side effects including nausea, vomiting, somnolence, voiding difficulties, and hemodynamic instability that is often inherent to GA and central neuraxial anesthesia
2. Patients who undergo surgery under a PNB (without GA) may meet criteria to bypass or be exposed to an abbreviated stay in the PACU/recovery room. Expeditiously discharged to the floor or to home (in the case of outpatient surgery). Improve the early transition into physical therapy if prescribed
3. Patients with compromised or unstable cardiovascular disease may undergo surgery under a PNB without experiencing significant hemodynamic compromise
4. Patients who have infections or hemostatic abnormality (coagulation concerns), which could contraindicate central neuraxial blockade, may be appropriate candidates for surgery under PNB
5. Potential time savings in the OR and/or OR turnover time is possible when a PNB is conducted outside of the OR environment; if there is a functioning PNB preoperatively, then there should be NO induction or emergence time in the OR
6. PNB combined with a GA can facilitate a lighter plane of GA and minimize or avoid the use of opioids that will expedite emergence and recovery with fewer patient side effects
7. Patients can often position themselves on the OR table with little risk to the loss of their airway with minimal stressful effort with a preoperatively placed PNB
8. Patient, surgical, and nursing satisfaction results because PNB provides superior pain control with minimal side effects
9. PNB anesthesia/analgesic techniques will permit opioid-sparing anesthesia and minimize or eliminate the side effect profiles associated with IV/PO opioid administration

PNB, peripheral nerve block; PACU, postoperative acute care unit; IV, intravenous; PO, per os; OR, operating room.

Table 20.3 Disadvantages/limitations to peripheral nerve block and ways to overcome the limitations.

Inadequate training and/or lack of experience	Knowledge of neural elements to be blocked, relationship to vascular, muscular, and other structures along with their motor and sensory innervation must be known.
Anxiety related to PNB success (PNB is not 100% successful in attaining surgical anesthesia)	Establish educational programs toward improving RA skills
Potential delay in the onset of surgical anesthesia and the duration of postoperative analgesia	Knowledge of local anesthetic pharmacology (onset and duration of action) will direct selection of the most appropriate local anesthetic drug(s), volume, and concentration
Complications associated with the placement of PNB and the drug(s) utilized	Knowledge of errors, complications, and possible side effects in techniques and drug(s) will help to avoid the complications and make managing them more successful should they occur
PNB is more labor intensive toward both patient education and PNB technique/placement	Designate a monitored space outside the OR to facilitate PNB placement well ahead of the scheduled surgery. Dissemination of patient education brochures with descriptions of PNB, side effects, possible complications, and merits (ahead of scheduled surgery)

PNB, peripheral nerve block; OR, operating room.

Among clinicians, RA has experienced a tremendous renaissance of interest over the past several years. Identification of a few reasons for the renewed enthusiasm is due to: (1) improvements toward suggested RA techniques and protocols, (2) advancements in technology to improve patient safety, (3) interest in the role that efficacy of techniques may play toward outcome-based measures, (4) anatomical and pharmacologic studies permitting more formalized use of RA, and (5) the overall "value added" of successfully performed RA on appropriately selected surgical and medical patients.

Table 21.4 serves as a useful foundation to enhance the clinical starting point of understanding for the most commonly performed PNBs and displays the most clinically relevant indications and suggestions for PNBs utilized in the perioperative setting. This summary will enable the reader to better understand one of the alternatives to the care of the majority of patients undergoing peripheral extremity surgery. Table 20.4 is by no means meant to be an all-inclusive guide to PNB placement, but is intended to act as a foundation for understanding the drugs (local anesthetics), skills, and concerns of the regional anesthesiologists.

For RA to remain an option in the armamentarium of the anesthesiologist, the techniques should have a high success rate, short latency to surgical anesthesia/analgesia, capability of providing prolonged postoperative analgesia, minimal side effect profile, and low risks to the patient. To improve success and minimize latency, the local anesthetic must be deposited close to the nerve(s) or nerve bundle(s). Methods of ensuring proximity of the needle to the nerve or nerve plexus are eliciting paresthesia, locating the peripheral nerve with a peripheral nerve stimulator (PNS), and using appropriate end points and/or using ultrasound-guided RA needle placement for PNB. Identifying human anatomy landmark techniques and ultrasound-directed techniques (see Chapter 22) to locate anatomical landmarks may also be used both for PNBs and for neuraxial techniques. Spinal and epidural anesthesia success and proficiency demand an understanding of the anatomy of the spinal cord and of the surrounding structures, as well as anatomical landmark techniques for successful placement.

Table 20.4 Peripheral nerve blocks matched to appropriate surgical procedure and local anesthetic selection.

Peripheral nerve block type	Indications	Problems and contraindication	Local anesthetic(s)	Onset (min)	Anest (h)	Analg (h)
Interscalene brachial plexus block	Shoulder, arm, elbow surgery	Phrenic and/or recurrent laryngeal nerve block, dyspnea, Horner's syndrome	3% 2-chloroprocaine (+HCO3 +epinephrine)	5–10	1.5	2
			1.5% mepivacaine (+HCO3)	10–20	2–3	2–4
			1.5% mepivacaine (+HCO3+epinephrine)	5–15	2.5–4	3–6
			2% lidocaine (+HCO3)	10–20	2.5–3	2–5
			2% lidocaine (+HCO3+epinephrine)	5–15	3–6	5–8
			0.5% ropivacaine	15–20	6–8	8–12
			0.75% ropivacaine	5–15	8–10	12–18
			0.5% bupivacaine (+epinephrine)	20–30	8–10	16–18
Supraclavicular brachial plexus block	Arm, elbow, forearm, hand surgery	Pneumothorax, missed ulnar nerve	3% 2-chloroprocaine (+HCO3+epinephrine)	5–10	1.5	2
			1.5% mepivacaine (+HCO3)	10–20	2–3	2–4
			1.5% mepivacaine (+HCO3+epinephrine)	5–15	2.5–4	3–6
			2% lidocaine (+HCO3)	10–20	2.5–3	2–5
			2% lidocaine (+HCO3+epinephrine)	5–15	3–6	5–8
			0.5% ropivacaine	15–20	6–8	8–12
			0.5% bupivacaine (+epinephrine)	20–30	8–10	16–18
Infraclavicular brachial plexus block	Elbow, forearm, hand surgery	Pneumothorax	3% 2-chloroprocaine (+HCO3 +epinephrine)	5–10	1.5	2
			1.5% mepivacaine (+HCO3+epi)	5–15	2.5–4	3–6
			2% lidocaine (+HCO3+epinephrine)	5–15	3–6	5–8
			0.5% ropivacaine	15–20	6–8	8–12
Axillary brachial plexus block	Forearm and hand surgery		1.5% mepivacaine (+HCO3+epinephrine)	5–15	2.5–4	3–6
			2% lidocaine (+HCO3+epinephrine)	5–15	3–6	5–8
			0.5% ropivacaine	15–20	6–8	8–12
Femoral nerve block	Anterior thigh and knee surgery	Relative contraindication with femoral vascular grafts	3% 2-chloroprocaine (+HCO3)	10–15	1	2
			3% 2-chloroprocaine (+HCO3+epi)	10–15	1.5–2	2–3
			1.5% mepivacaine (+HCO3)	15–20	2–3	3–5
			1.5% mepivacaine (+HCO3+epinephrine)	15–20	2–5	3–8
			2% lidocaine (+HCO3+epinephrine)	10–20	2–5	3–8
			0.5% ropivacaine	15–30	4–8	5–12
			0.75% ropivacaine	10–15	5–10	6–24
			0.5% bupivacaine (or levo-bupivacaine)	15–30	5–15	6–30

Table 20.4 (Continued)

Block	Indication	Considerations	Local anesthetic			
Sciatic block (posterior approach)	Surgery on the knee, tibia, ankle, and foot		3% 2-chloroprocaine (+HCO$_3$)	10–15	2	2.5
			1.5% mepivacaine (+HCO$_3$)	10–15	4–5	5–8
			2% lidocaine(+HCO$_3$)	15–20	5–6	5–8
			0.5% ropivacaine	10–20	6–12	6–24
			0.75% ropivacaine	10–15	8–12	8–24
			0.5% bupivacaine (or l-bupivacaine)	15–30	8–16	10–48
Popliteal block (intertendinous)	Corrective foot surgery, foot debridement, and Achilles tendon repair		3% 2-chloroprocaine (+HCO$_3$)	10–15	1	2
			3% 2-chloroprocaine (+HCO$_3$+epinephrine)	10–15	1.5–2	2–3
			1.5% mepivacaine (+HCO$_3$)	15–20	2–3	2–5
			1.5% mepivacaine (+HCO$_3$+epinephrine)	15–20	2–2	3–8
			2% lidocaine (+HCO$_3$+epinephrine)	10–20	2–5	3–8
			0.5% ropivacaine	15–30	4–8	5–12
			0.75% ropivacaine	10–15	5–10	6–24
			0.5% bupivacaine (or l-bupivacaine)	15–30	5–15	6–30
			1.5% mepivacaine (+HCO$_3$+epinephrine)	10–20	2–3	3–4
Lumbar plexus block	Hip, anterior thigh, and knee surgery	Hemodynamic effects, patient anticoagulation	2% lidocaine (+HCO$_3$+epinephrine)	10–15	2–3	3–4
			0.5% ropivacaine	15–25	3–5	8–12
			0.75% ropivacaine	10–15	4–6	12–18
			0.5% bupivacaine (+epinephrine)	15–25	4–6	12–18
			0.5% l-bupivacaine (+epinephrine)	12–25	4–6	12–18
Ankle block	Surgery on foot and toes		1.5% mepivacaine (+HCO$_3$)	15–20	2–3	3–5
			2% lidocaine(+HCO$_3$)	10–20	2–5	3–8
			0.5% ropivacaine	15–30	4–8	5–12
			0.75% ropivacaine	10–15	5–10	6–24
			0.5% bupivacaine (or levo–bupivacaine)	15–30	5–15	6–30
Intravenous regional block (Bier block)	Hand and/or foot surgery	Mixing with epinephrine, duration	0.5% lidocaine 50 ml			
			2% lidocaine 15 ml			
			0.20% ropivacaine			
			0.25% bupivacaine			

PNB, peripheral nerve block; epi, epinephrine; Anest, anesthesia; Analg, analgesia; min, minutes; h, hours.

Infection, patient refusal, pre-block neurologic compromise to intended site, patient positioning and allergic reactions are contraindications to PNB placement.

Infection, hematoma, bleeding, nerve injury, patient discomfort, failed or partial block, paresthesia, and intravascular injection are possible with all of the above.

Despite major improvements over the last decade in our understanding of acute postoperative pain pathophysiology, there is a continuous push to optimize and improve perioperative pain management. In this context, there has been much attention given to the relationship between analgesic efficacy and opioid-sparing effects. This is based upon the well-documented side effects of opioids on postoperative recovery and the lack of sufficient efficacy on mobilization-induced pain (Liu et al. 2005, Kehlet 2005). As a result, it was hypothesized more than 15 years ago that a combination of different non-opioid analgesics might increase analgesic efficacy with simultaneous reduction of side effects due to different side effect profiles of the analgesics used (Liu et al. 2006). The evidence from several controlled prospective case series with multimodal combinations combined with adjustment of the overall perioperative care program has demonstrated the multimodal approach to be worthwhile. There is also a need to investigate procedure-specific approaches since different analgesics may have different effects and side effects in different types of surgery.

Prevention of venous thromboembolism remains a crucial component of patient care following major surgery. The risk factors for thromboembolism include trauma, immobility/paresis, malignancy, previous thromboembolism, increasing age (over 40 years), pregnancy, estrogen therapy, obesity, smoking history, varicose veins, and inherited or congenital thrombophilia. There is a trend toward initiating thromboprophylaxis in close proximity to surgery. However, early postoperative (and intraoperative) dosing of low molecular weight heparin (LMWH) was associated with an increased risk of neuraxial bleeding and bleeding at a peripheral site where a PNB or PNB catheter had been placed. It has been demonstrated that the risk of bleeding complications is increased with the duration of anticoagulant therapy. The interaction of prolonged thromboprophylaxis and previous PNB placement or neuraxial instrumentation, including difficult or traumatic needle insertion, is unknown.

Practice guidelines or recommendations summarize evidence-based reviews. However, the rarity of spinal hematoma and hematologic complications associated with PNB techniques make a prospective-randomized study difficult to perform, and there is no current laboratory model. As a result, the consensus statements developed by the American Society of Regional Anesthesia and Pain Medicine (ASRA) represent the collective experience of recognized experts in the field. Recommendations for neuraxial blockade in the presence of anticoagulant therapy are present on the ASRA web site (www.asra.com) (see Table 20.5 for summary), and similar guidelines for the various PNBs are in the process of being developed.

Perioperative complications in the anticoagulated patient (prophylactic or therapeutic levels) may be reduced by allowing the local anesthetic effect to wear off prior to instituting continuous postoperative infusions, using low-dose local anesthetic and/or opioid infusions when appropriate, and performing ongoing evaluation of the patient's neurologic status during the postoperative period. The patient should be monitored closely for early signs of cord compression such as complaints of back pain or an increase in intensity of motor or sensory blockade, and particularly if there is development of new paresis subsequent to neuraxial techniques. In the instance of PNB placement, one much search and evaluate for evidence of peripheral hematoma formation, especially in anatomical locations where applying pressure may prove difficult. If spinal hematoma is suspected, the treatment of choice is immediate decompression laminectomy. Recovery is unlikely if surgery is postponed for more than 8–12 h.

In the last decade there has been a growing interest in the use of bedside 2D ultrasonography (US) to assess neuraxial and peripheral nerve anatomy and to aid in the performance

Table 20.5 Neuraxial techniques in patients receiving anticoagulants.

	Guidelines	Additional notes
Unfractionated heparin	*Subcutaneous heparin:* -If possible, delay dosing until after neuraxial technique *Intravenous heparin:* Discontinue **1 h** before and after needle placement -Discontinue **2–4 h** prior to catheter removal -Avoid resuming for minimum of **1 h** after catheter removal	-Neuraxial bleeding may be increased in debilitated pts, after prolonged therapy -Evaluate platelet count in patients receiving heparin for >4 days prior to neuraxial block or catheter removal
Low molecular weight heparin (LMWH)	-Avoid neuraxial block for minimum of **10–12 h** after last LMWH dose *Postoperative twice daily dosing:* First LMWH dose should be delayed for **24 h** -Remove any catheter before LMWH therapy, then hold therapy for at least **2 h** *Postoperative once daily dosing:* First LMWH dose should be delayed **6–8 h** -Catheters may be maintained, but should be removed **10–12 h** after last LMWH and subsequent LMWH dosing delayed for **2 h**	-If evidence of blood with needle or catheter placement, LMWH therapy should be delayed for **24 h** -Higher doses of LMWH will require at least **24 h** prior to needle placement -Twice daily dosing increases risk of hematoma development
Fondaparinux (Arixtra)	-Avoid indwelling catheters -Avoid traumatic needle placement	-Utilize neuraxial techniques with extreme caution
Warfarin (Coumadin)	-Discontinue **4–5 days** prior to needle placement -Ensure **INR <1.5** prior to needle placement or catheter removal	-Monitor PT/INR -Neurologic testing at least **24 h** after catheter removal if **INR <1.5**
Antiplatelet agents	*-Clopidogrel (Plavix)* discontinue **7 days** prior to needle/catheter placement *-Ticlopidine (Ticlid)* discontinue **14 days** prior to needle/catheter placement *-Eptifibatide (Integrilin)* and *Tirofiban (Aggrastat)* **AVOID** neuraxial anesthesia	-Aspirin/NSAIDs: Carries **NO current risk** when used alone -Careful preoperative assessment: alterations of health, history of easy bleeding/bruisability, female gender, increased age
Direct thrombin inhibitors (DTIs)	-Hirudin-based, bivalent DTIs including *Bivalirudin (Angiomax)*, *Lepirudin (Refludan)*, and *Desirudin (Iprivask)*, risk of bleeding complications unknown -Univalent DTIs including *Argatroban* and *Dabigatran (Pradaxa)*, risk of bleeding complications unknown	-Monitor aPTT, PT -Many have prolonged half-lives and are difficult to reverse without blood component administration
Herbal medications	-Discontinue **5–7 days** prior to needle placement	-Agents of particular concern include ginger, ginkgo, ginseng, garlic, feverfew, and vitamin E

of neuraxial and PNB interventional procedures. US can assist the practitioner in delivering local anesthetic to the target site, while minimizing complications by avoiding vital structures such as blood vessels and pleura. The evidence for safety over traditional nerve block and neuraxial techniques has yet to be established conclusively; however, studies have shown US-guided nerve blocks to have equivalent efficacy (Marhofer and Chan 2007). This chapter will describe various RA techniques and associated components of the procedures, but will not discuss US-guided PNB or US neuraxial nerve block techniques.

Some of the pharmacokinetics of local anesthetics used in RA are outlined in Table 20.4. Sodium permeability leads to the development of action potentials along nerve membranes, but local anesthetics prevent this permeability in peripheral neurons and stop the propagation of action potential (producing local anesthesia). Local anesthetics bind and block voltage-gated sodium channels in nerve membranes. Local anesthetics also play a role in inflammation, immune responses to malignancy and infection, microcirculation, coagulation, and postoperative gastrointestinal function.

Local anesthetics differ in potency, duration of action, onset, and resolution of effect. They can be divided into three main classes: (1) short duration of action and low potency, such as chloroprocaine and procaine; (2) intermediate duration of action and moderate potency such as lidocaine, procaine, and mepivacaine; and (3) prolonged duration of action and high potency such as bupivacaine, tetracaine, levo-bupivacaine, ropivacaine, and etidocaine.

Local anesthetics with the rapid onset of action include lidocaine, chloroprocaine, mepivacaine, and etidocaine, and those with prolonged duration of action include tetracaine, ropivacaine, and bupivacaine. Lipid solubility of a local anesthetic is strongly associated with its potency – more lipid soluble local anesthetics are more potent. Although it must be remembered in regional anesthesia that only a small fraction of local anesthetic molecules actually bind to sodium channels, while the other local anesthetic molecules have nonspecific binding.

Local anesthetics have differential sensory nerve block capacity that can differentially inhibit sensory over motor nerve fibers as seen with bupivacaine and ropivacaine. Smaller myelinated nerve fibers such as the A delta and non-myelinated C-fibers are more sensitive to local anesthetic effect than larger myelinated nerve fibers such as A beta and A alpha fibers.

Additives (vasoconstrictors, typically epinephrine) mixed with local anesthetics are capable of altering the action of onset, adequacy of anesthesia, and duration of anesthesia. Other additives that have been used along with local anesthetics for regional anesthesia are clonidine, dexmedetomidine, ketorolac, buprenorphine, and opioids.

Local anesthetic toxicity may be manifested in the central nervous system (CNS), as cardiovascular system toxicity, allergy, and methemoglobinemia. CNS depression, seizures, and respiratory arrest are possible toxic effects of local anesthetics and significant cardiovascular toxicity (seen most commonly with bupivacaine which binds more strongly to the cardiac sodium channels and for longer duration than lidocaine) can also occur with increasing local anesthetic plasma levels. Local anesthetics can inhibit calcium and potassium channels in the heart, but only at very high concentrations. Benzocaine and prilocaine cause methemoglobinemia.

Treatment of local anesthetic toxicity such as severe methemoglobinemia is with methylene blue (1 mg/kg) and oxygen. Seizures (CNS) may be terminated with thiopental 1–2 mg/kg, propofol 0.5–1 mg/kg, and midazolam 0.05–0.1 mg/kg, and, in addition, the airway often needs to be secured. In cardiac arrest secondary to local anesthetic toxicity that is unresponsive to standard therapy (CPR), intravenous administration of a lipid such as intralipid 20% is recommended. Initially, intralipid (20%) administration of 1 ml/kg is given over 1 min and may be repeated twice more at 3- to 5-min intervals. An infusion at a rate of 0.25 ml/kg/min may be initiated until hemodynamic stability is restored.

Neuraxial Anesthesia

Neuraxial anesthesia including spinal, epidural, and caudal anesthesia are commonly referred to as conduction or regional anesthesia. Spinal anesthesia is produced by injection of local anesthetic solutions into the lumbar subarachnoid space. Epidural anesthesia results when local anesthetic solutions are placed into the epidural space, often at the lumbar and thoracic levels. Caudal anesthesia is produced by injection of local anesthetics into the epidural space by introducing a needle through the sacral hiatus. Each neuraxial technique may be performed either as single injection or as a continuous catheter technique. Caudal anesthesia is more commonly performed in the pediatric population. Preoperative preparation does not differ from that for general anesthesia. Efficacy of duration, level obtained, and intensity of neuraxial block may be enhanced with the addition of adjuncts (e.g., epinephrine, opioids) to the local anesthetic solutions and by patient position immediately subsequent to local anesthetic injection.

The use of thromboprophylaxis in the perioperative period may conflict with neuraxial techniques in which maintaining hemostasis integrity is essential. A host of anticoagulants have been approved, both oral and parenteral, for use in a wide range of disorders. Neuraxial anesthesia, often used for orthopedic surgery (both for anesthesia and analgesia), should be performed with an optimal coagulation status. When thromboprophylaxis is needed, it remains necessary to keep in mind the pharmacology of the drug(s) used and to follow time interval recommendations in order to minimize the risk of related bleeding complications (Table 20.5).

Mechanism of Action

Neuraxial anesthesia results in selective anesthesia for the surgical site. Local anesthetics injected into the proper space will result in sodium channel blockade, with nerve transmission interruption along nerve roots. Blockade of neural transmission in the posterior nerve root fibers interrupts somatic and visceral sensation, whereas blockade of anterior nerve root fibers prevents efferent motor and autonomic outflow. The level and onset of neuraxial anesthesia obtained should be documented accordingly: (1) sympathetic nervous system is usually blocked first and tested by ability to discriminate temperature change and observation of hemodynamic effects, (2) level of sensory anesthesia is evaluated by ability to discriminate for sharpness, and (3) skeletal muscle strength is evaluated by testing the reduction in foot and knee movement power.

Sensory and Motor Blockade

Local anesthetics acting on the nerve roots block painful stimuli and produce profound skeletal muscle relaxation to the dermatome level achieved.

Autonomic Blockade

Interruption of efferent autonomic transmission at the spinal nerve roots can produce sympathetic and some parasympathetic blockade.

Indications

As primary anesthesia and/or postoperative pain relief (analgesia).

Clinical Uses
Surgical

Lower abdominal and pelvic surgery, including inguinal, urogenital, and rectal procedures. Lower extremity, caesarean section, and lumbar spinal surgery may also be performed under spinal anesthesia. Upper abdominal (e.g., cholecystectomy) and lower thoracic procedures may be performed with a spinal or an epidural, although it may be difficult to achieve a sensory level adequate for patient comfort while avoiding the complications of a high block.

Supplemental and/or Postoperative Analgesia
All of the surgeries indicated above along with selected thoracic and cardiac procedures.

Technique
Preparation
Mask and cap, sterile gloves, gauze pads, chloroprep, prefabricated spinal or epidural kit.

Needles
Typically a 17 g Tuohy for epidural/caudal and 22–27 g pencil point for single shot spinal.

Agents
Chloroprocaine, lidocaine, ropivacaine, bupivacaine, tetracaine.

Surface Anatomy and Landmarks
Spinal Anesthesia
Spinal anesthesia can be performed with the patient in a sitting or a lateral decubitus position. Principal landmarks include the spinous processes (midline) and the iliac crests (Fig. 20.1). A line connecting the highest point on each of iliac crests corresponds to the L4 vertebrae (midline). Interspace above the line represents L3–L4 and below the line indicates L4–L5. Since the spinal cord ends at L1–L2 in adults, interspaces of L3–L4 or L4–L5 are most commonly selected as the needle insertion site. The interspaces (palpable depression) between the spinous processes above and below the level to be used are palpated; the skin is then

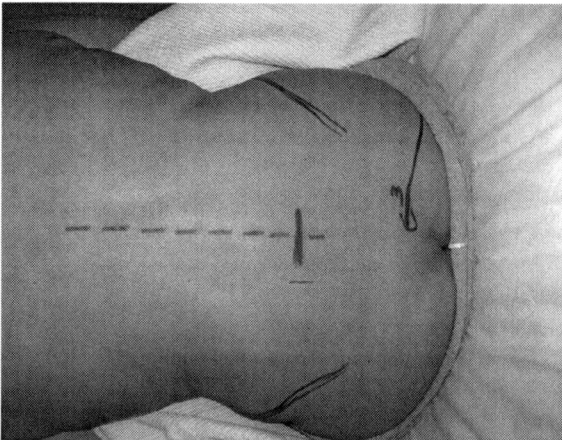

Figure 20.1 Spinal and epidural anesthesia/analgesia. *Dashed lines* in the midline indicate the palpable spinous processes. *Right* and *left* lateral arcs represent the iliac crests. *Line #1* is the L4 lumbar interspace.

prepped in sterile fashion and anesthetized by infiltration at the selected site. A spinal needle is introduced in the midline, remaining perpendicular in all directions to the patients, back (parallel to the spinous processes). The following structures are encountered in route to the subarachnoid space as the needle is deliberately and slowly inserted – skin, subcutaneous tissue, supraspinous ligament, interspinous ligament, epidural space, dura, then arachnoid mater, and finally the subarachnoid space, confirmed by appearance of CSF. Needle is stabilized on the patient's back and then connected to syringe containing local anesthetic; after confirming free flow of CSF (no blood), the syringe contents are injected.

Complications

If blood-tinged CSF continues to flow through the spinal needle, it should be removed and inserted at a different interspace. Additional issues include hypotension, bradycardia, postspinal headache, high spinal, nausea, urinary retention, backache, hypoventilation, and adverse neurologic consequences (rare).

Epidural Anesthesia

Epidural anesthesia is instituted with the patient in sitting or lateral decubitus position. Skin prep of the back is performed with antiseptic solution and the Tuohy (or another type) needle is inserted through a local anesthetic skin wheal placed at a selected interspace (lumbar or thoracic) using the landmarks described above for midline spinal anesthesia (Fig. 20.1). A method for identifying the epidural space during placement of epidural anesthesia is a sudden loss of resistance encountered (reflecting negative pressure) as the Tuohy needle penetrates through the ligamentum flavum. A technique to identify the epidural space is to connect a glass syringe with a freely movable plunger to the Tuohy needle. With either slow and continuous pressure or small incremental movements advance the needle attached to the syringe into and through the ligaments until a loss of resistance is detected as pressure on the plunger of the syringe is exerted. The syringe is then withdrawn from the positioned and stable Tuohy needle to check for evidence of CSF or blood flow. A test dose of 3 ml of local anesthetic solution containing epinephrine (1:200,000) is injected through the needle (for single shot), unless a catheter is to be placed through the needle, in which case the test dose may be injected through the catheter. A sterile plastic catheter is advanced 2–4 cm into the epidural space permitting repeated and/or continuous local anesthetic injection. Evidence of intravenous injection and/or subarachnoid blockade is observed following test dose injection. After a negative test dose, the needle is removed, epidural catheter is secured, and incremental boluses of local anesthetic can be administered.

Complications

Complications are similar to those described for spinal anesthesia, but with the added potential for accidental dural puncture and local anesthetic toxicity. Formation of an epidural hematoma is a rare, but potentially devastating concern.

Caudal Epidural Anesthesia

Caudal anesthesia can be performed with the patient in a lateral, prone, or jackknife position. The sacral hiatus is palpated and identified between the sacral cornua that are positioned about 5 cm cranial to the coccyx tip. A skin wheal with 1% lidocaine is raised between the sacral cornua following antiseptic skin preparation. The needle is positioned 90° to the skin and advanced through the sacrococcygeal ligament contacting the sacrum resulting in a "pop" sensation. The needle is withdrawn slightly as the perpendicular needle angle is reduced to 20–30° to the skin, directed cephalad, and then advanced about 2 cm into the caudal canal. The stylet is withdrawn to check for CSF or blood flow, and confirmation of proper needle placement can be made with a 5 ml injection of air through the needle (skin crepitation will be felt if needle placed erroneously into subcutaneous tissue). A test dose of 3 ml of local anesthetic solution containing epinephrine (1:200,000) is injected and observed for signs of subarachnoid or IV injection (similar to epidural anesthesia). A caudal catheter can be placed in a similar fashion as described for epidural anesthesia using a 17-gauge Tuohy needle.

Complications
Infection, subarachnoid injection, increased failure rate (up to 10%) secondary to abnormalities of anatomy within the caudal canal.

Pitfalls and Pearls
Pitfalls
Relative and absolute contraindications of neuraxial blockade:

- Patient refusal
- Deformities of the back and spine
- Coagulation status during the perioperative period (concern for hematoma development and neurologic symptoms)
- Severe hypovolemia
- Elevated intracranial pressure
- Sepsis or infection at the site of intended injection
- Severe stenotic valve heart disease or ventricular outflow obstruction

Pearls
- If bone is contacted superficially, a midline needle is likely hitting the lower spinous process.
- Contact with bone at a deeper depth usually indicates that the needle is in the midline and hitting the upper spinous process or directed lateral to the midline and hitting a lamina.
- Loss of resistance in the epidural space can be confirmed with loss of resistance to air/saline, or both.

Pudendal Nerve Block
Pudendal nerve block can be used to supplement pain relief during the second stage of labor. The S2–S4 nerves give off branches to the pudendal nerve that pass between the pyriformis and coccygeal muscles. The nerve exits the pelvis through the greater sciatic foramen and reenters it again through the lesser sciatic foramen. The nerve then divides into three nerves: inferior rectal nerve which innervates the anal and perianal regions; dorsal nerve of the penis

or the clitoris innervating the dorsum of the penis or clitoris; and perineal nerve which supplies muscles of the urogenital triangle, posterior 2/3 of the labia majora or posterior 2/3 of the scrotum in males.

Technique
Preparation
Arrange sterile towels, sterile gloves, gauze pads, syringes, and needles for local infiltration and nerve block placement.

Dose
20 ml syringes of local anesthetic.

Needles
20 g 6.0 in. needle for skin infiltration and a 22 g 5 cm short bevel insulated stimulation needle.

Agents
2% lidocaine.

Surface Anatomy and Landmarks
Landmarks
The pudendal nerve may be blocked by a transvaginal approach (A) or transperineal approach (B).

A. With the patient in the lithotomy position, the ischial spine is bracketed transvaginally by a hand in the vagina. A 20 g 6 in. needle is then inserted through the vaginal mucosa through the sacrospinous ligament and beyond the ischial spine. After negative aspiration, 10 cc of preservative-free lidocaine is injected and then another 3–4 cc can be injected as the needle is withdrawn to block the inferior rectal nerve.
B. The ischial tuberosity is identified with the patient in the lithotomy position. With aseptic technique, a 6-in. needle is inserted at a point that is 1 in. lateral and 1 in. posterior to the tuberosity and the needle is directed toward the ischial spine. After negative aspiration, a total of 10 cc of lidocaine is injected with another 3–4 cc of lidocaine injected as the needle is withdrawn to block the inferior rectal nerve.

Upper Extremity Blocks
The brachial plexus consists of the anterior rami of roots C5–C8 and T1. There also may be minor contributions from either C4 and/or T2. The roots then divide to form the three trunks (superior, middle, and inferior). The trunks further divide into three anterior and three posterior divisions as they pass over the first rib and dive below the clavicle. The six divisions then develop into the lateral, medial, and posterior cords as they pass into the axilla. The five primary terminal nerve branches finally formed include musculocutaneous, radial, axillary, median, and ulnar nerves (Figs. 20.2a, b). The brachial plexus typically travels with a vascular supply that is contained within a neural vascular bundle along a large portion of

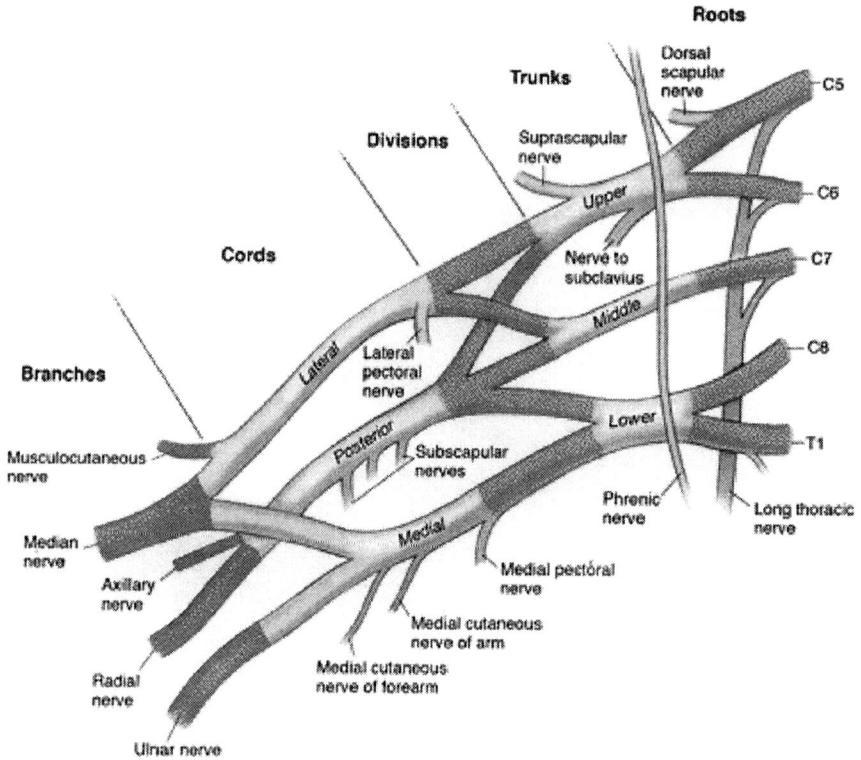

Figure 20.2   (a) and (b) Diagram of the brachial plexus.

the path of the brachial plexus from its origin to the terminal nerve branches. The associated vascular supply within the bundle is often helpful in targeting the various brachial plexus components and individual nerves.

Interscalene Block

The interscalene block targets the brachial plexus at the level of the trunks or roots and is used for surgeries performed on the shoulder and lateral aspect of the upper arm. Innervation of the shoulder and many of the nerves affected by an interscalene nerve blockade are identified in Table 20.6.

Indication

Indications include primary anesthesia and/or postoperative pain management with or without a continuous catheter for shoulder and shoulder joint, lateral two-third of clavicle, and proximal humerus surgeries. Arm and forearm surgeries with an interscalene block do not often provide adequate coverage of the ulnar nerve distribution (C8-T1) and are therefore not completely useful for surgeries of the lower arm, wrist, or hand. Lack of appropriate blockade of the ulnar nerve distribution subsequent to an interscalene block may be circumvented by

Axillary	Infradavicular	Supraclavicular	and	Interscalene
Branches	Cords	Divisions	Trunks	Roots
Musculocutaneous	Lateral	Anterior Posterior	Superior	C4 C5
Axillary				C6
Median	Posterior	Anterior Posterior	Middle	C7
Radial			Inferior	C8
Ulnar	Medial	Anterior Posterior		T1

Figure 20.2 (Continued)

Table 20.6 Innervation of the shoulder and interscalene nerve blockade.

Nerve	Motor of the shoulder	Sensory of the shoulder	Joint of the shoulder
Brachial plexus	All	All except cephalad cutaneous parts innervated by supraclavicular n. (C3–C4)	
Upper lateral brachial cutaneous (from the axillary n.)		Lateral side of shoulder and skin overlying the deltoid	
Intercostobrachial		Anterior and medial skin of shoulder and posterior upper arm	
Supraclavicular (C3, C4)		Skin over upper deltoid/shoulder	Acromioclavicular joint
Subclavius	Subclavius m.		Sternoclavicular joint
Dorsal scapular	Rhomboid and levator scapulae m.		
Long thoracic	Serratus anterior m.		
Suprascapular	Supraspinatus and infraspinatus m.		Shoulder joint
Axillary, suprascapular, subscapular	Deltoid and teres minor m.	Skin of the shoulder over inferior deltoid	Shoulder joint

using larger local anesthetic volumes or supplemental blockade of the ulnar nerve at a more distal location of the upper extremity.

Technique
Preparation
Arrange sterile towels, sterile gloves, gauze pads, marking pen, antiseptic solution, peripheral nerve stimulator, syringes, and needles for local infiltration and nerve block placement.

Dose
20–40 ml syringes of local anesthetic.

Needles
25 g 1.5 in. needle for skin infiltration and 22 g 3 or 5 cm short bevel insulated stimulation needle.

Agents
3% chloroprocaine, 2% lidocaine, 0.5% ropivacaine, 0.5% bupivacaine.

Surface Anatomy and Landmarks
Landmarks
Landmarks include posterior and lateral borders of the sternal and clavicular heads of sternocleidomastoid m., C6 tubercle, interscalene groove formed by the middle and anterior scalene m., upper border of cricoid cartilage, and clavicle (Fig. 20.3).

The patient should be positioned supine with their head turned away from the side to be blocked. The arms are to remain relaxed at the patient's side. A line drawn laterally from

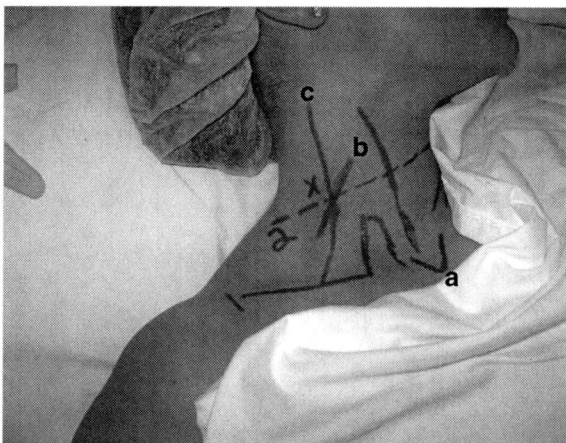

Figure 20.3 Surface landmarks for the classical interscalene approach to the brachial plexus. (a) Sternal notch, (b) external jugular vein, and c sternocleidomastoid muscle. *Line #1* identifies the clavicle. *Dashed line #2* indicates the C6 vertebral process and is the line/path along which to follow in search of the appropriate muscle response. *X* marks the needle entry site.

the cricoid cartilage in the direction toward and past the posterior border of the sternoclei-domastoid (SCM) muscle demarcates the C6 transverse process. This line will serve as the path to take when searching for the appropriate muscle twitch. The bony tubercle of the transverse process of C6 often can be palpated along this line. The posterior border of the SCM muscle is also marked and bisects the previously drawn line. The posterior border of the SCM can more easily be palpated by instructing the patient to raise their head off the table by flexing at the neck. Then the interscalene groove is marked (this will later serve as the nerve block needle insertion site) by palpating for the groove immediately behind and deep to the posterior border of the SCM muscle at a point along the C6 transverse process line drawn previously. A 22-gauge 3–5 cm b-bevel needle is connected to a nerve stimulator set at 1.0 mA (activate nerve stimulator subsequent to subcutaneous needle placement) and inserted at the mark of the interscalene groove. The needle is then directed perpendicular to the skin following shallow local infiltration and skin cleansing. The perpendicular orientation of the needle to the skin will mimic a caudal, posterior, and medial direction. The needle is inserted until an appropriate motor twitch of the deltoid or biceps muscle is obtained at a stimulation of between 0.2 and 0.5 mA or until a paresthesia to the arm or thumb is elicited. The muscle twitch typically occurs superficially at a depth of 1–2 cm (up to 3 cm in obese patients). Approximately 20–40 ml of local anesthetic is injected following a negative aspiration for blood/CSF. It is important to aspirate frequently during delivery of the anesthetic in small aliquots. A continuous single orifice catheter may be inserted to provide continuous infusion of local anesthetic, although securing such a catheter into the interscalene groove may prove to be difficult with this conventional approach.

Pitfalls and Pearls
Pitfalls

Several side effects from an interscalene block are possible, including infection. The phrenic nerve and the sympathetic chain are located in the region of the cervical nerve roots. Patients may complain of dyspnea because the phrenic nerve is affected in 90–100% of interscalene blocks, resulting in an ipsilateral diaphragmatic paralysis. Therefore, in patients with respiratory compromise (such as severe chronic obstructive pulmonary disease (COPD)), blocking the diaphragm may not be a tolerable side effect. In addition, Horner's syndrome is common from blockade of the stellate ganglion sympathetic chain, which can result in ipsilateral myosis, ptosis, and anhidrosis. Nasal stuffiness and blockade of the recurrent laryngeal nerve may occur, causing hoarseness as a result of an interscalene block.

A complication that may occur is a pneumothorax, as the cupola of the lung may be located in the vicinity of the C6 tubercle (rare). This complication must be considered if the patient develops chest pain or cough, even hours after performing an interscalene block. One severe complication would be an intravascular or intraarterial injection (the external jugular vein often transverses the interscalene groove, and the vertebral artery is just anterior to the cervical roots) as inadvertent injection of as little as 1–3 ml of local anesthetic into the vertebral artery may result in seizure activity. Another possible complication is injection of local anesthetic into the intervertebral foramina that may result in a high epidural or spinal anesthesia that requires immediate intervention.

Pearls

Twitches from the following muscles provide a similar success rate: pectoralis, deltoid, triceps, biceps, and any twitch of hand or forearm. The external jugular vein crosses close to the insertion site for this classical approach to the interscalene block. Shoulder surgery entails massive nociceptive input, and an interscalene block may provide relief of the deep somatic pain and reflex muscle spasm.

Clinical Uses
Surgical
- Arthroscopic shoulder surgery and arthroplasty of the shoulder
- Rotator cuff repair, arthrolysis, and acromioplasty of the shoulder
- Proximal humerus surgery, humerus open reduction and internal fixation (ORIF)

Postoperative Analgesia
For all the surgeries indicated above.

Supraclavicular Block

A supraclavicular block targets the brachial plexus at the level of divisions for upper extremity surgery and primarily covers the axillary, musculocutaneous, and radial nerves with possible delay of median nerve distribution blockade. If this block is performed for shoulder surgery, then the addition of a separate superficial cervical nerve block is needed.

Indication

As primary anesthesia and/or postoperative pain management with or without a continuous catheter for humerus (distal), elbow, forearm, hand, or wrist surgeries.

Technique
Preparation

Arrange sterile towels, sterile gloves, gauze pads, marking pen, antiseptic solution, peripheral nerve stimulator, syringes, and needles for local infiltration and nerve block placement.

Dose
20–40 ml syringes of local anesthetic.

Needles
25 g 1.5 in. needle for skin infiltration and a 22 g 5 cm short bevel insulated stimulation needle.

Agents
3% chloroprocaine, 2% lidocaine, 0.5% ropivacaine, 0.5% bupivacaine.

Surface Anatomy and Landmarks
Landmarks

Landmarks include sternocleidomastoid m., anterior and middle scalene m., clavicle, first rib, and subclavian artery (Fig. 20.4a, b). In the classic approach, the patient is positioned supine or semi-sitting with their head turned away from the side to be blocked. The arms are to remain relaxed at the patient's side. The brachial plexus is approached with the clavicle first identified and the midpoint marked (Fig. 20.4a). Following skin cleansing and local

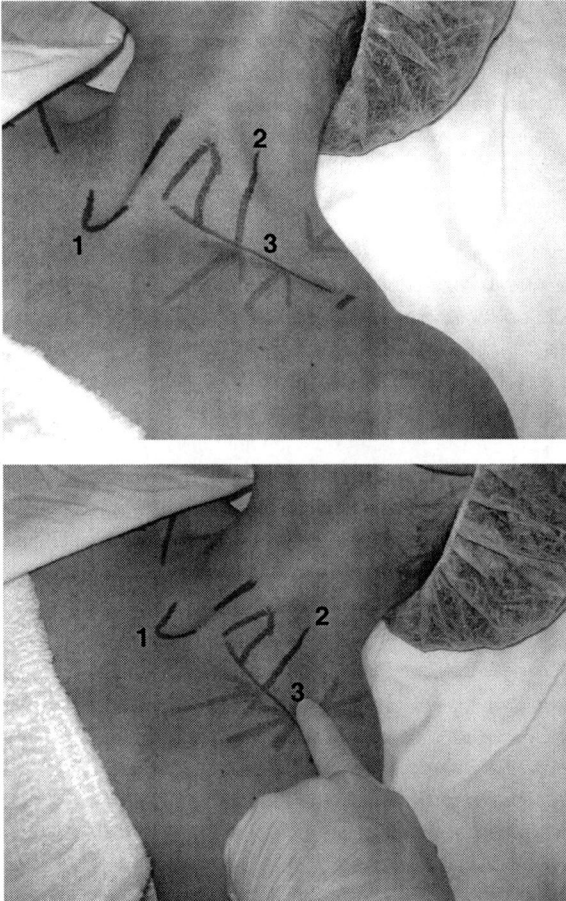

Figure 20.4 (a) and (b) Landmarks for the supraclavicular approach to the brachial plexus. (a) *Line #1* sternal notch and *line #2* sternocleidomastoid (SCM) muscle. *Line #3* identifies the clavicle. *Single medial arrow* indicates the lateral portion of the SCM muscle attachment to the clavicle. *Parallel arrow* (pointing cephalad) is approximately one-thumb width (2.5 cm) lateral to the medial *arrow* and provides a margin of safety away from the pleura dome. (b) *Line #1* sternal notch, *line #2* sternocleidomastoid (SCM) muscle, and *line #3* the clavicle. *Single arrow* pointing caudad identified the point on needle entry. This point is located cephalad to the palpating finger positioned above *line #3*, marking the clavicle. *Arrows* on each side of the palpating finger identify the direction of the advancing needle that is aligned parallel to the body midline.

infiltration, a 22-gauge 5 cm b-bevel needle is connected to a nerve stimulator set at 1.0 mA (activate nerve stimulator subsequent to subcutaneous needle placement) and inserted one-finger width cephalad to the mid-clavicular point which is 2.5 cm lateral to the SCM muscle attachment of the clavicle (Fig. 20.4b). The needle is then directed caudally after penetrating 2–5 mm perpendicular through the skin. Typically the first rib will be contacted by the needle at a depth of about 2–4 cm; the needle is then "walked off" the first rib until a paresthesia to the arm or thumb is elicited or an appropriate muscle twitch is obtained at a stimulation between 0.2 and 0.5 mA. The appropriate needle response should occur above the clavicle and under the palpating finger. Caution should be used not to direct the needle medially toward the cupola of the lung. After appropriate nerve stimulation, including flexion or extension of the wrist or digits, 20–40 ml of local anesthetic are injected in incremental doses following a negative aspiration for blood. Alternatively, a continuous single orifice catheter may be inserted to provide continuous infusion of local anesthetic.

Pitfalls and Pearls
Pitfalls
Several side effects from supraclavicular blockade may occur. Since the cupola of the lung is at the level of a supraclavicular block, one complication that may occur is a pneumothorax (0.5–6% incidence), depending on the experience and skill of the anesthesiologist. This complication must be considered if the patient develops chest pain or cough, even hours after performing a supraclavicular block. There is an increased risk of pneumothorax if the needle is allowed to be directed medially, which may result in contact with the pleura. Therefore, outpatients with severe lung disease may not be appropriate candidates for this block. Blockade of the ulnar nerve distribution may be spared or delayed. Another possible side effect is phrenic nerve or sympathetic chain block with the supraclavicular approach (less common than with an interscalene block). Infection, hematoma, bleeding, nerve injury, and intravascular injection (subclavian vessels are in the region of a supraclavicular approach to the brachial plexus) are also potential problems.

Pearls
The brachial plexus at the supraclavicular level is cephaloposterior and lateral to the subclavian artery, and paresthesia or muscle stimulation may be elicited before block needle contacts the first rib. When blocking the brachial plexus at the supraclavicular level, the middle trunk (median nerve) is more posterior to the artery and spread of the local anesthetic to this area may be prolonged. If the ulnar nerve distribution is missed with this block, a supplemental ulnar nerve block may be necessary. Also, a superficial cervical plexus block should be added for shoulder surgery as this approach often misses the skin overlying the shoulder. Block of the intercostobrachial nerve in the axilla is necessary if a tourniquet will be used and placed on the upper arm.

Clinical Uses
Surgical
- Humerus surgery (including ORIF)
- Elbow surgery

- Wrist and hand surgery
- Upper extremity proximal arteriovenous (AV) fistula surgery

Postoperative Analgesia
For all the surgeries indicated above.

Suprascapular Block
The fibers of C5 and C6 nerve roots and some contribution from the C4 nerve root form the suprascapular nerve that passes through the suprascapular notch under the coracoclavicular ligament.

Indication
A suprascapular block is useful for the diagnosis and treatment of pain and surgery involving the shoulder girdle and shoulder joint pain. It may also be used for treatment of "frozen shoulder" adhesive capsulitis or complex regional pain syndrome type I.

Technique
Preparation
Arrange sterile towels, sterile gloves, gauze pads, marking pen, antiseptic solution, syringes, and needles for local infiltration and nerve block placement.

Dose
20–40 ml syringes of local anesthetic.

Needles
25 g 1.5 in. needle for skin infiltration and a 22 g 5 cm short bevel insulated stimulation needle.

Agents
3% chloroprocaine, 2% lidocaine, 0.5% ropivacaine, 0.5% bupivacaine.

Surface Anatomy and Landmarks
Basic landmarks for performance of a suprascapular nerve block include the spine of the scapula, and the scapula is then palpated laterally to identify the acromion. With the patient in the sitting position, 25-gauge 3.5 in. needle is inserted at the junction of the spine of the scapula and the acromion in an inferior direction toward the scapula. Once it encounters the body of the scapula, the needle is walked off superiorly and laterally until it enters the suprascapular notch. Once a paresthesia is elicited, the needle should not be advanced any further. If a paresthesia is not encountered, the needle is then advanced another half an inch until it crosses the coracoclavicular ligament. After negative aspiration, 10 cc of a local anesthetic solution is slowly injected.

Table 20.7 Infraclavicular branches (at the level of the cords).

Nerve	Motor	Sensory	Joint
Lateral pectoral	Pectoralis major m.		
Medial pectoral	Pectoralis minor and part of pectoralis major m.		
Medial brachial cutaneous		Skin over the upper medial side of arm	
Medial antebrachial cutaneous		Skin over medial portion of forearm	
Upper subscapular	Superior portion of the subscapularis m.		
Lower subscapular	Inferior portion of the subscapularis m. and teres major m.		
Thoracodorsal	Latissimus dorsi m.		
Axillary	Teres minor, deltoid m.	Skin overlying the inferior deltoid	Shoulder joint
Musculocutaneous	Coracobrachialis, biceps brachii, brachialis m.	Branches form the lateral antebrachial cutaneous n. covering the skin	Elbow joint, proximal radioulnar joint
Ulnar	Flexor carpi ulnaris, ulnar portion of flexor digitorum profundus, and most small muscles of the hand	Medial skin over hand, fifth digit, and medial half of the fourth digit	
Median	All flexor muscles in the forearm except for flexor carpi ulnaris, ulnar portion of flexor digitorum profundus, and the five hand muscles	Skin over the anterior (palmar) hand into digits first–third, lateral half of the fourth digit	Radioulnar joint (distal and proximal)
Radial	Triceps brachii, brachioradialis, anconeus, extensor muscles of the forearm	Skin over lateral posterior hand and lateral thumb; branches to the lower lateral brachial and posterior antebrachial cutaneous covering lateral skin over the lower arm, forearm, and elbow	Elbow joint, radioulnar joint (distal and proximal)

Infraclavicular Block

The infraclavicular block targets the brachial plexus at the level of the cords below the clavicle and is most commonly used for surgery distal to mid-humerus. Table 20.7 identifies innervation from the nerves affected by an infraclavicular block. The infraclavicular block insertion site is quit useful for placement and securing of a catheter for continuous postoperative analgesia.

Indication

As primary anesthesia and/or postoperative pain management with or without a continuous catheter for elbow, forearm, wrist, and hand surgeries.

Technique
Preparation

Arrange sterile towels, sterile gloves, gauze pads, marking pen, antiseptic solution, peripheral nerve stimulator, syringes, and needles for local infiltration and nerve block placement.

Dose

30–40 ml syringes of local anesthetic.

Needles

25 g 1.5 in. needle for skin infiltration and 20 or 21 g, 5–10 cm short bevel insulated stimulation needle.

Agents

3% chloroprocaine, 2% lidocaine, 0.5% ropivacaine, 0.5% bupivacaine.

Surface Anatomy and Landmarks

Landmarks

Surface landmarks include pectoralis major and minor muscles, subscapularis and teres major muscles, serratus anterior m., humerus, scapula, clavicle, and the coracoid process (Fig. 20.5). The patient is positioned supine with the head turned to the contralateral side and arm to be blocked at the patient's side or flexed at the elbow and resting on the abdomen. Local skin infiltration and skin preparation are performed. A 10 cm, 21-gauge b-bevel needle is connected to a nerve stimulator set at 1.0 mA (activate nerve stimulator subsequent to subcutaneous needle placement) and initially inserted perpendicularly through the skin 2 cm medial and 2 cm caudad to the coracoid process. The needle is then directed in a vertical parasagittal plane (aimed toward the axilla) until an appropriate muscle twitch is obtained at a stimulation of between 0.2 and 0.5 mA or a paresthesia to the distal upper extremity is elicited. A muscle twitch at the wrist or hand (not the musculocutaneous nerve distribution) is considered appropriate for injection. Approximately 30–40 ml of local anesthetic is injected after negative aspiration for blood and aspiration performed frequently (∼3–5 cc) during anesthetic delivery in small aliquots. Depth of the brachial plexus during an infraclavicular

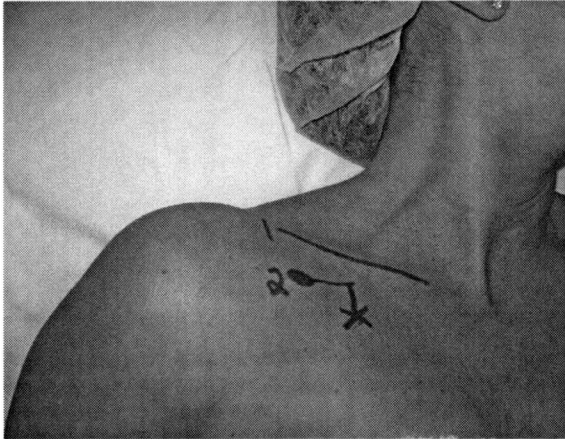

Figure 20.5 Coracoid approach landmarks for the infraclavicular brachial plexus block. *Line #1* identifies the clavicle and *line # 2* indicates the coracoid process marked as a *blue dot*. *X* identifies the needle insertion site that is positioned 2 cm lateral and medial to the coracoid process.

block may vary from 2 to 8 cm (average 4 cm) depending on body habitus. A continuous single orifice catheter may be inserted to provide continuous infusion of local anesthetic.

Pitfalls and Pearls
Pitfalls
A potential problem of an infraclavicular block can be discomfort as the pectoral muscles are pierced by the block needle, so appropriate subcutaneous infiltration with 1% lidocaine and patient sedation is helpful. The first twitches elicited when advancing the needle is motor response of the pectoral muscles so the needle must be advanced further (aiming toward the axilla) until obtaining a distal upper extremity twitch response. A deltoid (axillary nerve) or biceps (musculocutaneous nerve) motor response should not be accepted as these nerves often branch from the brachial plexus earlier and would not provide reliable brachial plexus blockade. Another possibility is phrenic nerve or sympathetic chain effect from the infraclavicular approach, but less commonly than with an interscalene or supraclavicular approach to the brachial plexus. Intravascular injection, infection, hematoma formation, nerve injury, and pneumothorax may also occur.

Pearls
A benefit of this block is supine patient positioning and permitting the patient to keep their arm in any neutral or comfortable position. Catheter position is easily maintained for prolonged postoperative analgesia at this site as compared to other approaches of the brachial plexus.

Clinical Uses
Surgical
- Distal humerus surgery, including ORIF
- Elbow surgery, epicondylitis
- Wrist and hand surgery
- Forearm surgery, including distal AV fistula surgery

Postoperative Analgesia
For all the surgeries indicated above.

Axillary Block
An axillary block targets the brachial plexus at the level of the terminal nerve branches appropriate for surgeries of the distal upper extremity. Multiple techniques are described for this block including transarterial, paresthesia seeking, and nerve stimulator approaches.

Indication
As primary anesthesia and/or postoperative pain management with or without a continuous catheter for forearm, hand, and wrist surgeries.

Technique
Preparation
Arrange sterile towels, sterile gloves, gauze pads, marking pen, antiseptic solution, peripheral nerve stimulator, syringes, and needles for local infiltration and nerve block placement.

Dose
30–40 ml syringes of local anesthetic.

Needles
25 g 1.5 in. needle for skin infiltration and a 22 g, 3 or 5 cm short bevel insulated stimulation needle.

Agents
3% chloroprocaine, 2% lidocaine, 0.5% ropivacaine, 0.5% bupivacaine.

Surface Anatomy and Landmarks
Landmarks
Landmarks include axilla, axillary artery, and humerus (Fig. 20.6). Imagining the upper arm (just distal the axillary hair pad) in cross-sectional view, the musculocutaneous nerve is typically found outside the neural vascular bundle and in the 9–12 o'clock position embedded in the coracobrachialis muscle; the median nerve is usually located (within the neural vascular bundle) in the 12–3 o'clock quadrant (above the pulse of the axillary artery). The ulnar nerve is often located in the 3–6 o'clock position and radial nerve (below the pulse of the axillary artery) varied in the 6–9 o'clock position, both branches within the neural vascular bundle.

The patient is positioned supine with their head neutral or turned away from the side to be blocked. The arm to be blocked is abducted 90° at the shoulder and flexed 90° at the elbow. Axillary artery is palpated and its course marked followed by skin preparation and local skin

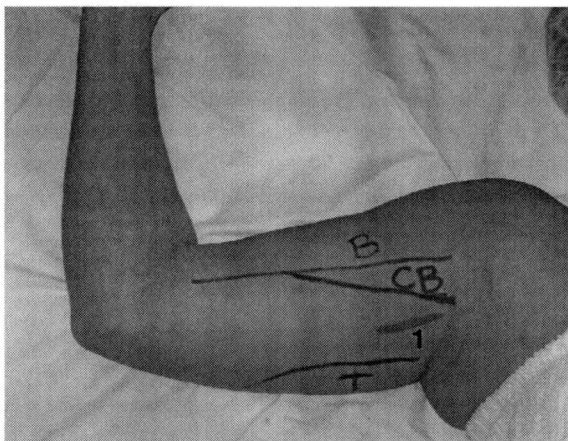

Figure 20.6 Landmarks for the approach to the axillary brachial plexus block. *B* biceps muscle, *T* triceps muscle, *CB* coracobrachialis muscle. *Line #1* indicates pulse of the axillary (brachial) artery.

infiltration. A 22-gauge 3–5 cm b-bevel needle is connected to a nerve stimulator set at 1.0 mA (activate nerve stimulator subsequent to subcutaneous needle placement) and while palpating the axillary artery, the needle is inserted in the distal axilla aimed 30–45° to the skin directed toward the axilla directly overlying the palpable artery. The needle is inserted searching for appropriate motor response at a stimulation of between 0.2 and 0.5 mA or eliciting a paresthesia to the wrist, hand, or thumb. A consistent muscle twitch of the wrist and hand reflecting ulnar, radial, and/or median nerve stimulation is appropriate for injection. A total of approximately 30–40 ml of local anesthetic is injected following a negative aspiration for blood and again aspirating frequently during delivery of the anesthetic in small aliquots. Keeping in mind the clockwise arrangement of the three nerves within the neural vascular bundle (ulnar, radial, and median), each quadrant should have local anesthetic injected in order to insure the blockade of each terminal nerve branch. Local anesthetic should be injected in at least two locations around the artery (superficial and deep) and within the neural vascular bundle to increase success of the block. A continuous single orifice catheter may be inserted to provide continuous infusion of local anesthetic. The musculocutaneous nerve branches early (higher in the axilla) from the brachial plexus and passes into the coracobrachialis muscle, therefore the musculocutaneous nerve must usually be blocked outside the neurovascular bundle within the belly of the coracobrachialis muscle. Musculocutaneous nerve blockade is achieved by inserting the block needle into and through the coracobrachialis muscle until contacting the humerous and then pulling back a few millimeter off the periosteum prior to injection.

Pitfalls and Pearls
Pitfalls
Intravascular injection (with possible local anesthetic toxicity), hematoma formation, nerve injury, and infection are potential complications of an axillary block. Positioning of the extremity for this block (abducting the arm, especially if there is a shoulder injury) may prove difficult.

Pearls
An axillary block lacks the same risk of pneumothorax compared to other approaches of the brachial plexus. If a tourniquet of the upper extremity is to be used, the additional blockade of the medial brachial cutaneous and intercostobrachial nerves within the axilla must be performed to provide anesthesia of the skin overlying the medial upper arm.

Clinical Uses
Surgical
- Elbow surgery, including epicondylitis
- Forearm surgery, including distal AV fistula surgery
- Wrist surgery, including posterior synovial cyst removal, carpal tunnel release, and Colles' fracture repair
- Hand surgery, including Dupuytren's contracture release

Postoperative analgesia
For all the surgeries indicated above.

Radial Nerve Block

A brachial plexus block can be supplemented or "rescued" with a radial nerve block for surgeries in the distribution of the radial nerve or in the instance when a brachial plexus block may have spared the radial nerve distribution. The radial nerve is formed by fibers from C5-T1 spinal nerve roots and passes between the medial and the long heads of the triceps muscle, giving off a motor branch to the triceps and then inferiorly giving off sensory branches to the upper arm. At the level of the lateral epicondyle, between the lateral epicondyle and musculospiral groove, the radial nerve divides into superficial and deep branches. The superficial branch gives sensory innervations to dorsum of the wrist, dorsal portion of index and middle fingers, and dorsal aspect of a portion to the thumb. Extensors of the forearm obtain most of the motor innervations from the deep branch of the radial nerve.

Technique
Preparation
Arrange sterile towels, sterile gloves, gauze pads, marking pen, antiseptic solution, peripheral nerve stimulator, syringes, and needles for local infiltration and nerve block placement.

Dose
5–10 ml syringes of local anesthetic.

Needle
25 g 1.5 in. needle for skin infiltration.

Agents
3% chloroprocaine, 2% lidocaine, 0.5% ropivacaine, 0.5% bupivacaine.

Surface Anatomy and Landmarks
Landmarks
Radial nerve block can be performed at the humerus (A), at the elbow (B), and at the wrist (C):

A. A point 3 in. above the lateral epicondyle of the humerus is identified on the musculospiral groove between the heads of the triceps muscle. A 25 g 1.5 in. needle is inserted until a paraesthesia is elicited in the distribution of innervation of the radial nerve. When there is no persistent paresthesia, 7–10 cc of local anesthetic is injected following negative aspiration.
B. Lateral margin of biceps tendon at the crease of the elbow is identified. In a sterile fashion a 25 g 1.5 in. needle is inserted lateral to the biceps tendon at the crease and directed in a superior–medial direction. When a paresthesia is elicited and subsequent to negative aspiration, a total of 7–10 cc of local anesthetic is slowly injected.
C. With the patient in a supine position and operative arm adducted, identify the flexor carpi radialis tendon by asking the patient to flex the wrist. After aseptic preparation of the

wrist, a 25 g 1.5 in. needle is inserted perpendicularly lateral to the flexor carpi radialis tendon, medial to the radial artery at the level of the distal radial prominence. Subsequent to eliciting a paresthesia, the needle is aspirated, and, when there is no persistent paresthesia and no blood to aspiration, a total of 3–4 cc of local anesthetic is injected.

Intercostobrachial and Median Cutaneous Nerve Block

These blocks are usually performed to decrease tourniquet pain and augment a brachial plexus block. Fibers from the C8 and T1 nerve roots form the medial cutaneous nerve. Fibers of the second intercostal nerve form the intercostobrachial nerve that has communication with the median cutaneous nerve. Both of these nerves exit the axilla outside the brachial plexus sheath parallel to the triceps muscle.

Technique
Preparation
Arrange sterile towels, sterile gloves, gauze pads, marking pen, antiseptic solution, syringes, and needles for local infiltration and nerve block placement.

Dose
5–10 ml syringes of local anesthetic.

Needles
21 g 4 in. needle for skin infiltration.

Agents
3% chloroprocaine, 2% lidocaine, 0.5% ropivacaine, 0.5% bupivacaine.

Surface Anatomy and Landmarks
Landmarks
To block the intercostobrachial and medial cutaneous nerve, have the patient positioned supine and the operative arm abducted 90°. The anterior axillary line and superior margin of the biceps muscle are identified. Then following aseptic technique, a needle is inserted in full length (4 in.) at this point and placed subcutaneously, directed from the biceps to the triceps muscle. Subsequent to negative aspiration, 5–10 cc of local anesthetic is injected as the block needle is being withdrawn creating a subcutaneous skin wheal.

Median Nerve Block

A brachial plexus block can be supplemented or "rescued" with a median nerve block for surgeries in the distribution of the median nerve or in the instance when a brachial plexus block may have spared the median nerve distribution. Fibers from C5-T1 spinal roots make up the median nerve. The nerve traverses the anterior-superior part of the axillary artery before exiting the axilla along with the brachial artery. The median nerve lies medial to the brachial artery at the level of the elbow and gives off a number of motor branches to the flexor muscles of the forearm. It lies in between the tendons of the palmaris longus muscle and the flexor carpi radialis in a deeper plane at the level of the wrist. The median nerve provides sensory innervation to part of the palmar surface of the hand, radial portion of ring finger, palmar surface of the thumb, index and middle finger, radial surface of the ring finger, and distal dorsal surfaces of index and middle fingers.

Technique
Preparation
Arrange sterile towels, sterile gloves, gauze pads, marking pen, antiseptic solution, peripheral nerve stimulator, syringes, and needles for local infiltration and nerve block placement.

Dose
5–10 ml syringes of local anesthetic.

Needle
25 g 1.5 in. needle for skin infiltration.

Agents
3% chloroprocaine, 2% lidocaine, 0.5% ropivacaine, 0.5% bupivacaine.

Surface Anatomy and Landmarks
Landmarks
Median nerve block at the elbow (A) and median nerve block at the wrist (B):

A. With the patient in a supine position and arm adducted to the patient's side with elbow placed in a slightly flexed position, the brachial artery pulsations at the level of the elbow are palpated. A 25 g 1.5 in. needle is inserted at a point medial to the brachial artery and advanced in a superior–medial direction. Paresthesia is usually elicited at about half to three-quarters inch depth. Then when there is no persistent paresthesia, 5–7 cc of local anesthetic is injected.
B. For this block, the patient is placed in a supine position and the arm is adducted completely to the side of the patient and the elbow is maintained in a slightly flexed position. Palmaris longus tendon is identified while having the patient make a fist and flex the wrist. A 25 g 1.5 in. needle is inserted in a sterile fashion medial to the tendon, and in a slightly superior trajectory (just below the crease of the wrist), elicit a paresthesia. Following the paresthesia which usually occurs at a depth of 0.5 in. and after negative aspiration in the absence of persistent paresthesia, a total of 3–5 cc of local anesthetic solution is injected.

Ulnar Nerve Block
A brachial plexus block can be supplemented or "rescued" with an ulnar nerve block for surgeries in the distribution of the ulnar nerve or in the instance when a brachial plexus block may have spared the ulnar nerve distribution. Fibers from the spinal roots of C6-T1 form the ulnar nerve. The ulnar nerve is inferior and anterior to the axillary artery above the axilla and exits the axilla along with the brachial artery. At the level of the elbow, the ulnar nerve lies between the medial epicondyle of the humerus and the olecranon process, before continuing downward between the heads of the flexor carpi ulnaris and further downward along with the ulnar

artery. It divides into a dorsal and palmar branch at a point approximately 1 in. proximal to the crease of the wrist. Sensation to the dorsum of the hand, the dorsum of the little finger, and the ulnar half of the ring finger is provided by the dorsal branch. The sensation to the ulnar aspect of the palm of the hand, the ulnar half of the ring finger, and the palmar aspect of the little finger is provided by the palmar branch of the ulnar nerve.

Technique
Preparation
Arrange sterile towels, sterile gloves, gauze pads, marking pen, antiseptic solution, peripheral nerve stimulator, syringes, and needles for local infiltration and nerve block placement.

Dose
5–10 ml syringes of local anesthetic.

Needles
25 g 1.5 in. needle for skin infiltration.

Agents
3% chloroprocaine, 2% lidocaine, 0.5% ropivacaine, 0.5% bupivacaine.

Surface Anatomy and Landmarks
Landmarks
Basic considerations for the ulnar nerve block at the elbow (A) and ulnar nerve block at the wrist (B) are discussed below:

A. The arm is abducted to 85–90° with the patient in a supine position. The landmarks identified are the medial epicondyle of the humerus and the olecranon process, in between which lies the ulnar nerve sulcus. In an aseptic fashion a 25 g 1 in. needle is inserted in a slightly cephalad direction to elicit paresthesia, which is usually observed at a depth of 0.5 in. After negative aspiration and in the absence of persistent paresthesia, a total of 5–7 ml of local anesthetic is slowly.

B. Ulnar nerve block at the wrist is usually performed in the supine position with the arm fully adducted and the wrist slightly flexed. The flexi carpi ulnaris tendon is identified and in an aseptic fashion, a 25 g 1 in. needle is inserted at the level of the styloid process on the radial side of the tendon in a slightly cephalad direction. A paresthesia is usually elicited at a depth of about half an inch and after negative aspiration (in the absence of persistent paresthesia), a total of 3–5 cc of local anesthetic is injected.

Digital and Metacarpal Nerve Block
Fibers of the median and ulnar nerves give rise to the common digital nerves. Common digital nerves divide as they reach the distal palm after passing along the metacarpal bones. Volar digital nerves run along the ventrolateral aspect of the fingers alongside the digital vein and artery providing most of the sensation to the fingers. Fibers from the ulnar and radial nerves form the smaller dorsal digital nerves and supply the dorsum of the fingers up to the proximal joints.

Technique
Preparation
Arrange sterile towels, sterile gloves, gauze pads, marking pen, antiseptic solution, syringes, and needles for local infiltration and nerve block placement.

Dose
5 ml syringes of local anesthetic.

Needles
25 g 1.5 in. needle for skin infiltration.

Agents
3% chloroprocaine, 2% lidocaine, 0.5% ropivacaine, 0.5% bupivacaine.

Surface Anatomy and Landmarks
Landmarks
Digital nerve block (A) and metacarpal nerve block (B):

A. With the patient in the supine position, the arm is placed in an abducted position and the elbow slightly flexed. In a sterile fashion a 25 g 1.5 in. needle is used on each side of the base of the digit to be blocked from the dorsal to the palmar aspect of the finger. A total of 1–2 cc of local anesthetic is slowly injected after negative aspiration.
B. In an aseptic fashion, a 25 g 1.5 in. needle is inserted on either side of the metacarpal bone proximal to the metacarpal head from the dorsal all the way to the palmar surface of the hand. After negative aspiration 1–2 cc of local anesthetic is slowly injected and pressure is applied at the injection site after removal of the needle to prevent the formation of hematomas.

Intravenous Regional Anesthesia (Bier Block)
This block can be used for surgery involving the hand, forearm, or elbow. Examples include manipulation of forearm fractures, excision of wrist ganglia, and palmar fasciotomy. Local anesthetics diffuse from blood vessels to the surrounding soft tissues and nerves and provide anesthesia to the extremities when the circulation of the extremity is occluded with the aid of a tourniquet.

Technique
Preparation
Arrange sterile towels, sterile gloves, gauze pads, Esmarch bandage, antiseptic solution, syringes, and needles for local infiltration and nerve block placement.

Dose
20 ml syringes of local anesthetic.

Needles
25 g 1.5 in. needle for skin infiltration.

Agents
3% chloroprocaine, 0.5% lidocaine, 0.5% ropivacaine.

Surface Anatomy and Landmarks
Landmarks
The extremity to be anesthetized is elevated to drain blood as much as possible (gravity effect) subsequent to inserting an intravenous catheter as far distal in the extremity as possible. The intravenous catheter will later be used for injection of local anesthesia of the extremity to be anesthetized. A double bladder tourniquet is applied over a cotton padding that has been wrapped around the arm as far proximal as possible. The Esmarch bandage is used to exsanguinate the extremity of blood by circumferentially wrapping around the entire extremity beginning from the most distal portion up to the previously placed double bladder tourniquet while the extremity remains elevated. The most proximal bladder of the double tourniquet is then inflated to 100 mm Hg above the systolic blood pressure of the patient. The Esmarch bangade is then removed and preservative-free lidocaine, 0.5% up to a total of 30–50 cc, is injected into the previously placed intravenous catheter for surgical anesthesia.

For chronic pain conditions, drugs such as bretylium, reserpine, and methylprednisolone with lower concentrations of lidocaine may be injected for pain relief. For surgeries requiring longer periods of time (greater than 40–60 min) and to reduce tourniquet pain, the distal cuff can be inflated over the anesthetized area and the proximal cuff then deflated following confirmation of inflation of the distal bladder on the double tourniquet. It is recommended that at least 30 min elapse following the initial injection of lidocaine prior to slowly releasing the double bladder tourniquet. Release of the tourniquet can be done safely by deflating the tourniquet to just below the patient's systolic pressure for a few seconds, followed by quick reinflation. This is done repeatedly to permit slow wash out of the local anesthetic while constantly observing the patient for any signs of local anesthetic toxicity. Bier block is most commonly performed for surgery involving the upper extremity, but may also be used for surgeries of the lower extremity.

Femoral Nerve Block
Femoral nerve is the largest branch of the lumbar plexus and derived from the posterior divisions of L2–L4 lumbar nerves. Femoral nerve supplies innervation to the lower extremity as indicated in Table 20.8 (supplies anterior portion of the thigh and the medial portion of the calf). Subsequent to fusion of nerve roots, the femoral nerve descends laterally between the psoas and iliacus muscles to enter the iliac fossa. It enters the thigh by going underneath the inguinal ligament just lateral to the femoral artery and gives motor branches to the iliacus, sartorius, quadriceps femoris, and pectineus muscles. It also provides sensory innervation to the skin of the anterior thigh and to the skin over the knee joint.

The saphenous nerve is a continuation of the femoral nerve as it passes distal to the foot on the medial portion of the leg. This nerve is the largest branch of the femoral nerve and is derived predominately from L3 and L4 nerve roots. The nerve travels with the femoral artery in the Hunters canal as it moves toward the knee and then to the foot.

Table 20.8 Femoral nerve innervation of the lower extremity.

Motor	Sensory
Sartorius muscle	Anteromedial thigh (from inguinal ligament to the knee)
Quadriceps muscle (knee extension)	Medial aspect of leg (saphenous branch)
Articular branches to hip and knee	

Indications

As primary anesthetic and/or postoperative pain management with or without a continuous catheter.

Clinical Uses

Surgical

Postoperative analgesia for all the following surgeries:

- Anterior thigh surgery
- Arthroscopic knee surgery
- Surgical repair of midfemoral shaft fractures
- Long saphenous vein stripping

Supplemental (in Combination with an Obturator and Sciatic Nerve Block)

- Total knee replacement
- Tibia plateau fracture repair
- Total ankle replacement (saphenous nerve distribution)
- Above and below knee amputation
- Ankle surgery (saphenous nerve distribution)

Technique

Preparation

Arrange sterile towels, sterile gloves, gauze pads, marking pen, antiseptic solution, peripheral nerve stimulator, syringes, and needles for local infiltration and nerve block placement.

Dose

20–40 ml syringes of local anesthetic.

Needles

25 g 1.5 in. needle for skin infiltration and 5 or 10 cm short bevel insulated stimulation needle.

Agents

3% chloroprocaine, 2% lidocaine, 0.5% ropivacaine, 0.5% bupivacaine.

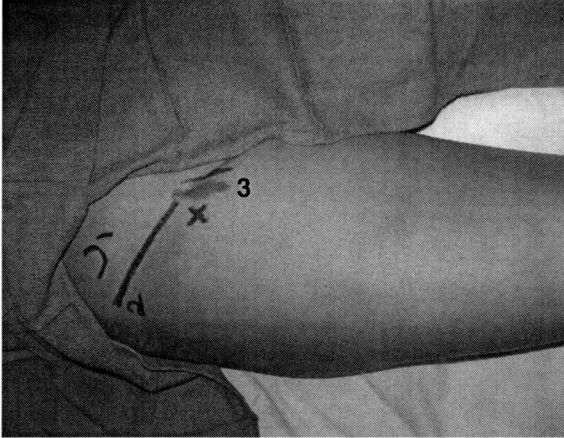

Figure 20.7 Anatomical landmarks for the classical approach to the femoral nerve block. The anterior superior iliac spine that is the attachment of the inguinal ligament is identified as *line #1*. The inguinal crease is identified as *line #2* and the femoral artery (FA) is identified as *line #3*. The needle insertion site (*X*) is located just below the inguinal crease and 1–2 cm lateral to the FA.

Surface Anatomy and Landmarks

Femoral crease, femoral artery, inguinal ligament, pubic tubercle, and anterior superior iliac spine (Fig. 20.7). Patient is placed in supine position and a line is drawn from the anterosuperior iliac spine to the pubic tubercle. The femoral artery is identified as it passes below this line by feeling for the pulsation. A point is marked on the skin 1–2 cm lateral to the femoral artery pulsation and approximately 1–2 cm below the previously drawn anterosuperior iliac spine to the pubic tubercle line. Subsequent to aseptic precautions, a skin wheal is raised with the infiltrating needle at the point marked. The stimulating needle is connected to the nerve stimulator set at 1.0 mA and inserted through the skin wheal at 45–60° angle to the skin and directed cephalad. Quadriceps muscle is watched for appropriate twitching and the current decreased to a range between 0.2 and 0.5 mA while maintaining a consistent muscle twitch. Maximizing the quadriceps muscle twitch can be obtained by small, gentle, organized, and deliberate movement of the needle in medial and lateral directions until consistent quadriceps muscle stimulation is obtained between 0.2 and 0.5 mA. Confirm a negative aspiration for blood and then inject the chosen local anesthetic through the needle.

Saphenous Nerve Block at the Knee

To perform this block, the patient is placed in the lateral position with the operative leg slightly flexed. In an aseptic fashion, a 25 g 1.5 in. needle is slowly advanced through a point in front of the posterior ridge of the medial condyle, toward the medial condyle of the femur. At a depth of 0.25–0.5 in., a paresthesia is sometimes obtained in which the needle should be slightly withdrawn. In the absence of persistent paresthesia and after negative aspiration a total of 5 cc of local is injected.

Saphenous Nerve Block at the Ankle

To perform this block, the patient is placed in a supine position with the operative leg extended. Identify the extensor longus tendon by having the patient extend the big toe against resistance. With an aseptic technique a 25 g 1.5 in. needle is inserted at a point just medial to the tendon at the skin crease of the ankle. After negative aspiration a total of 7–8 cc of local is slowly injected with the needle aiming toward the medial malleolus.

Pitfalls and Pearls
Pitfalls

- Intravascular injection
- Hematoma
- Paresthesia
- Presence of femoral vascular grafts is a relative contraindication

Pearls

- If no response to the nerve stimulator is obtained, then the needle is moved either medial or lateral from the initial insertion site in a logical and sequential manner. The changes should occur by 0.5 cm increments
- A sartorius muscle twitch alone is usually not acceptable, but by passing the needle deeper to this twitch will often evoke a patella twitch which is acceptable
- If bone is contacted (pubic bone) the needle has been inserted too deep

Lateral Femoral Cutaneous Block

The posterior division of the L2 and L3 nerves forms the lateral cutaneous nerve that passes below the ilioinguinal nerve at the anterior superior iliac spine and then passes below the inguinal ligament. The lateral cutaneous nerve then divides into the anterior branch that supplies sensory innervation over the anterolateral thigh and the posterior branch that supplies sensory innervation to the lateral thigh from the knee to just above the greater trochanter.

Technique
Preparation

Arrange sterile towels, sterile gloves, gauze pads, marking pen, antiseptic solution, syringes, and needles for local infiltration and nerve block placement.

Dose

10 ml syringes of local anesthetic.

Needles

25 g 1.5 in. needle for skin infiltration.

Agents

3% chloroprocaine, 2% lidocaine, 0.5% ropivacaine, 0.5% bupivacaine.

Surface Anatomy and Landmarks

Landmarks include femoral crease, inguinal ligament, and anterior superior iliac spine. With the patient in the supine position, the anterior superior iliac spine is identified by palpation. Under an aseptic technique, 25 g 1.5 in. needle is advanced at a point 1 in. medial to the anterior superior iliac spine and just below the inguinal ligament. As the needle passes through the fascia, a pop can often be felt. After negative aspiration a total of 5–7 cc of local is injected in a fan-like fashion.

Obturator Nerve Block

The obturator nerve is derived from the posterior branches of L2–L4 nerves. This nerve enters the thigh through the obturator canal along with the obturator vessels and then divides into anterior and posterior branches. The anterior branch of the obturator provides sensory innervation to the hip joint, a cutaneous branch to the medial aspect of the distal thigh, and motor branches to the superficial hip adductors. The posterior branch gives off an articular branch to the posterior knee joint and motor innervation to the deep hip adductors.

Technique
Preparation

Arrange sterile towels, sterile gloves, gauze pads, marking pen, antiseptic solution, peripheral nerve stimulator, syringes, and needles for local infiltration and nerve block placement.

Dose

20–40 ml syringes of local anesthetic.

Needles

25 g 1.5 in. needle for skin infiltration and 22 g 3 in. short bevel insulated stimulation needle.

Agents

3% chloroprocaine, 2% lidocaine, 0.5% ropivacaine, 0.5% bupivacaine.

Surface Anatomy and Landmarks

Landmarks include femoral crease, femoral artery, inguinal ligament, and pubic tubercle. In performance of this block, a 22 g 3 in. needle is inserted perpendicular to the skin 1 in. lateral and 1 in. inferior to the pubic tubercle until the superior pubic ramus is identified/contacted. The needle is then directed inferiorly and laterally about 0.75–1 in. deeper to place the needle in the obturator canal. After negative aspiration a total of 10–15 cc of local is slowly injected.

Sciatic Nerve Block

Sciatic nerve originates from the lumbosacral plexus (L4, L5, S1, S2, and S3) and is the largest nerve of the lower extremity. The sciatic nerve innervates the lower extremity as indicated in Table 20.9.

Indications

As the primary anesthetic and/or postoperative pain management with or without a continuous catheter.

Table 20.9 Sciatic nerve innervation of the lower extremity.

Motor	Sensory
Biceps femoris and ischial head of adductor magnus muscle	Posterior aspect of the thigh
Semitendinous and semimembranous muscles	The entire leg except the medial aspect of lower leg
Articular branches to hip and knee	

Clinical Uses
Surgical
- Foot and ankle surgery (not effective for sensory distribution on the medial portion of ankle or foot)
- Short saphenous vein stripping
- Surgery below the knee and posterior thigh (spares sensory on medial calf)

Supplemental (in Combination with a Femoral Nerve Block, May Also Require An Obturator or Lumbar Plexus Blockade)
- Total knee replacement
- Tibia plateau fracture repair
- Total ankle replacement
- Above and below knee amputation
- Ankle surgery

Postoperative Analgesia
For the surgeries indicated above.

Technique
Preparation
Arrange sterile towels, sterile gloves, gauze pads, marking pen, antiseptic solution, peripheral nerve stimulator, syringes, and needles for local infiltration and nerve block placement.

Dose
20–30 ml syringes of local anesthetic.

Needles
25 g 1.5 in. needle for skin infiltration and 10 or 15 cm short bevel insulated stimulation needle.

Agents
3% chloroprocaine, 2% lidocaine, 0.5% ropivacaine, 0.5% bupivacaine.

Surface Anatomy and Landmarks (Classical Approach of Labat)
Landmarks
Landmarks include greater trochanter (GT), posterior superior iliac spine (PSIS), and the sacral hiatus (SH) (Fig. 20.8).

The patient lies in a lateral decubitus position with the side to be blocked non-dependent. The knee of the non-dependent leg is flexed 45–60° so as to rest the plantar portion of the foot or ankle on the knee of the dependent limb. Mark the palpable location of the GT, PSIS, and the SH. Then draw two lines, one connecting the PSIS to the GT and another connecting the SH to the GT. At the midpoint of the line between the PSIS and the GT, another 4–5 cm long perpendicular line is drawn which should approximate the line between the SH and the GT; this point will serve as the block needle insertion site. Subsequent to aseptic precautions, a local anesthetic skin wheal is raised with the infiltrating needle at the point marked. A 10 or 15 cm short bevel insulated needle is connected to the nerve stimulator set at 1.0 mA and introduced through the skin wheal perpendicular to the skin. Appropriate muscle twitch responses include the lower leg and/or foot that remains consistent as the current on the nerve stimulator is decreased to a range of 0.3–0.5 mA. If appropriate and sustained muscle twitches are not obtained, then the needle is withdrawn to the skin and reintroduced in a logical and sequential fanwise fashion in a path perpendicular to the course of the sciatic nerve in the hip. Following confirmation of negative aspiration for blood, inject the chosen local anesthetic through the needle once an appropriate and sustained muscle twitch is obtained.

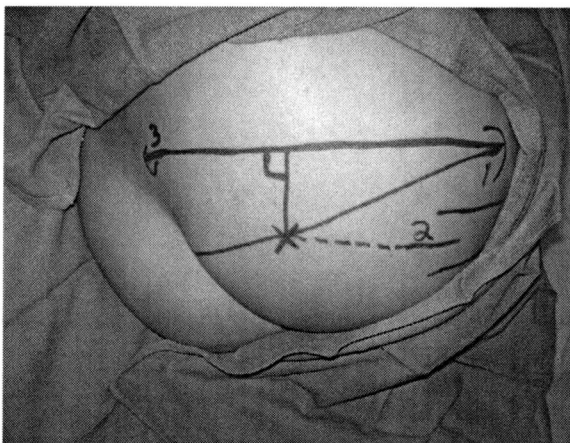

Figure 20.8 Posterior anatomical landmarks for the classical approach (Labat's) to the sciatic nerve block. The greater trochanter (GT) is identified as #1 and a straight line is drawn from the midpoint of the GT (1) to the posterior superior iliac spine (3). A 4–5 cm long second line is drawn caudomedially perpendicular to the midpoint between these two landmarks (1 and 3) and will serve as the needle insertion site (X). Another line is drawn connecting the midpoint of the GT (1) to the sacral hiatus which should bisect the X (needle insertion site) and serve as a cross-check for proper needle insertion. The dashed line (2) represents the furrow formed between the long head of the biceps femoris muscle and the medial edge of the gluteus maximus muscle. This dashed line (2) represents the course of the sciatic nerve toward the leg and should intersect at the needle insertion site (X) serving as another cross-check for proper needle placement.

Pitfalls and Pearls
Pitfalls
- Patient discomfort secondary to large muscle group twitching
- Local anesthetic toxicity must be considered when combining additional PNBs
- Infection
- Paresthesia
- Hematoma

Pearls
- Adequate patient positioning is key to the successful block
- Systematic redirection of the needle is necessary until the appropriate twitch response is obtained
- Twitches of the quadriceps muscle often occur, but the needle should be advanced deep to this response

Lumbar Plexus Block

The lumbar plexus is formed from nerve roots of L1–L4 with variable involvement from T12. The lumbar plexus travels within the psoas muscle and supplies motor and sensory innervations to the lower abdomen and proximal lower extremity as indicated in Table 20.10. Lumbar plexus block depends on placement of local anesthetic in the facial plane of the psoas muscle where the roots of the plexus are located. There are four major branches composing the lumbar plexus: genitofemoral nerve, lateral femoral cutaneous nerve, femoral nerve, and obturator nerve.

Table 20.10 Lumbar plexus innervation to the lower extremity.

Motor	Sensory
Quadriceps muscle	Skin of anteromedial thigh and medial aspect of the leg below the knee to the foot
Adductor muscles of the hip (obturator distribution)	Variable cutaneous distribution to the medial aspect of thigh and knee
Articular branches to hip and knee	Cutaneous distribution from the lateral femoral cutaneous and genitofemoral

Indications
As the primary anesthetic and/or postoperative pain management with or without a continuous catheter.

Clinical Uses
Surgical
- Acetabular fracture
- Anesthesia for the entire lumbar plexus distribution including the saphenous nerve below the knee, hip, knee, and anterolateral/medial thigh

Supplemental (in Combination with Sciatic Nerve Block)

- Total hip replacement
- Total knee replacement
- Anterior cruciate ligament repair
- Amputation of any component of the lower extremity

Postoperative Analgesia

For above-mentioned surgeries.

Technique
Preparation

Arrange sterile towels, sterile gloves, gauze pads, marking pen, antiseptic solution, peripheral nerve stimulator, syringes, and needles for local infiltration and nerve block placement.

Dose

25–35 ml syringes of local anesthetic.

Needles

25 g 1.5 in. needle for skin infiltration and 10 cm short bevel insulated stimulation needle.

Agents

3% chloroprocaine, 2% lidocaine, 0.5% ropivacaine, 0.5% bupivacaine.

Surface Anatomy and Landmarks

Landmarks include iliac crests, midline of spinous processes of L2–L5, posterior superior iliac spine (Fig. 20.9). The patient is placed in a lateral decubitus position with a slight pelvic forward tilt, and the side to be blocked is nondependent. The foot of the extremity to be blocked should be positioned over the dependent leg so twitching of the patella and/or quadriceps muscle can easily be seen. The lumbar midline is identified starting at L4 spinous process and then draw a horizontal line connecting the tips of the palpable spinous processes from L1 to L5. A parallel line is then drawn 4–5 cm lateral to the midline on the non-dependent side (parasagittal line). Palpate the iliac crest (usually originating from the posterosuperior iliac spine) and draw a vertical line from the level of the highest point on the iliac crest down to the midline (bicrestial line). The intersection of the bicrestial line with the parasagittal line determines the site of insertion of the stimulating needle (approximately at the level of L4–L5). The skin is anesthetized by infiltrating local anesthetic subcutaneously after cleaning with an antiseptic solution. After connecting the 10 cm short bevel insulated needle to a nerve stimulator set at 1.5 mA, the needle is inserted through the skin wheal perpendicular to the skin and advanced slowly in search of visible quadriceps muscle twitch or contact of the transverse process. If the needle comes in contact with the transverse process (indicates proper needle orientation), it is withdrawn to the skin then redirected 5–10° caudally or cranially and again advanced until consistent twitching of the quadriceps muscle is obtained (6–8 cm depth) while decreasing the current of the nerve stimulator to 0.5–1.0 mA. After confirming

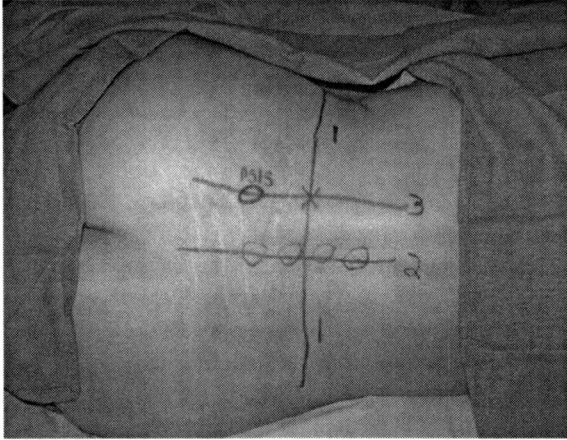

Figure 20.9   Anatomical landmarks for approach to the lumbar plexus block. *PSIS* posterior superior iliac spine. *Vertical line #1* (bicrestal line) connects the right and *left* iliac crests, *line #2* indicates the midline and the *circles* on *line # 2* represent the palpable spinous processes, *line #3* (parasagittal line) is parallel to the *line #2* and 4–5 cm lateral to *line #2*. *Line #3* should bisect *line #1* at 90° and connect to the PSIS while remaining parallel to *line #2*.

negative aspiration for blood, local anesthetic is injected slowly with repeated aspiration for blood after every 3–5 ml of injected solution.

Pitfalls and Pearls
Pitfalls
- Infection
- Position patient so as to avoid spinal rotation
- Hematoma
- Patient discomfort associated with twitching of large muscle groups
- Increased risk of local anesthetic toxicity
- Hemodynamic consequences (unilateral sympathectomy)
- Nerve injury
- Quadriceps muscle stimulation at currents less than 0.5 mA may indicate needle tip placement within a dural sleeve permitting spread of local anesthetic solution toward the epidural or subarachnoid space potentially resulting in a high spinal or epidural blockade
- Takes longer for effectiveness to take effect

Pearls
- If twitching of paravertebral/paraspinal muscles is observed, then the needle needs to be introduced deeper
- Twitching of hamstrings means that the needle is introduced to caudally
- Flexion of thigh (stimulation of the psoas muscle) indicates that the needle is inserted too deep

- Needle contacts bone (transverse process at 4–6 cm depth), but NO twitches are seen; redirect the needle 5° caudally or cranially after withdrawing back to the skin
- Needle placed deep (≥10 cm), but without proper quadriceps stimulation; then withdraw needle to skin and confirm protocol defined in surface anatomy and landmarks

Popliteal Nerve Block (Sciatic Nerve Block in Popliteal Region)

The sciatic nerve is a bundle consisting of the tibial and common peroneal nerves contained in an epineural sheath. A popliteal nerve block will block components of the sciatic nerve (tibial and common peroneal) at the level of the popliteal fossa where the two branches typically diverge. The common peroneal nerve gives sensory innervation to the inferior portion of the knee joint and lateral and posterior portion of the upper calf. The tibial nerve is a branch of the sciatic nerve and provides sensation to the posterior portion of the calf, the medial plantar surface, and heel of the foot. The tibial nerve at the knee lies just below the popliteal fossa and runs between the two heads of the gastrocnemius muscle and then passes deep to the soleus muscle. It divides into the lateral and medial plantar nerves as it turns medially between the Achilles tendon and medial malleolus. Dermatome distribution of the lower extremity innervated by the popliteal nerve block is indicated in Table 20.11.

Table 20.11 Popliteal nerve innervation to the lower extremity.

Motor	Sensory
Branches to the knee joint (common peroneal)	Cutaneous branches that form the sural nerve
Superficial and deep peroneal nerves (terminal branches of the common peroneal)	
Medial and lateral plantar nerves (terminal branches of the tibial nerve)	Collateral branches of the tibial nerve give rise to cutaneous sural nerves
Muscular branches to the calf and articular branches to the ankle (tibial nerve)	

Indications

As primary anesthetic and/or postoperative pain management with or without a continuous catheter.

Clinical Uses

Surgical

- Foot and ankle surgery (sensory on the medial part of the foot and ankle innervated by the saphenous nerve)
- Anesthesia of the distal two-third of the lower extremity
- Short saphenous vein stripping

Supplemental (in Combination with Femoral Nerve Block)

- Tibial plateau fracture repair
- Total ankle replacement

- Below knee amputation
- Ankle surgery

Postoperative Analgesia
For above-mentioned surgeries.

Technique
Preparation
Arrange sterile towels, sterile gloves, gauze pads, marking pen, antiseptic solution, peripheral nerve stimulator, syringes, and needles for local infiltration and nerve block placement.

Dose
35–40 ml syringes of local anesthetic.

Needles
25 g 1.5 in. needle for skin infiltration and 5 or 10 cm short bevel insulated stimulation needle.

Agents
3% chloroprocaine, 2% lidocaine, 0.5% ropivacaine, 0.5% bupivacaine.

Surface Anatomy and Landmarks
Landmarks
Popliteal fossa crease, tendons of biceps femoris muscle, and tendons of semitendinosus and semimembranosus muscles (Fig. 20.10). Patient is placed in prone position with both feet

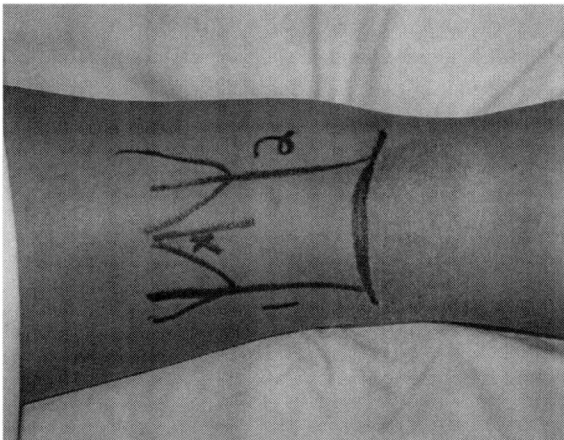

Figure 20.10 Landmarks for the intertendinous approach of the popliteal block. Sciatic nerve is positioned between the tendons of the biceps femoris (BF) muscle laterally (1) and the semitendinosus/semimebranosus (ST/SM) muscle medially (2). The needle insertion site (X) is marked lateral to the midline between BF and ST/SM muscle tendons and approximately 7–10 cm cephalad to the popliteal crease.

extending, to the ankles, beyond the block table. Anatomical landmarks of the biceps femoris tendon (laterally), semimembranosus tendon (medially), and semitendinosus tendon (medially) can be accentuated by having the patient flex the leg at the knee. The needle insertion sight is marked 7–10 cm above the popliteal fossa crease and slightly lateral to the midpoint between the medial and lateral tendon surface landmarks. Antiseptic solution cleanses the skin followed by subcutaneous local anesthetic infiltration. The short beveled insulated needle is attached to a nerve stimulator set at 1.0 mA and inserted perpendicular through the skin wheal or at a 45–60° angle to the skin and aimed cephalad toward the ipsilateral shoulder. The goal is consistent stimulation of the either common peroneal or tibial nerves (toes or foot twitch) as the current is decreased to between 0.2 and 0.5 mA. Correct needle placement will achieve a foot twitch of either dorsiflexion or eversion (common peroneal nerve) or plantar flexion and/or inversion (tibial nerve) at the ankle. After negative aspiration for blood the local anesthetic is injected with frequent aspiration (every 3–5 cc) to check for blood.

Alternative approaches to individually block each the tibial (A) and common peroneal (B) nerves are described as follows:

A. Patient is placed in the prone position, and the apex of the triangle at the convergence of semitendinosus and the biceps femoris tendons/muscles is identified. The base of the triangle is the skin crease of the knee. In an aseptic fashion at the center of the apex a 22 g 1.5 in. needle is inserted perpendicularly until a paresthesia in the distribution of the tibial nerve is elicited. The needle is withdrawn slightly and in the absence of any persistent paresthesia following negative aspiration, 8 cc of local is injected slowly. Tibial nerve block at the ankle is performed with the patient in the lateral position and the operative leg slightly flexed. In an aseptic fashion a 25 g 1.5 in. needle is inserted between the medial malleolus and the Achilles tendon toward the posterior tibial artery. After a depth of 0.5–0.75 in., a paresthesia can be elicited. The needle is withdrawn about 1 mm and in the absence of persistent paresthesia and negative aspiration, a total of 6 ml of local is injected.
B. To perform this block, the patient is placed in the lateral position and the leg is flexed. A 25 g 0.5 in. needle is inserted at a point just below the fibular head and is advanced slowly toward the neck of the fibula until paresthesia is elicited. The needle is then withdrawn slightly, and local anesthetic solution is injected.

Pitfalls and Pearls
Pitfalls
- Infection
- Hematoma
- Local anesthetic toxicity
- Vascular puncture
- Nerve injury
- Prolonged onset time
- Inadequate skin anesthesia (commonly delayed) despite good evidence of motor blockade
- Uncomfortable for some patients to be in the prone position
- Isolated twitches of the calf muscle is unacceptable
- Patients require instructions to avoid injury to the insensate lower extremity

Pearls
- Stimulation of tibial nerve to obtain plantar flexion is most reliable (especially for those patients with peripheral neuropathy in which stimulation at 0.7 mA or below is acceptable)
- Rely on the tendon surface landmarks rather than subjective interpretations of the popliteal triangle

Ankle Block

Innervations to the ankle involves five major nerve branches of the foot as indentified in Table 20.12. An ankle block is basically an infiltration block. Peripheral nerves blocked during an ankle blockade are derived from the terminal branches of the sciatic nerve (deep and superficial peroneal and sural nerves) and one from the distal branch of the femoral nerve (saphenous nerve). Motor blockade is not often needed for surgeries carried out under the influence of an ankle blockade.

Table 20.12 Nerve innervation to the ankle.

		Cutaneous innervation	Cutaneous innervation
Femoral n.		Medial ankle and foot (saphenous n.)	
Sciatic n.	Tibial n.	Lateral and posterior half of ankle above and below the lateral malleolus (sural n.)	
		Posterior tibial n.	Anterior two-third on plantar surface of foot (plantar n.)
			Posterior one-third on plantar surface of foot and entire heal (calcaneal n.)
	Common peroneal n.	Dorsal surface of foot (superficial peroneal n.)	
		Area between great toe and second toe (deep peroneal n.)	

The deep peroneal nerve is derived from the common peroneal nerve that is a continuation of the sciatic nerve. The common peroneal nerve obtains fibers from the posterior branches of L4, L5, S1, and S2 nerve roots. It descends behind the head of the fibula and after crossing the fibula tunnel the nerve divides into the superficial and deep peroneal nerves. The deep peroneal nerve provides innervation to the space between the first and the second toes and the adjacent dorsal area.

The superficial peroneal nerve, a branch of the common peroneal nerve, descends down along with the extensor digitorum longus muscle dividing into terminal branches above the ankle. The sensory innervation is to most of the dorsum of the foot and also to the toes except in between the first and the second toes.

The sural nerve is a branch of the posterior tibial nerve. It passes around the lateral malleolus from the posterior calf to provide innervation to the posterior lateral aspect of the calf, lateral surface of the foot, fifth toe, and also the plantar surface of the heel.

Indications

As primary anesthetic and/or postoperative pain management. Surgical procedures of the foot (well suited for surgery not requiring high-tourniquet pressure).

Clinical Uses
Surgical

Foot surgery.

Postoperative Analgesia

Foot surgery.

Technique
Preparation

Arrange sterile towels, sterile gloves, gauze pads, marking pen, antiseptic solution, syringes, and needles for local infiltration and nerve block placement.

Dose

20 ml syringes of local anesthetic.

Needles

25 or 22 g 5 cm short bevel needle.

Agents

2% lidocaine, 0.5% ropivacaine, 0.5% bupivacaine.

Surface Anatomy and Landmarks

Landmarks include medial malleolus, lateral malleolus, Achilles tendon, tendons on dorsal surface of foot (Fig. 20.11a–c). It may be helpful to place the patient in the prone position initially (blockade of the posterior tibial and sural nerves) and then have the patient assume the supine position (saphenous, superficial, and deep peroneal nerves). The ankle block may also be performed with the patient in the supine position, but the leg should be placed on a padded and elevated support for circumferential access of the ankle. The entire ankle is first prepped in sterile fashion with an antiseptic solution. Three separate injection sites around the ankle may block all five nerve branches. The superficial peroneal, deep peroneal, and saphenous nerves can be blocked by inserting the needle between the tendons of the extensor hallucis longus and the anterior tibial muscles (extensor digitorum longus tendon) on the dorsum of the foot. The anterior tibial artery may be palpated and the deep peroneal nerve located immediately lateral to the pulsation. Subsequent to negative aspiration for blood, infiltrate 5 cc of local anesthetic solution in the area to block the deep peroneal nerve (Fig. 20.11a). From the same approach, subcutaneously advance the needle first laterally (superficial peroneal nerve) and then medially (saphenous nerve) to the respective malleoli and inject 3–5 cc of local in each direction (Fig. 20.11b). Second injection site for blockade of the posterior tibial nerve should position the needle to be inserted at the cephalic border of the medial malleolus, just medial to the Achilles tendon, and advanced until eliciting a paresthesia or contact of posterior portion of the medial malleolus (Fig. 20.11c). If a paresthesia is obtained, then inject 5–7 cc of local after negative aspiration for blood or slightly (approximately 1 mm) remove the needle tip contact from the periosteum before injecting. The third injection site will position the block needle lateral to the Achilles tendon at the cephalic border of the lateral malleolus to block the sural nerve. The needle is advanced until contact with the lateral malleolus or obtaining a paresthesia and then injecting 5–7 cc of local upon withdraw (approximately 1 mm) of the block needle from contact with the lateral malleolus.

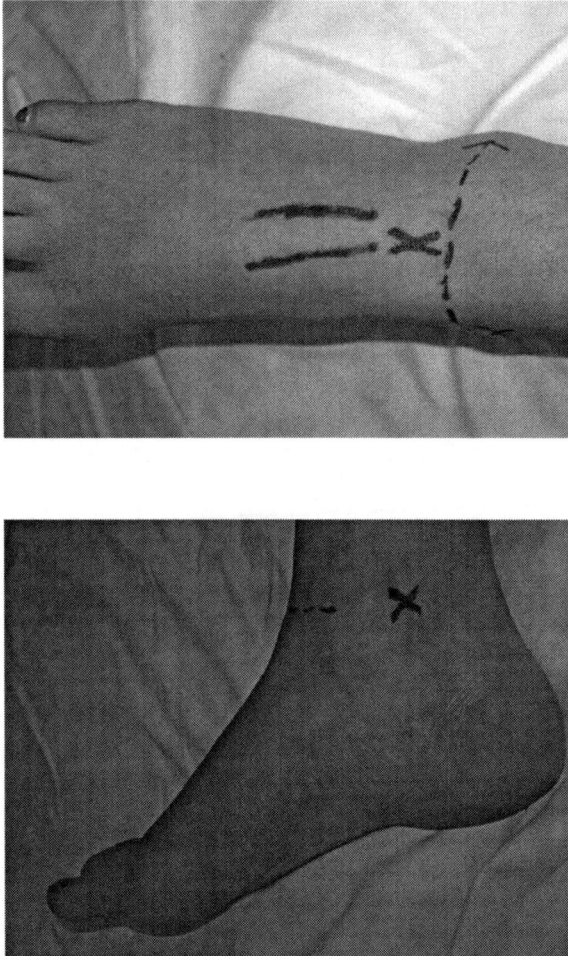

Figure 20.11 (a–c) Landmarks for the approach of the ankle block. (a) Block of the deep peroneal nerve. Needle insertion site (*X*) is just lateral to the extensor hallucis longus tendon and deep to the retinaculum. *X* is distal to the *blue dashed line* connecting the lateral and medial malleolus. (b) Posterior tibial nerve block. Midway between the Achilles tendon and the medial malleolus identifies the needle insertion site (*X*). Deep to the retinaculum and posterior to the tibial artery (*X*) is where the local anesthetic is to be injected. (c) Sural nerve block. *Dashed line* connecting the lateral and medial malleolus is pointing toward the lateral malleolus.

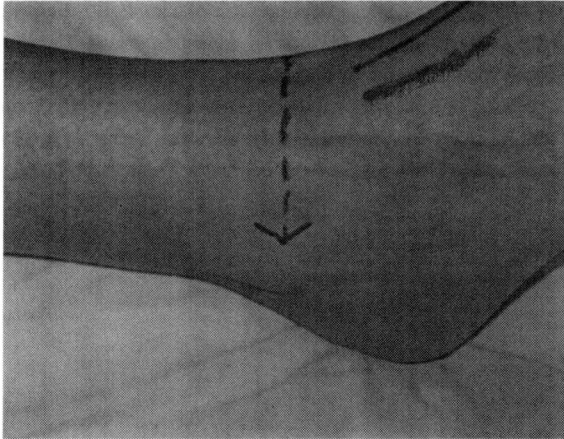

Figure 20.11 **(Continued)**

Pitfalls and Pearls
Pitfalls
- Infection
- Hematoma
- Vascular puncture
- Nerve injury
- Painful due to pressure from local injection

Pearls
- Patient can be well sedated as the block is considered a volume and diffusion-type block
- Patients are usually able to ambulate following surgery that may permit shortened or bypass PACU stay with effective analgesia

Metatarsal and Digital Nerve Blocks for the Foot
The plantar digital nerves are derived from the posterior tibial nerve and provide sensation to most of the plantar surface.

Metatarsal Nerve Block
In a sterile fashion a 25 g 1.5 in. needle is inserted proximal to the metatarsal head adjacent to the bone of the toe to be blocked. The needle is advanced from the dorsal surface to the plantar surface since the plantar digital nerve is on the dorsal side of the flexor retinaculum. A total of 3 cc of local is injected after negative aspiration.

Digital Nerve Block
In a sterile fashion a 25 g 1.5 in. needle is inserted at the base of the toe adjacent to the bony portion of the digit that has to be blocked. Following negative aspiration a total of 3 cc of local per digit is injected.

Case Scenario
Thomas Halaszynski, DMD, MD, MBA

Ben is a 48-year-old man who has sustained a traumatic injury to his left ankle after being hit by a car while riding his bicycle. He also suffered a burn injury to his left calf secondary to lying on the hot pavement subsequent to his accident. His medical history is significant for aortic stenosis (asymptomatic), and past surgical history is significant for both cervical and lumbar posterior fusion. He has a documented difficult intubation during his lumbar fusion surgery. He is scheduled for open reduction and internal fixation (ORIF) of **left** ankle and excision of the eschar on the left calf with a split thickness skin graft from **his** right thigh. As an anesthesiologist, you are requested to assess this patient for the surgery.

What are your concerns regarding the anesthetic options for Ben?
The stress response to anesthesia and surgery could lead to an increased oxygen demand. Typically, there is limited coronary reserve in patients with aortic stenosis (AS). Even in the absence of coronary artery disease (CAD), patients with AS may experience angina, and CAD frequently coexists with AS. Decreased preload and reductions in afterload may affect the cardiac output in patients with AS. Therefore, regular sinus rhythm (60–70 beats/min) and adequate venous return are necessary for cardiac function in patients with AS. Inadequate coronary and cerebral perfusion may result from adverse effects on heart rate and cardiac filling volumes due to a decrease in sympathetic activity. For these reasons, AS has been considered a relative contraindication to neuraxial anesthesia, but currently the medical literature has no concrete evidence in the support of such a statement.

On the other hand, general anesthesia can pose difficulties with regards to airway management. Difficult and prolonged intubation attempts can lead to increased myocardial oxygen demand and concurrent hypoxia. The effect of general anesthetic drugs can have substantial effects on myocardial contractility, sympathetic tone, and peripheral vascular resistance.

Could you elaborate on the hemodynamic effects of neuraxial blockade?
The cardiovascular effects of neuraxial blockade with local anesthetics may lead to decreases in both arterial blood pressure and heart rate. The vertebral level or height attained with a neuraxial block will determine the degree of sympathectomy. Typically, a sympathectomy will extend for several dermatomes above the sensory level achieved with a spinal anesthetic (2–6 levels) and at the sensory level (or 1–2 dermatomes above) for an epidural. Sympatholysis achieved with a neuraxial block results in both arterial and venous dilation. The venodilation effects predominate due to venous pooling (about 75% of blood volume).

Within the context of Ben's preexisting conditions, what are the advantages of regional or peripheral nerve block?

Regional sympathectomy is created by the local anesthetic used during the performance of regional/peripheral nerve block. Major hemodynamic changes seldom result from a regional sympathectomy of an extremity nerve block. Patients with a disease process in which a sympathectomy from a neuraxial block is unsafe may undergo an extremity nerve block without significant hemodynamic instability.

The anterior rami of lumbar nerves (L1–L4), with possible contribution of branches from L-5 and T12, forms the lumbar plexus. A lumbar plexus block technique employs injection of local anesthetic into the psoas compartment (between the psoas major and the quadratus lumborum muscles) and will anesthetize the hip and anterolateral thigh. A side effect of the lumbar plexus block is the possible spread of local anesthetic to the lumbar sympathetic chain, resulting in a unilateral sympathectomy.

What are the anesthetic options for Ben?

Anesthetic options to be discussed with this patient would involve neuraxial blockade, general anesthesia, a single regional anesthetic or combination of different techniques. Postoperative pain management issues will also need to be addressed.

(a) General Anesthesia and PCA Postoperative Pain Relief:

The advantages of this technique are being in control of the situation (for the anesthesiologist), patient comfort, and avoiding potential complications of regional anesthetic techniques such as incomplete nerve blockade which might warrant conversion to GA. Disadvantages include hemodynamic instability during induction and recovery and a potential for difficult airway. Yet another problem is respiratory depression and hypoxia due to opioid with accompanying myocardial ischemia.

(b) Neuraxial Blockade:

A carefully controlled spinal aimed at a sensory block up to T10 level can reduce the hemodynamic consequences due to sympathetic blockade and is beneficial in providing a stress-free anesthetic with an added benefit of postoperative pain relief the duration of which can be prolonged with a long-acting opioid. An epidural catheter technique has the extra benefit of slow titration of the neuraxial blockade. However, a high level of blockade is not ideal for the patient with AS.

A neuraxial opioid only, without the local anesthetic, will seem to be an attractive due to the lack of sympathetic effects. The downside of this technique is lack of ability to provide perfect surgical conditions for the surgeon, and the patient may experience excessive touch, pressure, and movements.

(c) Bilateral Lower Extremity Regional Anesthetic Techniques:

This can provide near perfect anesthetic conditions for both the patient and the surgeon; the analgesia can be extended to cover the postoperative period if a catheter technique is used. There is no accompanying sympathetic blockade and avoid hemodynamic and respiratory effects of GA. It is also capable of reducing the stress response to surgery which is beneficial in patient with AS and a difficult airway. The disadvantage is multiple injection, potential for local anesthetic overdose or underdose (when the given total local anesthetic dose is divided into multiple individual nerve blocks).

Describe the advantages of regional anesthesia?
Regional anesthesia can provide some benefits to the patient undergoing orthopedic surgery. It can significantly reduce the incidence of deep venous thrombosis and surgical blood loss. Other factors to consider include reducing postoperative nausea and vomiting, reductions in opioid analgesic requirements and their potential adverse side effects, prolonged postoperative analgesia, expedited and improved postoperative recovery, earlier and improved compliance with any physical therapy, earlier discharges from both the PACU and the hospital, reductions in postoperative cognitive dysfunction, better patient satisfaction, and overall improved long-term advantages with an aim on reducing morbidity. Whether the chosen intraoperative anesthetic technique can reduce or decrease pulmonary complications is not clear, but regional anesthesia may still be a good option in patients with impaired pulmonary function.

Regardless of the anesthetic choice, informed consent should be obtained and include patient acceptance, selection of an anesthetic method compatible with the surgery, nature of the drugs involved (local anesthetics, sedatives, analgesics, etc.), and possible side effects should be explained. Inform the patient that complete anesthesia at all stages of the perioperative period cannot be guaranteed, reassure the patient that they will receive adequate relief of pain and anxiety, and identify alternative anesthetic choices that may be made necessary. It is important to understand that failure of regional anesthesia is possible in which case a general anesthetic would be administered.

After you have explained all the available options, Ben chose a combined femoral and sciatic nerve block. He also requested sedation during his surgery. You perform sciatic and femoral nerve blocks under ultrasound guidance. Two catheters are inserted near these nerves to provide postoperative analgesia. Ben undergoes the surgery successfully and he is satisfied with the pain relief he experiences after the surgery.

References

Ballantyne JC, Carr DB, deFerranti S, et al. The comparative effects of postoperative analgesic therapies on pulmonary outcome: cumulative meta-analyses of randomized, controlled trials. Anesth Analg. 1998;86:598–612.

Block BM, Liu SS, Rowlingson AJ, et al. Efficacy of postoperative epidural analgesia: a meta-analysis. JAMA 2003;290:2455–63.

Goldman L, et al. Multifactorial index of cardiac risk in noncardiac surgical patients. N Engl J Med. 1977;297:845.

Jorgensen H, Wetterslev J, Moiniche S, et al. Epidural local anaesthetics versus opioid-based analgesic regimens on postoperative gastrointestinal paralysis, PONV and pain after abdominal surgery. Cochrane Database Syst Rev. 2000;CD001893.

Joshi GP, Bonnet F, Shah R, et al. A systematic review of randomized trials evaluating regional techniques for postthoracotomy analgesia. Anesth Analg. 2008;107:1026–40.

Kehlet H. Postoperative opioid sparing to hasten recovery: what are the issues? Anesthesiology 2005;102:1083–5.

Liu SS, Block BM, Wu CL. Effects of perioperative central neuraxial analgesia on outcome after coronary artery bypass surgery: a meta-analysis. Anesthesiology 2004;101:153–61.

Liu SS, Richman JM, Thirlby RC, Wu CL. Efficacy of continuous wound catheters delivering local anesthetic for postoperative analgesia: a quantitative and qualitative systematic review of randomized controlled trials. J Am Coll Surg. 2006;203:914–32.

Liu SS, Strodtbeck WM, Richman JM, Wu CL. A comparison of regional versus general anesthesia for ambulatory anesthesia: a meta-analysis of randomized controlled trials. Anesth Analg. 2005;101:1634–42.

Liu SS, Wu CL. Effect of postoperative analgesia on major postoperative complications: a systematic update of the evidence. Anesth Analg 2007;104:689–702.

Marhofer P, Chan VW. Ultrasound-guided regional anesthesia: current concepts and future trends. Anesth Analg. 2007;104:1265–1269.

McDonald SB. Is neuraxial blockade contraindicated in the patient with aortic stenosis? Reg Anesth Pain Med. 2004 Sep–Oct;29(5):496–5.

Richman JM, Liu SS, Courpas G, et al. Does continuous peripheral nerve block provide superior pain control to opioids? A meta-analysis. Anesth Analg. 2006;102:248–57.

Rigg JR, Jamrozik K, Myles PS, et al. Epidural anaesthesia and analgesia and outcome of major surgery: a randomised trial. Lancet 2002;359:1276–82.

Torsher L, et al. Risk of patients with severe aortic stenosis undergoing noncardiac surgery. Am J Cardiol. 1998;81:448–52.

Wu CL, Cohen SR, Richman JM, et al. Efficacy of postoperative patient-controlled and continuous infusion epidural analgesia versus intravenous patient-controlled analgesia with opioids: a meta-analysis. Anesthesiology 2005;103:1079–88.

Wu CL, Hsu W, Richman JM, et al. Postoperative cognitive function as an outcome of regional anesthesia and analgesia. Reg Anesth Pain Med. 2004;29:257–68.

Chapter 21

Principles of Ultrasound Techniques

Thomas Halaszynski, DMD, MD, MBA

Introduction

Surgery of the upper and lower extremity presents anesthesiologists with an alternative to general anesthesia (GA), that being regional anesthesia (RA). RA is most often performed for postoperative analgesia, but RA may also be utilized as the primary technique for intraoperative anesthesia under certain circumstances and with certain patients. For years, neuraxial techniques (spinal or epidural) have been used as the sole regional anesthetic of choice for the lower limb. The advent of low molecular weight heparins (i.e., enoxaparin, fondaparinux) and the potential risk for the development of neuraxial hematomas have limited neuraxial technique use and have led to a much higher use of peripheral nerve blocks (PNBs) in everyday practice. Since the mid-2000s, great improvements have been made in equipment used to perform PNB, including stimulating peripheral nerve catheters and the use of ultrasound to guide in the placement of RA and to assist in the identity of nerves and nerve plexus (Marhofer et al. 2007).

Recent literature continues to show a growing body of evidence supporting the benefits of RA versus GA with respect to mortality, morbidity, postoperative analgesia, and functional recovery in certain surgical scenarios. Additional potential benefits of RA include increased operating room efficiency, improved pain control, and decreased incidence of chronic pain syndromes (Ballantyne et al. 1998, Beattie et al. 2001, Wu et al. 2004, Urwin et al. 2000). In one meta-analysis, Rodgers et al. (2000) showed a reduction in mortality of 33% with a significant decrease in the incidence of myocardial ischemic events, respiratory depression, rate of deep vein thrombosis (DVT) formation, and blood loss. Adequate pain management following surgery using a multimodal technique, including the use of cycloxygenase-2 inhibitors (COX-2 inhibitors), pregabalin or gabapentin, central neuraxial blockade, and PNB plays an important role in the management of acute postoperative pain and possibly the prevention of subsequent chronic pain syndromes (Reuben and Buvanendran 2007, Kehlet et al. 2006). Development of chronic pain syndromes following surgery shows some correlation to the severity of acute pain experienced during the immediate perioperative period (e.g., phantom limb syndrome).

However, the benefits of RA must be weighed against the possible negative aspects of RA that include consumption of operating room resources, potential patient discomfort, block failures, nerve injury, and toxic reactions to local anesthesia. Many of the negative aspects

N. Vadivelu et al. (eds.), *Essentials of Pain Management*,
DOI 10.1007/978-0-387-87579-8_21, © Springer Science+Business Media, LLC 2011

of RA stem from the fundamental fact that these procedures have traditionally been performed without the ability to visualize needle insertion, adjacent blood vessels, and the spread of local anesthesia. In the past decade, there has been a valuable shift in the administration techniques of RA. Anesthesiologists can now visualize (in real time) neural anatomy, needle movement, collateral structures, and the perineural spread of local anesthesia. This is all possible secondary to the use of an "old" technology: ultrasound.

Described in this chapter are the commonly performed ultrasound-guided PNB that are used for some of the common upper and lower limb surgeries. The chapter will also include some of the new developments in this fast-growing area of RA and describe how to perform these blocks in every day practice. Basic principles for clinicians learning ultrasound-guided RA (USGRA) must be remembered and are keys to success in initial acquisition and refinement of skills for USGRA. A basic understanding of anatomy is required in order to utilize the ultrasound machine as a tool in the performance of RA. As Gaston Labat in 1928 stated, "*Anatomy is the foundation on which the edifice of regional anesthesia is built.*" Some of the common tips or basic rules that serve as a guide for trainees are identified in Table 21.1.

Table 21.1 Basic guidelines for ultrasound-guided regional anesthesia (USGRA).

1. Proper ergonomics (position the patient, bed, and US machine to the proper height and position) will reduce operator fatigue
2. Know both applied and gross anatomy (use a nerve stimulator for confirmation when initially starting USGRA)
3. Optimize ultrasound image(s) of block area anatomy prior to PNB placement and identify footprint of US probe on patient's skin prior to proceeding
4. Recommended as a primary technique is to insert the PNB needle "in-plane" to the US probe
5. Visualize the PNB needle at all times and do not advance needle if needle tip cannot be visualized
6. Move head (eyes) or one hand at a time. Avoid movement of head or either hand simultaneously (helps to avoid a moving target and assists with orientation)
7. Stabilize the US hand and needle hand on the patient and grasp the US probe close to its base (extend the fingers of the US hand on the patient for added stability)
8. If needle visualization on US screen is lost, look at your hands, US probe, and the PNB needle (to confirm alignment) before repositioning
9. Follow nerve structure course (proximally and distally) a short distance, in order to confirm its identification as a nerve. Veins usually collapse and arteries do not when pressure is applied with the US probe
10. Visualize PNB needle tip and pertinent surrounding structures before LA injection. Surrounding tissues move upon LA injection (STOP if tissues do not move as PNB needle tip may be in a blood vessel). Be aware of proper injection pressure to avoid intraneural injections and aspirate frequently to assist in identifying intravascular injections

US, ultrasound; USRA, ultrasound-guided regional anesthesia; PNB, peripheral nerve block; LA, local anesthetic.

An understanding of nerve innervation of the surgical site is a prerequisite for a successful RA plan, and a grasp of perineural anatomy is needed to guide a needle to the site for local anesthetic injection with the least trauma and risk of complications from errant needle pass(es). Perineural anatomy and the ultrasound appearance of various tissue types are necessary to correctly locate local anesthetic injections for successful RA. With experience, ultrasound pattern recognition is developed and typical anatomy is rapidly identified. Anatomic expertise is fundamental to the development of ultrasound proficiency, but the regular use of ultrasound imaging teaches the practitioner a great deal about human anatomy and its variations.

The science of pain medicine has made great strides with regards to postoperative pain management, but many patients fail to receive these basic treatment protocols (Apfelbaum et al. 2003). Typically, physicians often base their perioperative pain management plan on the use of a single analgesic agent, usually an opioid. There is now abundant evidence that a multimodal approach to pain management is beneficial for patients (Kehlet and Dahl 2003, Kehlet and Wilmore 2002). The many benefits of multimodal analgesia are derived from the fact that using multiple agents blocks pain pathways at different sites and that the effects of these analgesic agents are not only additive but also often synergistic. This allows the use of lower doses of analgesics and thus reducing the dose-dependent side effects of any one single agent.

One aspect of multimodal analgesia protocols includes performance of PNB and, if possible, use of an indwelling nerve catheter (typically remains in place for 2–4 days postoperatively) to extend the beneficial effects of the nerve and nerve plexus blockade. Single-shot nerve blocks eventually wear off according to the pharmacokinetics and pharmacodynamics of the local anesthetic agents used (e.g., typically late at night following discharge from the one-day surgical center), and this can result in a period of severe pain because the patients may have no opioids within their system. The presence of an appropriately placed peripheral nerve block catheter(s) and a continuous infusion of local anesthetics may avoid this problem.

Deep vein thrombosis (DVT) poses a serious threat to patients undergoing general surgery and orthopedic procedures. A multitude of anticoagulant techniques and drugs are used, often dictated by the preference of the surgeon, with no uniform evidence-based criteria in which to optimize DVT prophylaxis. For use with a variety of anticoagulants in the presence of regional techniques, guidelines have been developed and presented by the American Society of Regional Anesthesia (ASRA) (Horlocker et al. 2003). These ASRA guidelines were intended for neuraxial techniques, but are often extrapolated to use with PNB. It is important to remember that these are guidelines and that when deciding whether to perform RA in the presence of potential coagulation issues, the clinician needs to balance the risk of a regional technique versus the risk imposed by GA. Based on the guidelines, a PNB should not be performed on a patient with suspected coagulation issues. As an example, a PNB should not be performed within 12 h of the last dose of low molecular weight heparin (LMWH) if a standard prophylactic dose (LMWH, 40 mg) has been used. With higher doses of LMWH, such as 1 mg/kg, waiting a period of 24 h should be necessary prior to nerve block placement. In the presence of LMWH, PNB catheters can be used, but should be removed 2 h prior to the next dose of LMWH administration. The ASRA guidelines for patients receiving platelet inhibitors suggest that clopidogrel should be stopped for 7 days prior to a major nerve block placement, whereas ticlopeidine would delay the placement of RA for 10 days. Other non-steroidal anti-inflammatory drugs (NSAIDs) and aspirin can be safely used in the presence of PNB.

Logistics and equipment needs for the performance and placement of regional anesthesia and PNB need to be considered. To perform these PNBs with a degree of efficiency and consideration of patient safety, it is important to have the appropriately developed protocols and readily available supplies and equipment. A preoperative block area with full monitoring and resuscitation equipment is one model that has been established. Complications associated with RA, some of them being life threatening, may follow the initiation of regional techniques, thus mandating the availability of resuscitative equipment. Recent studies indicate that 20% intralipid can be of benefit during resuscitation from negative cardiovascular events following the inadvertent intravascular injection of higher doses/concentrations of local anesthetics (especially bupivacaine) (Weinberg 2006a, b).

The presence of another assigned health-care provider (anesthesia attending, resident, Certified Registered Nurse Anesthetist (CRNA), or anesthesia assistant) in the preoperative block area can help with maintaining appropriate patient turnover and can also lead

Table 21.2 Drugs and equipment needed to perform regional anesthesia.

- Insulated stimulating needles (1, 2, 4, and 6 in.)
- Stimulating and nonstimulating PNB catheters
- Infusion pumps
- Ultrasound machine(s) with software specifically designed for regional anesthesia
- Sterile sheaths for ultrasound probes
- PNB stimulators
- Long-acting local anesthetics
    ropivacaine (0.5 or 0.75%)
    bupivacaine (0.5%)
    for postoperative analgesia
        ropivacaine (0.1 or 0.2%)
        bupivacaine (0.125 or 0.25%)
- short-acting local anesthetics
    mepivacaine (1.5%)
    lidocaine (2%)
    for postoperative analgesia only
        mepivacaine (0.75%)
        lidocaine (1%)
        epinephrine to make 1/400,000 solution
- Steri-strips, tincture of benzoin, and tagederm for securing PNB catheters
- Marker pens for identifying anatomical landmarks
- Resuscitative drugs
    midazolam for sedation and management of seizures
    20% intralipid can be of benefit for the management of local anesthesia-induced arrhythmias
    thiopental for management of resistant seizures
- Resuscitative equipment
    oxygen
    ambubag and airway supplies
    endotracheal tube and laryngoscope equipment

PNB, peripheral nerve block.

to improved educational training and experience of assigned health-care providers (example: residents) (Martin et al. 2002). Table 21.2 represents the standard and minimum equipment, supplies, and drugs necessary when performing regional anesthesia.

Follow-up of patients with single-shot and PNB catheters is essential and necessary for the monitoring of efficacy, efficiency, and patient safety and satisfaction. The acute pain service (APS) or an anesthesiologist can readily assume this responsibility. The APS can also make important decisions about adjustment to infusion rates, the addition of adjuvants for pain management, and timing of PNB catheter(s) removal for patients admitted to the hospital (especially with reference to the administration of anticoagulants).

Medicine is an ever-changing science and as new research and clinical experience broaden, that knowledge, changes in techniques and approaches are required. One of the most exciting advances in technology in relation to RA has been the introduction of anatomically based ultrasound imaging. Real-time viewing of the target nerve structures, the block needle trajectory, and local anesthetic spread, as well as critical structures to avoid, can better ensure success and safety in RA. USGRA is a quantum leap in technology; however, ultrasound visualization still generates indirect images which are subject to individual interpretation depending on one's experiences and training and where that training and experience were obtained. Additionally, it is important to obtain a good knowledge base of the physics on ultrasonography as well as to learn tools for avoiding imaging artifacts and other common mistakes. Literature on ultrasound imaging and guidance in RA is increasing, thus maintaining up-to-date versions of this information is necessary. Readers are advised to consult other sources of current literature related to the physics of ultrasonography and specific RA techniques used in clinical practice.

Basic ultrasound terminology is described in Table 21.3. Some basic clinical pearls for USGRA have been developed by utilization and application of the physics of the ultrasound machine(s). Structures of interest can be imaged either on the short axis (cross section) or on the long axis. A short-axis view becomes a long-axis view when the probe is turned 90° in either direction. In general, regional anesthesiologists prefer to image nerves and blood vessels on short axis because the operator has a simultaneous anterior–posterior and lateral–medial perspective. In the long-axis view, the lateral–medial perspective can be lost.

Two techniques are described in the literature with respect to needle insertion (Sites and Brull 2006). The needle can be inserted using an "in-plane" approach where the needle is inserted parallel to footprint of the ultrasound transducer such that it is visualized in long axis and allowing full needle visualization (Figs. 21.1a and 21.1b). Alternatively, the needle can be inserted perpendicular to the ultrasound transducer footprint, generating a short-axis view of the needle identified as "out-of-plane" (Figs. 21.2a and 21.2b). The major drawback

Table 21.3 Ultrasound terminology.

1. Ultrasound: sound waves that are at a frequency of 20,000 cycles/s or Hertz (Hz) or higher (most transducers used for UGRA are between 7 and 15 million Hz or 7–15 megahertz (MHz))

2. Ultrasound waves are produced when an electrical signal is placed across a piezoelectric crystal that forces the crystal to vibrate (vibration is then conducted through the body). Ultrasound waves are characterized by a specific wavelength and frequency Relationship between these variables:
$c = (\lambda)(f)$, where c = the propagation velocity (presumed to be 1540 m/s in the human body). Therefore, if c is held constant, then to increase the frequency of an ultrasound wave, the wavelength would have to proportionately decrease. (This concept is at the core of UGRA since different frequency probes are used for different blocks)

3. Ultrasound attenuation (a) and resolution (b): (a) Attenuation is the loss of ultrasound wave energy as it travels through tissue. Generally, a lower frequency wave will attenuate less at a given distance in comparison to a higher frequency wave. Thus, the lower frequency ultrasound wave will penetrate deeper into the patient and (b) axial resolution, or the ability to identify two or more points in space (one lying in front of the other), is between one and two wavelengths. This means that the lower frequency (larger wavelength) ultrasound beam will penetrate deeper but will lack the resolution of the higher frequency and smaller wavelength beam

4. Concepts of impedance (a) and reflection (b) form the "images" for UGRA. (a) Impedance can be referred to as the tendency of a medium to conduct ultrasound. When a sound wave travels through an object and contacts an adjacent object with different acoustic impedance, a demarcation is formed (e.g., would be nerve tissue surrounded by adipose tissue). (b) Reflection occurs at interfaces between objects with different acoustic impedances. The larger the difference in acoustic impedances, then the greater the reflection. Objects that are highly reflective are displayed as white or hyperechoic (fascial planes, bones, and some nerves). Objects that weakly reflect ultrasound waves are darker or hypoechoic (muscle, fat, and some nerves). Blood vessels are anechoic and appear black

5. Muscle is typically hypoechoic with internal striation, and the shape of various muscles and the characteristic appearance of fascial layers separating muscles produce specific pattern that becomes recognizable at each ultrasound site

6. Bone reflects ultrasound waves resulting in a bright, hyperechoic edge with shadowing (no image) deep to that edge

7. Veins and arteries are hypoechoic, round, or oval in short axis. Veins are readily collapsible with probe pressure and have respiratory variation in diameter while arteries are pulsatile; color-flow Doppler may be employed to help identify vascular structures

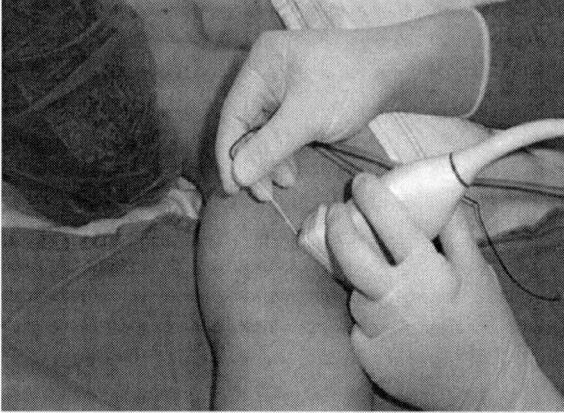

Figure 21.1a Photograph demonstrating suggested ultrasound probe and needle position for an in-plane technique.

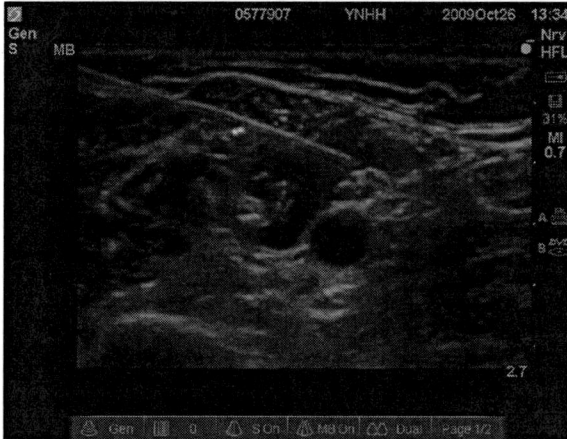

Figure 21.1b Ultrasound image demonstrating anatomy of the axillary brachial plexus with needle approaching the brachial plexus in-line with the ultrasound probe.

to this out-of-plane approach is that a short-axis view of a block needle appears as a small hyperechoic dot on the screen that can sometimes be difficult to see. In addition, the operator is often then unable to confirm the exact location of the needle tip.

Ultrasound by the anesthesiologist is used for anatomical evaluation and to facilitate the performance of RA: both neuraxial and peripheral nerve blocks. Ultrasound technology is useful in patients with obscure anatomical landmarks, in patients with coagulopathy and neural pathology, and in patients suffering extremity trauma. Ultrasound provides an opportunity to visualize individual anatomical variations, and USGRA is typically performed by anesthesiologists and pain specialists in a procedure room or within the operating room. Table 21.4 identifies 10 steps of USGRA for improved RA success, efficacy, and patient

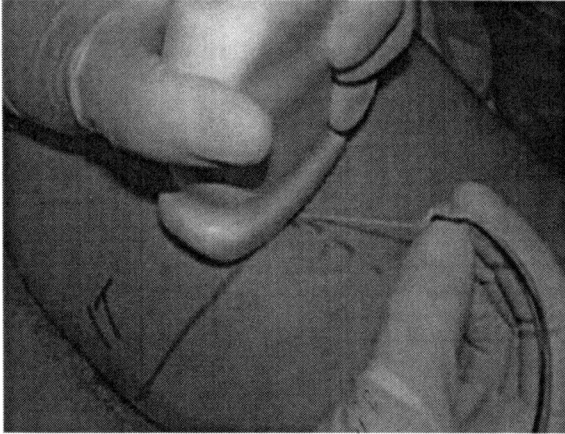

Figure 21.2a Photograph demonstrating probe placement and needle insertion point with needle position for an out-of-plane technique.

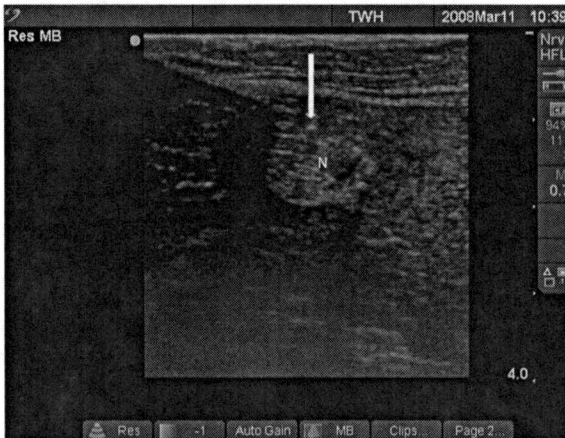

Figure 21.2b Out-of-plane needle approach where needle tip (17G Tuohy) is visualized in transverse view and appears as a hyperechoic dot (*arrow*) on the ultrasound image. The target 'nerve' (*N*) is imaged in short axis.

safety. These fundamental steps should be followed during all RA procedures that utilize this technology.

Peripheral Nerve Blocks of the Upper Extremity

In the following descriptions, standard anatomic axes or planes will be used throughout for consistency, with the three primary descriptive planes: horizontal, coronal, and sagittal. Probe angulation is further described in the cephalad–caudad, medial–lateral, and anterior–posterior directions. The most common ultrasound orientation for nerve (and blood vessel) visualization will be in the short-axis (view in transverse or cross section) view. A long-axis (view in longitudinal section) view of nerves may be used to distinguish a putative nerve

Table 21.4 Steps to ultrasound-guided regional anesthesia (USRA).

1. Visualize key landmark structures (muscles, fascia, blood vessels, and bone)
2. Identify nerves and nerve plexus on short-axis imaging
3. Confirm normal anatomy and recognize anatomical variation(s)
4. Plan the safest and most effective needle approach
5. Use aseptic needle insertion techniques
6. Follow the needle under real-time visualization as it is advanced toward the target
7. Consider a secondary confirmation technique such as nerve stimulation
8. When needle tip is presumed to be in the correct position, inject a small volume of a test solution
9. Make necessary needle adjustments to obtain optimal perineural spread of local anesthesia
10. Maintain traditional safety guidelines of frequent aspiration, monitoring, patient response, and assessment of resistance to injection

from other structures, but short axis is most commonly employed during needle placement, whether the needle is introduced either in-plane or out-of-plane with the ultrasound beam.

The ultrasound appearance of peripheral nerves in the brachial plexus seen in short axis with high-frequency linear transducers can be described as multiple, round, hypoechoic areas seen within a hyperechoic stroma corresponding to nerve fascicles with intervening connective tissue separating the fascicles. In long axis, the fascicular pattern of nerve tissue is seen as longitudinal, discontinuous hypoechoic tubules separated by hyperechoic lines. High-frequency probes have better axial resolution to discriminate this fascicular pattern. Tendons have the closest ultrasound appearance to nerves, but can be distinguished from them by a smaller and more homogeneous fibrillar pattern, described as a fine pattern of alternating hyperechoic and hypoechoic areas in short axis (Silvestri et al. 1995). In addition, tendons can be seen to evolve to muscle when followed proximally or distally and display a greater tendency to anisotropy.

The proximal portions of the brachial plexus above the clavicle have different sonographic appearances than the terminal nerves, with roots and trunks seen in short axis as round or oval hypoechoic structures with a hyperechoic rim and few internal reflections (Cash et al. 2005). This is presumably due to the fact that the roots and trunks are oligo- or mono-fascicular on histologic exam, with less interfascicular connective tissue to produce the hyperechoic acoustic reflection seen in terminal nerves of the brachial plexus.

Interscalene Brachial Plexus Block

Ultrasound guidance for accurately depositing local anesthetic at the level of the cervical roots and trunks of the brachial plexus has many advantages secondary to the abundance of vascular, neurological, and pleural structures that may be entered inadvertently using blind techniques. An easy method of identifying and then following the brachial plexus at this level starts by first visualizing the subclavian artery (SA) immediately posterior to the clavicle by holding the probe between the base of the neck and the clavicle (Fig. 21.3). The probe is then moved from lateral to medial until the pulsation of the SA is visualized. Further medial movement also brings the subclavian vein (SV) into view and its junction with the innominate vein.

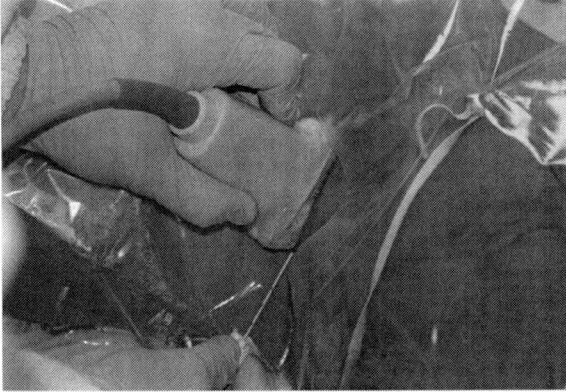

Figure 21.3 Photograph demonstrating suggested initial ultrasound probe position for ultrasound-guided interscalene block.

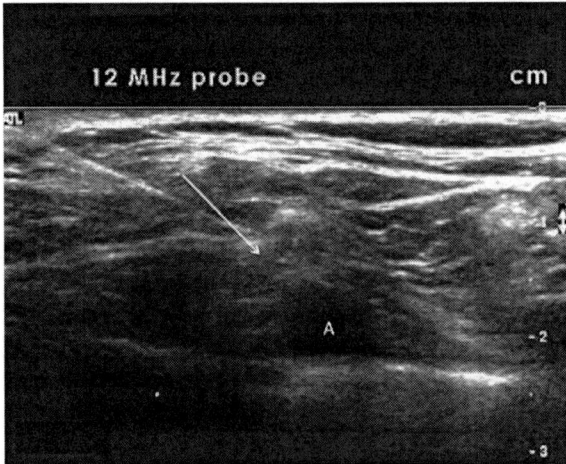

Figure 21.4 Ultrasound image demonstrating anatomy of the supraclavicular brachial plexus. The *arrow* identifies the nerve plexus and A indicates the subclavian artery.

Once the SA is seen, the brachial plexus can be easily seen as a group immediately lateral to the artery (Fig. 21.4).

Once visualizing the brachial plexus in the supraclavicular region, it becomes straightforward to trace the anatomical structures to find the interscalene brachial plexus. The easiest way to do this is to follow the anterior scalene muscle as it passes first medial and then over the SA. The anterior scalene muscle is then followed more cephalad into the neck and the brachial plexus trunks followed by the brachial plexus roots can be seen lying anterior to the scalenus medius muscle and posterior to the anterior scalene muscle. A transverse view of the interscalene brachial plexus is demonstrated in Fig. 21.5a.

Another method of finding the interscalene brachial plexus is to hold the ultrasound probe in the horizontal plane at the laryngeal or cricoid level (transverse process of C6). The

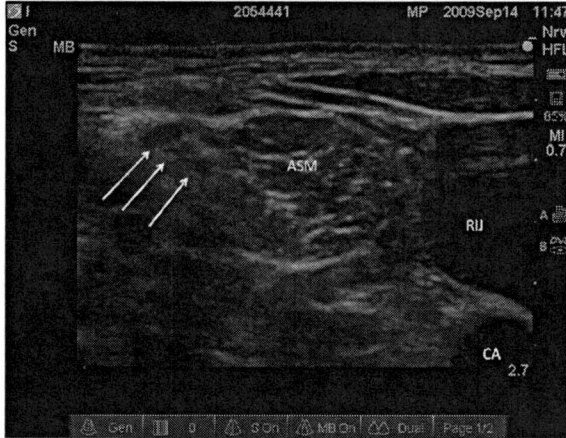

Figure 21.5a Interscalene brachial plexus and its anatomical relations as seen with ultrasound in the transverse plane. *ASM* anterior scalene muscle, *CA* carotid artery, *RIJ* right internal jugular vein, *arrows* identify the roots/trunks of the brachial plexus and the target for deposition of local anesthetic.

probe is inclined somewhat caudad to produce an ultrasound beam that cuts across the roots of the brachial plexus that inclines inferiorly and anteriorly from their origin at the transverse processes. The most recognizable structure anteriorly is the pulsatile common carotid artery (CA) and its companion internal jugular (IJ) vein usually anterior and lateral to the carotid. The IJ may be collapsed or vary in diameter with respiration. The sternocleidomastoid muscle (SCM) is a characteristic muscular structure (hypoechoic with striations) just deep to the subcutaneous layer with a tapered posterior edge, and the anterior and middle scalene muscles are deep to the SCM and posterior to the CA. The cervical roots of C5 through C7 are oligofascicular and hypoechoic round or oval structures which become apparent with slight changes in the caudad inclination of the probe or with movement of the probe in the cephalad or caudad direction (Fig. 21.5b).

Ultrasound-guided interscalene block is most easily performed using the transverse view of the brachial plexus. The roots and trunks of the brachial plexus can be seen stacked from lateral to medial with the C5–C6 roots or superior trunk visible most laterally. The needle can be advanced either in-plane or out-of-plane with the probe. The needle tip can be placed within the interscalene groove in order to obtain local anesthetic spread around the brachial plexus. The in-plane approach permits the needle shaft to be visualized throughout insertion using a posterior approach to the plexus in the long axis and is the most commonly preferred technique (Figs. 21.3 and 21.5b).

An indwelling PNB catheter technique is possible using the described method, but catheter fixation may be somewhat more difficult than that of an infraclavicular technique (described below). Using a Tuohy needle, a catheter can be inserted 1–2 cm past the needle tip, initial local anesthetic bolus given, and infusion initiated. "Hydrodissection" may be accomplished prior to catheter placement by local anesthetic administration through the Tuohy needle under ultrasound in order to visualize the local anesthetic spread within the plexus. A common side effect of this PNB technique is the occurrence of Horner's syndrome secondary

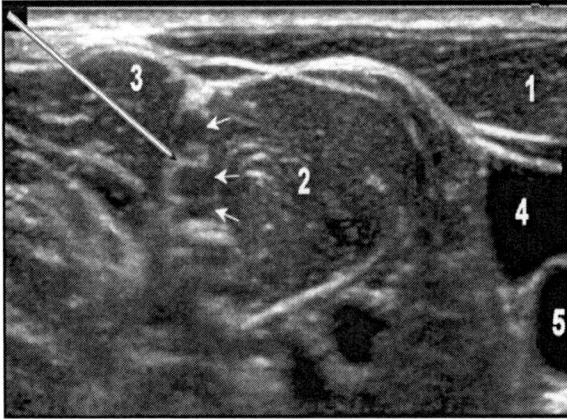

Figure 21.5b Interscalene block. Interscalene brachial plexus and its anatomical relations as seen with ultrasound in the transverse plane. Interscalene anatomy in the transverse plane at the C6 level with the needle (in-line) identifying the plexus. *1* sternocleidomastoid muscle, *2* anterior scalene muscle, *3* middle scalene muscle, *4* internal jugular vein, *5* carotid artery, *arrows* aimed at trunks of brachial plexus.

to the proximity of the sympathetic chain at this level. In addition, phrenic nerve blockade may be as frequent as 100%. Other potential complications include infection, hematoma, local anesthetic toxicity, patient discomfort, neurologic injury, and failed block.

Supraclavicular Brachial Plexus Block

Probe placement for supraclavicular block is near the sagittal plane by visualizing the subclavian artery (SA) immediately posterior to the clavicle and holding the probe between the base of the neck and the clavicle (Fig. 21.3). The probe is angled slightly medially but mainly caudad, and the probe is rotated on its axis with its anterior edge more medial than its posterior to produce the best short-axis view of the pulsatile SA (Fig. 21.6a). A bright, hyperechoic line is seen deep to the artery which is reflected ultrasound from the first rib and the pleura of the lung deep to the rib. A cluster of hypoechoic round structures resembling a "grape cluster" is identified lateral, posterior, and superior to the artery and often extends down to the rib or may be more horizontal in orientation. It is uncommon to see three distinct trunks, but rather to see fascicles within those trunks or divisions at this level. Posterior to the fascicles, the middle scalene muscle can be identified and the anterior scalene muscle found anterior and medial to the SA. Superficial to the supraclavicular brachial plexus will be the omohyoid muscle and often the pulsatile superficial cervical or suprascapular arteries that arise from the thyrocervical trunk. Occasionally, the clavicular anatomy limits optimal movement of the linear ultrasound probe, and a probe with a smaller head/footprint may be necessary for better visualization of the artery, nerves, and rib or pleura prior to needle placement.

The ultrasound supraclavicular technique is an efficient and very effective block of the brachial plexus that blocks all trunks/divisions quickly and typically with a lower volume of local anesthetic than required for most other brachial plexus approaches (Winnie and Collins 1964). The confined nature of the brachial plexus at this point between the first rib

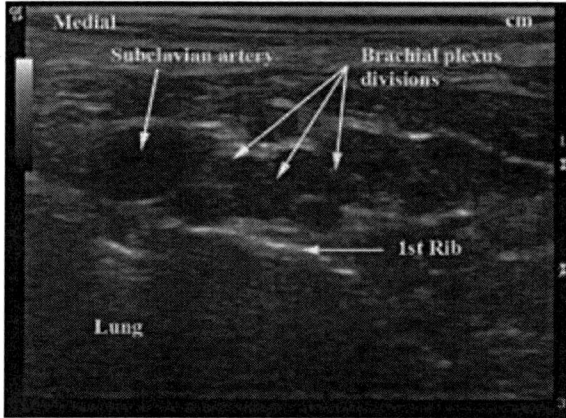

Figure 21.6a   Supraclavicular ultrasound anatomy. The brachial plexus at this level (divisions) appears as hypoechoic circles/ovals in a cluster just lateral to the subclavian artery.

and the clavicle allows for easier localization/spread and restriction of local anesthetic flow to intended targets.

With approaches other than USGRA of the brachial plexus in the supraclavicular area, there is a somewhat higher risk of pneumothorax (approx. 0.5–3%) that can often be delayed in presentation (Franco and Vieira 2000). A pneumothorax is a major deterrent to practitioners who may wish to send patients home following an ambulatory surgical procedure in which a supraclavicular block was placed. In addition, with a technique other than USGRA together with the pulsatile nature of the SA, the ulnar nerve distribution of the brachial plexus is often spared an effective block secondary to poor diffusion of the local anesthetic posterior and caudally within the neurovascular bundle. The use of ultrasound appears ideal in this circumstance, because the first rib, pleura, and SA are readily visible and can be easily avoided provided the practitioner maintains vigilance in keeping the block needle tip in vision under ultrasound during the entire procedure of PNB placement (Fig. 21.6b).

USGRA of a supraclavicular block usually has the PNB needle inserted in-plane with the ultrasound probe so that the needle tip is constantly visualized and inadvertent puncture of the pleura is minimized (Fig. 21.6b). Usually a high-frequency (>10 MHz) linear array probe is used for most brachial plexus approaches (with the possible exception of an infraclavicular nerve block) to allow increased resolution of the superficial brachial plexus structures. The needle is typically inserted at a point lateral to the probe and directed toward inferior and medial portion of the plexus between the first rib and the artery. Needle movement and local anesthetic spread should be directed to the middle and lower trunks/divisions of the plexus by placing the needle tip close to the first rib prior to local anesthetic injection. Typically, an USRA supraclavicular technique requires 20–30 ml of local anesthetic to produce a successful block. Smaller volumes may provide successful anesthesia, and this is currently being studied.

An indwelling PNB catheter technique is possible using the described method with a Tuohy needle, but catheter fixation may be somewhat more difficult than that of an infraclavicular technique (described below). A common side effect of this PNB technique is the occurrence of Horner's syndrome secondary to the proximity of the sympathetic chain at

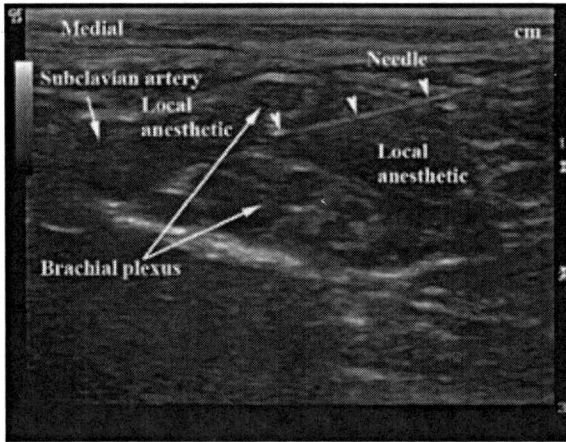

Figure 21.6b Supraclavicular ultrasound anatomy. Image demonstrates anatomy of the supraclavicular brachial plexus with needle approaching the brachial plexus in-line with the ultrasound probe. Note the local anesthetic spread around the nerve plexus.

this level. In addition, phrenic nerve blockade may be as frequent as 60%. Other potential complications include pneumothorax (previously mentioned), infection, hematoma, local anesthetic toxicity, patient discomfort, neurologic injury, and failed block.

Infraclavicular Brachial Plexus Block (USRA Below the Clavicle)

Anatomy of the infraclavicular brachial plexus (Fig. 21.7a) and perineural structures changes in a progressive and predictable fashion from the apex in the anatomic axilla (brachial plexus divisions and cords) at the first rib through to the base of the axilla (brachial plexus cords and branches). Probe placement from medial to lateral demonstrates the changes in anatomy and is relevant to performance of the infraclavicular block. The ultrasound probe is placed close to the sagittal plane and may be slightly rotated on its axis with the caudal edge more medial than the cephalad edge to obtain the best transverse view of the pulsatile axillary artery (AA) (Fig. 21.7b). The AA is more superficial medially, and the axillary vein is identified caudad and medial to the AA. The axillary vein may be collapsible or seen to vary in size with respiration. A significant amount of hypoechoic fat surrounds the axillary contents. At the medial aspect of the clavicle, the pectoralis major and pectoralis minor form two distinct muscular layers superficial to the artery. The rib and pleura can be identified as a hyperechoic structure deep to the AA with anechoic air deeper still. All three cords of the plexus are typically cephalad to the artery as is their position crossing the first rib. These brachial plexus elements (cords) are seen as hyperechoic structures with a fibrillar pattern (Fig. 21.7c).

At the midpoint of the clavicle, but still medial to the coracoid process, the lung is positioned deeper than the infraclavicular portion of the brachial plexus. The medial cord begins to pass posterior to the AA as it twists around it to eventually rest medial to the AA further distally. The posterior cord moves closer to the posterolateral edge of the AA and will ultimately rest posterior to the artery. The lateral cord is readily identifiable using ultrasound as the most superficial hyperechoic structure lateral and superficial to the AA. The medial and posterior cords sometimes can be more difficult to distinguish as they are positioned at an

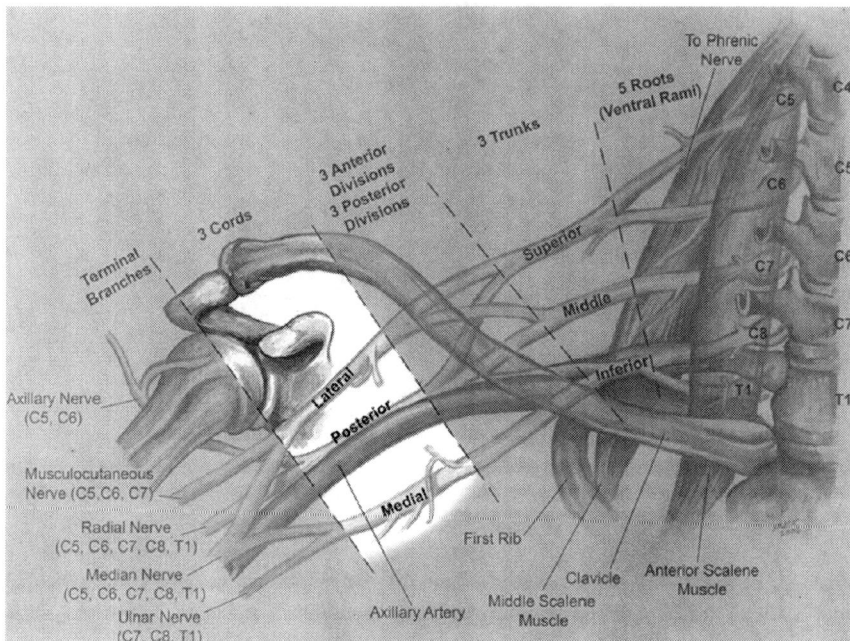

Figure 21.7a   The cords of the brachial plexus are named according to there relationship around the axillary artery: lateral, medial, and posterior.

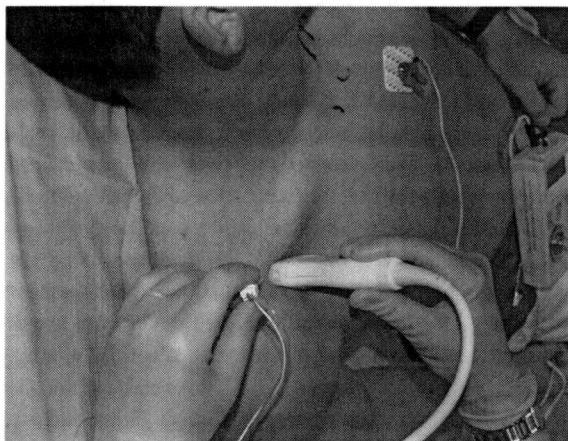

Figure 21.7b   Photograph demonstrating ultrasound probe and needle orientation for an infraclavicular brachial plexus block.

increased depth, and shadowing artifact from the AA often occurs. Bigeleisen et al. (2006) demonstrated that abduction of the upper arm brings the cords of the brachial plexus into a more superficial position in the infraclavicular region facilitating ultrasound visualization.

At the lateral aspect of the clavicle directly inferior to the coracoid process, the lung is not usually seen, the pectoralis minor may not be seen, and the axillary vessels and cords

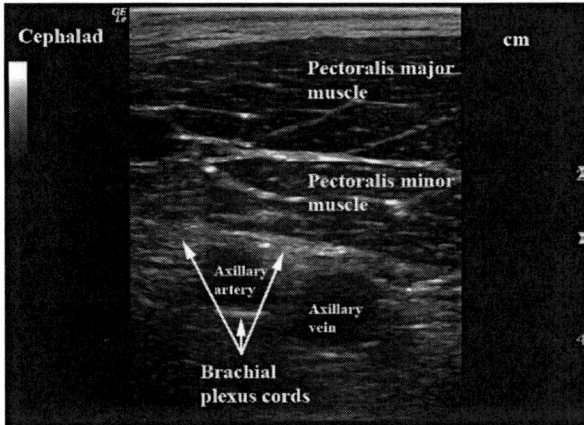

Figure 21.7c   Ultrasound anatomy of the infraclavicular (cords) brachial plexus.

of the plexus are deeper than at the other two sites previously described (interscalene and supraclavicular). The description of the anatomy of the cords in relation to the AA at this point is the most common configuration, but the infraclavicular plexus may have significant variability that may be identified by an ultrasound exam. The depth of the plexus structures and the AA lying anterior to two of the cords may make it difficult to determine the position of the posterior and medial cords (lateral cord remains relatively easy to visualize because of the superficial location). Imaging of the neurological structures in the parasagittal plane is easier to obtain by moving laterally. Moving further laterally from midline reduces the chance of pneumothorax, but the cords lie further apart and therefore there is a greater chance of slow onset or failure to anesthetize the medial cord.

The infraclavicular approach to the brachial plexus has increased in popularity since its initial description in 1981. To achieve a successful infraclavicular block with the nerve stimulator technique, a distal motor end point is required and to seek such a twitch sometimes can be time consuming, and the multiple needle passes required can be painful and increase the risk of complications. The use of ultrasound for infraclavicular block has significant potential to reduce complications compared to other infraclavicular approaches to the brachial plexus. Blockade of all three cords of the brachial plexus may often be achieved with a single injection, and the risk of pneumothorax is considerably less than with blind supraclavicular approaches (parasthesia or nerve stimulation techniques). Fixation of a continuous infraclavicular catheter on the anterior chest wall is the most stable and comfortable for the patient compared to other brachial plexus catheter sites.

Secondary to the depth of the brachial plexus at the coracoid level (4–6 cm), it is often advantageous to use a lower frequency probe (5–10 MHz) of either the linear or the curved array type. The needle is inserted in-line with the US probe and advanced until the needle tip lies at the 9 o'clock position (superolateral) to the AA. The lateral cord is often identified and can be stimulated in this position. The posterior and medial cords lie deeper and often posterior (posterior and medial) or posterior and inferior (medial cord) to the AA at this point. Currently the best method of performing ultrasound-guided infraclavicular block is with the infraclavicular neurovascular structures in a cross-sectional view and the PNB needle

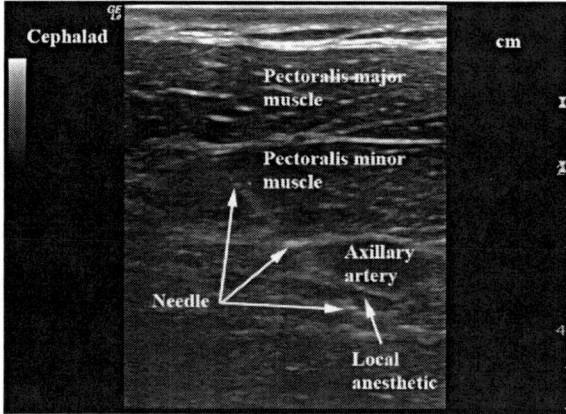

Figure 21.7d Ultrasound of anatomy and block needle of an infraclavicular brachial plexus block. Note the increased difficulty to easily image the block needle as well as some local anesthetic spread.

inserted with an in-plane approach (Figs. 21.7b and 21.7d). It is suggested to place two boluses of local anesthetic with one beside the lateral cord at the 9 o'clock position of the AA and the second injection posterior to the AA at the 6 o'clock position. Care must still be taken to avoid over insertion of the needle since the pleura can still lie within 8 cm or shallower, especially with more medial approaches.

An indwelling infraclavicular catheter may be easily inserted by placing the catheter tip just posterior to the AA followed by local anesthetic bolus and infusion (Fig. 21.7e). A complication of this PNB technique is the occurrence of a hematoma, and would be difficult to apply manual pressure. Other potential complications include pneumothorax (reduced risk

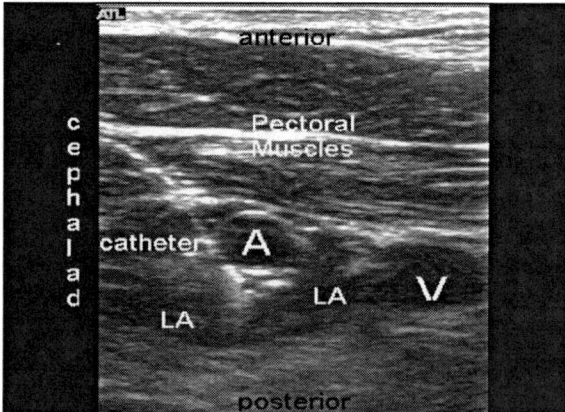

Figure 21.7e Ultrasound image of an infraclavicular indwelling catheter. Note the more hyperechoic local anesthetic solution surrounding the morehyperechoic nerve structures at the 3 o'clock position (medial cord), 6:30 position (posterior cord), and 8 o'clock position (lateral cord) around the axillary artery.

with proper technique), infection, local anesthetic toxicity, patient discomfort, neurologic injury, and failed block.

Axillary Brachial Plexus Block (USRA Below the Clavicle)

Axillary block of the brachial plexus remains a commonly performed means of anesthetizing the plexus, despite the requirement of placing multiple injections in order to facilitate complete anesthesia of all four nerves supplying the forearm and hand (musculocutaneous, median, radial, and ulnar nerves). Blockade of the axillary brachial plexus was successful by elicitation of parasthesia, transvascular (vascular landmark-guided) approach, or peripheral nerve stimulator-guided techniques. With the introduction of the ultrasound, brachial plexus block in the axilla has gained popularity.

In order to best visualize the sonoanatomy of the brachial plexus at the level of the axilla, the ultrasound probe is placed at the junction of the arm and the chest wall in the horizontal plane perpendicular to the axis of the humerus and the axillary vessels (Fig. 21.1a). With mild-to-moderate probe pressure, the axillary veins are collapsed and the pulsatile AA can be readily identified. With relaxation of probe pressure, one or often several axillary veins are identified superficial and deep to the AA. With some probe position variability, terminal branches (median, ulnar, radial) of the brachial plexus are identified as hyperechoic fascicular structures with the median nerve generally superficial and lateral to the AA, the ulnar nerve superficial and medial to the AA, and the radial nerve usually deep to the AA around the 5 o'clock position to the AA (the radial can be traced distally between the long head of triceps and humerus before passing around the spiral groove). The typical appearance of muscle tissue is evident in the biceps and coracobrachialis muscles lateral to the artery and the long head of the triceps medially (Fig. 21.8a). With small changes in ultrasound probe orientation/inclination caudad or cephalad, the hyperechoic musculocutaneous nerve can be seen within the coracobrachialis muscle (Fig. 21.8b). Typically the hyperechoic bony edge of the

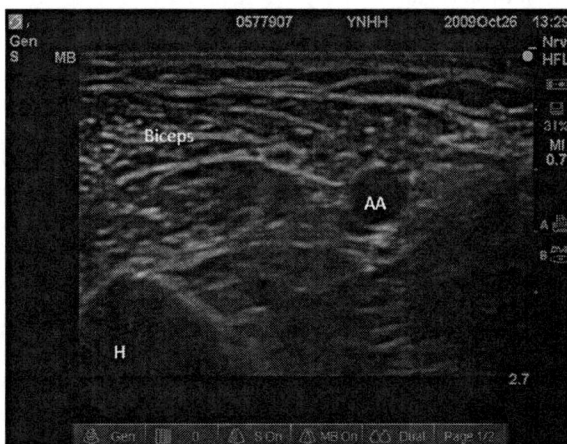

Figure 21.8a Ultrasound anatomical view in the transverse plane demonstrating the anatomical relations of the axillary brachial plexus. H humerus, AA axillary artery.

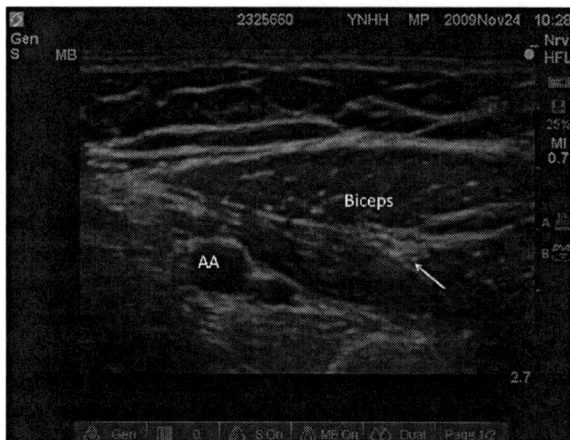

Figure 21.8b **Ultrasound demonstrating the orientation of the musculocutaneous nerve in the axilla.** *Arrow* **pointing to the musculocutaneous nerve in cross section,** *AA* **axillary artery.**

humerus can be seen deep to the axillary sheath, but probe penetration is usually set at a shallower depth than needed to see the humerus in order to magnify the view of the vessels and nerves in the axilla.

Ultrasound use can greatly facilitate performance of axillary brachial plexus block because all four nerves are readily visible around and in proximity to the AA – the median nerve (anterior/lateral to AA): when at the apex of the axilla the contributions from the medial and lateral cords can be seen uniting; the radial nerve (typically deep and medial to AA): a branch to the triceps can occasionally be identified separate from the radial nerve arising from its deep and medial side; the ulnar nerve (typically medial/superficial to AA): can be located medial to the axillary vein, but can also lie on the lateral aspect of the vein adjacent to the AA; and the musculocutaneous nerve: traced from the lateral cord high in the axilla and followed into the belly of the coracobrachialis muscle as it passes into the upper arm. Using ultrasound, axillary plexus nerves can be easily identified by confirming with nerve stimulation (appropriate muscular twitch) and/or tracing the nerves into the arm to follow their anatomical path to the elbow.

Ultrasound-guided axillary plexus block typically positions the probe in a transverse plane, and needle orientation is an in-plane technique (Fig. 21.1a). The block needle is passed from lateral to medial across the axilla (identifying the needle shaft and tip along its trajectory) in order to identify and surround each nerve with local anesthetic (Figs. 21.8c and 21.8d). Both ultrasound and nerve stimulation can be used to place the needle tip close to the nerve and confirm by electrical stimulation. As confidence increases with identification of individual nerves, there may be less need for nerve stimulation. The goal is to surround each nerve with local anesthetic by a dynamic process of real-time needle tip movement. For each nerve of the plexus, up to 10 ml of local anesthetic solution is used, but less (4 ml of local anesthetic) if ideal circumferential local anesthetic spread is visualized around each nerve.

The radial nerve may be difficult to locate or be obscured by ultrasound reflections from the AA because of its position posterior to the axillary vessels. However, it is helpful to define

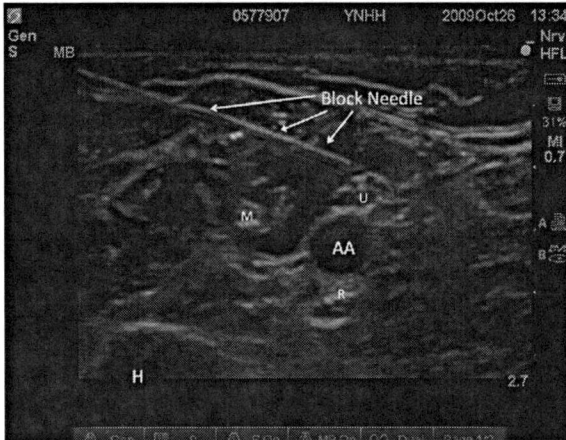

Figure 21.8c Ultrasound of axillary brachial plexus block. Image demonstrating suggested block needle position for ultrasound-guided axillary block. *H* humerus, *AA* axillary artery, *M* median nerve, *R* radial nerve, *U* ulnar nerve. Note the location of local anesthetic (hypoechoic) spread within the axillary sheath.

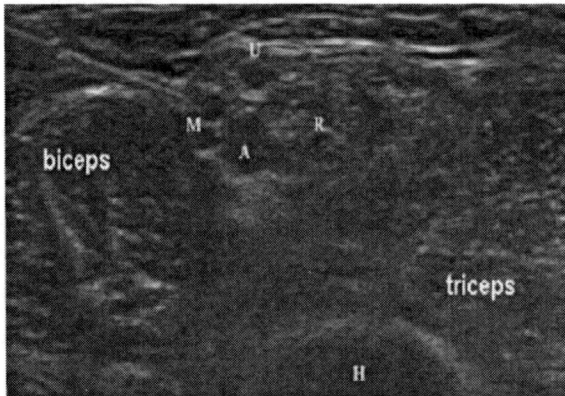

Figure 21.8d Ultrasound of axillary brachial plexus block. Sonogram demonstrating anatomy of the axillary brachial plexus with needle approaching the brachial plexus in-line with the ultrasound probe. *H* humerus, *A* axillary vessels, *U* ulnar nerve, *R* radial nerve, *M* median nerve.

the muscular and vascular anatomy initially and then look for a hyperechoic structure posterior to the artery or vein, especially upon injection of local anesthetic. The nerves may also be followed into the upper and lower arm and confirmed by their typical anatomic paths. The musculocutaneous nerve usually can be followed high in the axilla as it divides from the lateral cord and followed in the muscular septa between biceps and coracobrachialis muscles.

Peripheral Nerve Blocks of the Lower Extremity

Femoral nerve block provides anesthesia/analgesia to the anterior thigh, including the flexor muscles of the hip and extensor muscles of the knee. Historically this block was also known as the "3-in-1 block," suggesting that the femoral, lateral femoral cutaneous, and obturator nerves could be blocked from a single injection at the femoral crease. However, it has been demonstrated that the femoral and lateral femoral cutaneous nerves can be reliably blocked by a single injection, but the obturator nerve is often missed. The femoral nerve block is an ideal block for surgeries of the hip, knee, or anterior thigh and can be combined with a sciatic nerve block for near complete lower extremity analgesia. Complete analgesia of the leg can be achieved by adding an obturator nerve block.

Dorsal divisions of the anterior rami of L2–L4 form the femoral nerve (largest terminal branch of the lumbar plexus). Femoral nerve travels through the psoas muscle, then descends caudally into the thigh (via the groove formed by the psoas and iliacus muscles), entering the thigh beneath the inguinal ligament. Femoral nerve divides into an anterior and posterior branch after emerging from the ligament. It is usually located lateral and posterior to the femoral artery at this level. The anatomic location of the femoral nerve makes this block one of the easiest to master because the landmarks are easily identified, patient's remains supine, and the nerve depth is superficial.

Sciatic nerve supplies motor and sensory innervation to the posterior aspect of the thigh as well as the entire lower leg (except for sensory to the medial leg below the knee, which is supplied by the saphenous nerve, a terminal branch of the femoral nerve). The sciatic nerve, formed from the ventral rami of spinal nerves L4–S3, forms most of the sacral plexus (L4–S4) and is the largest nerve in the human body. Since the sciatic nerve is so large, it can be blocked at several different locations along the lower extremity.

The sciatic nerve is actually two nerves in close apposition, tibial and common peroneal (fibular) nerves. These nerves usually separate at the mid-thigh (75%), although separation as proximal as the pelvis and as distal as the popliteal crease may occur. Sciatic nerve leaves the pelvis via the greater sciatic foramen, travels under the gluteus maximus, and continues distally toward the posterior thigh between the greater trochanter and the ischial tuberosity. The sciatic nerve supplies motor innervation to the posterior thigh muscles as well as all muscles of the leg and foot. It also provides sensory innervation to the skin of most of the leg and foot (except for medial leg below the knee).

The popliteal block of the sciatic nerve is typically performed at a more distal location immediately cephalad to the popliteal fossa. Posterior or lateral approaches to the sciatic nerve at this level anesthetize the same dermatomes distal to PNB placement. The posterior approach may be technically easier than the lateral block, as the needle depth is shallower, making it more comfortable for the patient. Because the popliteal block of the sciatic nerve is performed more distal than the subgluteal (posterior) or anterior (medial thigh) approaches to the sciatic nerve, attention to both components of the sciatic nerve (tibial and common peroneal) is necessary to ensure adequate anesthesia and analgesia.

In the following descriptions, standard anatomic axes or planes will be used throughout for consistency, with the three primary descriptive planes: horizontal, coronal, and sagittal. Probe angulation is further described in the cephalad–caudad, medial–lateral, and anterior–posterior directions. The most common ultrasound orientation for nerve (and blood vessel) visualization will be in the short-axis (view in transverse or cross section) view. A long-axis (view in longitudinal section) view of nerves may be used to distinguish a putative nerve from other structures, but short axis is most commonly employed during needle placement, whether the needle is introduced either in-plane or out-of-plane with the ultrasound beam.

Femoral Nerve Block

When performing femoral nerve blockade, the ultrasound probe is placed in the inguinal crease. This flexion line is closest to the horizontal plane, but the medial edge of the probe is more caudad than the lateral edge (Fig. 21.9a). A slight caudad inclination of the probe may provide the best short-axis view of the femoral nerve, artery, and vein (Fig. 21.9b). Pulsatile femoral artery is the easiest structure to identify, and the collapsible femoral vein is positioned medial to the artery. The profunda femoris artery usually arises from the lateral side of the common femoral artery from 2.5 to 5 cm below the inguinal ligament, so it may sometimes be seen on ultrasound at the inguinal crease. Lateral to the femoral artery, the curved surface of the iliacus muscle (fascia iliaca) can be identified inclining posteromedially, and the femoral nerve appears as a hyperechoic, ovoid structure with the same posteromedial inclination as the iliacus muscle (Fig. 21.9b). The femoral nerve is apposed to the anteromedial surface of the iliacus, just deep to its fascia iliacus. Further medial and posteriorly, the tendon of the iliopsoas complex can be identified and is also hyperechoic and fibrillar in appearance. Medial to the femoral vein are superficial muscular layers consisting of the pectineus laterally and the adductor longus medially. Posterior (deep) to both superficial muscle layers is the adductor brevis muscle, and the anterior and posterior branches of the obturator nerve lie on the anterior and posterior surface of this muscle at the level of the inguinal crease. The lateral femoral cutaneous nerve enters the thigh just medial to the anterior superior iliac spine and is a purely sensory nerve. The obturator nerve enters through the superomedial aspect of the obturator foramen, enters the medial side of the thigh and divides into an anterior branch, which lies between the short adductor, external obturator, long adductor, and pectineus muscles and a posterior branch, which pierces the external obturator muscle, lies above the great and short adductor muscles.

Femoral nerve block, or the so-called 3-in-1 block, is a regional anesthetic technique used to block the femoral, lateral femoral cutaneous, and obturator nerves by a single injection

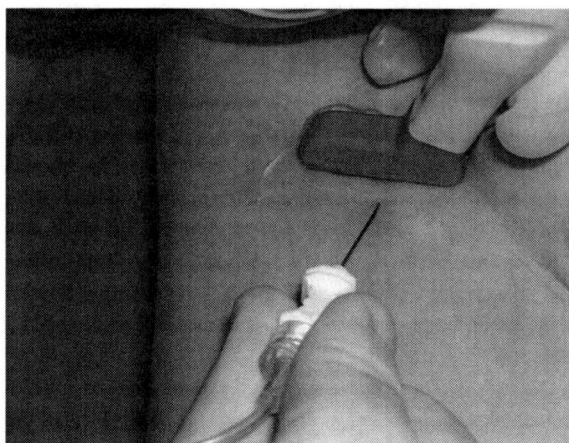

Figure 21.9a Ultrasound probe orientation for femoral nerve blockade. Note medial–lateral orientation of probe to optimize cross section of femoral anatomy below. The needle orientation in the photo is showing an out-of-plane technique, but an alternative would be an in-plane technique with the block needle parallel to the ultrasound probe in a lateral–medial orientation.

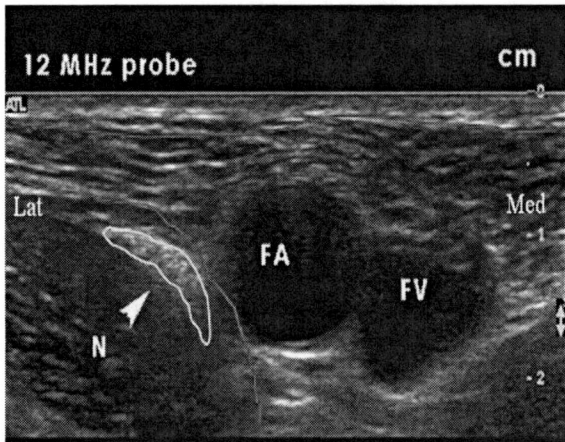

Figure 21.9b Ultrasound image of femoral anatomy. *FA* femoral artery, *FV* femoral vein, *N* (with *arrow*) identifying the femoral nerve, *Med* medial, *Lat* lateral, *top red line* fascia latta, *curved (lower) red line* fascia Iliacus.

of local anesthetic lateral to the femoral vessels and caudal to the inguinal ligament. This block concept remains controversial because all three nerves are rarely anesthetized with this single injection technique (blockade of the obturator nerve is often spared). With the use of ultrasound, a 7.5 MHz linear array transducer made it possible to visualize the femoral nerve and the relevant adjacent structures (vessels, muscles, ligaments) and to inject local anesthetic under control. Results of this described ultrasound guided femoral nerve blockade may now permit real-time visualization of local anesthetic spread, resulting in blockade of the femoral nerve as well as local anesthetic spread lateral and slightly medial to the femoral nerve for blockade of the lateral femoral cutaneous and the anterior branch of the obturator nerve (Fig. 21.9c). A significantly faster sensory block (onset time reduced) and improved quality of anesthesia of all three nerves could be achieved in comparison to the traditional nerve stimulation method.

Indications for an ultrasound femoral block include surgical procedures in the sensory distributions of the femoral, lateral femoral cutaneous, and anterior branch of the obturator nerve. A femoral nerve block together with a sciatic nerve block (described below) may provide anesthesia/analgesia for surgical procedures of the majority of lower extremity surgeries. The ultrasound-guided femoral block is a simple technique, but good anatomical knowledge is necessary for optimal performance of this block. In many surgical indications, only a femoral nerve block is necessary and since the femoral nerve is a superficial structure just distal to the inguinal ligament, a high-frequency linear ultrasound probe (>10 MHz) is adequate for optimal visualization.

The sonographic view of the femoral nerve is different from all other nerve structures because it has divided into a number of terminal branches at the level of the distal inguinal ligament. Therefore, the typical ultrasound appearance represents several distal sensory and motor branches of the femoral nerve (Fig. 21.9d). Femoral nerve block needle orientation can be performed in the long-axis or short-axis (Fig. 21.9a) orientation to the probe, but is most easily performed in the short axis using a 50-mm short bevel needle. Once the fascia iliaca

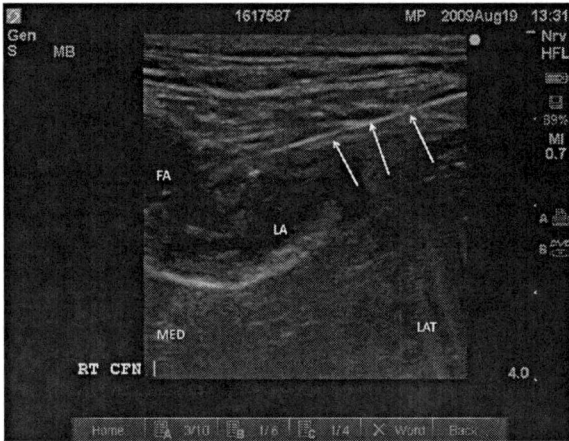

Figure 21.9c Ultrasound image of a femoral block. Note the spread of local anesthetic (hypoechoic) around the femoral nerve. *FA* femoral artery, *LA* local anesthetic, *MED* medial, *LAT* lateral, *arrows* identify the block needle.

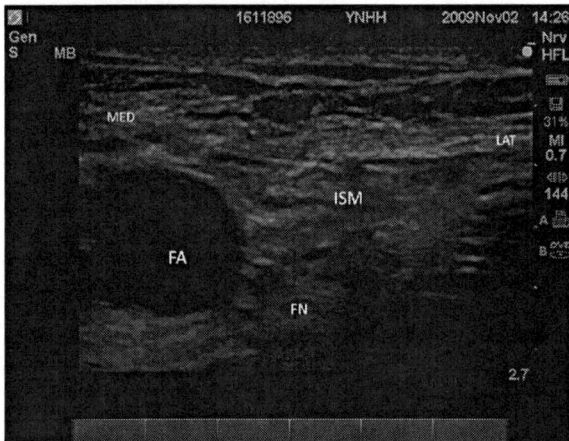

Figure 21.9d Ultrasound of the femoral nerve and surrounding structures. Note the mixed natured appearance (white–gray–black) of the nerve just lateral to the femoral artery. *FA* femoral artery, *FN* femoral nerve, *ISM* iliopsoas muscle, *LAT* lateral, *MED* medial.

is pierced, the femoral nerve block can be performed with typically 20 ml of local anesthetic. There is little information about the optimal volume of local anesthetic for ultrasound-guided femoral nerve block although it is possible in the future that the volume required for adequate block will decrease. Higher volumes (>20 ml) are likely required to ensure blockade of the lateral femoral cutaneous nerve of the thigh and the anterior branch of the obturator nerve via proximal spread of the local anesthetic.

Sciatic Nerve Block (Proximal)

The sciatic nerve is the largest nerve in the human body. It is composed of the tibial and peroneal segments and is derived from L4-S3 anterior rami. The sciatic nerve runs through the greater sciatic foramen to the gluteal region deep to gluteus maximus muscle. Most of the conventional approaches for sciatic nerve blockade at this level are relatively deep and therefore not attractive for ultrasonography in much of the adult surgical population. Once the sciatic nerve enters the dorsal side of the thigh between the caudal border of the gluteus maximus and the biceps muscles, its position is more superficial, appears as an oval or flat hyperechoic structure, is more easily seen with current ultrasound technology, and is an easier block to perform under ultrasound guidance. Posterior cutaneous nerve of the thigh is in a medial position relative to the sciatic nerve at the subgluteal level. Distally, the sciatic nerve components (tibial and common peroneal) run between the semitendinosus (medial) and the biceps femoris muscle (lateral) where division into the two end branches can be observed at 5–10 cm superior to the popliteal crease and lateral and more superficial to the popliteal vessels (artery and vein).

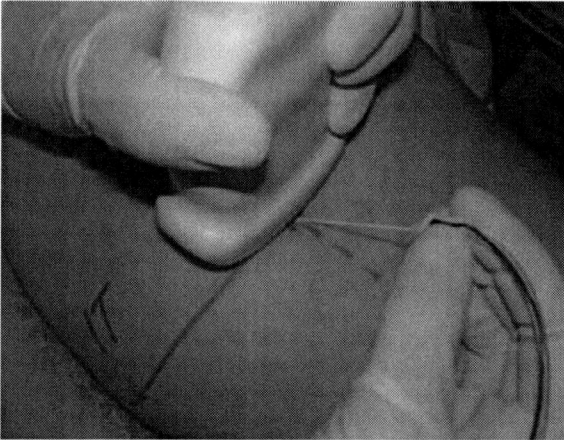

Figure 21.10a   Ultrasound probe position for subgluteal approach to the sciatic nerve. Stimulating nerve block needle is positioned out-of-plane in relation to the ultrasound probe. *IT* ischial tuberosity.

With the patient positioned in the semi-lateral to lateral decubitus position (typically), the ultrasound probe is placed to scan in the horizontal plane between the ischial tuberosity and the greater trochanter of the femur (Fig. 21.10a). Subcutaneous fat and the gluteus maximus muscle are superficial to the sciatic nerve, and the nerve is usually a flattened or ovoid hyperechoic structure at this level and somewhat closer to the ischial tuberosity than to the femur. The conjoint tendon of the long head of the biceps muscle, tendon of the semitendinosus muscle and tendon of the semimembranosis muscle insert on the ischial tuberosity which may make it difficult to distinguish from the sciatic nerve since there appearance in the transverse plane may all seem similar (Fig. 21.10b).

Ultrasound visualization and blockade of the sciatic nerve is a theoretically attractive technique that should be possible in clinical practice due to the large size of this nerve. However, this block may be challenging for two reasons: first, the depth and distinctive

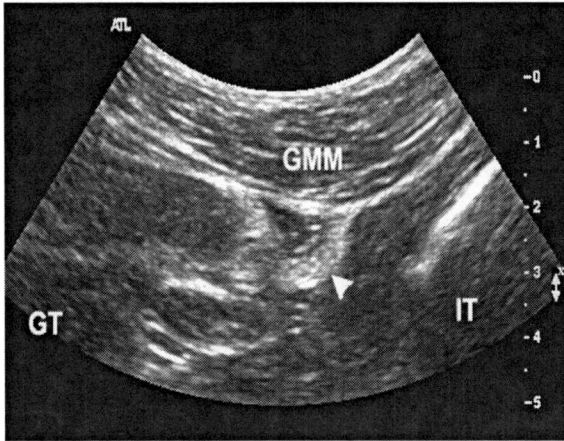

Figure 21.10b   Ultrasound image of the subgluteal approach to the sciatic nerve. *GMM* gluteus maximus muscle, *GT* greater trochanter, *IT* ischial tuberosity, *arrow* identifying the sciatic nerve.

anisotropy, where appropriate ultrasonographic visualization is only possible when the ultrasound beam is perpendicular to the nerve and the lack of adjacent vascular structures to guide approximation of anatomical nerve location; second, in obese individuals the depth of the nerve is increased and the superficial adipose layer creates a hyperechoic layer that impedes visualization of deeper nerve structures. Therefore, when performing a sciatic nerve block, two major considerations must be considered: the choice of an appropriate needle insertion site (including the necessity to block the posterior cutaneous nerve of thigh) and the best level to visualize the nerve pending the body habitus of the patient.

Usually the best ultrasound image of the proximal sciatic nerve can be achieved in the subgluteal region (described above). At the subgluteal level the sciatic nerve lies in a more superficial position and can be identified between the gluteus maximus and biceps muscles and superficial to the quadratus femoris and adductor magnus muscles between the two boney landmarks of the greater trochanter and ischial tuberosity (Fig. 21.10c). At this level, the sciatic nerve appears as round to oval to flat and only moderately hyperechoic structure. The sciatic nerve is often easier to find more distal as a hyperechoic structure medial to biceps femoris in the popliteal region and then followed cephalad to the subgluteal region.

When performing a subgluteal approach to the sciatic nerve, a curvilinear ultrasound probe is most often used in adults. Depending upon the depth of the sciatic nerve, ultrasound probe frequencies between 2 and 5 MHz are appropriate for optimal visualization. With the patient placed either in the supine position with the hip flexed to 90° or in the lateral or prone position, the block can be performed with a 50- to 70-mm short bevel needle and a needle insertion point with an out-of-plane technique in the transverse plane (Fig. 21.10a). Currently, larger volumes of local anesthetic are being used for ultrasound-guided blockade of the sciatic nerve (20–30 ml); however, these volumes may decrease as appropriate evidence for efficacy and safety continues to be determined. In thinner adults and in pediatric patients, it is often possible to use an in-plane technique and this facilitates the approach of the needle

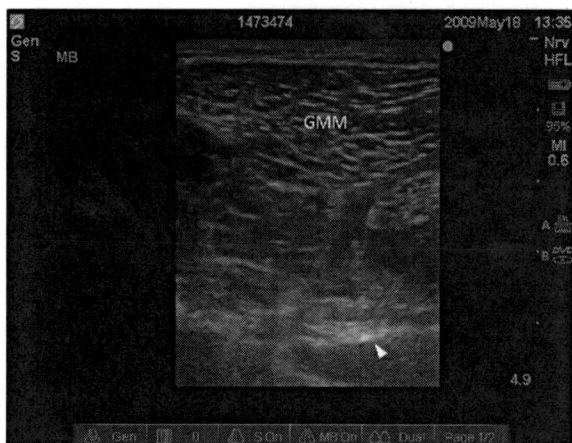

Figure 21.10c Ultrasound image of the sciatic nerve in the subgluteal area. *GMM* gluteus maximus muscle, *arrow* identifies the sciatic nerve.

both deep and superficial to the nerve to obtain optimal local anesthetic spread around the sciatic nerve.

Popliteal Nerve Block (Distal Sciatic)

This is a peripheral nerve block of the sciatic nerve performed more distal in the leg proximal to the popliteal crease. With the patient in the supine or prone position, the ultrasound probe is placed to scan in the transverse plane on the posterior surface of the popliteal fossa 5 cm or more proximal to the popliteal flexion crease of the knee (Fig. 21.11a). Subtle inclination of the ultrasound probe in the caudad or cephalad direction may be needed to produce ideal visualization of the nearly round, hyperechoic sciatic nerve or sciatic nerve components (Fig. 21.11b) (within this proximity of the popliteal crease, the sciatic nerve will often take on the appearance of separate tibial and common peroneal nerve branches). The sciatic nerve is surrounded by a large amount of fat, and, laterally, the typical muscular pattern of the biceps femoris can be recognized with its medial surface concave toward the nerve. Medial to the nerve, the muscle/tendon of the semimembranosus is identifiable, with its lateral surface convex toward the nerve. The ultrasound view of the sciatic nerve at the popliteal site is often so distinct as to allow discrimination of the peroneal and tibial nerve components, and these components will separate as the ultrasound probe is slid caudad along the popliteal fossa (Fig. 21.11c). At, or just proximal to the popliteal flexion crease of the knee, scanning for the popliteal artery pulsation at this site can help locate the tibial nerve since the tibial nerve is typically immediately lateral to the popliteal vein(s) and artery. Once the tibial nerve is identified, it can be followed cephalad by sliding the probe (still in the transverse plane) until the peroneal nerve is seen to join the tibial nerve on its lateral side (Fig. 21.11c). In addition to imaging the sciatic nerve in the transverse plane just described, asking the patient to dorsiflex and/or plantarflex the foot produces a rotation of the nerve components allowing for easier nerve confirmation/identification ("seesaw" sign) (Schafhalter-Zoppoth et al. 2004).

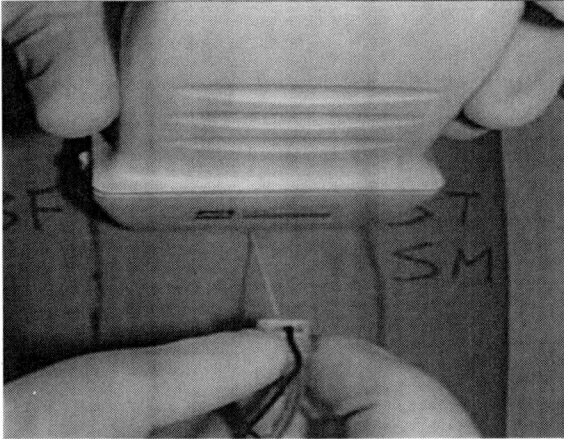

Figure 21.11a   Photograph demonstrating ultrasound probe placement and needle insertion point for sciatic nerve block in the popliteal fossa. *ST* and *SM* semimembranosus and semitendenosus muscle tendons, *BF* biceps femoris muscle tendons. Nerve block needle is in an out-of-plane orientation.

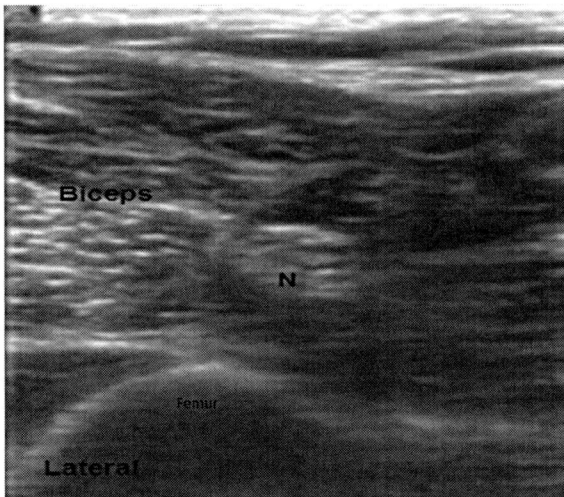

Figure 21.11b   Ultrasound image of sciatic nerve in the popliteal fossa. Note the biceps muscle/tendon lateral to the nerve (*N*). The femur bone can be identified by the hyperechoic arched image within the sonogram.

The optimal selection for distal sciatic nerve blockade depends on the best ultrasound visualization of the nerve. This site typically occurs just proximal to sciatic nerve division into tibial and peroneal nerve branches and with the probe positioned in the transverse plane of the popliteal fossa. The popliteal sciatic nerve block can be performed with either an in-plane (Fig. 21.11d) or an out-of-plane technique (Fig. 21.11a). In both techniques, the patient can remain in a supine position with flexed hip and knee (keeping the tib–fib portion of the

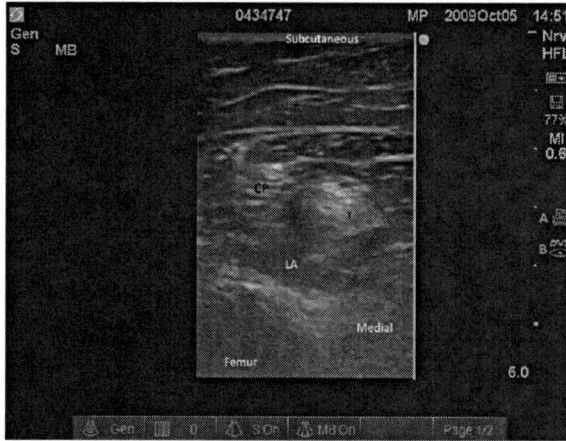

Figure 21.11c Ultrasound image of sciatic nerve components in the popliteal fossa. The common peroneal (*CP*) and the tibial (*T*) nerves become more defined subsequent to injection of local anesthetic (*LA*).

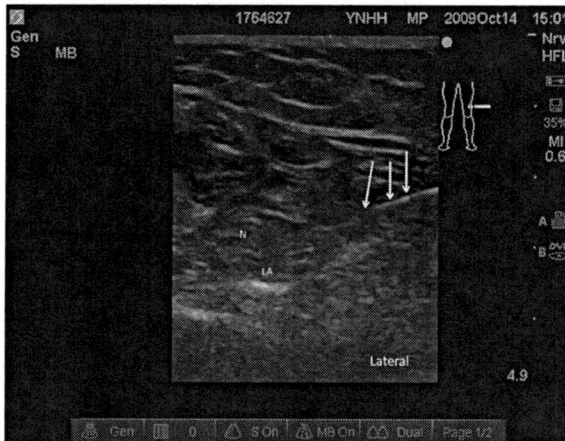

Figure 21.11d Sonogram of "in-plane" popliteal sciatic nerve block. Note the spread of local anesthetic (*LA*) that is spreading around the nerve (*N*). *LA* local anesthetic, *N* nerve, *arrows* identify the peripheral nerve block needle.

operative leg parallel to the floor with blanket or pillow support), in the lateral position with straightened lower limb or in the prone position (slightly flexed hip and knee). By using the in-plane technique, ultrasound image illustrated in Fig. 21.11d, the puncture site is above the biceps muscle with a 70- to 80-mm short bevel needle. The block needle tip should be placed both above and then below the sciatic nerve to achieve an optimal spread of local anesthetic and reliably sufficient sciatic nerve block.

Case Scenario

Sreekumar Kunnumpurath, MBBS, MD, FCARCSI, FRCA, FFPMRCA

Ronan is a 45-year-old truck driver who is scheduled for right shoulder reconstruction. He has been admitted in your hospital for the last week following a road traffic accident. During this accident, he sustained extensive damage to his right shoulder joint along with fractures of ribs and lung contusion. At the time of admission to the emergency department, it was noted that he had developed pneumothorax and this was treated with the insertion of a chest tube. The surgeon is keen to proceed with the surgery as early as possible. His pain control has been an issue because he could not tolerate morphine secondary to severe nausea.

Over the week, his pneumothorax resolves and he is currently on acetaminophen and ibuprofen along with codeine phosphate PRN that he uses occasionally for fear of side effects. The surgeon has specifically requested you to anesthetize this patient as you are well known for your proficiency in regional anaesthesia.

Summarize the issues regarding anesthesia and pain management for this patient?
Regarding anesthetic management, Ronan is recovering from a recent pneumothorax and so a general anesthetic with positive pressure ventilation carries the potential risk of a further air leak into the pleural space. The second issue is managing postoperative pain. Using potent long-acting opioids such as morphine or hydromorphone in the form of PCA is not ideal as he had side effects due to these drugs. On the day before the scheduled surgery, you visit Ronan. After obtaining a detailed clinical history, you make a thorough clinical examination and go through the lab results and X-rays. This time you notice that the chest drain has been removed and the lungs have expanded back to normal without any evidence of residual air or fluid in the pleural cavity. His right shoulder has extensive soft tissue and bone injuries. All his laboratory values are within normal limits, except for the coagulation panel that shows an INR of 1.2.

What would be your anesthetic management for this patient?
There are two key issues in this situation. The first is a potentially for the recurrence the pneumothorax. This could be addressed by administering an effective brachial plexus block through the interscalene route combined with sedation if the patient is worried about being wide awake during the procedure. The second issue is managing postoperative pain in the presence of opioid intolerance, which could possibly be the result of high-opioid requirement in the presence of uncontrolled pain. This could be addressed by adapting a multimodal approach to pain management, namely extending the regional anesthetic technique for postoperative analgesia along with acetaminophen and NSAIDs. Opioid could be reserved for breakthrough pain by PRN administration together with an antiemetic.

You explain your anesthetic technique to Ronan. You describe how you are going to do the interscalene block. You mention that you are going to put a needle in his neck to inject local anesthetic solution and then leave a catheter near the nerve plexus. Ronan is very unhappy about your anesthetic plan. He tells you that he had an unpleasant experience with a nerve block which he had for his knee surgery about 10 years ago. More than the needle, he remembers and worries about electric shocks used by the anesthetist to stimulate and identify the nerves which were very painful and made his limb jerk uncontrollably. Moreover, the block did not work properly and he had to have a general anesthetic, and the postoperative pain was "bad" as well.

How will you explain the advantages of US-guided nerve block to Ronen?
You explain to Ronan that using electrical nerve stimulation for identification of individual nerves is probably outdated. Instead, you are going to use high-resolution ultrasound scanner to identify and block the individual nerve roots as they come out of the spinal canal. Advantages of US are the precision with which you can visualize and identify the needle, nerves, blood vessels, and other structures. It helps you to see the local anesthetic spread around the nerves. So there is less chance of any damage to nerves or pleura with the needle and less risk of injecting the local anesthetic into a blood vessel. You would be able to pass the specialized catheter under direct image guidance and leave it close to the nerve plexus for postoperative pain relief. US-guided techniques have higher success rates. The other advantage is that it is least distressing to the patient as he will not be experiencing any of the uncomfortable and painful shocks and muscle jerks.

You stress the importance of avoiding a general anesthetic and the need for an effective and side effect-free postoperative pain relief so that his recovery is hastened without any respiratory complication due to inadequate pain control. Ronan agrees for an ultrasound-guided interscalene block.

What are the disadvantages of ultrasound-guided nerve block?
Sometimes nerves and tendons may have similar echo patterns making their identification difficult. Bones can cast acoustic shadows under it, obscuring the view of underlying structures. On occasions, abnormal anatomy may confuse the operator. Proficiency in this technique will require training and practice. Moreover, the cost of the equipment such as the ultrasound scanner, specialized echogenic needles, and catheters is another drawback.

How can you overcome these difficulties?
Resolution of ultrasound can be increased by using higher frequency ultrasound waves. Penetration to visualize deeper structures can be increased by using lower frequencies (these two properties are in conflict). Penetration and resolution can be adjusted on the ultrasound machine. Echogenic needles have specialized patterns on their surface, thereby reflecting back the sound waves. One of the techniques to make catheters echogenic is to incorporate tiny air bubbles into them during fabrication, thereby creating air–surface interfaces.

Satisfied with your reasoning and explanation, Ronen undergoes surgery with a successful ultrasound-guided interscalene brachial plexus block. A catheter is passed for continuous infusion of local anesthetic for postoperative analgesia. You administer target-controlled propofol infusion to keep him sedated during the procedure.

References

Apfelbaum JL, Chen C, Mehta SS, Gan TJ. Postoperative pain experience: results from a national survey suggest postoperative pain continues to be undermanaged. Anesth Analg. 2003;97:534–40.

Ballantyne JC, Carr DB, et al. The comparative effects of postoperative analgesic therapies on pulmonary outcome: cumulative meta-analyses of randomized, controlled trials. Anesth Analg 1998;86:598–612.

Beattie WS, Badner NH, Choi P. Epidural analgesia reduces postoperative myocardial infarction: a meta-analysis. Anesth Analg. 2001;93:853–8.

Bigeleisen P, Wilson M. A comparison of two techniques for ultrasound guided infraclavicular block. Br J Anaesth. 2006;96:502–7.

Cash CJC, Sardesai AM, et al. Spatial mapping of the Brachial plexus using three-dimensional ultrasound. Br J Radiol. 2005;78:1086–94.

Franco CD, Vieira ZE. 1,001 subclavian perivascular brachial plexus blocks: success with a nerve stimulator. Reg Anesth Pain Med. 2000 Jan–Feb;25(1):41–6.

Horlocker TT, Wedel DJ, et al. Regional anesthesia in the anticoagulated patient: defining the risks (the second ASRA Consensus Conference on Neuraxial Anesthesia and Anticoagulation). Reg Anesth Pain Med. 2003;28:172–97.

Kehlet H, Dahl JB. Anaesthesia, surgery, and challenges in postoperative recovery. Lancet 2003;362:1921–8.

Kehlet H, Jensen TS, Woolf CJ. Persistent postsurgical pain: risk factors and prevention. Lancet 2006;367:1618–25.

Kehlet H, Wilmore DW. Multimodal strategies to improve surgical outcome. Am J Surg. 2002;183:630–41.

Marhofer P, Chan VW, Marhofer P, Chan VWS. Ultrasound-guided regional anesthesia: current concepts and future trends. Anesth Analg. 2007;104:1265–9.

Martin G, Lineberger CK, MacLeod DB, El-Moalem HE, Breslin DS, Hardman D, D'Ercole F. A new teaching model for resident training in regional anesthesia. Anesth Analg. 2002;95:1423–7.

Reuben SS, Buvanendran A. Preventing the development of chronic pain after orthopaedic surgery with preventive multimodal analgesic techniques. J Bone Joint Surg. 2007;89: 1343–58.

Rodgers A, Walker N, Schug S, McKee A, Kehlet H, van Zundert A, Sage D, Futter M, Saville G, Clark T, MacMahon S. Reduction of postoperative mortality and morbidity with epidural or spinal anaesthesia: results from overview of randomised trials. BMJ 2000;321:1493.

Schafhalter-Zoppoth I, Younger SJ, et al. The "seesaw" sign: improved sonographic identification of the sciatic nerve. Anesthesiology 2004;101:808–9.

Silvestri E, Martinoli C, et al. Echotexture of peripheral nerves: correlation between US and histologic findings and criteria to differentiate tendons. Radiology 1995;197:291–6.

Sites, BD, Brull, R. Ultrasound guidance in peripheral regional anesthesia: philosophy, evidence-based medicine and techniques. Curr Opin Anaesthesiol. 2006;19:630–9.

Urwin SC, Parker MJ, Griffiths R. General versus regional anesthesia for hip fracture surgery: a meta-analysis of randomized trials. Br J Anaesth. 2000;84:450–5.

Weinberg G. Lipid infusion resuscitation for local anesthetic toxicity: proof of clinical efficacy. Anesthesiology 2006a;105:7–8.

Weinberg G. Lipid rescue resuscitation from local anaesthetic cardiac toxicity. Toxicol Rev. 2006b;25:139–45.

Winnie AP, Collins VJ. The subclavian perivascular technique of brachial plexus anesthesia. Anesthesiology 1964;25:353–63.

Wu CL, Hurley RW, Anderson GF, Herbert R, Rowlingson AJ, Fleisher LA. Effect of postoperative epidural analgesia on morbidity and mortality following surgery in medicare patients. Reg Anesth Pain Med. 2004;29:525–33.

Chapter 22

Labor Pain Management

Ferne Braverman, MD

Introduction

Childbirth is usually highly anticipated and a happy experience. However, it can be accompanied by severe pain; Melzack demonstrated that only the pain of causalgia or digit amputation exceeds that of labor (Melzack 1975). He also demonstrated that the severity of pain varied greatly among women (Melzack et al. 1984) and 30–75% of parturients characterized their pain as severe or intolerable. Painless labor is a reality for only a small minority of women. It is thus fortunate that pain relief in labor is accepted as part of the childbirth experience. The American College of Obstetrics and Gynecology (ACOG) emphasizes in their committee opinion #118 that, "maternal request is a sufficient justification for pain relief during labor."

Labor pain is actually the result pain stimuli which include intermittent uterine contraction pain (which is felt in the abdomen and/or back), continuous back pain, and cervical and vaginal pain related to cervical dilatation and movement of the fetus through the birth canal (Fig. 22.1). The severity of pain may be increased with occipit posterior presentation and dystocia. Primiparous labor is more painful than subsequent labors. Augmentation or induction of labor with oxytotic drugs is reported to result in increased labor pain (Lowe 1987). Cultural expectations also affect the maternal response to labor pain.

Mechanisms of Labor Pain

In the first stage of labor (onset of labor until full cervical dilatation, i.e., 0 to 10 cm) the distension of the cervix results in pain related to the activation of mechanoreceptors. Uterine contraction can result in myometrial ischemia, releasing potassium, histamine, serotonin, and bradykinins which stimulate chemoreceptors. This pain is experienced primarily during contractions as this is when the chemoreceptors and mechanoreceptors are stimulated.

Afferent impulses are transmitted by the nerves that accompany the sympathetic nerves and terminate in the dorsal horn of the spinal cora. These afferent nerves pass through the paracervical region; from there the visceral afferents pass through the pelvis by means of the inferior hypogastric, middle hypogastric, and superior pelvic plexes. They then enter the lumbar sympathetic chain, enter the white rami communicants at the T10, T11, T12, and L1 spinal nerves, and pass through the posterior roots to synapse in the dorsal horn.

In early labor, pain is referred primarily to the T11 and T12 dermatomes. As labor progresses, pain is also referred to T10 and L1 dermatomes. Visceral pain associated with

N. Vadivelu et al. (eds.), *Essentials of Pain Management*,
DOI 10.1007/978-0-387-87579-8_22, © Springer Science+Business Media, LLC 2011

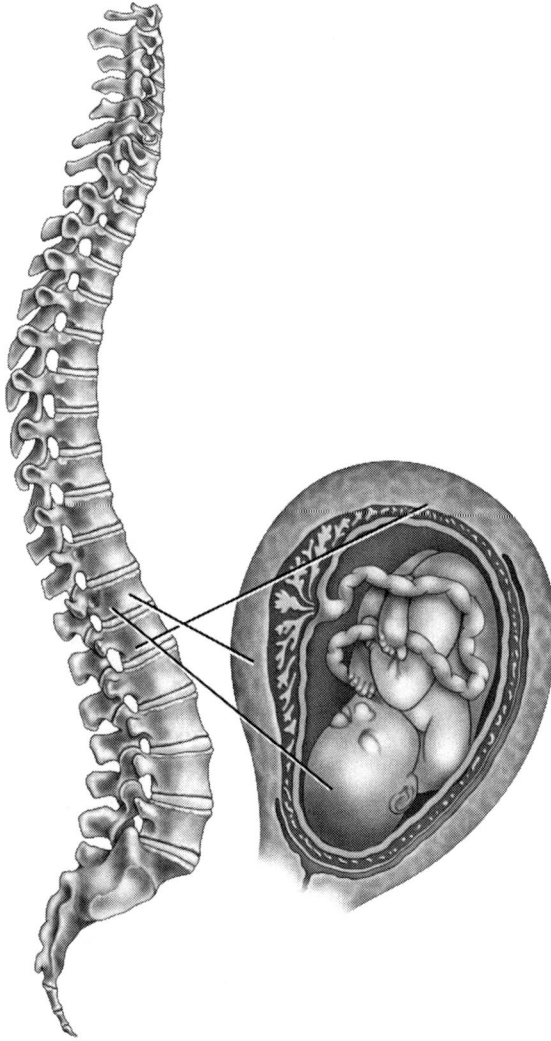

Figure 22.1   Labor pain results from uterine contraction, cervical dilatation, and vaginal and peroneal distention.

contractions and cervical dilatation can be alleviated with (1) segmental epidural blockade of T10–L1; (2) bilateral paravertebral blocks at the T10, T11, T12, and L1; (3) bilateral paracervical blocks; (4) bilateral lumbar sympathetic blocks; or (5) spinal opioid administration.

The somatic component of labor pain results from the distension of the vagina, the pelvic floor, and the perineum. These impulses are transmitted primarily through the pudendal nerves. The perineum also receives innervation from the ilioinguinal nerve, the genital branch of the genitofemoral nerve, and the posterior femoral cutaneous nerve. Somatic pain occurs late in the first stage of labor and into the second stage (full dilatation to delivery of the fetus). It is primarily related to the decent of the presenting part. This late first stage is

Table 22.1 Regional techniques for analgesia in labor.

Visceral pain (T10–L1) (stage 1 of labor)
• Bilateral paracervical blocks (associated with fetal bradycardia, therefore, rarely used)
• Bilateral lumbar sympathetic block
• Intrathecal opioids

Somatic pain (transition and stages 2 and 3 of labor)
• Bilateral pudendal nerve blocks
• Saddle block (spinal anesthesia)
• Low caudal epidural block (S2–S4)

All pain (T10–S4) (stages 1, 2, 3)
• Epidural (lumbar or caudal)
• Combined spinal epidural
• Continuous spinal

"transition," during which both somatic and visceral pain may be significant. Descent of the presenting part distends, and may tear, the vagina and perineal tissue, resulting in severe pain. The unanesthetized parturient will have the uncontrollable urge to valsalva (i.e., "push") at this time. The interval between onset of fetal descent and delivery has been described as the most painful period of labor (Table 22.1).

Effects of Labor Pain

Respiratory
As labor pain becomes severe, the unmedicated patient's minute ventilation increases by >75% in first stage and 150–300% during second stage of labor. This results in maternal hypocarbia and alkalosis. These changes lead to uteroplacental and fetoplacental vasoconstriction and a leftward shift of the maternal oxyhemoglobin dissociation curve, potentially resulting in fetal hypoxemia. Effective regional analgesia will markedly diminish maternal hyperventilation. Oxygen consumption increases by 40% in stage 1 and 75% in stage 2. This is attenuated, but not eliminated by regional analgesia. Parenteral opioid administration does not effectively prevent hyperventilation, in contrast to regional anesthesia. Most mothers and fetuses are not adversely affected by the respiratory changes occurring with labor. However, in patients with marginal uteroplacental function effective regional analgesia may be advantageous.

Cardiovascular
During pregnancy cardiac output rises gradually, reaching 150% of the pre-pregnant value by term. Labor results in a further increase in cardiac output, from an increase in both stroke volume and heart rate. With each contraction, auto-transfusion results in an additional 10–20% increase in cardiac output. Analgesia, with the resulting attenuation of the heart rate increase will alleviate but not eliminate the increase in cardiac output associated with labor.

Further increase in cardiac output occurs immediately postpartum and is a result of sustained uterine contraction and auto-transfusion. This is attenuated by regional analgesia only when it is associated with sympathetic vasodilatation.

Humoral

Anxiety, pain, and stress increase maternal catecholamine levels during labor and may lead to decreased uterine activity, prolonged labor, and abnormal fetal heart rate (FHR) patterns. Parenteral opioids do not appear to significantly blunt this catecholamine surge. However, epidural analgesia or spinal opioid analgesia does significantly decrease these levels (Howell et al. 2001). This effect is more dramatic in patients with pre-eclampsia.

Effect of Pain on the Progress of Labor

Pain is an expected part of labor and its effect on the course of labor is controversial. Dysfunctional labor, which many suggest is more painful, does appear to normalize in some patients with the provision of analgesia.

Options for Pain Management

The amount of pain experienced by women in labor is hard to predict. Some have tolerable pain while others may benefit from some form of analgesia. Many non-medical techniques can help deal with the pain of labor. The choice of analgesic techniques is between the patient, obstetrical caregiver, and when applicable the anesthesiologist. Again, both the ACOG and the American Society of Anesthesiologists (ASA) jointly opine that maternal request is sufficient medical indication for pain relief during labor. It is only the choice of analgesic that is made in conjunction with the medical team providing care to the patient.

The following discussion reviews options for labor analgesia, including nonmedicated and medicated pain relief methods. Nonpharmacologic analgesia techniques include prepared childbirth (LaMaze), aromatherapy, hypnotherapy, acupuncture, and transcutaneous electrical stimulation. Pharmacologic techniques include systemic analgesia, regional analgesia, and nerve blocks.

Nonpharmacologic Techniques

Prepared Childbirth

There is considerable evidence that preparation for childbirth can significantly modify the pain experience. Fear, fatigue, and anxiety can all enhance pain perception, thus good antenatal education may modify the experience, but it will not lead to "painless childbirth." Labor support and relaxation and breathing techniques form the basics for this technique. The continuous presence of a midwife or female support person (doula) has been shown to decrease the severity of pain reported. Relaxation techniques and/or self-hypnosis can relieve anxiety and tension and thus modify the pain experience. These techniques should be encouraged for all pregnant women.

Aromatherapy

Aromatherapy may promote stress relief in labor. There is no pain relief but a reduction in stress may allow the patient to better tolerate the pain of labor.

Acupuncture

There is evidence to support the use of acupuncture in other areas of medicine and recently for the treatment of backache in pregnancy (Wang et al. 2005). There are few reports of its use in labor, but those available suggest a beneficial effect on pain in labor. It is theorized that acupuncture works by interrupting or inhibiting pain impulses to the brain or by the stimulation of endorphin production.

Hypnotherapy

Hypnotherapy attempts to modify pain through post-hypnotic suggestion. Patients must take classes over 4–5 weeks to develop skills for this therapy. It requires significant prelabor preparation for success and with some patients, the level of hypnotic state required to tolerate pain may impact recall of the birth.

Transcutaneous Electrical Stimulation

Transcutaneous electrical stimulation (TENS) has been used to treat surgical and chronic pain. For labor, the placement of electrodes will be on the lower back or suprapubic area, through which a low current is passed results in a non-painful sensation at the electrodes. This current is thought to prevent pain impulse transmission to the brain and may stimulate endorphin production.

It is important to realize that the maternal satisfaction and relaxation obtained by the above techniques is not necessarily related to the degree of analgesia obtained. These techniques have no or minimal adverse effects and should be encouraged for all women, especially those with uncomplicated labors (Eappen and Robbins 2002).

Pharmacologic Analgesic Techniques

Pharmacologic techniques ordered or administered by the obstetrician or midwife include systemic opioid analgesia, paracervical blocks, and pudendal blocks.

Systemic Analgesia

A variety of opioid analgesics have been used to reduce the pain of labor. All opioid analgesics given in equianalgesic doses have similar advantages and disadvantages. The choice of opioid is often institutional preference. These medications are ordered by the obstetrician or midwife and administered by the patient's nurse. The advantages of systemic opioid analgesia for labor are ease of administration, low cost, maternal acceptance, and lack of the need for obstetrician or anesthetist presence. The disadvantages are failure to provide adequate analgesia, maternal side effects, and placental transfer of medication to the fetus.

Maternal side effects include altered respiration (hypoventilation between contractions), reduced gastric motility, nausea and vomiting, sedation, dysphoria, and inadequate analgesia. Fetal effects include loss of heart rate variability, neonatal respiratory depression, and a lower likelihood of successful breastfeeding. Systemic opioids can be administered intramuscularly, subcutaneously, intravenously, or using intravenous patient-controlled analgesia (IV-PCA) (Table 22.2).

Paracervical Block

The paracervical ganglion is located posterolateral to the cervico-uterine junction. Infiltration of the posterolateral aspect of the vaginal fornix will provide adequate analgesia for the first stage of labor in the majority of patients. The ganglia are located at the 4 and 8 o'clock positions, submucosally in the vaginal vault. Fetal badycardia may occur in approximately 40%

Table 22.2 Systemic opioids for labor analgesia.

Drug	Dose/interval	IV/PCA
Meperidine	25–50 mg IV q 2–3 h	a
Morphine	5 mg IV q 23 h	CI 0.2 mg/h PCA 0.5–1 mg q 6 min 4 h lockout 30 mg
Fentanyl	25–50 μg IV q 1–2 h	CI 25 μg/h PCA 10 μg q 6 min 4 h lockout 500 μg
Nalbuphine	10–20 mg IV q 3–4 h	a
Butorphanol	1–2 mg IV q 4 h	a

[a] These medications are not administered by IV-PCA.
IV=intravenous; PCA=patient-controlled analgesia.

of the cases, likely related to fetal absorption of local anesthetic. The duration of the block is 30–60 min. Doses of 0.125% bupivacaine, 1% lidocaine, and 3% chloroprocaine have all been used. Chloroprocaine is associated with the lowest incidence of side effects. This block is only effective for the first stage of labor. Because of the frequency of fetal bradycardia, it should not be used in the presence of a non-reassuring FHR pattern.

Pudendal Nerve Block

The pudendal nerve innervates the lower vagina, perineum, and vulva. Block of this nerve will relieve the pain of the second stage of labor. The nerve is blocked at the pudendal canal, just lateral and inferior to the sacrospinal ligament. Ten milliliters (ml) of 0.5% bupivacaine, 1% lidocaine, or 3–2% chloroprocaine is injected bilaterally. Complications are rare, most common are failure of the block and systemic toxicity from inadvertent intravascular injection. When successful, this block supplements analgesia in patients who received paracervical or lumbar sympathetic blocks for the first stage of labor.

Regional Analgesia

Regional analgesia is administered by anesthesiologists. This includes epidural, spinal, and combined spinal epidural analgesia. Also administered by the anesthesiologists is the lumbar sympathetic block, which, although effective, is rarely used in obstetrics. The aim of these interventions is to provide excellent regional analgesia with little or no motor block. This is achieved with the use of neuraxial opioids (spinal or epidural) combined with very low concentrations of local anesthetics. As with any anesthetic, the anesthesiologist, when consulted, will take a history, perform a focused physical examination, and obtain consent for the procedure.

Lumbar Sympathetic Block

Uterine and cervical afferent fibers join the sympathetic chain at L2 and L3. Blockade at this level will provide analgesic for the first stage of labor.

The block is placed by passing a 22 gauge needle 6–8 cm lateral to the L2 vertebra, angled at 30–45% off the saggital toward the vertebral body. The needle is directed just anterolateral to the vertebral body and 10–15 ml of 0.375–0.50% bupivacaine is injected. This is repeated on the contralateral side.

This block is used most commonly for managing the pain of the first stage of labor when epidural or spinal analgesia is precluded by previous spine surgery. Because it is useful for pain relief during stage one of labor, it is of limited use for obstetrical analgesia.

Epidural Analgesia

Epidural labor analgesia was first introduced in the 1940s, when a single dose of local anesthetic was administered into the caudal epidural space. Epidural analgesia is now provided via a lumbar epidural catheter. It is the analgesic technique used for the majority of women in the United States who request analgesia in labor.

The technique for epidural analgesia virtually always involved the insertion of an epidural catheter into the epidural space. This space is accessed by a midline or paramedian approach and identified by "loss of resistance" to air or saline. When the needle tip is in the ligamentum flavum, there is resistance to the injection; this resistance is lost when the epidural space is entered. Once the space is identified, the epidural catheter is inserted through the needle, leaving 2–4 cm within the space. The needle is removed and the catheter is secured to the mother's back (Fig. 22.2).

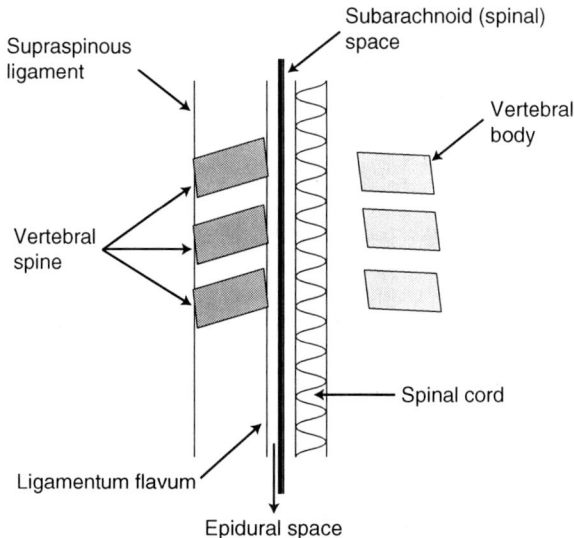

Figure 22.2   Anatomy of spinal and epidural anesthesia.

For the past 20 years, anesthesiologists have used a combination of opioid and local anesthetic for labor analgesia. This combination allows for excellent pain relief with minimal or no motor block. We see no difference in the labor outcomes between patients receiving epidural labor analgesia with these solutions and those receiving other analgesic techniques (Wong et al. 2005).

Epidural "mixtures" are listed in Table 22.3 and can be administered as intermittent doses by continuous infusion or using patient-controlled epidural analgesia.

Side effects of epidural analgesia are few. Epidural local anesthetics can cause sympathetic blockade and hypotension. Administration of intravenous fluids, pressors, or a combination

Tables 22.3 Epidural labor analgesia.

Loading dose
Bupivacaine 0.125% 10 ml with hydromorphone 100 μg or fentanyl 50 μg or sufentanil 10 μg
Ropivicaine 0.75% 10 ml with hydromorphone 100 μg or fentanyl 15 μg or sufentanil 10 μg
Infusion
Bupivacaine 0.0625–0.125% or ropivacaine 0.075–0.125%
With hydromorphone 3 μg/ml or fentanyl 2 μg/ml or sufentanil 2 μg/ml

thereof can treat the side effects. The low-dose local anesthetic (LA) opioid combinations used currently cause minimal hemodynamic disturbance. Since concentrated LA solutions may cause motor blockade, it can be avoided or minimized by using the lowest concentration, compatible with adequate analgesics. Epidural opioids may cause nausea, vomiting, and/or pruritis (itching). These side effects be treated with antiemetics and/or low-dose nalbuphine. Other complications of the epidural technique include a failed or inadequate block, dural puncture, intravascular injection, infection, or neurological complication. Fetal complications may include a transient change in the FHR pattern. In some cases, epidural analgesia may improve placental blood flow (i.e., in patients with pre-eclampsia).

Combined Spinal Epidural Analgesia

The combined spinal epidural analgesia (CSE) technique was first described approximately 60 years ago and came into favor approximately 20 years ago. Most commonly, the technique is performed by inserting an epidural needle into the epidural space, then inserting a long spinal needle into the subarachnoid space. Then, the spinal medication is injected and the epidural catheter is inserted through the epidural needle, once the spinal needle is removed. CSE offers the certainty and speed of onset of spinal analgesia with the flexibility and continuity of an epidural catheter. The major disadvantage is the additional potential for complications introduced by the deliberate dural puncture.

The spinal component usually consists of a small dose of fentanyl (12.5–25 μg) combined with 0.5–1.0 mg of bupivacaine made up to a volume of 1 ml with saline. This combination will provide 60–90 min of analgesia with little or no motor blockade. The epidural infusion may be started immediately or when the patient complains of returning pain. Most anesthesiologists will consider CSE for patients requesting very early epidural analgesia (≤1 cm cervical dilatation) or for those requesting analgesia late in the first stage of labor.

Spinal Analgesia

The use of "single shot" spinal analgesia alone and not as part of a CSE technique is most useful in the late stages of labor when delivery is imminent or to provide rapid analgesia for a mother who has "lost control," thus allowing her to "regroup" and cooperate for epidural catheter placement. The main consideration for single shot spinal analgesia is the limited duration of analgesia (60–90 min; Table 22.4) and the risk of post-dural puncture headache. The headache risk can be reduced by using a small gauge (24–25 g) pencil point needle (Sprotte®; B. Braun Medical Inc., Bethlehem, PA) rather than those with cutting tips. The incidence of headache should be ≤2% and, if it occurs, should be mild.

Table 22.4 Spinal opioids for labor.

Opioid	Dose
Fentanyl	10–25 μg in 1 ml normal saline
Sufentanil	2–5 μg in 1 ml normal saline

Bupivacaine, 0.5–1 mg may be added to the solution.

A "saddle block" or a low spinal anesthetic with a local anesthetic may be used to provide anesthesia in the perineal area (hence "saddle block") for stages 2 and 3 of labor, especially when assisted vaginal delivery is performed (forceps/vacuum). Most commonly used is 5–7 mg of hyperbaric bupivacaine with 10–25 μg of fentanyl administration in the sitting position, with the patient then placed immediately into the lithotomy position with the head of the bed approximately 45° upright. This helps ensure a "saddle block" distribution of anesthesia.

A continuous spinal catheter technique may be considered in some cases. This is achieved using a standard epidural kit. This technique may be used when an inadvertent dural puncture occurs with the epidural needle. More commonly it is used in patients in whom one may need a rapid onset of surgical anesthesia for operative delivery when a general anesthetic is ill advised (e.g., a morbidly obese patient or a patient with a history of malignant hyperthermia).

Controversies

The major controversy with respect to the management of labor pain is whether or not invasive analgesic techniques negatively impact the course or outcome of labor. Also, issues related to successful breastfeeding and analgesia continue to be raised.

With respect to regional analgesia and the course of labor, studies have shown that epidural labor analgesia with low-dose local anesthetic/opioid combination does not impact the course or affect the outcome of labor (Wong et al. 2005). Epidural or CSE may lengthen the duration of stage 1 of labor, but this is not clinically significant. Further, studies have suggested that spinal opioid analgesia may actually speed the duration of stage 1 of labor.

Successful breastfeeding is dependant upon multiple maternal and neonatal factors. There is no definitive evidence that any type of labor analgesia either positively or negatively impacts breastfeeding success.

Case Scenario

Suneil Ramessur, MBBS, BSc (Hons), FRCA, DipHEP

You are on call for labor and delivery floor. You are called to see Ann, a 30-year-old G0P0 who wishes to discuss her pain relief options with you. Over the phone, the midwife tells you that Ann is 2 cm dilated and "does not seem to be in too much pain."

What factors do you think will be important when considering Ann's pain relief options?

You will need to consider both her medical situation and psychological state. Remember that pain is subjective and the way that different people demonstrate their pain can vary greatly. While the opinion of an experienced midwife is valuable, if a patient says she is in pain, then assume that she is. Feeling "in control" can reduce pain, and this patient may want to know what options are available to her if she feels that her pain is getting out of control. You will need to address what preconceptions and beliefs she has about labor pain. Some women have a great fear of an epidural while others may believe that opting for medical pain relief is somehow a failure on their part. Addressing her fears and beliefs is vital.

When you arrive, you meet Ann and her partner. Ann is adamant not to have an epidural and confesses this is because she has read it could leave her "paralyzed." You learn that she had hoped for a home birth but, due to an abnormal lie of the fetus, she had to be admitted to the hospital. She wants to know about other "less invasive" methods to control pain.

What should you say?

It is clear that Ann's labor is not going according to the plan she had hoped for. You should be sensitive to her desire for non-invasive analgesia. You can discuss breathing techniques that she and her partner can use. Focusing on deep breathing during the contraction, with a supportive partner, has been demonstrated to reduce labor pain scores. You can also discuss the use of a transcutaneous electrical nerve stimulator (TENS) machine. While using TENS, pads are applied to her back and she can control the intensity and frequency of the stimulation. There are various kinds available, but generally they constantly stimulate at a low intensity and have a boost button that can be activated by the patient during a contraction.

The other options are aroma therapy, acupuncture, and hypnotherapy. Ann decides to try deep breathing technique to control her pain. They seem content with this and you leave, having reassured them that you can return if things get out of hand again. Three hours later you are called back. She is progressing slowly and her pain has worsened. She is not coping and is very tearful when you enter the room. She says that she thinks she is a "failure for not being able to handle this." She asks if she can have a cesarean section just to make it all stop.

What can you offer that may help Ann now?

The validity of informed consent in a patient who is in great distress, such as Ann, is considered controversial by some. For this reason it is important to document clearly what you have discussed and, if possible, to include the partner in the discussion. Ultimately though, only the patient can consent for any form of treatment.

You can offer her the option of intramuscular or intravenous analgesia with opioids such as such as nalbuphine, meperidine, or even morphine. However, sedating side effects are a concern, and these medications increase the risk of nausea and vomiting and respiratory depression. You will need to explain that a small amount of the drug may cross the placenta and affect the fetus, but this is not a major problem and can be managed.

You will need to directly approach her fear of paralysis when you offer an epidural. You can explain that the risk of paralysis when one crosses the road is similar to that of becoming paralyzed from an epidural in labor (i.e., virtually zero). You will also need to explain other possible consequences of epidural placement:

- Post-dural puncture headache (PDPH)
- Failed/patchy block
- Bruising around site of injection, bleeding, and infection
- Risk of permanent nerve injury 0.6/100,000
- Risk of temporary nerve injury
- Increased likelihood of assisted/instrumental delivery
- Weak legs
- Need for a urinary catheter
- Fall in blood pressure
- Need to monitor the fetus continuously and regular blood pressure checks
- Risk of allergic reaction or local anesthetic toxicity

Ann and her partner agree to have the epidural now. All her laboratory studies are normal and she does not have any signs of pre-eclampsia. You place a large bore IV cannula and commence fluid infusion before you site the epidural. You insert it without complication and after 20 min she is virtually pain free, except that she is still experiencing some "low-down pressure." You explain that you can treat this with a further dose of local anesthetic, but she may experience greater leg numbness and it may reduce the effectiveness of her pushing the fetus later. However, as she is still only 6 cm dilated she opts to have the extra top-up and soon falls asleep. Four hours later you are asked to see her as she has a forceps delivery and sustains a third degree vaginal tear. She now has to go to the operating room to have it repaired.

What are the anesthetic options for her repair?
If the epidural is working well bilaterally, you can "top up" with a more concentrated local anesthetic solution. As this is a repair of a vaginal tear, only a saddle block is required. If she were having a manual removal of the placenta, she would need a much higher block – to about T6/T7. If the epidural were patchy or had failed, one option would be to replace it, remove it and place a spinal anesthetic, or induce general anesthesia.

References

Eappen S, Robbins D. Nonpharmacological means of pain relief for labor and delivery. A review. Int Anethesiol Clin. 2002;40(4):103–14.

Howell CJ, Kidd C, Roberts W, et al. A randomized controlled trial of epidural compared with nonepidural analgesia in labour. BJ Obstet Gynecol. 2001;108:27–33.

Lowe N. Parity pain during parturition. J Obstet Gynecol Neonatal Nurs. 1987;16:340–6.

Melzack R, Kinch RA, Dobkin P, et al. Severity of labour pain: influence of physical as well as psychological variables. Can Med Assoc J. 1984;130:579–84.

Melzack R. The McGill pain questionnaire: major properties and scoring methods. Pain 1975;1:277–279.

Wang SM, DeZinno P, Fermo L, et al. Complementary and alternative medicine for low-back pain in pregnancy: a cross-sectional survey. J Altern Complement Med. 2005;11:459–64.

Wong CA, Scovone BM, Peaceman AM, et al. The risk of cesarean delivery with neuraxial analgesia given early versus late in labor. New Engl J Med. 2005;352(7):718–20.

Section VII

Chronic Pain Management

Chapter 23

Neuropathic Pain

Gerald W. Grass, MD, FAAMA

Introduction

Few medical problems are more complex in nature and perplexing to effectively manage than pain. Pain, in its acute form, is necessary for survival and serves an important role in the way an organism interfaces with its environment by signaling real or impending harm. Occasionally, circumstances lead to activity in the pain-signaling pathway that is not beneficial to the organism and has no survival value. Injury to nerve fibers or their projections may cause conditions that are not usually perceived as painful to become excessively painful. Although most nerve injuries do not lead to clinically important and sustained pain, in some cases, even small degrees of insult can precipitate severe and unremitting pain. Neuropathic pain exists when a nerve responds to an injury in a typical fashion and then continues to respond and signal pain long after the injurious stimulus is removed.

Neuropathic pain is widely recognized as a challenging condition to treat and reaching an accurate diagnosis of a patient with neuropathic pain requires a precise and clinically relevant definition of this condition. In an effort to address this issue, the International Association for the Study of Pain (IASP) introduced the term neuropathic pain in 1994 and defined it as "pain initiated or caused by a primary lesion or dysfunction in the nervous system (Mersky 1994, Bouhassira et al. 2008)." Unfortunately this definition lacks both precision and specificity. The IASP has recently revised its definition and states that neuropathic pain is a direct consequence of diseases that affect the somatosensory system (Treede et al. 2008). Although the new definition is more precise, it falls short of providing the practitioner with a clinically relevant framework to aid in diagnosis.

Furthermore, it is important to realize that neuropathic pain is not a single entity, nor a disease in and of itself, but rather a heterogeneous manifestation of multiple and varied disorders affecting the nervous system, particularly the somatosensory components. Common causes of neuropathic pain include diabetes, viral infections, chemical insults, cervical and lumbar radiculopathies, trigeminal neuralgia, complex regional pain syndrome, amputation, multiple sclerosis, and spinal surgery or injury. Although primary disease factors, as those described above, may initiate pain mechanisms, it is the molecular and structural reorganization of the pain pathways and not the disease factors that are responsible for chronic neuropathic pain.

N. Vadivelu et al. (eds.), *Essentials of Pain Management*,
DOI 10.1007/978-0-387-87579-8_23, © Springer Science+Business Media, LLC 2011

Epidemiology

The prevalence of neuropathic pain in the general population currently is estimated to be between 3.3 and 8.2% (Bouhassira et al. 2008, Torrance et al. 2008, Gustorff et al. 2008). The wide variability in these estimates is related to the challenges of measuring different neuropathic pain conditions.

As one might expect, the prevalence of neuropathic pain is markedly higher among patients with diseases known to cause neuropathic pain, such as diabetes (40–50%) (Veves et al. 2008), HIV infections (38–62%) (Simpson et al. 2006, Cherry et al. 2006, Morgello et al. 2004), and multiple sclerosis (27.5%) (Osterberg et al. 2005), as well as those with known or suspected neuronal injury such as trigeminal neuralgia, glossopharyngeal neuralgia, and postherpetic neuralgia. However, it is less well recognized that neuropathic pain has been reported after a range of different types of common surgical procedures such as thoracotomy, inguinal hernia repair, and mastectomy. In one of the largest studies conducted to date investigating neuropathic pain following thoracic surgery, Maguire et al. found that at 1 year following video-assisted thorascopic surgery (VATS), 57% of patients experienced neuropathic pain symptoms that significantly interfered with their daily activities (Maguire et al. 2006). Similarly, Poobalan et al. reported that as many as 30% of patients experienced neuropathic pain following open repair of an inguinal hernia and that a similar number following laparoscopic repair reported chronic neuropathic pain symptoms (Poobalan et al. 2001, Poobalan et al. 2003). Even less well known is the fact that many women experience significant chronic neuropathic pain following common surgical procedures on the breast including lumpectomy, breast augmentation, and mastectomy (Vadivelu et al. 2008). Postmastectomy pain syndrome (PMPS) which has recently been identified as a distinct, chronic pain syndrome, including characteristic neuropathic symptoms of paroxysmal pain at the surgical site, chest wall, upper arm, and shoulder following surgery, may affect as many as 20% of women undergoing these surgical procedures (Carpenter et al. 2008).

Ongoing research indicates that the prevalence of neuropathic pain is increasing. This may in part be due to the increasing number of surgical procedures being performed, but perhaps more importantly because the population is aging and several neuropathic pain syndromes including painful diabetic neuropathy and postherpetic neuralgia are more common in the elderly. In addition, cancer patients are living longer and many of the treatments used in the management of cancer including chemotherapy are known to cause neuropathic pain contributing to the increasing incidence of this challenging pain syndrome.

Mechanisms of Neuropathic Pain

In terms of the experience of pain, it must be remembered that noxious stimuli are not just passively conducted from the periphery to the central nervous system as a large number of mechanisms serve to attenuate, magnify, and extend the organism's perception and experience of pain. The current understanding of the pathogenesis of neuropathic pain suggests that multiple mechanisms appear to mediate the symptoms of neuropathic pain including, but not limited to, temporal and spatial summation, recruitment of inactive neurons, peripheral and central sensitization, phenotypic switching, and central neuronal reorganization. Although a systematic review of the pathophysiological mechanisms underlying neuropathic pain is beyond the scope of this chapter, they have been reviewed extensively within recent years by others in the field (Baron 2000, Besson 1999, Pace et al. 2006, Pasero 2004, Waxman 2006).

Normal activity in the peripheral nervous system involves a reciprocal balance between neuronal excitation and inhibition. Pain arises when the balance shifts toward excitation, and inhibition is altered. Damage to peripheral nerves results in hyperexcitability in the primary afferent nociceptors (*peripheral sensitization*) that leads to hyperexcitability in central neurons (*central sensitization*) and the generation of spontaneous impulses within the axon, as well as the dorsal root ganglion of the peripheral nerves. When the nerve is able to repair itself, the sensitization resolves; however, if the nerve is unable to effect this repair or the insult continues, continued sensitization and altered processes in nociceptors lead to further generation of spontaneous symptoms.

Unresolved peripheral nerve injury causes a multitude of changes in gene transcription and activation of various kinases and proteins involved in the transmission and amplification of noxious stimuli, including enhanced N-methyl-D-aspartate (NMDA) receptor activity (Wilson et al. 2005, Ultenius et al. 2006). At the cellular level these alterations can lead to the formation of new channels, upregulation of certain receptors and downregulation of others, and altered local or descending inhibition which are some of the biological features that can contribute to hyperexcitability, factors assumed to be a sine qua non for chronic pain (Waxman et al. 2000, Matthews et al. 2007, Cummins et al. 2007).

It is the altered expression of these channels that results in neurons becoming hyperexcitable and generating ectopic activity, which is thought to lead to the genesis of spontaneous and paroxysmal pain. Beyond this, neuronal hyperexcitability has a wide spectrum of secondary manifestations including expansion of neuronal receptive fields, change of modality to which neurons respond, recruitment of silent neurons or circuits, and a neuronal reorganization in the dorsal horn and within the central nervous system.

Additionally, non-neuronal cells, which consist of microglia, astrocytes, and oligodendrocytes, also become activated in the spinal cord on the side of a nerve injury in both the dorsal and ventral horns (Coyle 1998). These cells may then begin to express purinergic receptors which allow them to be activated by various neurotransmitters including adenosine triphosphate (ATP) and following activation, release various proinflammatory and pronociceptive cytokines, such as interleukin-1 (IL-1), tumor necrosis factor alpha (TNF-α), and neurotrophins, including brain-derived neurotrophic factor, which in turn modulate and/or amplify nociceptive transmission contributing to the sensitization and maintenance of neuropathic pain (Coyle 1998, Hains and Waxman 2006, Zhao et al. 2007, Terayama et al. 2008).

It is not entirely unexpected that a genetic component may also contribute to the individual experience of neuropathic pain and may contribute to the diverse phenotype of individuals with apparently similar lesions, some of whom develop chronic neuropathic pain and many others do not. In the past many genes have been identified that contribute to the development of non-neuropathic pain conditions; however, only one gene, thus far – GTP cyclohydrolase 1 (*GCH1*) – has been implicated specifically in neuropathic pain (Tegeder et al. 2006). In a recent investigation, Campbell et al. (2009) analyzed the association of five *GCH1* single nucleotide polymorphisms (SNPs) with ratings of pain induced by the use of high concentration (10%) topical capsaicin applied to the skin of 39 normal human volunteers (Campbell et al. 2009). Each of the *GCH1* polymorphisms was associated with lower pain ratings. When combined, three of the five accounted for a surprisingly high 35% of the inter-individual variance in pain ratings. They conclude that SNPs of the *GCH1* gene previously identified profoundly affect the ratings of pain induced by capsaicin. While these recent data suggest a "protective" (i.e., less pain) haplotype in the GTP cyclohydrolase (GCH1) gene, other research has failed to confirm this association and this remains an area of active ongoing investigation (Kim and Dionne 2007).

It is, therefore, not surprising that given the multiplicity of cellular alterations occurring subsequent to nerve injury, a host of neuroplastic changes take place in which the somatosensory information can be distorted in several ways secondary to the reorganization of all of the structures participating in the transduction, transmission, and translational processing of noxious information.

Clinical Presentation

Many physicians, including primary care physicians and other non-pain specialists, will encounter patients with neuropathic pain. The clinical spectrum of neuropathic pain ranges from barely discernable to severely disabling and as previously mentioned is caused by a wide range of disease processes listed in Table 23.1.

Generally speaking, a key feature usually seen in patients with neuropathic pain is that they exhibit persistent or paroxysmal pain that is independent of a stimulus. This stimulus-independent pain is often described by the patients as "shooting," "lancinating," "electric

Table 23.1 Classification of neuropathic pain by disease and anatomical site.

Peripheral	Spinal	Brain
Neuropathies	*Trauma*	*Trauma*
• Diabetic neuropathies	• Spinal cord injury	*Surgical lesions*
• HIV/AID-induced neuropathies	• Syringomyelia	*Vascular*
• Chemotherapy-induced neuropathies	• Arachnoiditis	• Infarction
• Hereditary neuropathies	• Surgery	• Hemorrhage
• Toxin-induced neuropathies	*Vascular*	• AV malformation
• Idiopathic neuropathies	• Infarction	*Multiple sclerosis*
Herpes zoster	• Hemorrhage	*Neoplasms*
• Post-herpetic neuralgia	• AV malformation	*Parkinson's disease?*
Neuronal injuries/dysfunction	*Neoplasms*	*Epilepsia?*
• Carpal tunnel syndrome	*Other*	
• Cubital tunnel syndrome	• Multiple sclerosis	
• Tarsal tunnel syndrome	• HIV/AIDS	
• Trigeminal neuralgia	• Neural tube defect	
• Glossopharyngeal neuralgia	• B12 deficiency	
• Complex regional pain syndrome 1, 2		
Amputations		
• Phantom limb pain		
• Post-mastectomy pain syndrome		
Plexopathies		
Radiculopathies		
• Herniated disc disease		
• Post-laminectomy syndrome		
• Arachnoiditis		
Avulsions		
Neoplasms		

shock like," or "burning" in quality and may be accompanied by "pins-and-needles sensations" and occasionally intractable itching. Often these symptoms are not confined to a single peripheral nerve dermatome, myotome, or sclerotome and are usually most pronounced distally. Typically, patients may state that the pain is worse at night or during periods of cold, damp weather and is exacerbated by movement of the affected body part. Spontaneous activity of nociceptive C fibers and sensitization of the dorsal horn neurons are thought to be responsible for persistent "burning" pain. Similarly, spontaneous activity in large myelinated A fibers (which normally signal innocuous sensations) is related to stimulus-independent paresthesias and, following central sensitization, to dysesthesias and pain.

In addition, patients with neuropathic pain may also experience stimulus dependent or *evoked pain* which has two key features; *hyperalgesia* and *allodynia*. Hyperalgesia is an increased pain response to a suprathreshold noxious stimulus and is the result of abnormal processing of nociceptive input. Allodynia is the sensation of pain elicited by a non-noxious stimulus and can be produced in two ways: by the action of low-threshold myelinated A beta fibers on an altered central nervous system and by a reduction in the threshold of nociceptive terminals in the periphery. Stimulus-evoked hyperalgesias are commonly classified into subgroups on the basis of modality, i.e., mechanical, thermal, or chemical. Mechanical hyperalgesias are further classified as brush-evoke (dynamic), pressure-evoked (static), and punctate hyperalgesia. Patients may complain, for example, that a simple pinprick or venipuncture is an exquisitely painful experience (*hyperalgesia*) or that light touch or the touch of articles of clothing or bed sheets at night is experienced as painful (*allodynia*).

Associated autonomic nervous system complaints such as abnormal sweating, impotence, orthostatic hypotension, and gastrointestinal symptoms are frequent. Also patients may note that the affected limb or body part feels "swollen," "cold," or "changes color."

Specific Neuropathic Pain Syndromes

The presence of neuropathic pain, whether of peripheral or central origin, continues to present a significant burden to individuals and society by increasing disability, reducing productivity, and diminishing the quality of life all with concomitant increases in healthcare resource utilization and costs.

Peripheral Syndromes

Painful peripheral neuropathies represent a debilitating neurologic problem, as well as a challenging diagnostic and therapeutic management issue. The examples cited below do not represent an exhaustive review, but do provide a useful resource and an impetus for the recognition and evaluation of these syndromes and their contribution to the overall burden of neuropathic pain.

Painful Polyneuropathies

Diabetic Peripheral Neuropathy

Diabetic peripheral neuropathy is a late complication of diabetes mellitus resulting from decreased blood flow and high blood sugar levels. Population-based studies indicate that diabetic neuropathies are common among patients with diabetes, affecting up to 66% of patients with insulin-dependent diabetes mellitus and 59% of patients with noninsulin-dependent diabetes mellitus. Several types of diabetic neuropathy have been identified including focal and multifocal neuropathies such as cranial, truncal, focal limb, and amyotrophic neuropathy, as well as generalized symmetric polyneuropathies that are not necessarily limited to sensorimotor pathways, but may also include autonomic neuropathies of the cardiovascular, gastrointestinal, and/or genitourinary systems.

The sensory neuropathies, frequently referred to as distal symmetric sensorimotor polyneuropathies, may be further characterized as either acute or chronic. The acute form is considered relatively rare while the chronic form is the more common. A variant of distal symmetrical sensorimotor polyneuropathy known as painful diabetic polyneuropathy (DPN) has been reported to be present in up to 10% of patients with diabetes.

Patients with DPN frequently describe their pain in various terms such as burning, prickling ("pins and needles"), lancinating, shooting ("like an electric shock"), cramping, aching, and frequently report contact hypersensitivity (allodynia) and "dead feeling" (numbness) in their legs. Walking is described by some patients as the sensation of walking barefoot on "pebbles" or "scalding sand." The spectrum of severity is wide with some patients presenting with mild symptoms in a toe or two, while others may have continuous painful symptoms involving both legs and extending to the upper limbs.

Diabetic cohort studies indicate that the prevalence of painful diabetes polyneuropathy increases with age, duration of diabetes, and worsening of glucose tolerance.

Human Immunodeficiency Virus

The presence of human immunodeficiency virus (HIV) is often associated with several different types of neuropathies including distal symmetrical polyneuropathy (DSP), inflammatory demyelinating polyneuropathy (IDP), progressive polyradiculopathy (PP), mononeuropathy multiplex (MM), autonomic neuropathy, and diffuse infiltrative lymphocytosis syndrome (DILS). These neuropathies may occur as a direct result of the disease process but may also be secondary to treatment, as many of the drugs used in the management of HIV patients are known to be neurotoxic, especially the antiretrovirals, although the antibacterials, anticancer drugs, and other agents may also be contributory factors.

Distal symmetrical polyneuropathy is the most common HIV-associated neuropathy and is frequently observed in individuals with advanced immunosuppression. The prevalence of HIV-related neuropathy varies but may be as high as 30–38% of HIV-positive patients. Various other forms of HIV-related neuropathy are less prevalent with MM present in 11% of individuals with HIV, IDP present in 4%, and PP, autonomic neuropathy, and monoradiculopathy present in 1% of patients.

Although evidence of peripheral neuropathies may be present in the earliest stages of HIV infection, they are frequently observed in nearly all patients with end-stage HIV. In addition, it has been suggested that painful polyneuropathy occurs in up to 50% of patients with acquired immunodeficiency syndrome (AIDS), with the highest rates of polyneuropathy found among patients in palliative care settings.

Post-herpetic Neuralgia

Acute herpes zoster, commonly called shingles, is an acute viral infection that primarily affects the posterior spinal root ganglia of spinal nerves or ganglia of the cranial nerves may be similarly affected. The causative agent, varicella zoster, belongs to a DNA group of viruses that is host specific. The same virus produces varicella or chickenpox in children and young adults.

The acute infection is initially characterized by a prodromal phase that is associated with pain and paresthesias in the affected dermatome. Hours to days later, a papular rash appears and progresses to vesicles, then pustules, and finally crusts and heals 3–4 weeks later. In some patients, the pain persists weeks to months or years after the rash has healed leading to the term postherpetic neuralgia (PHN). Studies have demonstrated that there are three phases of PHN: acute, subacute, and chronic. The acute phase occurs with the onset of the rash and lasts for approximately 30 days, the subacute phase lasts for 1–3 months after the onset of the rash, and the chronic phase, or PHN, lasts for 3 months or longer after the onset of the rash.

The persistent pain associated with PHN is variable in nature and can be characterized as any of the following: (1) burning background pain with fluctuating severity; (2) sudden, sharp shooting pain; and (3) mechanical or thermal allodynia (pain produced by non-noxious stimulus). As a result of this severe, often debilitating pain, a patient's quality of life is often adversely affected. In addition to interfering with activities of daily living, PHN may lead to fatigue, insomnia, anxiety, and depression. Because of the severity and complexity of the disease, treatment is initiated at the onset of the rash and may be necessary months to years later.

Risk factors for PHN include prodromal symptoms and severity of pain at the onset of the rash. The most significant risk factor for the development of PHN is age, as the incidence of PHN increases with age. While studies have demonstrated the overall incidence ranges from 10 to 27%, the incidence for individuals over the age of 50 is 40% and 75% for those over the age of 75.

Painful Mononeuropathies

Amputation

Phantom limb syndrome (PLS) is a broad classification that refers to a variety of sensory phenomena felt after limb amputation and that may vary in frequency, duration, and intensity. These phenomena include phantom limb sensations, which are the perception that the limb is still present; stump pain, which refers to pain perceived at the location of existing body parts in the region of amputation; and phantom limb pain, which is pain perceived in the absent limb.

Phantom limb pain is uncommon when considering the general population. Consequently, characterization of the epidemiology of phantom limb pain has generally been restricted to the population of patients experiencing amputation. Epidemiologic studies on PLS within amputee populations have consistently reported a high prevalence of phantom limb sensations ranging from 66 to 80% of patients reporting phantom limb sensations 1 year after amputation.

Of the phantom limb sensations, phantom limb pain may occur during the first year after amputation in 50–85% of patients. Chronic pain following amputation is either stump pain or phantom pain or both. Phantom limb pain is frequently described as a paroxysmal burning, crushing, and twisting in the missing part. It peaks within the first month following surgery and may fade slowly as it "telescopes" toward the stump. Patients who experience extremity pain prior to surgery are more likely to develop post-amputation phantom pain and preemptive analgesia with sensory blockade may reduce the incidence of phantom pain. Although the pain may improve, particularly with respect to frequency and duration, it often remains chronic over the course of months or years, either with no improvement or an increase in pain.

Carpal Tunnel Syndrome

Carpal tunnel syndrome (CTS) is one of the most commonly encountered neuropathies in clinical practice and is described as an uncomfortable condition of the wrist and hand that is precipitated by repeated flexion and extension of the wrist causing increased pressure on the median nerve. Although CTS is commonly considered a condition of repetitive movement that may be related to particular occupations, it is also associated with medical conditions including diabetes, rheumatologic and thyroid disorders. CTS symptoms include pain that may radiate up the forearm, numbness, tingling, and reduced sensation in the hand and wrist and the symptoms often worsen at night or after use of the hand. The symptoms usually begin in the dominant hand, although in more than half the cases, the disorder is bilateral.

Clinical examination reveals decreased sensation over the palmar aspect of the thumb through the ring finger. Atrophy of the thenar muscles can occur as a late sign of median nerve neuropathy. Two common physical diagnosis tests, Tinel's sign and Phalen's test, help to confirm the diagnosis. Tinel's sign refers to distal paresthesias produced by percussion of the median nerve either proximal to the flexor retinaculum in the wrist or distally at the base of the palm. Phalen's test is performed by acute flexion of the wrist for 60 s.

Because carpal tunnel syndrome is usually treated surgically, little is known about its natural history. In one clinical study which followed 12 patients with CTS who refused treatment between 4 and 9 years, 7 patients showed improved clinical symptoms and conduction studies over several years, bringing the universally accepted procedure of surgical treatment into some question.

Trigeminal and Other Cranial Neuralgias

Trigeminal neuralgia (TN), also known as "tic douloureux," is a neuropathic pain condition affecting the facial area. The IASP defines TN as "a sudden, usually unilateral, severe, brief, stabbing, recurrent pain in the distribution of one or more branches of the fifth cranial nerve." Although etiologically it is most frequently associated with vascular compression of the trigeminal nerve, other causes are also observed; between 2 and 4% of cases are associated with multiple sclerosis (MS) and tumors as the underlying cause account for approximately 2% of cases.

Patients suffering from trigeminal neuralgia describe a paroxysmal pain pattern and these paroxysms, which may only last for a few minutes or seconds, are frequently triggered by non-noxious stimuli or normal activities such as talking, chewing, and swallowing. The pain spreads rapidly at the beginning of the attack, recedes slowly, and is commonly recurrent. It most frequently involves the second and third divisions of the trigeminal nerve (V_2 and V_3), but can include or be limited to the first division (V_1) as well.

The epidemiology of TN has been described in several large population studies, with an annual age- and gender-adjusted incidence of 4.7–8 per 100,000. The incidence is higher in females, with female to male ratios of 1.7–2.2:1, and an incidence that increases with age, peaking at around 70 years.

Glossopharyngeal Neuralgia

Glossopharyngeal neuralgia (GPN) refers to a syndrome affecting the ninth cranial nerve that is similar to TN in that it is characterized by paroxysms of excruciating pain lasting seconds to minutes in duration. As with TN, GPN may be idiopathic but is also associated with MS, although probably to a lesser extent than TN. However, in contrast to TN, the pain in GPN is generally localized to the posterior pharynx, tonsillar fossa, and base of the tongue, often with radiation to the external auditory canal or the neck. Its onset is often related to specific trigger factors affecting the throat including swallowing, drinking cold liquids, sneezing, coughing, talking, and clearing the throat.

Glossopharyngeal neuralgia is probably the least well-characterized neuropathic pain condition with respect to pain quality/severity and patient burden. Similarly, its epidemiology is poorly characterized with limited data that suggest the incidence is estimated to be approximately 0.8/100,000 population. The reported peak age of onset is between 70 and 79 years, with similar incidence rates for men and women. The left side was predominantly affected (53%) and bilaterality was noted in 25% of cases.

Central Syndromes
Spinal Cord

Spinal cord injury (SCI) can be broadly defined as damage to the spinal cord that results from direct injury to the spinal cord itself or indirectly by damage to the bones and soft tissues and vessels surrounding the spinal cord. In epidemiologic reviews of SCI, the annual incidence of SCI in various countries throughout the world varies from 15 to 40 per million of the population.

While SCI can be caused by trauma or disease, in the United States almost half (47.5%) of reported SCIs were caused by motor vehicle accidents since the year 2000, with falls being the next most common cause (27.9%), followed by acts of violence (13.8%, primarily gunshot wounds) and sports injuries (8.9%).

Chronic pain is commonly a debilitating feature in patients with SCI, often commencing within 6 months after the SCI and continuing throughout life with prevalence rates of up to 80% reported as long as 5 years after injury. The underlying pain mechanisms in SCI may be nociceptive or neuropathic. The site of pain may be either above, at, or below the level of the nerve injury, and while below-level pain is generally considered to be neuropathic, at- or above-level pain can also be neuropathic in origin.

Most evidence suggests that neuropathic pain begins shortly after SCI (likely within the first 8 weeks), with a reported prevalence of acute neuropathic pain of up to 80%. The prevalence of chronic central neuropathic pain ranges from 10 to 82%, although most studies report prevalence estimates between 40 and 70%.

Although there was no difference in central pain prevalence between patients with complete and incomplete SCI, below-level pain was more prevalent among quadriplegics (50%) compared with paraplegics (32%). Pain severity was described as severe or excruciating in 48% of patients with below-level pain. Patients description of SCI-related pain vary with the majority reporting characteristics typical of neuropathic pain such as burning, shooting, or lancinating; however, a significant percentage also report nociceptive pain qualities suggestive of musculoskeletal or visceral pain.

Brain

Central Post-stroke Pain

Stroke is not only a leading cause of death, but also significantly contributes to long-term disability in both industrialized and developing countries. Central post-stroke pain (CPSP) is a sequelae of stroke that is characterized by neuropathic pain in areas of the body that have lost part of their sensory innervation by the stroke and has been considered by patients more distressing than other stroke sequelae. The IASP defines CPSP as pain following an unequivocal stroke episode, where a psychogenic, nociceptive, or peripheral neurogenic cause is considered highly unlikely. Although CPSP was originally termed "thalamic syndrome," it is now recognized that CPSP may also result from extrathalamic lesions and it is now known that this type of pain can occur following lesions located anywhere from the medulla to the cerebral cortex.

Only one prospective epidemiologic study of CPSP has been reported which found the 1-year prevalence of CPSP among stroke survivors was 8%. Patients may report the onset of pain as late as 2–3 years after a stroke, and while some patients reported pain immediately after a stroke.

Attempts to understand the mechanism of central pain have been largely based on clinical features, imaging studies, and neurophysiologic studies. Current hypothesis suggests that the most likely pain-driving mechanisms result after a disconnection or disinhibition of somatotopically organized somatosensory pathways resulting in hyperactivity in brainstem nuclei that mediate the polysynaptic portion of the pain pathway.

Complex Regional Pain Syndrome

Complex regional pain syndrome (CRPS) is a painful condition with clinical features that include pain, sensory, sudomotor, and vasomotor disturbances; trophic changes; and impaired motor function. Symptoms usually appear after an initiating noxious event such as trauma or surgery. The course varies from mild and self-limiting to chronic disease with a significant impact on daily functioning and quality of life.

The term "complex regional pain syndrome" was introduced to replace the terms "reflex sympathetic dystrophy and causalgia." CRPS type I was previously referred to as reflex sympathetic dystrophy and CRPS type II was known as causalgia. The terminology was changed because the pathophysiology of CRPS is not known with certainty. It was determined that a descriptive term such as CRPS was preferable to "reflex sympathetic dystrophy" which carries with it the assumption that the sympathetic nervous system is important in the pathophysiology of the painful condition.

CRPS type I typically follows an injury (usually of a hand or foot), most commonly after crush injuries, especially in a lower limb. It may follow amputation, acute MI, stroke, or cancer (i.e., lung, breast, ovary, CNS); no precipitant is apparent in about 10% of patients. CRPS type II is similar to type I but involves overt damage to a peripheral nerve.

At the present time no single hypothesis explains all features of CRPS and it shares common mechanisms that may be injury to central or peripheral neural tissue. While numerous theories have been proposed to explain the pathophysiology of CRPS, the exact mechanisms remain unclear. Most agree that CRPS is a neurologic disorder affecting both the central and peripheral nervous systems.

The initial signs and symptoms of CRPS may begin at the time of injury or be delayed for weeks. The clinical presentation is characterized by pain, frequently out of proportion to the injury, changes in cutaneous sensitivity (allodynia and hyperalgesia), autonomic dysfunction, trophic changes, and motor dysfunction. Autonomic dysfunction may manifest as edema of the affected part, sudomotor changes (hypo- or hyperhidrosis), changes in skin coloration (red or pale), and skin temperature differences. Cutaneous vasomotor changes (i.e., red, mottled, or ashen color; increased or decreased temperature) may be present and edema may be considerable and locally confined. Other symptoms such as trophic abnormalities (i.e., shiny, atrophic skin; cracking or excess growth of nails; bone atrophy; hair loss) and motor abnormalities (weakness, tremors, spasm, dystonia) may also be apparent upon clinical examination. Additionally, range of motion is often limited, sometimes leading to joint contractures.

CRPS occurs in approximately 1–15% of peripheral nerve injury cases. CRPS frequently occurs secondary to fractures, sprains, and trivial soft tissue injury. The incidence after fractures and contusions ranges from 10 to 30%. While some cases are associated with an identifiable nerve injury, many are not. Even "microtrauma" as might occur with an immunization may be responsible. The upper extremities are more likely to be involved than the lower.

The prognosis of CRPS varies and is difficult to predict. CRPS may remit or remain stable for years; in a few patients, it progresses, spreading to other areas of the body. The treatment is complex and often unsatisfactory, particularly if begun late and may include drugs, physical therapy, sympathetic blockade, psychological treatments, and neuromodulation.

Multiple Sclerosis

Pain is commonly reported in patients with multiple sclerosis (MS), and this pain can be of nociceptive or neuropathic origin and may sometimes have characteristics of both. The prevalence of pain in patients with MS has been variously reported to range from 50% to as high as 85%.

Pain descriptors in patients with MS are generally consistent with other central pain states and include tingling, burning, and aching, with the majority of MS patients (72%) reporting two or more pain qualities. Constant pain has been reported by 62–77% of patients and only 30% of these patients had pain-free periods that lasted minutes or hours.

The presence of central pain may occur as early as 7 years before the clinical onset of MS, and it has been suggested that such pain may be the first symptoms of MS. Alternatively, central pain may occur as many as 25 years after other symptoms emerge, although 57% of patients with central pain report onset within 5 years after MS onset and 73% report pain onset within 10 years of MS onset.

Assessment and Diagnostic Evaluation of Patients with Neuropathic Pain

The assessment and differential diagnosis of neuropathic pain syndromes is complex and challenging for the clinician. In patients presenting with chronic pain, the underlying pain mechanism or mechanisms are often difficult to diagnose and a distinction between noci-ceptive and neuropathic types of pain is sometimes challenging because conditions such as diabetes mellitus, cancer, and other neurological diseases can produce mixed pain pictures. It is important, of course, that the clinical assessment of a patient with suspected neuropathic pain focus on ruling out treatable conditions (e.g., spinal cord compression, neoplasm), con-firming the diagnosis of neuropathic pain, and identifying clinical features (e.g., insomnia, autonomic neuropathy) that might help individualize treatment. Crucial to any pain assess-ment is the clinician's acknowledgment that the patient is experiencing pain and that the pain is real. This validation of the patient's pain is critical in developing rapport with the patient and establishing a meaningful therapeutic relationship. Without this, any further steps in the care of the pain patient are unproductive, if not meaningless.

History

The first step in the diagnostic evaluation of any patient with neuropathic pain is the his-tory and physical examination. The pain history should note the pain location, time of onset, intensity, character, associated symptoms, and factors aggravating and relieving the pain, response to past treatments, comorbid conditions, and coping skills. Characteristic features of neuropathic pain should be sought and are important in differentiating it from any other source of pain, thereby differentiating nociceptive versus neuropathic pain thus serving as the primary evidence for a diagnosis of neuropathic pain. A guide to help in the assessment and evaluation of patients with a suspected neuropathic pain syndrome is presented in Table 23.2.

Positive symptoms that are typical of neuropathic pain include (1) paresthesias – non-painful, spontaneous sensory phenomena such as "pins-and-needles" sensation or tingling; (2) dysesthesias – unpleasant spontaneous or evoked sensory phenomena such as burn-ing; (3) hyperesthesia – increased sensitivity to stimuli, often with an unpleasant quality; (5) hyperpathia or hyperalgesia – exaggerated pain response elicited by a normally painful stimulus.

In addition, the effect of pain on quality of life and functional status issues is extremely important. Specific pain measures such as the Neuropathic Pain Scale, Neuropathic Pain Questionnaire, and the Pain Detect Questionnaire may be used to quantify the patient's pain as well as its effect on the quality of life. These tools share common features and in general have a similar accuracy rate of up to 80% (Bennett et al. 2007). These scales are particularly helpful for patients involved in clinical therapeutic trials and may be used to assess the effi-cacy of treatment regimens. It must be remembered that although these questionnaires aid in the identification of neuropathic pain syndromes and serve as reliable screening tools, they do not replace a detailed medical history and physical examination.

Physical Examination

The physical examination should be guided by the patient history. The goal of the physical examination is to characterize the pattern, symmetry, and distribution of abnormalities and to determine which modalities are involved (motor, sensory, autonomic). The examination should include a focused general medical examination and neurological assessment.

The general examination medical examination is an integral part of any diagnostic evalua-tion. One aspect of the general medical examination to be emphasized is the status of the skin, noting whether changes in skin color (red, pale, bluish, mottled), rashes, swelling, changes in

Table 23.2   A guide to the evaluation of patients with neuropathic pain.

History	Deep tendon reflexes
Pain intensity	• May be diminished or absent distal to involved nerves
• 0–10 rating scale (o = no pain, 10 = worst pain imaginable	*Sensory examination*
• Rate pain at the initial visit and at each subsequent visit to track treatment response	• Light touch, pin prick, vibration, and proprioception sense may be diminished or absent distal to involved nerves
Sensory descriptors	• Sensory abnormalities may extend beyond normal dermatomal, myotomal, and/or sclerotomal boundaries.
• Pain qualities: burning, electric, hot, cold, stabbing	• Dynamic allodynia (pain due to cotton lightly moving across the skin)
• Unusual sensations: "pins and needles," tingling, itching etc.	• Thermal allodynia (burning sensation in response to ice or alcohol on skin)
Temporal variation	• Pinprick hyperalgesia (exaggerated pain following light pinprick to skin)
• Neuropathic pain often become worse at the end of the day, with cold and/or damp weather	• Possible presence of Tinel's sign (distally radiating paresthesias upon percussion of damaged or regenerating nerve fibers)
• Suspect neoplastic process if the pain has progressively worsened over several months	*Skin examination*
Functional/psychological impact	• Alterations in temperature, color, sweating, hair, and/or nail growth suggestive of complex regional pain syndrome
• The effect of pain on sleep patterns, activities of daily living, work, and hobbies	• Residual dermatomal scars consistent with previous herpes zoster infection
• The effect of pain on mood, social and sexual functioning, suicidal ideation	• Characteristic skin changes consistent with diabetes mellitus
Previous treatment modalities	**Special tests**
• Neuropathic pain is resistant to NSAIDs and acetaminophen	*Computed tomography (CT) and magnetic resonance imaging (MRI) scans*
• Determine and document adequacy of dose titration for previously trailed drugs (dose reached, duration of treatment and drug stopped due to adverse effects of lack of efficacy)	• Facilitate specific diagnosis (e.g., disc herniations, nerve infiltration/compression by tumor)
Substance abuse history	*Electromyography and nerve conduction studies*
• Administer opioid screening tools (COMM or STOP)	• May provide objective evidence of nerve injury or dysfunction. Nerve conduction studies evaluate large fiber function, small-fiber neuropathy cannot be ruled out if results of NCS are normal
• Addiction history may affect decision to prescribe opioids.	*Three-phase nuclear medicine bone scan*

Table 23.2 (continued)

History	Deep tendon reflexes
• Consider safety of opioids, muscle relaxants, and/or hypnotics in the presence of alcohol use	• May aid in the diagnosis of complex regional pain syndrome. However, CRPS may be present despite negative study
• If substance abuse positive, consider earlier involvement with a psychologist, psychiatrist, or addiction specialist	*Clinical biochemistry*
Physical examination	• Perform tests to help identify cause of neuropathy; i.e., glucose tolerance test, thyroid function, vitamin B12 levels, CD 4+ T-lymphocyte count, etc.
Gross motor examination	
• Motor weakness may occur distal to involved nerves	
• Attempt to distinguish between true weakness and weakness secondary to pain.	

hair or nail growth, and temperature abnormalities are present or absent. In addition, attention should be paid to a musculoskeletal evaluation including the status of the joints, muscles, and ligaments noting any swelling, laxity, tenderness, and limitation of motion are present.

Several aspects of the neurological examination specific to neuropathic pain should be included while performing a standard neurological examination. These specific tests are part of the sensory examination and are helpful in confirming the presence or absence of neuropathic pain disorder. Traditional sharp–dull discrimination testing is not adequate and can be misleading in patients with neuropathic pain syndromes as it does not include testing for allodynia, hyperalgesia, or other positive sensory phenomena.

As previously mentioned, patients may present with positive and/or negative sensory symptoms. This means that stimuli such as light touch, pinprick, cold, warm, vibration, and two point discrimination may be perceived as either exaggerated or diminished. In patients with positive neuropathic symptoms, there are often correlative signs on the physical examination. Simple bedside tests, such as the use of von Frey filaments, a tuning fork, and pinprick testing, are helpful somatosensory tests. Allodynia, for example, may be elicited by lightly stroking the involved area or by testing with a cold instrument. Hyperalgesia or hyperpathia may be elicited during pinprick testing. These examination findings are important, because they are unique to patient with neuropathic pain.

Patients with neuropathic pain may experience motor symptoms and signs which could also be viewed as negative and/or positive motor signs and symptoms. Negative signs include hypotonia, decreased muscle strength, tremor, dystonia, and dyskinesia. Positive signs may include hypertonia, spasm, and exaggerated deep tendon reflexes.

Despite this, it is common for there to be relatively modest demonstrable clinical neurological deficits in patients with significant neuropathic pain, and in some conditions there may be a completely normal clinical examination. This is the rule in conditions such as trigeminal and glossopharyngeal neuralgia and it also occurs in many patients with post-herpetic neuralgia. In addition, some patients, particularly those with what appears to be small-fiber neuropathies or specific nerve injuries, may also have essentially normal clinical examinations and pain may be their only manifestation of neural dysfunction. It must be remembered, therefore, that a lack of significant physical findings does not exclude the diagnosis of neuropathic pain and should not be dismissed as psychogenic pain or as malingering.

Treatment Modalities

When considering treatment options for patients with neuropathic pain, it must be remembered that behavioral and psychiatric comorbidities are very common in patients with chronic pain and may be a consequence of delayed diagnosis or inappropriate treatment. In particular depression, anxiety disorders, and sleep disturbances are more common among patients with chronic or neuropathic pain than seen in the general population and may be accompanied or complicated by issues of substance abuse. It is, therefore, important that these factors be taken into consideration and appropriate consultation or referral be made to psychologists, psychiatrists, and addiction medicine professionals when indicated. Medical treatment is often the first-line therapy for neuropathic pain syndromes. Multiple mechanisms appear to mediate the symptoms of neuropathic pain, and current treatments as well as novel therapeutics are believed to interact with these mechanisms at different sites in the nervous system as outlined in Table 23.3.

Table 23.3 Symptom/mechanism-based treatment of neuropathic pain.

Symptom	Mechanism	Target	Drug
Spontaneous pain, paresthesias, neuroma hypersensitivity	Sodium-channel upregulation, redistribution, altered expression	Sodium channels sensitive to TTX Sodium channels resistant to TTX	Sodium-channel blockers Antiepileptics: carbamazepine, lamotrigine Antiarrhythmics: lidocaine, mexilitine, TCA's
Spontaneous pain	α_2 receptor expression, sympathetic sprouting	α_2 receptor antagonists, nerve growth factor/trKA	Phentolamine, guanethidine, nerve growth factor antagonists[a]
Spontaneous pain, hyperalgesia	Increased transmission, reduced inhibition	N-type calcium-channel receptors, also alpha$_2$, GABA, neurokinin 1, adenosine, P2X$_2$, kainite, CCK	Opiates, gabapentin, pregabalin, clonidine, TCA's, and SNRIs
Spontaneous pain, pressure hyperalgesia, thermal hyperalgesia, neurogenic inflammation	Peripheral sensitization	Neurokinin 1, sodium channels resistant to TTX, nerve growth factor, vanilloid receptor-1 desensitization	Capsaicin, neurokinin-1-R-antagonists, sodium-channel blockers, nerve growth factors
Tactile (dynamic) hyperalgesia, cold hyperalgesia, pinprick hyperalgesia	Central sensitization	NMDA receptors, neurokinin-1 receptors, neuronal nitric oxide synthase, protein kinase gamma	NMDA antagonists: ketamine, dextromethorphan, amantidine, memantine, neurokinin-1 receptor antagonists[a], neuronal nitric oxide synthase inhibitors[a]

[a]In clinical/preclinical development.

Table 23.4 Pharmacologic treatments for neuropathic pain

Topical agents	Lidocaine patch 5%[a], capsaicin
Antidepressants	
TCAs	Amitriptyline, nortriptyline, desipramine,imipramine, doxepin
SNRIs	Duloxetine[a], venlafaxine
Anticonvulsants	Carbamazepine[a], valproate, lamotrigine, toprimate, oxcarbazepine, gabapentin[a]pregabalin[a]
Opioids	Oxycodone, tramadol, morphine, fentanyl, hydromorphone

[a]FDA approved for use in various neuropathic pain syndromes.

The four major classes of medications for treating neuropathic pain syndromes are antidepressants, anticonvulsants, opioid analgesics, and topical agents (Table 23.4). Additionally, other adjunctive medications may be of benefit including antiarrhythmics, non-opioid analgesics, and NMDA antagonists.

Pharmacologic
Antidepressants
Tricyclic antidepressants (TCA) have been shown to be safe and effective in the treatment of neuropathic pain. Commonly used agents include amitriptyline, nortriptyline, imipramine, desipramine. These agents have been studied in double-blind, randomized controlled trials with results suggesting that each of them reduces pain independent of their effect on depression (Portenoy et al. 1984). TCAs are thought to exert their analgesic effect by inhibiting norepinephrine and serotonin reuptake in the central nervous system. Unfortunately, they also effect cholinergic, histaminergic, and adrenergic transmission, resulting in some limiting side effects. These include sedation, orthostasis, cardiac arrhythmia, and urinary retention which may limit their usefulness in certain patient populations, especially the elderly.

Since the introduction of tricyclic antidepressants, a number of newer generation of antidepressants have been developed. The selective serotonin and norepinephrine reuptake inhibitors (SNRI) are among the newest class of antidepressants, and their ability to reduce pain in various neuropathic syndromes has also been examined.

Duloxetine (Cymbalta®; Eli Lily, Indianapolis, IN) has recently been approved by the Food and Drug Administration (FDA) for the treatment of diabetic neuropathic pain. Goldstein and coworkers (Allen 2008) reported on a randomized trial of 457 patients treated for 12 weeks with 20, 60, or 120 mg a day of duloxetine. The 60 and 120 mg a day doses demonstrated greater improvement than placebo in the 24-h average pain score beginning 1 week after randomization. Duloxetine has a similar pharmacology to venlafaxine in that it is a reuptake inhibitor for serotonin and norepinephrine. It differs from venlafaxine in that it is a norepinephrine reuptake inhibitor at lower doses. The clinical significance of this difference has yet to be demonstrated; however, there is clinical evidence that venlafaxine is also useful in the treatment of neuropathic pain syndromes (Guldiken et al. 2004, Yucel et al. 2005).

Anticonvulsants
The classic anticonvulsant agents phenytoin and carbamazepine have been used in the treatment of neuropathic pain since the 1960s. Anticonvulsants are thought to inhibit seizures

by multiple mechanisms, including functional blockade of voltage-gated sodium channels, functional blockade of voltage-gated calcium channels, direct or indirect enhancement of inhibitory gamma aminobutyric acid (GABA)-ergic neurotransmission, and inhibition of glutamatergic neurotransmission (Challapalli 2005). The result is that they reduce the neuronal hyperexcitability that is fundamental to seizure disorders.

Because neuropathic pain is also characterized by neuronal hyperexcitability (Artus et al. 2007), clinicians and researchers have reasoned that anticonvulsants might alleviate it through similar mechanisms of action. This supposition is supported by a substantial amount of empirical data on the clinical effectiveness of anticonvulsants in neuropathic pain, as well as multiple studies that have been the subject of recent systematic reviews (Dworkin et al. 2007, Stacey 2005).

Gabapentin, for example, is an α-2-delta subunit voltage-gated calcium-channel antagonist that has repeatedly demonstrated analgesic efficacy and improvements in mood and sleep in several randomized controlled trials (Gilron 2007, Finnerup et al. 2007). Similarly, pregabalin, a gabapentin analogue with a similar mechanism, higher calcium-channel affinity, and better bioavailability, has also been shown to be effective in several RCTs in diabetic peripheral neuropathy and postherpetic neuralgia (Finnerup et al. 2007). Other anticonvulsants, including valproate, lamotrigine, and topiramate, have had equivocal results (Finnerup et al. 2007).

Opioids

Consensus guidelines and systematic reviews consistently indicate that antidepressant agent and anticonvulsants represent the first-line treatments in the management of neuropathic pain (Argoff et al. 2006, Gilron et al. 2006, Finnerup et al. 2005). Unfortunately, these drugs provide effective analgesia in less than half of this patient population (Sindrup and Jensen 1999).

There has been considerable controversy surrounding the use of opioid analgesics for chronic non-malignant pain in general and neuropathic pain in particular. It is well known that there are short-term and potential long-term adverse effects associated with opioid analgesia. In the short term, opioids produce significant nausea and constipation in 20–30% of patients and somnolence and dizziness in another 10–20% (Eisenberg et al. 2005). Fortunately, some degree of tolerance to the side effects occurs over time and nausea and constipation can often be managed with anti-emetics and a bowel regimen, respectively. Analgesic tolerance, defined as the need for increasing doses of an opioid drug to maintain the same analgesic effect, is relatively uncommon in the clinical setting. Similarly, the risk of psychological dependence or addiction is relatively low in the absence of a past history of substance abuse (Gilron et al. 2006).

Complicating this picture further is a recent finding that suggests the long-term use of opioids may lead to the development of abnormal sensitivity to pain or paradoxical opioid-induced hyperalgesia which is likely NMDA receptor mediated (Brodner and Taub 1978). The role of NMDA antagonists to reverse this phenomenon is being investigated. Additionally, the chronic use of opioids induces various hormonal changes that may be clinically significant when used long term. Opioids act on the hypothalamic–pituitary–gonadal axis to increase prolactin and decrease gonadotrophic hormones which in turn decrease testosterone (Ballantyne and Mao 2003) which results in a decreased libido and predispose patients to osteoporosis. Recent evidence also strongly suggests that opioids may alter immune function and opioid-related receptors have been found to reside on immune cells (Makman 1994). However, pain itself can impair immune function and it is not clear that long-term opioid use leads to clinically significant immunosuppression.

Despite the shortcomings the use of opioids in the treatment of neuropathic pain has been firmly established (Allen 2008). A recent systematic review of eight high-quality RCT lasting up to 8 weeks demonstrated clinically important analgesia in neuropathic pain states (Eisenberg et al. 2005). Three trials involved morphine, three involved oxycodone and there were single trials testing methadone and levorphanol. All of these trials demonstrated significant benefit relative to placebo or a dose-dependent analgesic response and demonstrating a 20–30% reduction in pain intensity. RCTs in patients with postherpetic neuralgia given controlled-release oxycodone (Watson and Babul 1998, Watson et al. 2003) or controlled-release morphine (Raja et al. 2002) have shown a significant reduction in pain intensity with variable improvement in sleep and disability. Trials of controlled-release oxycodone in painful diabetic neuropathy showed a more consistent overall improvement in pain, sleep, and ability to function (Watson et al. 2003, Gimbel et al. 2003).

Methadone is a synthetic opioid analgesic that may be particularly helpful in the management of neuropathic pain because it has NMDA antagonist properties that can reverse a major generator of neuropathic pain. Methadone is also attractive because it has excellent oral bioavailability, duration of action of at least 8 h with repetitive dosing and very low cost. However, it has an elimination half-life of 24–36 h or longer, which requires close observation and careful dosing adjustments during the titration phase. There are two small randomized controlled trials demonstrating benefit from methadone in chronic neuropathic pain (Gagnon et al. 2003, Morley et al. 2003) and survey data suggest efficacy in mixed nociceptive-neuropathic pain conditions (Moulin et al. 2005).

Non-opioid Analgesic Agents

Another relatively recent addition to pain therapy armamentarium is tramadol (Ultram®; Ortho-McNeil-Janssen, Titusville, NJ), a centrally acting, synthetic, non-narcotic analgesic that has been available in the United States since 1995. Its two mechanisms of action are (1) low-affinity binding to mu opioid receptors and (2) weak inhibition of norepinephrine and serotonin reuptake. Tramadol is, therefore, a weak opioid agonist and mimics some of the properties of tricyclic antidepressants (TCAs). A recent double-blind, randomized, placebo-controlled trail in patients with painful diabetic neuropathy found that those receiving an average dose of 210 mg/day of tramadol had significant pain relief with better physical and social functioning compared with patients receiving placebo (Finnerup et al. 2005). Most frequently occurring side effects were headache, constipation, nausea, and somnolence.

Topical Agents

Topical analgesics for neuropathic pain are attractive treatment options because they deliver medication locally and are usually well tolerated. Topical lidocaine (5%) is a peripherally acting topical analgesic that exerts its effect by transdermally delivering small amounts of lidocaine sufficient to block sodium channels on small pain fibers but insufficient to interfere with normal conduction of larger sensory fibers. When applied to a painful area, it produces local analgesia, with minimal systemic absorption and, therefore, minimum risk of systemic side effects or drug–drug interactions. In double-blind randomized controlled studies the lidoderm patch was evaluated as an adjunctive add-on medication for the treatment of chronic peripheral neuropathic pain syndromes from various causes and found to be effective in reducing both ongoing pain and allodynia (Meier et al. 2003).

In addition to the FDA-approved 5% lidocaine patch, other topical treatments include capsaicin, a vanilloid compound isolated from chili peppers that is available in formulations that do not require a prescription. It is believed to elevate pain threshold through depletion of substance P from the membranes of c-nociceptive fibers and through induction of calcitonin gene-related peptide.

Nonpharmacologic
Physical Modalities
One of the simplest forms of non-invasive, nonpharmacological treatment for pain is transcutaneous electrical nerve stimulation (TENS). These devices have been used since the 1960s, following the development of the gate control theory of pain transmission put forth by Melzack and Wall (1965). TENS attempts to control pain by stimulating peripheral nerve afferents. By stimulating these afferents at different amplitudes and frequencies, TENS may activate descending inhibitory pain fibers and block input from afferents that are signaling neuropathic pain. This technique may produce reasonable short-term improvement in pain, but long-term efficacy is unlikely. Nevertheless, given its usefulness in short-term applications, TENS units are often used as adjuncts to help patients complete rehabilitation exercises that would otherwise be too painful (Meyler et al. 1994).

Psychological and Behavioral Modalities
Psychological factors such as mood, beliefs about pain, and coping style have been found to play an important role in an individual's adjustment to chronic pain. If pain persists over time, a person may avoid performing or engaging in regular activities for fear of further injury or increased pain. This can include activities such as work, social activities, or hobbies. As the individual withdraws and becomes less active, their muscles may become weaker, they may begin to gain or lose weight, and their overall physical conditioning may decline. This can contribute to the belief that one is *disabled*. As pain persists, the person may develop negative beliefs about their experience of pain (e.g., this is never going to get better) or negative thoughts about themselves (e.g., I'm worthless to my family because I can't work.). These types of thoughts, along with decreased participation in enjoyable and reinforcing activities, may lead a person to feel depressed and anxious.

One particular psychological treatment approach that has been found to be effective in helping patients to reduce pain, disability, and distress is cognitive behavioral therapy (CBT). CBT for chronic pain management involves modifying negative thoughts related to pain (e.g., this pain is going to kill me, I'm worthless because of the pain, I can't cope with this pain) and on increasing a person's activity level and productive functioning. This approach has been shown to be highly effective in promoting positive cognitive and behavioral changes in individuals with chronic pain.

Although there are no large-scale meta-analyses of CBT in the management of neuropathic pain, cognitive behavioral therapy has been found to be effective in patients who had chronic pain from various causes (Morley and Keefe 2007). The few trials that have been done indicate that CBT and other psychological techniques may also be helpful in some forms of neuropathic pain (Evans et al. 2003). Studies of chronic pain management suggest that a combination of psychological, pharmacological, and physical therapies, tailored to the needs of the individual patient, may be the best approach (Turk et al. 2008).

Alternative and Complementary Therapies

There has been a recognized increasing demand for and acceptance of complementary and alternative medicine (CAM) therapies in the United States. In a national survey published in the *Journal of the American Medical Association* (JAMA) in 1998, Eisenberg et al. found that the number of visits to alternative therapy centers was twice that of visits to primary care physicians and that the money spent on complementary and alternative medicine was nearly equal to out-of-pocket expenditures for conventional care (Eisenberg et al. 1998).

Most multidisciplinary pain centers have adopted some form of complementary and alternative medicine in an effort to treat neuropathic pain syndromes. Much of this effort has been prompted by patient demand for nonpharmacologic alternatives to treat pain. The complementary treatments often used include those listed in Table 23.5.

Table 23.5 Complementary and alternative medicine.

Acupuncture	Chiropractic	Yoga
Acupressure	Massage	Reiki
Moxibustion	Hypnosis	Therapeutic touch
Tai Chi	Guided imagery	Naturopathy
Herbal therapy	Biofeedback	Homeopathy
Qi Gong	Meditation	Prayer

Overall, the evidence is not fully convincing for most CAM treatments in providing significant benefit in relieving neuropathic pain. However, it must be pointed out that numerous methodological difficulties in assessing complex interventions relating to the design of adequate control groups, blinding, and a lack of sufficient funding may be some of the reasons for the small number of studies carried out thus far. Nonetheless, small studies have shown some positive benefit and should be viewed as encouraging and warranting further study.

Interventional Therapies

Patients with neuropathic pain who do not respond or do not have a sufficient response to conventional treatment may benefit from neuromodulation techniques. The gate control theory, introduced by Melzack and Wall in 1965, provided the theoretical foundation for the use of implanted electrical stimulation (Melzack and Wall 1965). Although the specific mechanism of action of SCS remains elusive, neural and neurochemical changes, perhaps resulting from stimulation in the dorsal roots, dorsal root entry zone, or dorsal columns, have been implicated.

The systems in current use employ a totally implantable impulse generator system that utilizes an implantable receiver and external transmitter. The system is flexible to accept multiple leads, depending upon the need for bilateral extremity stimulation or wider unilateral or axial coverage. Similarly, various electrode configurations exist, varying in the number and spacing of electrodes. It is also possible to take advantage of complex programming options to fine-tune or change stimulation patterns.

Prior to permanent placement, a test stimulation is performed. Generally, temporary percutaneous stimulator leads are used for this purpose. Once an appropriate stimulation pattern is obtained, most protocols require at least a 50% reduction in pain scores. The length of the trial period varies but usually ranges from 3 to 7 days in most centers.

Lead migration and breakage are common problems with long-term stimulation. Lead migration may produce unwanted paresthesias or diminish benefit in the original area of stimulation. This can sometime be overcome by reprogramming of the electrode but may require lead replacement. Serious infection, bleeding, and nerve injury are uncommon complications. Impulse generator failure is unlikely; however, fully implantable generators will require replacement, depending upon use and battery life. Other contraindications to implantation such as the presence of localized infection, systemic sepsis, severe immune suppression, and coagulopathies are similar to other implantable devices.

The most critical issues in patient selection consist of identifying a well-founded diagnosis and the presence of specific neuropathic or ischemic pain states. A multidisciplinary approach including a psychological evaluation is often recommended.

Treatment Strategy

Effective pain management in these cases requires ongoing evaluation, patient education, and reassurance. Diagnostic evaluation of treatable underlying conditions (e.g., spinal cord compression, herniated disc, neoplasm) should continue concurrently with ongoing pain management efforts. Patients should be provided with education regarding the natural history of their condition and realistic treatment expectations (e.g., current treatments are not curative and analgesia is rarely complete). Unfortunately, as much as we would like, no single drug or therapeutic modality works for all neuropathic pain states. Given the multiplicity of etiologic causes, diversity of pain mechanisms involved, and individual patient circumstances, treatment regimens must be individualized.

Treatments with the lowest risk of adverse effects should be tried first. Evidence supporting conservative nonpharmacologic treatments (e.g., physiotherapy, exercise, transcutaneous electrical nerve stimulation, CBT, acupuncture) is limited; however, given their presumed safety, nonpharmacologic treatments should be considered whenever appropriate. Simple analgesics (e.g., acetaminophen, NSAIDs) are usually ineffective in pure neuropathic pain but may help with a coexisting nociceptive condition (e.g., sciatica with musculoskeletal low back pain). Additionally, early referrals to a pain clinic for nerve blocks or other interventional therapy may be warranted in some cases to facilitate physiotherapy and pain rehabilitation.

Needless to say, neuropathic pain is best managed with a multidisciplinary approach; however, several different treatments can be initiated in the primary care setting and a simplified treatment algorithm is outlined in Table 23.6.

Despite the previously noted treatment limitations, it is important to remember that even a 30% pain reduction is clinically important to patients (Farrar et al. 2001). Other than analgesia, factors to consider when individualizing therapy include tolerability, other benefits (e.g., improved sleep, mood, and quality of life), low likelihood of serious adverse events, and cost-effectiveness to the patient and the healthcare system.

Table 23.6 Algorithm for the management of neuropathic pain.

Step 1	Pain assessment, history and physical examination, obtain release of information to review previous diagnostic studies and treatment records	
Step 2	Consider nonpharmacologic modalities - i.e., physiotherapies, psychological interventions such as cognitive behavioral therapy, bio/neuro-feedback, or early referral for nerve blocks in some cases to facilitate rehabilitation in complex regional pain syndromes.	
Step 3	Initiate first-line monotherapy (gabapentin or pregabalin or tricyclic antidepressant (TCA) or serotonin–norepinephrine reuptake inhibitor (SNRI)	
Response	*Ineffective or not tolerated*	*Partial treatment response*
Step 4	Switch to alternative first-line drug monotherapy (TCA or SNRI or gabapentin or pregabalin)	Consider adding first-line drug (TCA or SNRI or gabapentin or pregabalin)
Response	*Ineffective or not tolerated*	*Partial treatment response*
Step 5	Initiate monotherapy with tramadol or opioid analgesic, consider use of opioid risk screening tool, medication management agreement, and informed consent	Consider adding tramadol or opioid analgesic, consider use of opioid risk screening tool, medication management agreement, and informed consent
Response	*Ineffective or not tolerated*	
Step 6	Refer patient to pain specialty clinic for consideration of third-line drugs, interventional treatments, and pain rehabilitation programs	

Although little is known about whether the response to one drug predicts the response to another, combining different drugs may result in improved results at lower doses and with fewer side effects. However, if the first oral medication tried is ineffective or not tolerated, one might switch to alternate monotherapy. In the event that all of the first-line oral monotherapies tried are ineffective or poorly tolerated, we would then recommend initiating monotherapy with tramadol or an opioid analgesic.

Many patients with neuropathic pain currently receive drug combinations (Gilron and Bailey 2003), often in the absence of supportive evidence. Nevertheless, clinical experience suggests that poly-pharmacy may be helpful. For example, in a recent RCT, analgesia with a morphine–gabapentin combination was found to be superior to treatment with either drug alone (Gilron et al. 2005). Therefore, in the event of a partial response to any single drug, one could add an alternate drug. Future trials are needed to evaluate optimal drug combinations and dose ratios as well as safety, compliance, and cost-effectiveness. If none of the above treatments is effective or tolerated, referral to a pain clinic is warranted for consideration of third-line drugs, interventional treatments, and pain rehabilitation programs.

Summary

Neuropathic pain remains a clinical challenge for treatment. Any medication used to treat neuropathy must be weighed for benefits and risks before using. It may take several trials to find an effective medication or combination of medications. Patients may need support throughout the process. Neuropathic pain often requires a combination of medication and nonpharmacologic modalities in order to achieve adequate pain relief. Currently available therapies clearly show varying degrees of clinical efficacy, but it is hoped that future advances in this active field of investigation will further expand the clinicians' armamentarium of treatments for this challenging pain syndrome.

Case Scenarios

Gerald W. Grass, MD, FAAMA

Case 1: Tom

Tom, a 57-year-old man with a 15-year history of type 2 diabetes mellitus, presents to his primary care provider complaining of sensations of pain alternating with tingling and burning in both feet and ankles. The pain, which is consistently moderate to severe during the day, frequently worsens at night with occasional unpredictable spikes that he describes as "unbearable." These exacerbations do not correlate with any obvious activity nor do they occur at consistent times. The pain was initially limited to his feet, but during the past 6–9 months has spread to his ankles, sometimes experienced as a burning sensation and at other times as tingling. The pain interferes with his ability to walk, socialize with friends, and sleep.

What further information would you seek from the patient?
It is very important to gather information regarding his past medical problems and details of his medications.

Tom is a type 2 diabetic and overweight with a BMI of 32 kg/m². He is taking metformin 1,000 mg/day and hemoglobin A1c levels are consistently less than 6.5%. He sometimes uses Tylenol 1,000 mg TID or Motrin 600 mg TID for the discomfort but reports no relief. However, he exercises routinely despite the pain.

What do you look for in the physical examination?
The history is suggestive of neuropathic origins of pain. A local examination along with detailed neurological assessment is mandatory. Evaluation of the autonomic nervous system using appropriate tests is also important if you are planning an intervention under anesthesia.

Physical examination revealed normal skin color and temperature. Tom reports no vibration sensation at either great toe when tested with a 128 Hz tuning fork and demonstrates a decrease in vibratory sensation to his knees bilaterally. He experienced discomfort over the dorsum of both feet when tested with a cotton-tipped applicator and experienced the application of an alcohol wipe as a burning sensation. His ankle reflexes were absent bilaterally but present at the knees and upper extremities.

What is your diagnosis? How will you manage this patient?
Tom is suffering from painful diabetic neuropathy. The treatment could be initiated with a tricyclic antidepressant. Other options would be gabapentin and pregabalin.

Tom was started on duloxetine beginning at 30 mg daily, which was increased after 10 days to 60 mg daily. At a 1 month follow-up appointment, Tom reported some improvement in his symptoms, stating that the burning and tingling sensations had lessened, allowing him more mobility during the day but that he continued to have paroxysms of pain at night that frequently disturb his sleep. In discussion with his PCP, Tom agreed to add gabapentin to his medication regimen. He was started on 100 mg three times per day and titrated up to 400 mg three times per day over 30 days. At a 3-month follow-up visit Tom reported the pain as significantly better, he is able to lead an almost normal life. He now sleeps better and free of any night pains.

Case 2: Michael

Michael is a 47-year-old construction worker presenting for follow-up evaluation for complex regional pain syndrome (CRPS). While managing a construction site 3 years ago, Tom fell approximately 9 ft from a rooftop, sustaining a tibial plateau fracture to his right leg. He underwent an open reduction and internal fixation. His post-operative recovery and rehabilitation were going well until 3 months following the accident, when he began to experience excruciating pain in his entire right leg. He described the pain as intensely burning as if it were on fire and that the leg had become sensitive to the slightest touch. He was unable to sleep because of the pain he experienced when the bed linen would touch his leg and wake him up. He states that he also began to notice that the leg would swell and change color (sometimes reddish, other times mottled following exposure to cold) and that he no longer had any hair on his right leg. He was seen by a number of physicians and received numerous diagnoses until last year, when a neurologist diagnosed him with CRPS.

What are the possible conditions? How would you make the diagnosis?
The diagnosis of CPRS is clinical. Michael's problems started following the injury and the surgery that followed it – therefore it is likely CRPS type I. However, certain conditions can mimic it. These include neoplasms, arthritis (septic, degenerative, gout, SLE), avascular bone necrosis, conversion/self-harm, and dis-/non-use. Certain tests, such as quantitative sensory testing, autonomic function tests, temperature measurement, vascular flow measurements, and imaging studies (bone scintigraphy, bone densitometry, CT, MRI), can be performed to rule these out.

Michael tried various medications to control the pain including tramadol, duloxetine, carbamazepine, gabapentin, and oxycodone. He reports that none of these treatments sufficiently controlled his pain and he is not using them anymore. He was also seen by a pain specialist who performed several nerve blocks that helped with the pain but only temporarily. He is very frustrated with his condition, he states that he can no longer work because of the pain, and he is afraid that he will soon lose his home. He admits that he is irritable at times and feels depressed occasionally, but denies suicidal ideation. His medical history is otherwise unremarkable.

What is your next step?
You have to take a detailed history and perform a systematic physical examination in order to confirm the diagnosis of CRPS and to rule out other diseases. His conditions might have changed since he saw his previous attending physician. Depending on your assessment, you may need to order further investigations as necessary.

His average pain score is 6–7 on a scale of 0–10. It can go up to 10 "on a bad day" and at night. His physical examination is notable for edema of the right leg to the level of the knee, associated with red reticulation of the skin and apparent hair loss. The right leg and foot are cooler than the left, but popliteal and dorsalis pedis pulses are intact bilaterally. He has widespread allodynia and hyperalgesia on clinical examination with preservation of muscle mass, tone, and strength. Deep tendon reflexes are present in all extremities and found to be normal.

What are the options now available to help Michael?
Michael has been suffering from CRPS for the last few years. He has failed to respond to pharmacotherapy and other forms of treatment. He is in distress. Unfortunately, the available options are limited. Spinal cord stimulation is one option, but it is an invasive procedure. The other option is to undergo a pain management program which is not a cure in its own merit.

Following an extensive review of his past medical history, prior treatment regimens, results of investigations, and consultation with a psychologist, Michael agrees to a trial of neuromodulation with a spinal cord stimulator. One week later Tom is seen in the operating room by an interventional pain specialist who, under local anesthesia, inserts a percutaneous epidural electrode array and connects it to an external pulse generator. Tom is allowed to go home following the procedure and is asked to return in 5 days for follow-up. Five days later Tom returns to the office and reports that his pain is much better and that its intensity has been reduced by 70%. He is able to play with his children and work around the house. He reports that the swelling has subsided and the leg no longer changes color in the cold. He is pleased with the trial and is anxious to proceed to a permanent implantation.

Following permanent implantation of the spinal cord stimulator, Michael experiences a greater than 50% reduction is his pain intensity and is now able to perform all of his activities of daily living. He also reports being able to sleep much better at night.

References

Allen SC. Neuropathic pain – the case for opioid therapy. Oncology 2008;74(suppl 1):76–82.

Argoff CE, Backonja MM, Belgrade MJ, et al. Consensus guidelines: treatment planning and options. Diabetic peripheral neuropathic pain. Mayo Clin Proc. 2006;81(4 suppl):S12–25.

Artus M, Croft P, Lewis M. The use of CAM and conventional treatments among primary care consulters with chronic musculoskeletal pain. BMC Fam Pract. 2007;8:26.

Ballantyne JC, Mao J. Opioid therapy for chronic pain. N Engl J Med. 2003;349(20):1943–53.

Baron R. Peripheral neuropathic pain: from mechanisms to symptoms. Clin J Pain. 2000;16(2 suppl):S12–20.

Bennett MI, Attal N, Backonja MM, et al. Using screening tools to identify neuropathic pain. Pain 2007;127(3):199–203.

Besson JM. The neurobiology of pain. Lancet 1999;353(9164):1610–5.

Bouhassira D, Lanteri-Minet M, Attal N, Laurent B, Touboul C. Prevalence of chronic pain with neuropathic characteristics in the general population. Pain 2008;136(3):380–7.

Brodner RA, Taub A. Chronic pain exacerbated by long-term narcotic use in patients with nonmalignant disease: clinical syndrome and treatment. Mt Sinai J Med. 1978;45(2):233–7.

Campbell CM, Edwards RR, Carmona C, et al. Polymorphisms in the GTP cyclohydrolase gene (GCH1) are associated with ratings of capsaicin pain. Pain 2009;141(1–2):114–8.

Carpenter JS, Sloan P. Andrykowski MA, et al. Risk factors for pain after mastectomy/lumpectomy. Cancer Pract. 1999;7(2):66–70.

Challapalli V, Tremont-Lukats IW, McNicol ED, Lau J, Carr DB. Systemic administration of local anesthetic agents to relieve neuropathic pain. Cochrane Database Syst Rev. 2005(4):CD003345.

Cherry CL, Skolasky RL, Lal L, et al. Antiretroviral use and other risks for HIV-associated neuropathies in an international cohort. Neurology 2006;66(6):867–73.

Coyle DE. Partial peripheral nerve injury leads to activation of astroglia and microglia which parallels the development of allodynic behavior. Glia 1998;23(1):75–83.

Cummins TR, Sheets PL, Waxman SG. The roles of sodium channels in nociception: implications for mechanisms of pain. Pain 2007;131(3):243–57.

Dworkin RH, O'Connor AB, Backonja M, et al. Pharmacologic management of neuropathic pain: evidence-based recommendations. Pain 2007;132(3):237–51.

Eisenberg E, McNicol ED, Carr DB. Efficacy and safety of opioid agonists in the treatment of neuropathic pain of nonmalignant origin: systematic review and meta-analysis of randomized controlled trials. JAMA 2005;293(24):3043–52.

Eisenberg DM, Davis RB, Ettner SL, et al. Trends in alternative medicine use in the United States. 1990–1997: results of a follow-up national survey. JAMA 1998;280(18):1569–75.

Evans S, Fishman B, Spielman L, Haley A. Randomized trial of cognitive behavior therapy versus supportive psychotherapy for HIV-related peripheral neuropathic pain. Psychosomatics 2003;44(1):44–50.

Farrar JT, Young JP, Jr, LaMoreaux L, Werth JL, Poole RM. Clinical importance of changes in chronic pain intensity measured on an 11-point numerical pain rating scale. Pain 2001;94(2):149–58.

Finnerup NB, Otto M, Jensen TS, Sindrup SH. An evidence-based algorithm for the treatment of neuropathic pain. MedGenMed 2007;9(2):36.

Finnerup NB, Otto M, McQuay HJ, Jensen TS, Sindrup SH. Algorithm for neuropathic pain treatment: an evidence based proposal. Pain 2005;118(3):289–305.

Gilron I, Bailey JM. Trends in opioid use for chronic neuropathic pain: a survey of patients pursuing enrollment in clinical trials. Can J Anaesth. 2003;50(1):42–7.

Gilron I, Bailey JM, Tu D, Holden RR, Weaver DF, Houlden RL. Morphine, gabapentin, or their combination for neuropathic pain. N Engl J Med. 2005;352(13):1324–34.

Gagnon B, Almahrezi A, Schreier G. Methadone in the treatment of neuropathic pain. Pain Res Manage. 2003;8(3):149–54.

Gilron I. Gabapentin and pregabalin for chronic neuropathic and early postsurgical pain: current evidence and future directions. Curr Opin Anaesthesiol. 2007;20(5):456–72.

Gilron I, Watson CP, Cahill CM, Moulin DE. Neuropathic pain: a practical guide for the clinician. CMAJ 2006;175(3):265–75.

Gimbel JS, Richards P, Portenoy RK. Controlled-release oxycodone for pain in diabetic neuropathy: a randomized controlled trial. Neurology 2003;60(6):927–34.

Guldiken S, Guldiken B, Arikan E, Altun Ugur B, Kara M, Tugrul A. Complete relief of pain in acute painful diabetic neuropathy of rapid glycaemic control (insulin neuritis) with venlafaxine HCL. Diabetes Nutr Metab. 2004;17(4):247–9.

Gustorff B, Dorner T, Likar R, et al. Prevalence of self-reported neuropathic pain and impact on quality of life: a prospective representative survey. Acta Anaesthesiol Scand. 2008;52(1):132–6.

Hains BC, Waxman SG. Activated microglia contribute to the maintenance of chronic pain after spinal cord injury. J Neurosci. 2006;26(16):4308–17.

Kim H, Dionne RA. Lack of influence of GTP cyclohydrolase gene (GCH1) variations on pain sensitivity in humans. Mol Pain 2007;3:6.

Maguire MF, Ravenscroft A, Beggs D, Duffy JP. A questionnaire study investigating the prevalence of the neuropathic component of chronic pain after thoracic surgery. Eur J Cardiothorac Surg. 2006;29(5):800–5.

Makman MH. Morphine receptors in immunocytes and neurons. Adv Neuroimmunol. 1994;4(2):69–82.

Matthews EA, Bee LA, Stephens GJ, Dickenson AH. The Cav2.3 calcium channel antagonist SNX-482 reduces dorsal horn neuronal responses in a rat model of chronic neuropathic pain. Eur J Neurosci. 2007;25(12):3561–9.

Meier T, Wasner G, Faust M, et al. Efficacy of lidocaine patch 5% in the treatment of focal peripheral neuropathic pain syndromes: a randomized, double-blind, placebo-controlled study. Pain 2003;106(1–2):151–8.

Melzack R, Wall PD. Pain mechanisms: a new theory. Science 1965;150(699):971–9.

Mersky H, Bogduk N. ed. Classification of chronic pain. Seattle, WA: IASP Press; 1994. pp. 209–14.

Meyler WJ, de Jongste MJ, Rolf CA. Clinical evaluation of pain treatment with electrostimulation: a study on TENS in patients with different pain syndromes. Clin J Pain 1994;10(1):22–7.

Morgello S, Estanislao L, Simpson D, et al. HIV-associated distal sensory polyneuropathy in the era of highly active antiretroviral therapy: the Manhattan HIV Brain Bank. Arch Neurol. 2004;61(4):546–51.

Morley JS, Bridson J, Nash TP, Miles JB, White S, Makin MK. Low-dose methadone has an analgesic effect in neuropathic pain: a double-blind randomized controlled crossover trial. Palliat Med. 2003;17(7):576–87.

Morley S, Keefe FJ. Getting a handle on process and change in CBT for chronic pain. Pain 2007;127(3):197-8.

Moulin DE, Palma D, Watling C, Schulz V. Methadone in the management of intractable neuropathic noncancer pain. Can J Neurol Sci. 2005;32(3):340-3.

Osterberg A, Boivie J, Thuomas KA. Central pain in multiple sclerosis – prevalence and clinical characteristics. Eur J Pain. 2005;9(5):531-42.

Pace MC, Mazzariello L, Passavanti MB, Sansone P, Barbarisi M, Aurilio C. Neurobiology of pain. J Cell Physiol. 2006;209(1):8-12.

Pasero C. Pathophysiology of neuropathic pain. Pain Manage Nurs. 2004;5(4 suppl 1):3-8.

Poobalan AS, Bruce J, King PM, Chambers WA, Krukowski ZH, Smith WC. Chronic pain and quality of life following open inguinal hernia repair. Br J Surg. 2001;88(8):1122-6.

Poobalan AS, Bruce J, Smith WC, King PM, Krukowski ZH, Chambers WA. A review of chronic pain after inguinal herniorrhaphy. Clin J Pain. 2003;19(1):48-54.

Portenoy RK, Rapscak S, Kanner R. Tricyclic antidepressants in chronic pain. Pain 1984;18(2):213-5.

Raja SN, Haythornthwaite JA, Pappagallo M, et al. Opioids versus antidepressants in postherpetic neuralgia: a randomized, placebo-controlled trial. Neurology 2002;59(7):1015-21.

Simpson DM, Kitch D, Evans SR, et al. HIV neuropathy natural history cohort study: assessment measures and risk factors. Neurology 2006;66(11):1679-87.

Sindrup SH and Jensen TS. Efficacy of pharmacological treatments of neuropathic pain: an update and effect related to mechanism of drug action. Pain 1999;83(3):389-400.

Stacey BR. Management of peripheral neuropathic pain. Am J Phys Med Rehabil. 2005;84(3 suppl):S4-16.

Tegeder I, Costigan M, Griffin RS, et al. GTP cyclohydrolase and tetrahydrobiopterin regulate pain sensitivity and persistence. Nat Med. 2006;12(11):1269-77.

Terayama R, Omura S, Fujisawa N, Yamaai T, Ichikawa H, Sugimoto T. Activation of microglia and p38 mitogen-activated protein kinase in the dorsal column nucleus contributes to tactile allodynia following peripheral nerve injury. Neuroscience 2008;153(4):1245-55.

Treede RD, Jensen TS, Campbell JN, et al. Neuropathic pain: redefinition and a grading system for clinical and research purposes. Neurology 2008;70(18):1630-5.

Torrance N, Smith BH, Bennett MI, Lee AJ. The epidemiology of chronic pain of predominantly neuropathic origin. Results from a general population survey. J Pain. 2006;7(4):281-9.

Turk DC, Swanson KS, Tunks ER. Psychological approaches in the treatment of chronic pain patients – when pills, scalpels, and needles are not enough. Can J Psychiatry. 2008;53(4): 213–23.

Ultenius C, Linderoth B, Meyerson BA, Wallin J. Spinal NMDA receptor phosphorylation correlates with the presence of neuropathic signs following peripheral nerve injury in the rat. Neurosci Lett. 2006;399(1–2):85–90.

Veves A, Backonja M, Malik RA. Painful diabetic neuropathy: epidemiology, natural history, early diagnosis, and treatment options. Pain Med. 2008;9(6):660–74.

Vadivelu N, Schreck M, Lopez J, Kodumudi G, Narayan D. Pain after mastectomy and breast reconstruction. Am Surg. 2008;74(4):285–96.

Watson CP, Babul N. Efficacy of oxycodone in neuropathic pain: a randomized trial in postherpetic neuralgia. Neurology 1998;50(6):1837–41.

Watson CP, Moulin D, Watt-Watson J, Gordon A, Eisenhoffer J. Controlled-release oxycodone relieves neuropathic pain: a randomized controlled trial in painful diabetic neuropathy. Pain 2003;105(1–2):71–8.

Waxman SG. Neurobiology: a channel sets the gain on pain. Nature 2006;444(7121):831–2.

Waxman SG, Cummins TR, Dib-Hajj SD, Black JA. Voltage-gated sodium channels and the molecular pathogenesis of pain: a review. J Rehabil Res Dev. 2000;37(5):517–28.

Wilson JA, Garry EM, Anderson HA, et al. NMDA receptor antagonist treatment at the time of nerve injury prevents injury-induced changes in spinal NR1 and NR2B subunit expression and increases the sensitivity of residual pain behaviours to subsequently administered NMDA receptor antagonists. Pain 2005;117(3):421–32.

Yucel A, Ozyalcin S, Koknel Talu G, et al. The effect of venlafaxine on ongoing and experimentally induced pain in neuropathic pain patients: a double blind, placebo controlled study. Eur J Pain. 2005;9(4):407–16.

Zhao P, Waxman SG, Hains BC. Extracellular signal-regulated kinase-regulated microglia-neuron signaling by prostaglandin E2 contributes to pain after spinal cord injury. J Neurosci. 2007;27(9):2357–68.

Chapter 24

Ischemic and Visceral Pain

Robby Romero, MD, Dmitri Souzdalnitski, MD and Trevor Banack, MD

Ischemic Pain

Introduction

Ischemic pain is a distinct type of pain associated with decreased or complete cessation of blood flow rather than direct damage to tissues or neuropathic processes. The variety of pathological conditions which produce arterial or venous blood flow obstruction will be discussed. Ischemic pain is often intractable and requires acute intervention aimed at reperfusion of the ischemic tissues. This chapter describes various pain management tools which may be utilized for treatment of patients with chronic ischemic pain as adjuncts to reperfusion techniques for the most common condition associated with ischemic pain, peripheral arterial occlusive disease.

"Ischemia" is defined as deficient blood supply to a part of the body. Pain is defined as an unpleasant sensory and emotional experience associated with actual or potential tissue damage or described in terms of such damage. Therefore, the ischemic pain can be defined as an unpleasant sensory and emotional experience associated with impaired circulation of blood.

Pathophysiology

Ischemic pain can be viewed as a part of protective mechanisms used to alert the central neural system about impending or actual tissue injury and prompt a living system to respond to this injury. Ischemic pain is different from other types of pain so far that tissue hypoxia, rather than direct tissue or nerve damage, is a main cause of this pain. Namely, tissue hypoxia secondary to decreased blood supply, and resultant tissue acidosis, seems to be the main trigger of the complex pathophysiological reaction to this damage, part of which is pain. Ischemic pain is thought to be mediated by protons. An acid sensing ion channel (ASIC) that may be responsible for the detection and sensing of ischemia has been cloned about 10 years ago. It is expressed in dorsal root ganglia and is also distributed widely throughout the brain (Dubé et al. 2009). Not specific to the etiology of pain, some inflammatory and pain mediators, such as bradykinin, histamine, serotonin, acetylcholine, potassium ions, and adenosine, participate in pain triggering and conduction mechanisms. Additionally, studies of molecular mechanisms of ischemic pain led to the discovery of substance P almost 80 years ago. Substance P was found to be accumulated in ischemic tissues and quickly disappeared after reperfusion

N. Vadivelu et al. (eds.), *Essentials of Pain Management*,
DOI 10.1007/978-0-387-87579-8_24, © Springer Science+Business Media, LLC 2011

(Cervero 1994). A better understanding of pathophysiology of ischemic pain brought by basic studies should promote the development of more effective treatment modalities of this type of pain (Bonica 1990a).

Types of Chronic Ischemic Pain

Ischemic pain can be associated with acute problems such as acute coronary syndrome, arterial embolism, acute deep venous thrombosis, compartment syndrome, ischemic bowel, and other emergencies (Bonica 1990b). This section will outline essentials of pain management of the conditions associated with chronic ischemia. Common and some rare clinical conditions associated with chronic ischemic pain are listed in Table 24.1. Signs and symptoms of these conditions are listed in Table 24.2.

The most common condition associated with ischemic pain is arterial insufficiency. It is present in 5–15% of the adult population older than 55 years. One to two percent of the adult population suffers from critical limb ischemia (CLI), a subset of arterial insufficiency. Chronic CLI, defined as greater than 2 weeks of rest pain, ulcers, or tissue loss attributed to arterial occlusive disease, is associated with great loss of both limb and life. The immediate rescue interventions typically include anticoagulation followed by definitive therapy of acute arterial occlusion (thrombolysis, percutaneous transluminal angioplasty, open or endovascular thromb/embolectomy, or angioplasty). Therapeutic goals in treating patients with CLI after revascularization include reducing cardiovascular risk factors, relieving ischemic pain, healing ulcers, preventing major amputation, improving quality of life, and increasing survival. Traditionally, these aims were achieved through medical therapy, yet may still result in amputation. Nonetheless medical therapy includes local wound care and pressure relief, treatment

Table 24.1 Examples of clinical conditions associated with pain, produced by tissue ischemia.

Types of conditions	Examples
A variety of degenerative and inflammatory vascular conditions: arterial or venous ischemic diseases, microangiopathies, and lymphatic vessel diseases	Atherosclerosis obliterans Thromboangiitis obliterans Takayasu arteritis Giant cell arthritis Other vaculitides Reynold's phenomena/Raynaud's disease Sickle cell disease/priapism Chronic deep venous thrombosis Lymphoedema Diabetic calcyphylaxis Diabetic foot
Conditions affecting bones	Sickle cell disease Avascular necrosis of joints, especially shoulder, hip, or knee (joint "angina")
Conditions affecting muscles	Compartment syndrome Crush injury
Ophthalmologic conditions	Painful ophthalmoplegia Mucormycosis
Neuronal ischemia	Carpal tunnel syndrome

Table 24.2 Signs and symptoms of common and rare conditions associated with pain produced by tissue ischemia.

Condition	Symptoms and diagnosis
Arterial insufficiency	- Claudication (pain with walking)
Atherosclerosis obliterans	- Critical limb ischemia (pain at rest or the presence of ulcer on feet or gangrene); pain often worse at night
Buerger's disease (thromboangiitis obliterans)	- Ischemic signs and symptoms in toes and/or fingers: coldness, pain
Raynaud's phenomenon	- Ischemia of the fingers or toes and sometimes of the ears or nose, marked by severe pallor and pain
	- Frequently occurs following cold or emotional stimuli and is relieved by heat
Deep venous thrombosis	- Pain in affected leg, tenderness along the course of major veins
	- Leg pain on foot dorsiflexion (Hoffman sign)
	- Massive edema with cyanosis and ischemia (phlegmasia cerulean dolens)
Polyarteritis nodosa	Polymorphic skin rashes, persistent livedo reticularis, ischemia, or gangrene
Sickle cell anemia	- Bone pain caused by pressure in marrow and vascular occlusion
	- Visceral pain caused by ischemia (cholecystitis, spleen infarction/rupture, appendicitis, pancreatitis, bowel ischemia)
	- Back pain, chest wall pain
	- Acute chest syndrome
	- Hand and foot syndrome (dactylitis), painful swelling of hands and feet caused by ischemia
Priapism	- Penile erection that is painful and tender
	- Dark blood as well as acidosis on corporal blood gas analysis indicates ischemic (veno-occlusive) priapism
Compartment syndrome	- Pain with passive extension of the fingers is the most common sign of ischemia
	- Irreversible changes might be observed after 6–8 h of ischemia
Avascular (ischemic) necrosis of hip or femur	- Limping
	- Pain at rest, night pain ("bone migranes")
Painful ophthalmoplegia	- Pain, restriction of extraocular eye movements, proptosis, chemosis, and eyelid edema
Mucormycosis	- Slowly progressive, ischemic infarctions that cause necrosis of the skin, nasal mucosa, or palate
	- Common in immunocompromised or diabetic patients
	- Eyelid edema, proptosis, external ophthalmoplegia, fever, and pain.
Erythromelalgia	- Ischemic ulcers may be present and could lead to infection and gangrene
Vascular ulcers	- Pain may vary from nonexistent to extreme
	- Venous ulcers are most common around the middle of the ankle above the malleolus and may extend all the way around the leg

of infection, and aggressive therapy to modify atherosclerotic risk factors, for example, smoking cessation. Nowadays, pain medicine specialists become involved in the subacute care or rehabilitation of these patients because of unique palliative approaches available to them.

Pain Management Modalities for Patients with Peripheral Arterial Occlusive Disease

Traditional Approach

The traditional approach to management of ischemic pain includes administration of the opioids and non-steroidal anti-inflammatory drugs. A wide arsenal of oral and parenteral analgesics is used for patients with ischemic pain in perioperative period as a part of multimodal pain management. However, patients with ischemic type of pain, who are not candidates for a definitive treatment, are frequently experiencing intractable pain in spite of administration of these medications. The effectiveness of traditional analgesics is typically limited by their side effects frequently presenting before their analgesics effects. Therefore, other pain management modalities has been evolving to treat the ischemic pain, as discussed below.

Electrical Stimulation

Electrical stimulation for the relief of pain has progressed from an experimental treatment to being on the threshold of becoming a standard of medical practice. The most common approach, spinal cord stimulation (SCS), was proposed for lower limb ischemic pain treatment about 40 years ago. Clinical trials reported a pain reduction in up to 91% of patients. Pain relief, ulcer healing, and limb salvage seems to be greater in non-diabetic patients, in diabetics without autonomic neuropathy, and in patients with rest pain or ulcer more than in patients with gangrene. Pain relief obtained with SCS was maintained at follow-up while relief after medical treatment quickly disappeared. Implantation of an SCS device in a patient with critical limb ischemia dramatically improves quality of life, and pain relief, according to a recent study, might delay the appearance of ischemic skin lesions and amputation. While SCS could be costly, at advanced stages of the disease presumed long-term benefits could justify the cost. While tens of thousands of devices are implanted every year, the mechanism of action still escapes complete understanding (Foletti et al. 2007).

Other forms of electrical therapy, namely interferential currents and transcutaneous electrical nerve stimulation, can be part of rehabilitation and physical therapy program for patients recovering after definitive surgical treatment of ischemic pain.

Sympathectomy, Neuraxial, and Peripheral Nerve Blocks

Sympathectomy with radiofrequency ablation or chemical sympathectomy is reported to be effective for severe refractory ischemic pain. Reduction in pain, increased sleep, and low incidence of side effects have been reported with transdermal buprenorphine plus epidural (or intrathecal) infusion of morphine with ropivacaine or bupivacaine. Peripheral nerve block (PNB) with inpatients with chronic ischemic lower extremity pain showed that continuous PNB is an effective, safe, and comfortable modality for long-term use in the home setting for patients with intractable chronic pain.

Adjunctive and Experimental Therapies

There are reports about adjunctive and experimental therapies for ischemia-induced pain. Intravenous adenosine resulted in a reduction of intractable ischemic pain for several hours. A potent, dose-dependent analgesic effect of ketamine in ischemic pain was demonstrated about 10 years ago. However, apparently it has not received further development.

A study of sensory and affective ischemic pain discrimination after inhalation of essential oils led to the conclusion that aromatherapy may not elicit a direct analgesic effect but instead may alter affective appraisal of the experience and consequent retrospective evaluation of treatment-related pain. Hyperbaric oxygenation combined with streptokinase for treatment of arterial thromboembolism of the lower extremity resulted in regression of ischemic pain and prolongation of the survival time of tissues compromised by ischemia. One report suggests that hypnosis may serve as an efficacious adjunct to standard medical care in the management of peripheral arterial occlusive disease.

Summary

The pain specialist may offer some unique techniques for palliative management of intractable ischemic pain. Further basic and clinical studies are needed for better understanding of the nature of ischemic pain and developing of effective therapeutic approaches.

Visceral Pain

Definitions

The viscera are the organs of the digestive, respiratory, urogenital, endocrine systems as well as the spleen, the heart and great vessels, the hollow and multilayered walled organs studied in splanchnology (Jain and Morrison 1986). Visceral pain is pain that results from the activation of nociceptors of organs in the thoracic, pelvic, or abdominal cavities (Bonica 1990c). It is felt as a poorly localized aching or cramping sensation that may be referred to the surface of the body. Often the pain originates as a midline sensation that can be referred to a somatic region. Once localized, the presented pain can remain unchanged or progress with hyperalgesia (an increased response to a painful stimulus). The diffuse localization of true visceral pain is probably due to the low density of visceral sensory innervation and extensive divergence of the visceral input within the central nervous system (CNS).

Classifications

Visceral pain can be classified into three categories: (a) true visceral pain, (b) referred pain without hyperalgesia (segmental pain), and (c) referred pain with hyperalgesia (true parietal pain).

True Visceral Pain

Initially true visceral pain is felt during the first instance of the visceral sensation. Regardless of which viscera the pain originates from (esophagus, duodenum, gallbladder, heart, jejunum, pancreas, spleen, stomach), the location of presentation of the pain is constant (Fig. 24.1). The symptoms are poorly defined and usually described as deep, dull sensation. It can vary from slight to maximal intensity and is characteristically associated with marked autonomic phenomena, such as pallor, profuse sweating, nausea, vomiting, changes in blood pressure and heart rate, diarrhea, and changes in body temperature (Table 24.3).

Referred Pain

Referral (or superficialization) is one of the fundamental classifications of visceral pain. If a visceral sensation recurs or intensifies the pain evolves and will not be felt at a common location. The pain often is perceived in superficial somatic structures (i.e., skin, subcutaneous tissue, and muscle) of areas that differ according to the viscus and that are often remote from the primary source of the stimulus (Fig. 24.1 – right). Now, the sensation becomes sharper, qualitatively more similar to pain of somatic origin, much better defined and localized, and is no longer accompanied by marked autonomic phenomena. Two types of referred pain from viscera have been described: (1) without hyperalgesia and (2) with hyperalgesia.

Referred Pain Without Hyperalgesia

This type of pain is also called irradiated segmental pain. This pain is felt in areas of the same spinal segments of the stimulated viscus. The sensation can also extend to adjoining segments.

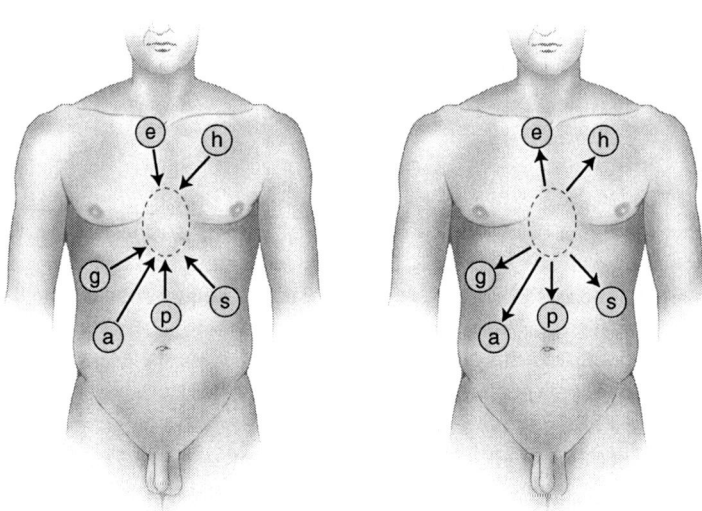

Figure 24.1 Phases of pain. *Left*, true visceral pain is always perceived in the same site (*shaded area*) whether it originates from the esophagus (*e*), heart (*h*), gallbladder (*g*), spleen (*s*), pancreas (*p*), or appendix (*a*). *Right*, referred pain from viscera is perceived in different areas according to the viscus of origin (*arrows*).

Additional stimuli exerted on the area of referral do not increase the painful symptoms, and the pain threshold is not decreased. Infiltration with local anesthetic in the site where pain is felt produces no effect.

Referred Pain with Hyperalgesia
This type of pain is also called true parietal pain (the term parietal is here used to indicate pain in parietal somatic structures including three tissues: skin, subcutaneous tissue, and muscle; the use is different from that reported by Bonica in which parietal pain refers to pain origi-nating from a disease of the parietal pleura or parietal peritoneum). Non-noxious stimulus on skin areas where referred pain exists can provoke pain. Stimulation of the skin area causes a sensation of greater pain than would typically be expected (allodynia) as well as lowering the pain threshold.

Anatomy and Physiology
Visceral Nociceptors
There have been many theories on the signaling of visceral receptors. The specific theory con-sists of a painful stimuli in viscera encoded in the activity of specific nociceptors that is similar to those described in the skin, muscles, and joints (i.e., receptors with no background activ-ity that respond only to high-intensity stimulation). The intensity theory consists of painful events in the viscera encoded in the discharge intensity of the same population of visceral receptors that is also responsive to non-painful events.

Table 24.3 Clinical features of pain.

Characteristic	Visceral pain [a]	Superficial somatic pain	Deep somatic pain
Site	Thorac abdominal, generally along the central axis and mainly in the low sternal and epigastric regions	Limited skin area	Structure involved, sometimes with a scleromeric or myomeric pattern with extension to the dermatomere
Spatial discrimination	Poorly discriminated, diffused	Perfectly discriminated, circumscribed	Fairly well discriminated, of medium diffusion
Quality	Dull, heavy, oppressive, tensive	Pricking, burning, depending on thestimulus	Piercing, cramplike, constrictive, lacerating, burning, heavy
Intensity	Slight to intolerable	Slight to intolerable	Slight to intolerable
Evolution in time	Continuous, subcontinuous, undulating, occasional (colic)	Immediate, continuous, subcontinuous, undulating	Continuous, subcontinuous, occasional
Duration	A few minutes to a few hours, after which pain stops or becomes "referred" (parietalized)	Variable in relation to the noxa	Variable in relation to the noxa
Emotional reaction	Severe anxiety, anguish, sense of impending death	Absent	Absent
Accompanying neurovegetative signs	Pallor, sweating, nausea, vomiting, brady- or tachycardia, pollakiuria, alvus disturbances	Generally absent	Pallor, sweating, nausea
Additional stimuli	Do not increase pain	Increases pain	Increases pain

[a]Clinical features of "true visceral pain" as opposed to those of superficial (i.e., skin) and deep somatic (i.e., muscles, ligaments, joints) pain. Adapted from Giamberberardino (1997).

Visceral Afferent Fibers

Sensory fibers in the viscera originate from the cranial and spinal nerves with the cell bodies located in the posterior root ganglia. Their distal processes mostly course along with sympathetic but also parasympathetic nerves, reaching the viscera while their central processes pass via the dorsal (and occasionally the ventral) roots. The density of innervation of the viscera by spinal afferents is small compared with the density of afferent innervation in the skin and probably also in many deep somatic tissues. As Ness and Gebhart state, "Numerically, visceral afferents have been estimated to compose 5–15% of the neuronal cell bodies in the dorsal root ganglia at the spinal segments receiving maximal visceral afferent input. The relative number of spinal neurons that respond to visceral afferent input at these same spinal segments is, however, estimated to be 56–75%, supporting the assertion that visceral afferent terminals are widely distributed in the spinal cord." Therefore, a few visceral afferent fibers can activate many neurons in the spinal cord through extensive functional divergence.

Viscerosomatic Convergence

The second-order neurons that receive visceral inputs are mostly located in laminae I and V of the dorsal horn as well as in the ventral horn of the spinal cord. Additionally, they are also activated by somatic inputs from (a) superficial dorsal horn (neurons with visceral and superficial somatic input), brain stem, and thalam1us and (b) deep dorsal horn and ventral horn (neurons with visceral and deep somatic input).

Viscerovisceral Convergence

In addition to viscerosomatic convergence there are viscerovisceral convergences in the spinal cord. An example is the convergence of inputs from the colon/rectum, bladder, vagina, and uterine cervix (as well as from the skin) or of inputs from the gallbladder and heart.

Pathophysiology

True Visceral Pain

Because the viscera have bilateral afferent supply, true visceral pain is often felt midline. Visceral organs not supplied by afferents bilaterally are the cecum, ascending colon, appendix, descending and sigmoid colon, kidneys, and ureters, whose innervation is unilateral or predominantly unilateral. Low density of sensory innervation to the viscera along with divergence of visceral input from the central nervous system results in poor localization and diffuse nature of visceral pain. The non-specificity of a visceral sensation is caused by the CNS viscerovisceral convergence.

Referred Pain Without Hyperalgesia

Early ideas of referred pain without hyperalgesia were founded on viscerosomatic convergence theory. This theory is based upon afferent fibers along with multiple peripheral branches supplying the somatic and viscera. However, the amount of converging peripheral fibers is limited which makes it unlikely that this theory alone can explain the result of referred pain. It is known that centrally there is a convergence of somatic and visceral afferent inputs as described by extensive electrophysiologic and anatomic studies for neurons in the spinal cord and higher centers. Using this information, it is possible that referred pain processing can result from processing in the CNS. The convergence-projection theory states that a message from the viscera would be interpreted by higher brain centers as coming from the somatic structure because of the mnemonic traces of previous experiences of somatic pain.

Referred Pain with Hyperalgesia

Further interpretation of referred pain with hyperalgesia is more complex than can be explained by the convergence-projection theory. Two predominant theories exist for the explanation of hyperalgesia one based upon central mechanisms and one by peripheral. The convergence-facilitation theory states that an abnormal visceral input would produce an "irritable focus" in the relative spinal cord segment, thus facilitating messages from somatic structures. Because of the central convergence of visceral and somatic fibers, this results in an increase in the visceral signaling as well as an increase in the normal somatic input centrally. The outcomes of these increased inputs are a more intense painful sensation than would typically be sensed. According to this theory, referred pain with hyperalgesia is mainly caused by central mechanisms.

The second theory postulates that pain-causing conditions develop in the periphery (i.e., the referral area), with subsequent excitation of pain receptors, because of several viscerocutaneous and visceromuscular reflexes that are triggered by the afferent visceral barrage. Referred pain with hyperalgesia can be produced by stimulation of the sensory afferents from the viscera and the efferent fibers would be triggered via a reflex arc. According to some authors, hyperalgesia and related phenomena at skin level are induced by sympathetic efferents, because an experimental, local anesthetic block of the sympathetic ganglia led to disappearance or marked decrease of referred pain, hyperalgesia, and dermographic skin alterations. In contrast, hyperalgesia in muscle is caused by somatic efferents in this view. These are responsible for a sustained contraction that in turn sensitizes muscular nociceptors and becomes a new source of pain.

Treatment

Visceral pain is often temporal in nature and does not require procedural intervention for pain. For more chronic visceral pain conditions produced from cancer, pain relieving choices can be employed. As mentioned previously the sympathetic nervous system is involved in the transmission of visceral pain. When sympathetic outflow to the viscera is blocked it is possible to experience pain relief. Taking these experiences into account sympathetic axis blockade has been used for ablation of visceral pain (Gofeld and Faclier 2006). It was not until the late 1940s when local anesthetic blockade of the splanchnic and celiac plexus was first advocated to relieve non-surgical abdominal pain. With the use of improved radiographic tools and an understanding of the risks and complications of the block, these techniques can be powerful tools in controlling visceral pain.

Non-opioids are often insufficient in relieving pain to an acceptable level in patients suffering from severe pain originating from the gastrointestinal tract. Opioids have been studied in the use in visceral pain models, and differences in opioid analgesia have been observed. One study compared morphine to oxycodone showed oxycodone has a superior effect on visceral pain than morphine indicating oxycodone may interact with different visceral opioid receptors compared to morphine. Ketamine, a N-methyl-D-aspartate (NMDA) receptor antagonist, is known to also bind to opioid receptors (Willert et al. 2004). Ketamine has the added benefit of counteracting spinal sensitization or windup phenomena experienced with chronic pain. In visceral pain models ketamine has been found to decrease the pain during visceral distention and prevent development of hyperalgesia and reverses induced hyperalgesia.

Case Scenario

Dr. Adam Fendius, BSc (Hons), MBBS, FRCA, DipIMC (RCSED), DipHEP

Arthur, a 64-year-old man, who is an obese, heavy smoker with diabetes, has a history of gradually increasing calf pain on walking. He had CABG surgery 6 years ago. Over the last 2 weeks, he has noticed the pain occurring more readily. The pain disappears after he has stopped walking for a few minutes, but resumes after he has walked even a short distance.

What questions would you like to ask?
It is important to determine the exact nature of the pain, as this will point to the cause, and therefore, potential treatment. You should ask whether the pain is characterized by tightness, burning, stinging "like pins and needles," electric shock, or dull ache. Also, you need to determine whether the pain occurs only when he walks or even when he rests, and whether he has any back pain, or pain in his hip or knee? Also, is it related to position

of the limb at rest or how quickly he walks? You could also administer the "Edinburgh Claudication Questionnaire."

What is your differential diagnosis?
For proper pain management in this setting, diagnosis is important, as there can be several causes of lower limb pain while walking. These include nerve entrapment syndromes such as sciatica and spinal canal stenosis, as well as deep vein thrombosis, musculoskeletal injury, and intermittent claudication due to peripheral vascular disease. The diagnosis might be confirmed by Doppler sonography of iliac and lower limb arteries.

Arthur tells you that the pain only comes when he walks and does not interfere with his sleep. He only has it in his calf and it feels like a "dull, aching, tightness." It is worse when he has to climb a hill or in cold weather. You decide this is most likely to be an ischemic pain, related to peripheral vascular disease, for which he has multiple risk factors.

How are you going to manage his current pain?
Primary intervention should include lifestyle advice to prevent deterioration of the intermittent claudication to ischemic rest pain and critical limb ischemia. He should be advised to stop smoking and you should optimize his diabetic control. He should attempt to lose weight through diet and exercise. In fact, he does not need to walk to do exercise and instead may use an arm exercise machine. Low-dose antiplatelet therapy such as aspirin or clopidogrel should be considered, and antihypertensive medications should be reviewed for optimal therapy. Cilostazol has also been shown to improve claudication pain. The use of pentoxyfilline and inositol is controversial. Evidence supports regular exercise at near maximum pain tolerance for a minimum of 6 months to increase his maximum walking and pain-free walking distance. The possibility of surgery or endovascular luminal revascularization should be borne in mind. As the pain is intermittent and of short duration, at this stage there is no indication for regular analgesia.

After a few months Arthur presents in your clinic again. His pain is now severe and he can hardly walk 50 yards without getting pain in his calf. He also tells you that he wakes up in the middle of the night with pain in his toes, which resolves if he places his foot on the floor.

What treatment will you offer him now?
As his symptoms have worsened it is likely that he will need surgery and will, therefore, need referral to a vascular surgeon or interventional radiologist. In the interim, to control any pain which is not relieved by dropping his foot to the floor, he is likely to require regular analgesia. His analgesic regimen should follow the **WHO analgesic ladder of simple analgesics followed by a weak opioid and then a strong opioid, as required.** Bearing in mind his comorbidities, NSAIDs may be contraindicated if his renal function is impaired, and opioid doses may need to be reduced accordingly.

Are there any other alternatives?
Lumbar sympathectomy has been advocated in the past, but probably has limited application in this setting. It can still be suggested for older patients with multiple comorbidities in whom surgery may not be recommended.

Unfortunately, despite revascularization surgery, Arthur develops severe complications and the graft fails, leading to acute ischemia. He is brought to hospital with a pale, pulseless, painful cold foot and calf several months after surgery.

What can you offer him now?
This man has acute ischemia and will need a vascular surgical consultation. Treatment options might include embolectomy, repeat revascularization, or amputation depending on the severity and duration of ischemia. Anticoagulation with heparin should be started and analgesia, including the use of strong opioids should be considered. Peripheral nerve block with or without a catheter is also an option and may help with perfusion by causing sympathetic blockade. However, this treatment remains controversial.

References

Bonica JJ. General consideration of acute Pain. In: Bonica JJ, editor. The management of Pain. Philadelphia, PA: Lea & Febiger; 1990a. pp. 159–79.

Bonica JJ. Applied anatomy relevant to Pain. In: Bonica JJ, editor. The management of pain. Philadelphia, PA: Lea & Febiger; 1990b. pp. 133–58.

Bonica JJ. General considerations of abdominal pain. In: Bonica JJ, editor. The management of pain. Philadelphia, PA: Lea & Febiger; 1990c. pp. 1146–85.

Cervero F. Sensory innervation of the viscera: peripheral basis of visceral pain. Physiol Rev. 1994;74:95–138.

Dubé GR, Elagoz A, Mangat H. Acid sensing ion channels and acid nociception. Curr Pharm Des. 2009;15(15):1750–66.

Foletti A, Durrer A, Buchser E. Neurostimulation technology for the treatment of chronic pain: a focus on spinal cord stimulation. Expert Rev Med Devices. 2007;4(2):201–14.

Giamberberardino MS, Vecchiet L. Pathophysiology of visceral pain. Curr Pain Headache Rep. 1997;23–33.

Gofeld M, Faclier G. Bilateral pain relief after unilateral thoracic percutaneous sympathectomy. Can J Anaesth. 2006;53(3):258–62.

Janig W, Morrison JFB. Functional properties of spinal visceral afferent supplying abdominal and pelvic organs with special emphasis on visceral nociception. In: Cervero F, Morrison

JFB, editors. Visceral sensation progress in brain research. Amsterdam: Elsevier; 1986. pp. 87–114.

Willert RP, et al. The development and maintenance of human visceral pain hypersensitivity is dependent on the n-methyl-d-aspartate receptor. Gastroenterology 2004;126;683–92.

Chapter 25

Fibromyalgia, Arthritic, and Myofascial Pain

Nalini Vadivelu, MD and Richard D. Urman, MD, MBA

Fibromyalgia

Fibromyalgia (FMS) is an idiopathic painful syndrome of a chronic nature and of unclear etiology. It is more prevalent in females with a ratio of 9:1 females to males. About 5 million people in the United States are thought to suffer from fibromyalgia. It is estimated to be present in 2–7% of the population in most countries and is a debilitating illness with resultant loss of work days and school days, disability, and functional impairment.

Fibromyalgia is often associated with somatic complaints and comorbidities. The wide range of comorbid conditions includes anxiety, depression, sleep disorders, paresthesia, morning stiffness, and cognitive problems. Care of these patients is a challenge, since it includes the restoration of both the physical and emotional well-being.

Symptoms

Fibromyalgia patients present with a myriad of symptoms, the most common being pain and soreness in the axial skeleton, peripheral joints, muscles, ligaments, and tissues. In addition, there can be complaints of disturbed sleep, psychological disorders, morning stiffness in the joints, and paresthesias. All these symptoms can lead to decreased movement, poor sleep, anxiety, and stress.

Etiology

The etiology of fibromyalgia is unclear, but evidence suggests that it is a heritable disorder. The etiology of fibromyalgia is now thought to be due to a combination of several factors associated with the presence of both chronic pain and affective disorders, similar to those postulated in irritable bowel syndrome, chronic fatigue syndrome, major depressive disorder, temperomandibular joint disorder, and tension and migraine headaches. The factors include genetic factors, aberrant pain processing in the central nervous system, abnormalities in the neuroendocrine system, and specific triggers in the environment.

Genetic relationships have been found between fibromyalgia and several genes, including genes encoding proteins in neurotransmitter signaling, catechol-O-methyltransferase, and dopaminergic signaling. Patients with fibromyalgia have enhanced sensitivity to several stimuli including heat, pressure, and sound. Patients with fibromyalgia have been noted to have lower pain thresholds than controls. The levels of central neurotransmitters such as serotonin,

N. Vadivelu et al. (eds.), *Essentials of Pain Management*,
DOI 10.1007/978-0-387-87579-8_25, © Springer Science+Business Media, LLC 2011

norepinephrine, and dopamine have been noted to be lower in patients with fibromyalgia as compared to rheumatoid arthritis or healthy controls. In addition, there are possibly elevated levels of excitatory amino acids, neurotrophins, and substance P in the cerebrospinal fluid (CSF) seen in patients with fibromyalgia. Some researchers have suggested that there may be activation in the neuroendocrine axis, namely the hypothalamic-pituitary-adrenal axis. There appears to be increased activity of the sensory inputs in these patients as well, contributing to increased pain perception.

Signs and Symptoms

The most common symptom is chronic pain, which can be localized or involve several muscle groups. The common areas of pain include the neck, middle and lower back, chest wall, arms, and legs. The intensity of the pain is variable and can increase with several triggering factors. These factors include stress, lack of sleep, exertion, surgery, and changes in the weather.

Other factors associated with fibromyalgia include fatigue and sleep disturbances such as reduction in delta sleep and nocturnal myoclonus. Fatigue has been seen in about 90% of cases studied. Cognitive deficits in memory and vocabulary are also seen in patients with fibromyalgia.

Conditions Associated with Fibromyalgia

Fibromyalgia is associated with a number of medical conditions. These include headaches, panic disorder, major depressive disorder, posttraumatic stress disorder, and generalized anxiety disorder.

Diagnosis

The foremost complaint of patients with fibromyalgia is pain. The American College of Rheumatology states that fibromyalgia is diagnosed when there is widespread pain involving three out of four quadrants of the body for at least 3 months in duration. The criteria for the diagnosis of fibromyalgia includes widespread pain encompassing the axial system and involving both sides of the body above and below the waist, and also includes the presence of tender points. Axial skeletal pain must be also be present, such as pain involving cervical or thoracic spine, anterior chest, and lower back.

Tender points are considered positive when pain is elicited by digital palpation with an approximate force of 4 kg/cm^2 and includes the presence of at least 11 out of 18 tender points located at nine pairs of specific sites, according to the definition of the American College of Rheumatology (Fig. 25.1). For a tender point to be considered "positive" the subject must state that the palpation was painful. Tender point sites include:

1. Low cervical, bilateral and anterior to C5–C7 interspaces.
2. Second rib, bilateral at the second costochondral junctions.
3. Lateral epicondyle, 2 cm distal to the epicondyles.
4. Knee, bilateral and proximal to the joint line at the medial fat pad.
5. Occiput, bilateral at the insertions of the subocciput muscles.
6. Trapezius, bilateral at the midpoint of the upper border of trapezius muscles.
7. Supraspinatus origins: bilateral, above the scapula spine near the medial border.
8. Gluteal: bilateral, in the anterior fold of the muscle in upper outer quadrant.
9. Greater trochanter: bilateral and posterior to the prominence of the trochanter.

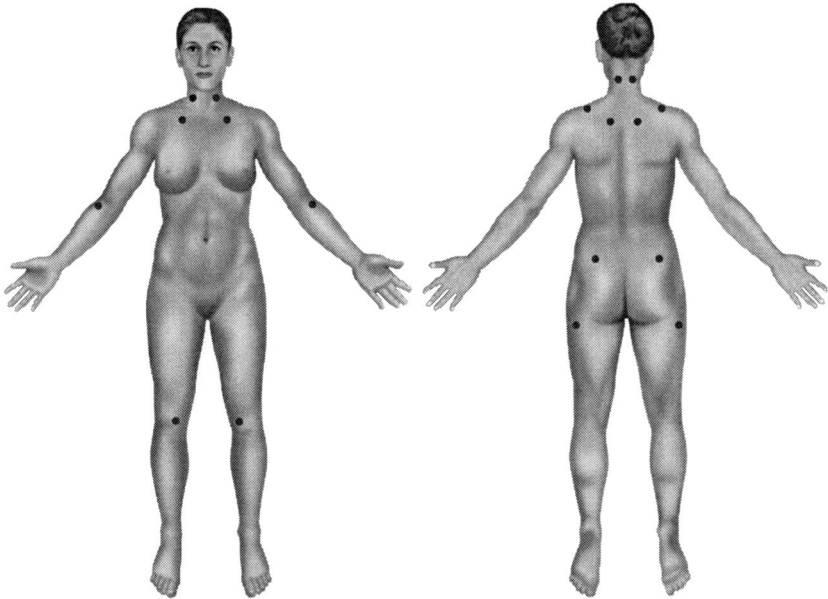

Figure 25.1 Common tender points associated with Fibromyalgia.

Despite these guidelines, the diagnosis of fibromyalgia still can be challenging, since there are many other conditions that have overlapping signs and symptoms.

These conditions include:

1. Rheumatologic disorders, such as systemic lupus erythematosus, Sjögren's syndrome, and ankylosing spondylitis.
2. Neurological disorders, such as myasthenia gravis and multiple sclerosis.
3. Peripheral neuropathic disorders.
4. Endocrine disorders, such as hypothyroidism and hyperthyroidism.
5. Myofascial pain syndrome.
6. Chronic fatigue syndrome.
7. Multiple chemical sensitivity syndrome.

It is important to remember that detailed medical evaluation and diagnosis by exclusion are important in order to distinguish fibromyalgia from these other conditions.

Assessment of Physical Activity in Fibromyalgia Patients

In addition to diagnosing fibromyalgia, it is important to assess physical activity in these patients, which will help guide treatment plans. A 10-question self-report questionnaire called the *Fibromyalgia Impact Questionnaire* can be a useful tool in assessing physical activity (Bennett 2005).

Management

Treatment of fibromyalgia should be multimodal and include control of:

1. Pain
2. Affective symptoms
3. Fatigue
4. Interventions to improve dysfunction

Multimodal therapies include the following components:

1. Education of the patient
2. Pharmacological therapies, including the use of tricyclic depressants, serotonin-norepinephrine reuptake inhibitors, selective serotonin reuptake inhibitors, tramadol, and anticonvulsants such as gabapentin
3. Alternative therapies such as acupuncture and herbal medications
4. Psychotherapy
5. Physical therapy
6. Treatment of anxiety, depression, and sleep dysfunction, as well as other comorbid conditions

Table 25.1   Effectiveness of pharmacological agents in the treatment of fibromyalgia

The FIQ Directions and Questions

Directions: For questions 1 through 3, please circle the number that best describes how you did overall for the past week. If you don't normally do something that is asked, cross the question out.

Question 1.

Were you able to:	Always	Most	Occasionally	Never
1. Do shopping ?	0	1	2	3
2. Do laundry with washer and dryer ?	0	1	2	3
3. Prepare meals ?	0	1	2	3
4. Wash dishes/cooking utensils by hand ?	0	1	2	3
5. Vacuum a rug ?	0	1	2	3
6. Make beds ?	0	1	2	3
7. Walk several blocks ?	0	1	2	3
8. Visit friends or relatives ?	0	1	2	3
9. Do yard work ?	0	1	2	3
10. Drive a car ?	0	1	2	3
11. Climb stairs ?	0	1	2	3

Question 2. *Of the 7 days in the past week, how many days did you feel good ?*

0   1   2   3   4   5   6   7

Question 3. *How many days last week did you miss work, including housework, because of fibromyalgia ?*

0   1   2   3   4   5   6   7

Table 25.1 (continued)

Directions: For the remaining items, mark the point on the line that beat indicates how you felt overall for the past week.

Question 4. *When you worked, how much did pain or other symptoms of your fibromyalgia interfere with your ability to do your work, including housework ?*

●___|___|___|___|___|___|___|___|___|___●
No problem   Great difficulty
with work   with work

Question 5. *How bad has your pain been ?*

●___|___|___|___|___|___|___|___|___|___●
No pain   Very severe
                                     pain

Question 6. *How tired have you been ?*

●___|___|___|___|___|___|___|___|___|___●
No tiredness   Very tired

Question 7. *How have you felt when you get up in the morning ?*

●___|___|___|___|___|___|___|___|___|___●
Awoke well   Awoke
rested   very tired

Question 8. *How bad has your stiffness been ?*

●___|___|___|___|___|___|___|___|___|___●
No stiffness   Very stiff

Question 9. *How nervous or anxious have you felt ?*

●___|___|___|___|___|___|___|___|___|___●
Not anxious   Very anxious

Question 10. *How depressed or blue have you felt ?*

●___|___|___|___|___|___|___|___|___|___●
Not depressed   Very depressed

Pharmacotherapy can be used to control the symptoms of pain, fatigue, and affective symptoms. Nonpharmacological therapies are used to increase functionality.

Pharmacotherapy

Serotonin and norepinephrine reuptake inhibitors (such as duloxetine) and tricyclic antidepressants are commonly used to treat fibromyalgia. Cyclobenzaprine has been shown to be effective as a muscle relaxant in treating some of the symptoms of fibromyalgia, but it did not reduce the tender points or fatigue associated with the disease. Another potential useful agent is pregabalin – an antiepileptic drug which binds to the alpha-2 delta subunit of the voltage-gated calcium channels. It is approved by the Food and Drug Administration (FDA) for the treatment of fibromyalgia. Of the selective serotonin reuptake inhibitors, fluoxetine has shown reduction in symptoms. Tramadol, a weak opioid, also has been used with some success in patients with fibromyalgia. However, the use of strong opioids in fibromyalgia has yet to be evaluated.

As described above, there are several pharmacological treatments that have been employed over the years for the treatment of fibromyalgia all showing varying levels of effectiveness. As first-line treatment, it is best to use medications that have strong evidence for effectiveness, such as serotonin–norepinephrine reuptake inhibitors (SNRIs), selective serotonin uptake inhibitors (SSRIs), and tricyclic antidepressants (Table 25.2). It is best to start with monotherapy and get at least a partial response before moving to multidrug therapy.

Table 25.2 Effectiveness of pharmacological agents in the treatment of fibromyalgia.

No evidence	Moderate evidence	Strong evidence
Corticosteroids	Tramadol with or without acetaminophen	Gabapentin
Benzodiazepines	Fluoxetine	Duloxetine
Opioids		Amitriptyline
NSAIDs		Pregabalin
		Cyclobenzaprine

Nonpharmacological Therapy

Nonpharmacological therapy includes several modalities. Important examples include exercise, cognitive behavioral therapy, patient education, acupuncture, massage therapy, and patient support groups.

Fibromyalgia is a major chronic pain syndrome which can lead to a significant decrease in overall function, long-term disability, and a decrease in the quality of life. Its pathophysiology is complex and is still under investigation. Recent research has shown the probability of central sensitization and exaggeration of "wind up" as part of pain processing in these patients. The definitive diagnosis of fibromyalgia is not clear-cut, because of the multiple overlapping pain syndromes which can be part of the differential diagnosis. Also, its nonspecific nature can lead to underdiagnosis. Thus, a multidisciplinary treatment approach appears to be the most appropriate and effective method.

Effectiveness of treatment in fibromyalgia

Fibromyalgia can present with a variety of symptoms and various treatments have been tried, all showing different levels of effectiveness. The more effective treatments appeared to include walking, warm baths, clonazepam, and acupuncture, followed by opioids such as oxycodone, tizanidine, and gabapentin. The lesser effective therapies include amitriptyline, trigger point injections, and duloxetine.

Myofascial Pain Syndrome (MPS)

Myofascial pain syndrome (MPS) is a syndrome that is different from fibromyalgia. It is characterized by trigger points which are localized hyperexcitable painful areas inside muscles or fasciae. These trigger points produce intense pain, which can be localized or referred. Restricted movement of muscles and the presence of taut bands and tender nodules are common features of MPS. The taut bands and tender nodules respond immediately to a trigger point injection. Effective local anesthetics include 0.5–2 cc of 0.5% of procaine, 0.25% of bupivacaine, or 1–2% of lidocaine.

Effectiveness of treatments in myofascial pain syndromes

More outcome studies and sensitivity analysis are necessary to statistically confirm the effectiveness of different modalities of treament in myofascial pain syndromes. There is a lack of clinical research to establish evidence-based guidelines for the treatment of myofascial pain. The commonly prescribed treatments are moderately effective, and the characterizations of the available treaments have often been rated to be insufficient.

Arthritis

The term arthritis means inflammation in the joints. Rheumatoid arthritis, osteoarthritis, and infectious arthritis are the most common forms of arthritis in humans. In osteoarthritis and rheumatoid arthritis, pain in the joints can be due to several causes. Arthritis can be inflammatory as seen in rheumatoid arthritis or noninflammatory such as in osteoarthritis. Arthritis can also occur because of concurrent diseases such as gout, infectious arthritis, and viral infections such as mumps and varicella.

Of the different types of arthritis, osteoarthritis is the most common form of arthritis with its incidence increasing with age. It is a degenerative disease of the joints, and it is sometimes also called hypertrophic osteoarthritis. Osteophytes, loss of articular cartilage, and hypertrophy of bone can all be seen as a result of altered hyaline cartilage. Osteoarthritis can be idiopathic (also called primary osteoarthritis) or can be due to a variety of causes such as genetic defects, congenital joint disease, and trauma (secondary osteoarthritis).

Osteoarthritis is a progressive condition with a gradual onset. Patients complain of morning stiffness in the joints that improves with the activities of daily living. In more advanced osteoarthritis, the pain in the joints increases with exercise and is typically relieved with rest. Joint effusions can occur along with muscle spasms.

Diagnosis

The diagnosis is made by signs and symptoms and also by an X-ray which can show narrowing of the joint space and show the presence of osteophytes.

Treatment

Osteoarthritis is a progressive disease and therefore exercise, stretching, and physical therapy are of foremost importance to maintain range of motion, functionality, and physical fitness in these patients. Medications used for the treatment of osteoarthritis include nonsteroidal anti-inflammatory drugs (NSAIDs), low-dose muscle relaxants, intra-articular injections of hyaluronic acid, and intra-articular corticosteroids. Surgical interventions such as laminectomy and osteotomy can be considered in advanced cases.

Rheumatoid Arthritis

Rheumatoid arthritis is characterized by a symmetrical inflammation of the joints with an insidious onset. Synovial thickening is common, and in advanced cases there may be destruction of the articular surfaces of the joint and flexor contractures and subcutaneous nodules. A late finding includes ulnar deviation of the fingers leading to a "swan neck" deformity. This is a result of the slipping of the extensor tendons off the metacarpophalangeal joints.

Differential Diagnosis

The differential diagnosis of rheumatoid arthritis includes systemic lupus erythematosus (SLE), systemic sclerosis, polyarteritis, polymyositis, ankylosing spondylitis, and osteoarthritis.

Diagnosis

X-ray findings in rheumatoid arthritis may include narrowing of joint space, periarticular osteopenia, juxtaarticular bony erosions, subluxation and gross deformity, and periarticular soft tissue swelling. Laboratory findings include antibodies to altered globulin called rheumatoid factors (RFs) and increased ESR.

Treatment

Nonpharmacological treatment of the rheumatoid arthritis includes rest, exercise, and nutritional adjustments. Pharmacological approaches include NSAIDs, salicylates, gold compounds, hydroxychloroquine, corticosteroids, and immunosuppressive drugs such as methotrexate, azathioprine, and cyclosporine (Table 25.3). Gold compounds are rarely used today. Advanced cases of rheumatoid arthritis may need a surgical intervention to improve function such as gait correction, hip surgery, and joint fusions.

Table 25.3 Pharmacological treatments of rheumatoid arthritis.

Mild RA	Moderate RA	Severe RA
NSAIDs	Hydrochloroquine	Sulfasalazine
Salicylates	Gold compounds	Methotrexate
		Cyclosporine
		Azathioprine
		Gold compounds

RA = rheumatoid arthritis; NSAIDs = nonsteroidal anti-inflammatory drugs.

Case Scenario

Jones Kurian, MD, MRCP, FRCA, DIP Pain Med

Philip is a 16-year-old university student and a swimming champion. He has just returned from a competition and now suffers from severe pain in his right shoulder. He had this pain even before attending the meet but now it has become "unbearable." He describes the pain as a dull and constant ache. It radiates along his neck and right arm. The pain is associated with a tingling sensation and is localized to the shoulder. You are requested to see him. Philip is worried about the future of his swimming career.

Outline your approach.

The pain could be arising from the underlying structures: muscles, bones, ligaments, and nerves. It could be coming from internal organs in the vicinity or a referred pain. It could be the result of trauma, tumor, or infection. The only positive finding elicited by your physical examination is tender points over his right trapezius and serratus anterior muscles. Philip jumps with pain when you press on these points and he says he is getting the typical pain and tingly sensation over his shoulder, chest, and neck when you press over the points.

You test the sensory and motor system and find it to be normal. In order to be thorough, you order routine investigations and X-ray of the shoulder which returns as normal. At this point you might consider a MR scan of the cervical spine to rule out any nerve root pathology. You diagnose myofascial pain syndrome of the trapezius and serratus anterior muscles.

What are your treatment options?

The simplest option is a repeated application of a cold spray over the tender point followed by gentle massage. An immediate favorable response to this will also serve as a feedback moment for patient education. This can be repeated in several sittings. Philip has a positive response to this treatment. You refer him to his physiotherapist. The physiotherapist teaches Philip better posture and relaxation techniques.

A month later Philip returns to see you. He mentions that although the physiotherapy and coolant spray and massage helped him, he is still getting pain. He is due to start training for the next swimming competition. He is again seeking your help.

What would you recommend?

The next step in the management of his discomfort would be to use more invasive techniques such as needling the trigger point. It could be done either alone or in combination with a local anesthetic. The local anesthetic can reduce the pain during the needling. Other drugs which have been used in combination include steroids and botulinum toxin type A (Botox).

Philip opts for Botox injection of the trigger point. The response seems to be very impressive. Following the injection he is pain-free for many weeks. He utilizes the pain-free interval to boost his fitness.

What are the other options for treating myofascial pain syndrome?

TENS and acupuncture could be tried for treating myofascial pain. TENS has the advantage of being noninvasive, simple, and easy to use.

References

Bennett R. The Fibromyalgia Impact Questionnaire (FIQ): a review of its development, current version, operating characteristics and uses. Clin Exp Rheumatol. 2005;23(Suppl. 39):S154–S162.

Chakrabarty S, Zoorob R. Fibromyalgia. Am Fam Physician 2007 Jul;76(2):247–54.

Gürsoy S, Erdal E, Herken H, Madenci E, Alaşehirli B, Erdal N. Significance of catechol-O-methyltransferase gene polymorphism in fibromyalgia syndrome. Rheumatol Int. 2003 May;23(3):104–7.

Hudson J, Pope HJ. The relationship between fibromyalgia and major depressive disorder. Rheum Dis Clin North Am. 1996 May;22(2):285–303.

Lawrence R, Felson D, Helmick C, Arnold L, Choi H, Deyo R, Gabriel S, Hirsch R, Hochberg M, Hunder G, Jordan J, Katz J, Kremers H, Wolfe F. Estimates of the prevalence of arthritis and other rheumatic conditions in the United States. Part II. Arthritis Rheum. 2008 Jan;58(1):26–35.

McBeth J, Silman A, Gupta A, Chiu Y, Ray D, Morriss R, Dickens C, King Y, Macfarlane G. Moderation of psychosocial risk factors through dysfunction of the hypothalamic-pituitary-adrenal stress axis in the onset of chronic widespread musculoskeletal pain: findings of a population-based prospective cohort study. Arthritis Rheum. 2007 Jan;56(1):360–71.

Raphael K, Janal M, Nayak S, Schwartz J, Gallagher R. Psychiatric comorbidities in a community sample of women with fibromyalgia. Pain 2006 Sep;124(1–2):117–25.

Russell I, Raphael K. Fibromyalgia syndrome: presentation, diagnosis, differential diagnosis, and vulnerability. CNS Spectr. 2008 Mar;13(3 suppl 5):6–11.

Tofferi J, Jackson J, O'Malley P. Treatment of fibromyalgia with cyclobenzaprine: a meta-analysis. Arthritis Rheum. 2004 Feb;51(1):9–13.

Wolfe F, Smythe H, Yunus M, Bennett R, Bombardier C, Goldenberg D, Tugwell P, Campbell S, Abeles M, Clark P. The American College of Rheumatology 1990 Criteria for the Classification of Fibromyalgia. >Report of the Multicenter Criteria Committee. Arthritis Rheum. 1990 Feb;33(2):160–72.

Chapter 26

Head, Neck, and Back Pain

May L. Chin, MD

Introduction

This chapter covers pain in the head, neck, and back regions. These are broad topics. Therefore, to be concise, the discussion in this chapter will focus on common presentations and findings in patients presenting with pain in these anatomical regions. Since back pain is one of the most common complaints among patients, this topic will be addressed first, followed by neck pain and pain in the head region. Headaches are covered in length in Chapter 27 and therefore will not be discussed under pain in the head section.

Back Pain

Low back pain is a common ailment. About 60% of patients suffer from low back pain which is second only to upper respiratory symptoms for physician visits (Deyo and Weinstein 2001). Back pain is often challenging for healthcare professionals in terms of diagnosis and treatment. In addition to enormous healthcare costs, back pain is one of the leading causes of disability and work loss, incurring huge costs to society. Men and women appear equally affected with low back pain. Risk factors associated with low back pain include a history of previous back pain, history of heavy lifting, bending, twisting, whole body vibration, obesity, poor job satisfaction, lower social class, and emotional distress.

Diagnosis of Low Back Pain

It is often difficult to pinpoint a specific anatomical diagnosis for most patients with isolated low back pain. The majority of low back pain is benign; in other words, the pain is musculoskeletal in origin. A careful history and physical examination (Tables 26.1, 26.2, and 26.3) can generally rule out serious causes of low back pain. A history of pain at night, fever, history of cancer and/or unexplained weight loss, loss of bowel or bladder control, and progressive neurological deficits may be associated with serious causes of low back pain and should prompt urgent evaluation of the patient (Table 26.4). It should be noted that serious causes of low back pain are rare compared to mechanical low back pain or leg pain (Table 26.5).

Anatomic Structures That Contribute to Back Pain
Muscles

Anatomic structures that can contribute to back pain and innervation of the lumbar spine are outlined in Table 26.6 and Fig. 26.1, respectively (Deyo and Weinstein 2001; Bogduck

N. Vadivelu et al. (eds.), *Essentials of Pain Management*,
DOI 10.1007/978-0-387-87579-8_26, © Springer Science+Business Media, LLC 2011

Table 26.1 History for back pain.

Pain
Location
Radiation
Severity
Quality (e.g., sharp, dull, associated numbness/paresthesia)
Frequency and duration (e.g., continuous, intermittent)
Relieving factors (e.g., lying supine, rest)
Exacerbating factors (e.g., bending over, coughing)
Weakness of extremity
Associated loss of bowel or bladder control
Therapy and effectiveness (e.g., analgesics, physical therapy)
Previous back surgery
Medical history
History of neoplasia
Significant weight loss
Fever
Systemic illness (e.g., diabetes)
Systemic infection (e.g., tuberculosis)
Psychosocial history
Occupation (e.g., employed/disability; operates heavy machinery/lifting)
Smoking, alcohol use, substance abuse

Table 26.2 Focused physical examination in a patient with back pain.

Inspection
    Posture, spine curvature, muscle atrophy
Gait
Lumbar spine, facet joints
    Paraspinous muscle tenderness, spasm
    Range of motion (flex, extend, lateral flexion, rotation)
Hip joints (range of motion)
Sacroiliac joints
Lower extremities
    Straight leg raise
    Reflexes
    Sensory testing
    Motor testing
    Peripheral pulses
Abdomen (rule out pulsatile mass/abdominal aneurysm)

1997). The posterior or dorsal rami of the spinal nerves supply the paraspinous muscles and the anterior or ventral rami innervate the others, including the quadratus lumborum and psoas. Pain can arise from muscle spasm, muscle strain, or sprain. Muscle spasm can also be triggered by pathology or trauma to surrounding anatomical structures such as a disk herniation, facet arthropathy, or trauma to the vertebral body.

Ligaments
Pain can arise from stretching the anterior and posterior longitudinal ligaments.

Table 26.3 Associated motor, sensory, and reflex changes with lumbar nerve root compression.

Nerve root	Reflex (decreased or absent)	Motor affected	Sensory/pain
L4	Patellar	Dorsiflexion (difficulty with heel walking)	Lateral thigh, medial aspect of ankle, ankle, big toe
L5	None	Dorsiflexion (ankle, big toe)	Over sacroiliac joint, lateral thigh and leg, dorsum of foot
S1	Achilles	Plantar flexion (difficulty walking on toes)	Over sacroiliac joint, posterior thigh and leg, heel, lateral foot

Table 26.4 "Red Flags" in medical history may be associated with serious causes of back pain.

- Cauda equina: loss of bowel or bladder control (incontinence, retention)
- Progressive neurological deficit(s)
- History of neoplasia
- Unexplained weight loss
- Fever
- Severe unrelenting pain
- Pain worse at night
- Intravenous drug abuse
- History of recent trauma

Vertebral Bodies
The periosteum is well innervated by nerve plexuses.

Intervertebral Disks
The outer annular fibers of the intervertebral disks but not the nucleus pulposus are well innervated.

Facet or Zygapophysial Joints
These joints are innervated by the medial branches from the posterior rami of the spinal nerve. Each joint is supplied by the medial branch from the posterior rami at the same level as well as the medial branch from the posterior rami one level above.

Sacroiliac Joints
The posterior rami of L4, L5, S1, and S2 innervate the sacroiliac joint.

Dura Mater
The dura mater has rich innervations, particularly on the ventral aspect and around the nerve root sleeves.

Table 26.5 Differential diagnosis of low back pain.

Mechanical low back or leg pain	Non-mechanical low back pain	Visceral disease
Lumbar strain/sprain	Neoplasia	Pelvic disease
Degenerative disease	Metastatic carcinoma	Endometriosis
Disk	Multiple myeloma	Pelvic inflammatory
Facet joints	Lymphoma, leukemia	disease
Herniated disk	Spinal cord tumors	Prostatitis
Spinal stenosis	Retroperitoneal tumors	Renal disease
Fractures	Infection	Nephrolithiasis
Compression (osteoporosis)	Osteomyelitis	Pyelonephritis
Traumatic	Diskitis	Vasular disease
Spondylolisthesis	Epidural abscess	Abdominal aortic
Congenital disease	Paraspinal abscess	aneurysm
Severe kyphosis	Shingles	Gastrointestinal disease
Severe scoliosis	Inflammatory arthritis	Pancreatitis
Transitional vertebrae	Ankylosing spondylitis	Cholecystitis
	Psoriatic spondylitis	
	Reiter's syndrome	
	Inflammatory bowel disease	
	Paget's disease	

Modified from Deyo (2001) – with permission.

Table 26.6 Anatomical sources of low back pain.

- Muscles
- Ligaments
- Vertebral bodies
- Disks
- Facet joints
- Sacroiliac joints
- Dura mater
- Nerve roots

Nerve Roots

Pain, numbness, and/or paresthesia can result from compression or irritation of a nerve root or the dorsal root ganglion.

Common Presentations of Back Pain

Once serious causes of back pain are ruled out, the next step is to determine if the patient has musculoskeletal back pain or nerve root pain. Back pain that is musculoskeletal or mechanical in nature varies with activity and presents predominantly in the lumbosacral area, buttocks, and thighs in a patient who is otherwise well or in stable health. Nerve root pain can arise from a prolapsed disk, spinal stenosis, or surgical scarring. The pain generally radiates to the foot or toes and may be associated with numbness or tingling and signs of nerve root irritation such as positive straight leg raising (Table 26.3).

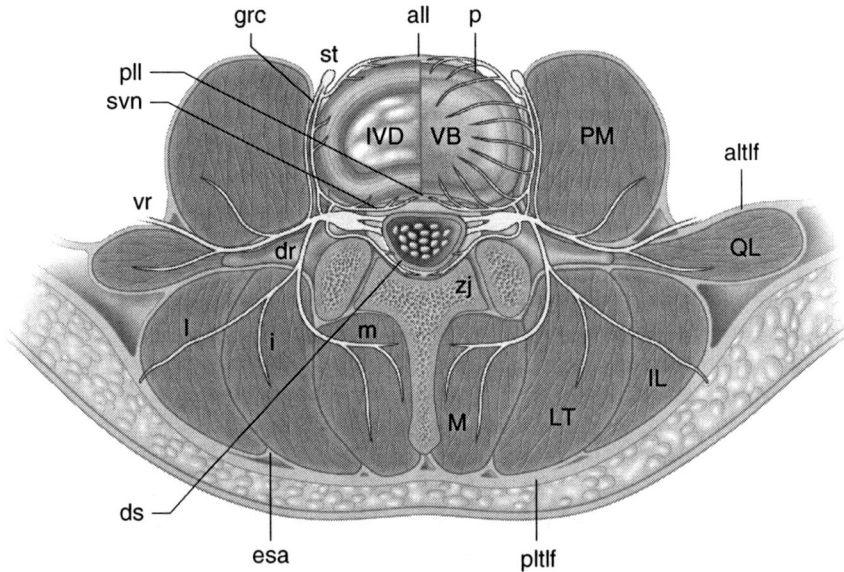

Figure 26.1 Innervation of the lumbar spine. VB-vertebral body, IVD-intervertebral disc, PM-psoas major, QL-quadratus lumborum, IL-iliocostalis lumborum, LT-longissimus thoracis, M-multifidus, p-periosteum, all-anterior longitudinal ligament, st-sympathetic trunk, grc-grey rami communicans, pll-posterior longitudinal ligament, svn-sinuvertebral nerve, vr-ventral ramus, dr-dorsal ramus, ds-dural sac, zj-zygapophysial joint, l-lateral branch, i-intermediate branch, m-medial branch, esa-erector spinae aponeurosis, altlf-anterior layer of thoracolumbar fascia, pltlf-posterior layer of thoracolumbar fascia. Modified from Bogduk 1997 – with permission.

Non-specific Acute Low Back Pain

This pain generally lasts 4–6 weeks. The vast majority of patients improve with conservative management which may include hot or cold packs and anti-inflammatory agents. It is unclear if these patients will benefit from muscle relaxants which often cause sedation. Patients should be encouraged to return to normal activities and should be reassured (after complete patient assessment) that there is no serious pathology. Patients may recover from non-specific back pain as quickly as within 2 weeks, although they should be warned that back pain often recurs. In view of this, physical therapy or manipulation therapy may be delayed until 3 weeks since many patients may improve on their own.

Subacute and Chronic Back Pain

If back pain has not resolved in 4–6 weeks, further workup including imaging studies may be helpful. Plain x-rays may demonstrate bone changes such as fractures. Although x-rays may show bone destruction, it may not be sensitive enough to pick this up early on. Computed tomography (CT) and especially Magnetic resonance imaging (MRI) are more sensitive than plain x-rays for the detection of soft tissue injury and disk pathology. MRI should be considered early on in patients where there is a high index of suspicion for neoplasm or an infection involving the spine. However, it should be noted that disk herniations, bulges, and degenerative changes are found just as commonly in asymptomatic patients and that such findings on an MRI may or may not be related to the patient's presenting back pain.

Myofascial Back Pain

Injury to muscles is a common cause of back pain. This may be related to increased activity or an acute injury. Trigger points or tender points may be palpated in the back. There are no neurological changes on examination. Muscle spasm may be noted, and tender or trigger points, which is diagnostic, palpated. Injection of trigger points, usually with local anesthetic is often helpful and may decrease discomfort and improve range of motion. For maximum benefit, it should be carried out in conjunction with physical rehabilitation.

Spinal Stenosis

If vascular claudication is ruled out, pain in the lower back and lower extremities exacerbated by walking may be diagnosed as neurogenic claudication. This is caused by lumbar spinal stenosis, which results in a narrowing of the central spinal canal and/or the neural foramina (Fig. 26.2) (Deyo and Weinstein 2001). Spinal stenosis is commonly seen in elderly patients in whom degenerative changes in the disks, facet joints as well as including osteophyte formation and thickening of the ligamentum flavum contribute to the narrowing. Spondylolisthesis also can cause these symptoms. Classically, the patient's symptoms are relieved by forward flexion (such as leaning on the grocery cart) and rest. Symptoms may occur in younger patients from congenital stenosis, although this is less common.

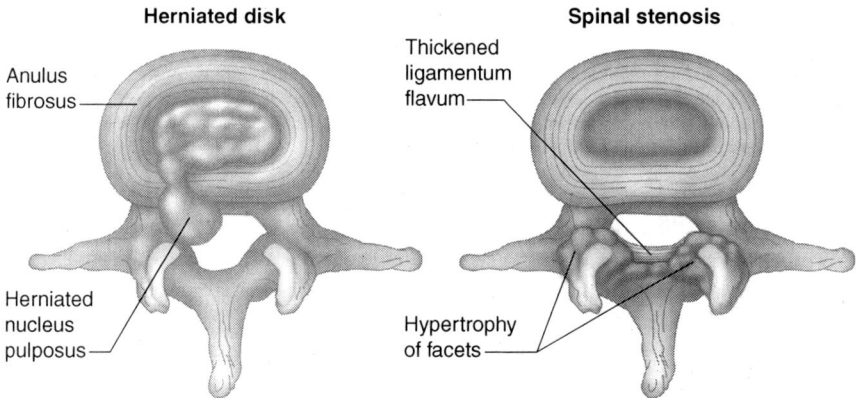

Figure 26.2   Herniated disk and spinal stenosis. Modified from Deyo 2001 with permission.

Patients with spinal stenosis may or may not demonstrate neurological changes on physical examination. Diagnosis is confirmed with MRI. Patients may be managed with analgesics and physical therapy. Epidural steroid injections may help. The disease can be progressive and surgery may be considered if pain is severe and disabling.

Discogenic Back Pain

The intervertebral disks separate each vertebral body. Each disk consists of a nucleus pulposus surrounded by an annulus fibrosus. Disk degeneration can lead to small tears in the annulus fibrosus, causing back pain which is usually non-radiating. Patients may present with a work history that involves repetitive motions, such as handling heavy machinery. MRI may show a desiccated disk. Provocative discography, although a controversial study, may help identify the disk (or disks) as the source of pain.

Facet Joint Pain

The facet joint is a synovial joint and therefore subject to osteoarthritis. The joint is well innervated and most likely contributes to back pain, although the extent to which it does so is unclear. The diagnosis of facet joint often can be controversial and difficult to isolate. Patients may present with non-specific back pain which may radiate to the buttocks or down the leg but not below the knee. The patient may have a normal neurologic examination and may exhibit paravertebral muscle tenderness and symptoms with lumbar rotation and flexion. Diagnosis of facet joint pain can be made with intra-articular injection of local anesthetic or block of the medial branch of the posterior rami at two levels.

Sacroiliac Joint Pain

Pain from the sacroiliac joint may be the source of pain in 10–15% of chronic low back pain patients. Patients may present with back pain with radiation to the buttock, the back of the thigh, and the groin. On examination pain is generally reproduced with pressure over the joint. There is no consistency between imaging findings and pain presentation. Injection of the joint with local anesthetic and steroid often provides relief.

Herniated Lumbar Disk

Patients with pain from disk herniation may experience this suddenly after an inciting event (such as lifting a heavy suitcase) or the onset of pain may be gradual (Fig. 26.2). The pain usually radiates down a leg to the foot or toes. There may be associated numbness and/or paresthesia. Physical examination demonstrating specific nerve root irritation or compression (Table 26.3) as well as a positive straight leg raise or a positive contralateral straight leg raise helps confirm the diagnosis. This can be further substantiated by MRI or CT.

Urgent or emergent surgery is indicated in the presence of cauda equina syndrome (loss of bowel or bladder control) and/or progressive neurologic deficits. Otherwise, patients should be treated conservatively in the initial month following the presentation of pain. Bed rest is not helpful and is generally discouraged. Epidural steroid injections may provide faster onset of pain relief, although relief may not be long lasting. Surgery to remove the disk may provide immediate relief, but long-term advantage of surgery over non-surgical management is not clear. Options to remove the disk range from standard laminectomy and discectomy to microdiscectomy, laser discectomy, and percutaneous discectomy.

Neck Pain

Just as with back pain, the cause of common neck pain is often not apparent. Neck pain of less than 3 months duration is considered acute neck pain, while neck pain that has been present for more than 3 months is generally considered chronic neck pain.

Neck pain can arise from the cervical spine and surrounding anatomical structures. These structures include the facet or zygapophysial joints, the intervertebral disks, the vertebral bodies, the anterior and posterior ligaments, the prevertebral muscles, and the posterior neck muscles. Serious but rare causes of neck pain include tumors (vertebral body, spinal cord) and infection (e.g., epidural abscess, meningitis, discitis, and osteomyelitis). Abnormal neurological findings associated with neck pain can be found in patients with cervical radiculopathy, cervical myelopathy, spinal cord tumor, and thoracic outlet syndrome (Carette 2005).

Risk factors for neck pain differ from those for back pain. There appears to be no consistent correlation between neck pain and psychological factors. The presence of degenerative disk disease, facet disease, the patient's socioeconomic status, history of smoking, and sitting for long periods at work do not appear to be risk factors for neck pain. The main risk factors appear to be occupational such as working with machines, previous injury, and report of stress at work. Interestingly, involvement in a motor vehicle accident does not pose an increased risk for chronic neck pain, but developing pain or symptoms after such an accident increases the risk of chronic neck pain by threefold.

Acute Neck Pain

The outcome of acute neck pain without neurologic deficits is generally favorable with 40 percent of patients recovering fully and 25% percent with mild residual symptoms only (Bogduk and McGuirk 2006a). It is often construed that patients in motor vehicle accidents who develop acute neck pain following whiplash are less likely, to recover disability perhaps due to other factors such as litigation or disability claims. On the contrary, both clinical and claims data have indicated that most patients recover over time following acute neck pain from whiplash.

Chronic Neck Pain

Most patients with common neck pain improve by 3 months. If pain persists beyond that, the patient has chronic neck pain. Unless there is a history of trauma, there are no known causes for chronic neck pain. With a history of trauma, chronic pain may arise from annular tears and from the facet joints which are subject to osteoarthritis (Bogduk and McGuirk 2006b).

Whiplash

This is a term for an event that occurs in a rear end collision in a motor vehicle accident, sometimes leading to in neck pain. Studies have shown that whiplash is not a flexion–extension or acceleration–deceleration injury as popular belief would have it. It appears that the cervical spine is subjected to a compression injury in which the trunk is forced upward into the cervical spine, resulting in possible strain and injury to the disk and facet joints. According to epidemiological data not all patients sustain injury, and most injuries are minor from which the majority of patients recover (Bogduk and McGuirk 2006c).

History of Neck Pain

Pain in the neck originates from anatomical structures innervated by the cervical spinal nerves at each level. These structures include the facet or zygapophysical joints, intervertebral disks, and muscles. As in back pain, a thorough history helps exclude serious causes of neck pain.

Onset and Duration of Pain

In a patient with an acute or sudden onset of severe neck pain, trauma or injury should be ruled out.

Site of Neck Pain

Pain in the upper neck is likely to originate from the upper cervical levels, commonly C2–3, and pain in the lower neck is most often C5–6 and C6–7 in origin. Patients may experience pain referred to the head from upper cervical segments; pain in the anterior aspect of the neck may be indicative of pathology in the throat.

Radiation of Neck Pain

Pain can radiate to the upper limb, referred to as radicular pain. Cervical radiculopathy is pain in the neck and an upper extremity associated with abnormal neurologic findings such as sensory loss, motor loss, or diminished reflex in a corresponding nerve root. Pain may be referred to various "zones" around the neck and shoulder, depending on the cervical level affected (Fig. 26.3).

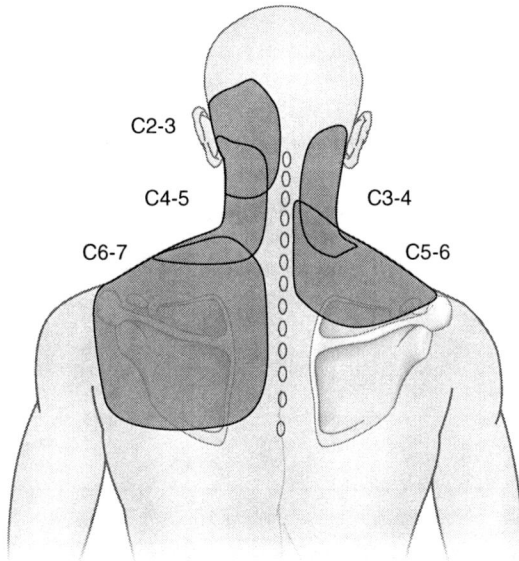

Figure 26.3 Pain may be referred to various "zones" around the neck and shoulder depending on the cervical level affected. From Bogduk 2006, with permission.

Severity and Characteristics of the Pain

Somatic pain is generally described as a dull, aching pain. Pain that is shooting or lancinating is usually indicative of a neurogenic origin. The level of pain reported by the patient is useful information. Severe acute neck pain requires urgent evaluation. In patients with chronic neck pain, assessment of the level of pain may be useful in guiding effectiveness of various treatment modalities. Factors that relieve or exacerbate pain may include specific patient or activities, although none are specific for any source of pain.

Medical History

A careful medical history including questions regarding systemic illness, unexplained weight loss, history of neoplasm, fever, infection, neurological changes including numbness and weakness in the extremities, and history of substance abuse is important to exclude serious causes of neck pain. Just as there are "red flags" with the assessment of low back pain, the same red flags should be emphasized in patients with neck pain. Infection, tumor, trauma (spinal cord, epidural hematoma, fractures) are serious causes that require urgent evaluation to be ruled out. Myelopathy may present as difficulty grasping, diffuse numbness in the hands, difficulty with balance, and problems with sphincter control such as urinary urgency or frequency.

Psychological History
Although common in patients with chronic low back pain, psychological factors do not appear to play as big a role. If psychosocial issues are present (e.g., stress, ability to work), they should be addressed. Patients who suffer whiplash injuries may have psychosocial issues related to anger at being a victim in an accident and should have these issues addressed.

Physical Examination
The cause of common neck pain is not usually determined on physical examination. Range of motion of the neck and areas of tenderness in the neck and shoulder girdle muscles are noted. In patients with neurologic symptoms, a neurological examination including motor, sensory, and reflex testing in upper and lower extremities may help narrow findings to specific nerve roots (Table 26.7). The presence of hyperreflexia, clonus, Babinski's sign, and abnormal gait may indicate myelopathy.

Table 26.7 Physical findings with cervical nerve root compression.

Disk	Nerve root	Pain	Motor weakness	Decreased sensation	Decreased reflex
C4–5	C5	Medial scapula, lateral arm to elbow	Deltoid, supraspinatus, infraspinatus	Lateral upper arm	Supinator
C5-6	C6	Lateral forearm, thumb, index finger	Biceps, brachioradialis, wrist extensors	Thumb and index finger	Biceps
C6-7	C7	Medial scapula, posterior arm, dorsum forearm, third finger	Triceps, wrist flexors, finger extensors	Posterior arm, third finger	Triceps
C7-T1	C8	Medial forearm, fifth finger	Thumb flexors, abductors, intrinsic hand muscles	Fifth finger	

Modified from Carette (2005) – with permission.

Imaging Studies in Neck Pain
With a history of trauma, cervical spine x-ray in an AP, lateral, odontoid view may be helpful. History suggestive of infection or tumor also warrants urgent x-ray of the cervical spine. Cervical spine x-ray is not generally indicated if the patient is alert, does not have neurological deficits, and does not have midline tenderness posteriorly. CT is best for bone changes and MRI is best for soft tissue evaluation. Both CT and MRI are not required initially in neck pain that appears uncomplicated.

Treatment of Neck Pain
Acute Neck Pain
The natural history for acute neck pain is recovery within 3 months. Reassure patient that serious causes, which are rare, are ruled out. Patient should be encouraged to maintain normal activities. The most effective treatment may be simple neck exercises to keep the neck

mobile and increase range of motion. If there is no improvement, patient should be further evaluated with imaging (e.g., MRI). There is no evidence that analgesics, non-steroidal anti-inflammatory agents, or muscle relaxants are effective in acute neck pain, although they are often prescribed. In general opioids are not indicated in acute neck pain. Studies have reported long-term relief in up to 60 of patients with cervical epidural steroid injections using the interlaminar or transforaminal approach. Rare but serious complications can occur with these injections, (particularly with the transforaminal approach), including spinal cord or brainstem infarction and death.

Chronic Neck Pain

In chronic neck pain, there is no solid evidence that the use of the following is effective: traction, use of cervical collar, TENS, acupuncture, botulinum toxin injections, conventional physical therapy, and manipulation therapy. Exercises appear to be as effective as manual therapy or physical therapy in reducing pain. There is evidence that percutaneous radiofrequency neurotomy for cervical facet pain provides pain relief for chronic neck pain. Pain from the facet joints can be diagnosed by diagnostic blocks of the medial branches that innervate the joints.

Surgical Management

In both presentations of acute and chronic neck pain, surgery is indicated when neurologic function is compromised (instability, spinal cord compression). The natural history of cervical radiculopathy is unknown. Few studies compare surgical and non-surgical management.

In patients with cervical radiculopathy without myelopathy, surgery is recommended if conservative treatment for 6–12 weeks is ineffective, there is progression of pain and dysfunction, and the MRI shows evidence of compression of the corresponding nerve root. The optimal timing of surgery is unclear.

Head Pain

There are multiple anatomical structures that contribute to the experience of pain in the head. It may be helpful to think of pain in the head as arising from various structures (Table 26.8), including musculoskeletal structures, neural structures, structures within the oral cavity (dental, periodontal), and from the eyes, ears, nose, and sinuses (DaSilva and Acquadro 2005).

Musculoskeletal Pain
Myofascial Disorders

This is a common presentation of pain in the orofacial region. Patients may present with diffuse aching pain affecting several muscle groups. Trigger points or tender points may be elicited and pain may radiate (e.g., masseter to the ear, temporalis to the frontal area). This type of pain presentation may be seen in patients with fibromyalgia and other systemic illnesses such as lupus erythematosus.

Table 26.8   Sources of head pain.

Musculoskeletal
    Myofascial disorders
    Temporomandibular muscle disorders
    Temporomandibular joint disorders
    Cervical facet pain (C2–3)
Neuropathic pain syndromes associated with the trigeminal nerve
    Trigeminal neuralgia
    Acute herpes zoster
    Post-herpetic neuralgias
Dental pain
Eyes, ears, nose, sinuses
Head and neck cancer

Temporomandibular Muscle Disorders

This describes pain arising from the muscles of mastication usually characterized by a dull, aching pain worsened by jaw movement. There may be tenderness to palpation of the muscles and tendons and limited range of motion of the jaw. Patients may have a history of bruxism.

Temporomandibular Joint Disorder

Pain from the temporomandibular joint (TMJ) can arise from abnormal joint movements or trauma, resulting in inflammation and joint effusion. The joint is useful painful to palpation. Pain may be associated with a painful click or crepitus during mouth opening which may be limited.

Treatment for Myofascial and Temporomandibular Disorders

For the above disorders, treatment strategies include patient education, use of analgesics such as non-steroidal anti-inflammatory drugs (NSAIDS), physical therapy or exercise programs, and use of occlusal splints. Patients with myofascial and temporomandibular muscle disorders may also benefit from a trial of muscle relaxants, tricyclic antidepressants, trigger point injections, botulinum toxin injections, and cognitive-behavioral therapy.

Pain from Cervical Spine

Pain from cervical structures referred to the head is called cervicogenic headache. It can be experienced in the occipital, parietal, frontal, or orbital regions. The sensory axons from C1, 2, and 3 converge on dorsal horn neurons that also receive afferent supply from the trigeminal nerve. Hence pain mediated by the C1, 2, and 3 nerves is perceived in areas supplied by the trigeminal nerve. A common cause of cervicogenic headache, particularly in patients after whiplash injury, is pain from the C2–3 facet joint mediated by the third occipital nerve. The source of pain can be diagnosed using controlled diagnostic blocks. Facet intra-articular injection with steroid and more so radiofrequency neurotomy is effective in relieving pain.

Neuropathic Pain Syndromes Associated with the Trigeminal Nerve

Trigeminal Neuralgia

The patient presents with sudden severe lancinating facial pain usually on one side, often triggered by chewing, talking, or touch. The patient is pain free between attacks, which can range from seconds to minutes. Patients may be pain free for months or years but each period of painful attacks may last weeks or months. V2 and V3 and rarely V1 of the trigeminal nerve are affected. MRI may demonstrate compression of the trigeminal tract or root by blood vessel or tumor. The average age of onset is 50 years. If trigeminal neuralgia presents in a young patient, multiple sclerosis should be ruled out.

Treatment

The drug of choice is carbamazepine. Other anticonvulsants are gabapentin, topiramate, oxcarbazepine. Baclofen and tricyclic antidepressants are useful adjuncts. Microvascular decompression of the trigeminal nerve can provide long-term pain relief in the majority of patients.

Acute Herpes Zoster and Post-herpetic Neuralgia (PHN)

Acute herpes zoster (AHZ; shingles) presents as pain usually in V1, distribution the ophthalmic division of the trigeminal nerve. The pain is spontaneous and is described as burning, aching or lancinating. There is associated hyperalgesia. Small cutaneous vesicles are seen during AHZ (acute phase) and scarring may be present during post-herpetic neuralgia (PHN). Post-herpetic neuralgia describes the persistence of pain after a month, when the vesicles have healed.

Treatment

The goal is to treat AHZ early with antiviral drugs and analgesics with the hope of decreasing the incidence of PHN. Tricyclic antidepressants, anticonvulsants, NSAIDS, and opioids are also useful for pain control. It is often challenging to treat pain in PHN. Tricyclic antidepressants, lidoderm patch 5%, and anticonvulsants are helpful.

Dental Pain

The mouth and the structures within are well innervated. Dental pathology probably accounts for the vast majority of pain that presents in the face. Pain can present locally, as a headache or in the eye. Sources of pain include the dental pulp (caries, fracture, or cracked tooth), inflammation (gingivitis), or abscess. Patients should be seen by a dentist for a thorough evaluation and treatment. Management of oro-dental pain is discussed in Chapter 33.

Pain in Eyes, Ears, Sinuses

Eye Pain

Patients may present with pain in the orbit that may or may not be associated with eye movement. Ocular pain and photophobia may be associated with corneal irritation or abrasions. Pain in the eye may also arise from increased intraocular pressure which occurs in glaucoma. Dental pain and temporal giant arteritis can be referred to the eye. Pain from the greater occipital nerve may be referred to the eye and face. If eye pathology is suspected, patients should be evaluated by an ophthalmologist.

Ear Pain

A common cause of ear pain is referred myofascial pain from neck and/or face muscles. Pain from ear infection (otitis media, otitis externa) can be a dull ache or severe sudden pain. There may or may not be associated discharge from the ears. Patients should be evaluated by ear, nose, and throat (ENT) specialists. If the patient has been thoroughly evaluated and continues to suffer from chronic pain, it may be reasonable to consider myofascial and neuropathic causes of pain because of the complex innervations by multiple cranial and cervical nerves in the periauricular area.

Sinus Pain

Pain from the sinuses can be bilateral or unilateral. The pain is often described as a pressure or as throbbing, made worse by palpation over the sinus. There is usually a history of chronic sinusitis or upper respiratory tract infections and allergies. The patient may benefit from an evaluation by an ENT specialist.

Head and Neck Cancer

Pain from tumor in the head and neck can present in a multitude of ways. The pain may arise from tumor growth and the resultant nerve compression and local invasion. Myofascial pain may present secondary to tumor growth in the surrounding tissues. However, the treatment of the tumor itself may give rise to pain. Surgical dissection may be associated with nerve damage; chemotherapy and radiation therapy may cause neuropathy. Patients are often fearful and anxious of their prognosis and this may contribute to an exaggerated pain response. Adjuvant analgesics such as anticonvulsants are often effective in relieving neuropathic pain. Trigger point injections and/or physical therapy may be helpful in managing myofascial pain. Management of patients with head and neck cancer may be complex. An interdisciplinary approach to the treatment of the disease not only addresses pain management but also takes into consideration psychological issues, nutritional issues if oral intake is affected, and cosmetic issues following extensive and disfiguring surgery.

Case Scenarios
Case 1: Andrew
Sreekumar Kunnumpurath, MBBS, MD, FCARCSI, FRCA, FFPMRCA

Andrew is 75-year-old man who has been very active until about a year ago. He used to play golf twice a week. One year ago, he slowly started to get persistent lower back pain which gradually began to worsen. A few months later he noted that he was getting pain in his thigh and to his dismay his neck was becoming painful too. Finally, he had to stop playing golf altogether. He was seen by his PCP who after a careful examination made a diagnosis of non-specific back pain. Andrew was started on acetaminophen and ibuprofen, which reduced his back pain to such an extent that he could play some golf again. However, a few months later during a routine checkup his PCP noticed edema of his ankles. On further investigation, he was found to have elevated blood urea and creatinine. Ibuprofen was promptly stopped with resulting recurrence of back and neck pain. Andrew was then prescribed regular codeine phosphate and diazepam before bedtime for insomnia. These medications made him constipated and sleepy during the day. Andrew again consulted his PCP, who suggested that he should see a pain specialist.

Outline your approach to Andrew's problems?
Majority of back pain cases have a benign etiology. Regardless, a detailed history and complete physical examination are necessary. The ankle edema could be directly linked to the NSAID use as it can cause water retention and heart failure as well as rise in creatinine. It is essential to rule out the existence of red flags which could be a warning of existing serious health problems.

During evaluation, Andrew describes his pain as a dull ache in the lower part of his back. It is present most of the time and radiates to his both thighs but not below the knees. On exam, he exhibits tenderness over the paravertebral area in the lumbar region and pain on flexion and rotation of lumbar spine. On examining the neck, he has trigger points in the trapezius muscles and the gluteus muscles. There are no sensory or motor deficits and nothing suggestive in his past medical history. Reports from the laboratory show mild renal impairment, and the provisional diagnosis of mechanical back pain is made. You order an MRI scan and the report states that Andrew has lumbar facet joint arthropathy and generalized degenerative disk disease.

Can you correlate neck pain and back pain?
We can consider the vertebral column as a complex, integrated unit made of bones, muscles, and ligaments. Damage to one component or misalignment between the individual components can lead to instability of posture and balance leading to the symptoms of pain spreading to other parts. Alternatively, the two could have totally unrelated pathologies.

What are your management options?
In general terms, it depends on the age, desired range of activities, and the attitude of the patient. In the case of Andrew, he wants to be able to play golf at least once a week. He cannot take NSAIDs. Regular physiotherapy and regular exercise could be helpful, but persistent pain could hinder this mode of treatment. TENS therapy might be helpful and this has the advantage of being simple, side effect free and could be used practically anytime during the day or night. An analgesic such as tramadol is another option. Interventions such as facet joint injections combined with physiotherapy could give short-term pain relief. A successful facet joint injection could be followed-up with RF ablation, which if successful, can provide long-term pain relief.

Andrew does not want to take any more pills because of their side effects. He would like you to do the facet joint injection.

What are the pros for Andrews's choice? What are the cons?
One advantage is that the facet joint injection can be used as a diagnostic test. If pain relief is achieved, the cause of the back pain could be attributed to facet joint arthropathy. If it gives immediate pain relief, steroid could be administered through the needle before it is withdrawn. A successful block can later be followed with RF ablation.

However, RF ablation is an invasive procedure with a success rate of about 50–70%. Though considered a safe procedure, the risks of infection, bleeding, intrathecal injection, and nerve damage are real. Following a good response to the injection, Andrew should be encouraged to mobilize actively.

How do you treat trigger points?
These could be dealt with at the time of facet joint injections. You can either inject them with bupivacaine or in combination with steroid. Back pain can arise from various structures at the same time. Treating one source can unmask pain from adjacent sources, which will need to be treated at a later time. Andrew has degenerative changes due to the natural aging process; the options to treat this are unfortunately limited. Hence, at a later stage he could be a potential candidate for a pain management program

Case 2: Gareth

Suneil Ramessur, MBBS, BSc (Hons), FRCA, DipHEP

Gareth, 40-year-old man, is referred to you with persistent pain and tingling around his neck and upper limbs. The pain started following a road traffic accident during which he sustained whiplash injury several months ago. He has tried various pain killers and physiotherapy without much benefit. The attending neurologist has requested you to see Gareth. A recent MRI of cervical spine is showing arthritic changes in the cervical facet joints.

Explain your approach to Gareth's problem?
Though the presentation and investigations indicate pain secondary to the whiplash injury and cervical facet joint arthropathy, it essential that a detailed first-hand history and clinical assessment are performed.

During your session with Gareth he reveals that he is a former intravenous drug abuser. Your examination reveals tenderness over the lower paracervical regions and trigger points of trapezius and sternocleidomastoid muscles on the right side. Gareth explains that his pain is a constant and dull ache and his sleep is disturbed due to the pain. He also mentions that there is an ongoing claim for compensation from the insurance company. You offer to inject the trigger points and perform a cervical facet joint injection. Gareth accepts this and undergoes the treatment.

A few weeks later Gareth is back to see you and states that the injections did not work. He wants to know why the pain is persisting. During your interview, Gareth admits that the court case is not going in his favor because of the past history of drug abuse.

What is your explanation?
In whiplash injury, pain course can be difficult to predict. Pain can persist for many years. There could be periods of remission and exacerbation. Regular medications and interventions such as physiotherapy, trigger point injections, and acupuncture have all been tried with variable success. Another interesting aspect of pain in such situations is that the ongoing litigation can have a profound psychological effect and can affect patient's

perception of pain. Pain is highly subjective and as a pain specialist you have to trust your patient in order to perform proper assessment and recommend appropriate treatment.

Gareth says he would like to try acupuncture as one of his friends has had some success with it.

What would you say to Gareth?
Pain experience is purely subjective. In situations like whiplash injury, there is no single measure that is 100% successful. In fact, a multimodal approach is often the favored path. You should always try to give a thoughtful consideration to the patient's beliefs and preferences. You agree that Gareth should try acupuncture, while continuing his medications, physiotherapy, and rehabilitation program.

Three weeks later Gareth is back to see you. He is looking very unwell. He tells you that his pain is now throbbing in nature and is constant. It is radiating to his neck and arm. He mentions that he is coughing up blood. You notice that his voice has become hoarse and there is a diffuse swelling over the right supraclavicular area.

What should you do now?
Since his symptoms are rapidly progressing, it would be prudent to arrange for an immediate investigation of his neck. An ultrasound or CT/MR scan would be an appropriate choice. It is possible that the pain may be due to a vascular abnormality. You should check his hemoglobin level and arrange for a vascular surgical consult. **You are soon informed that the CT scan demonstrates an aneurysm of the subclavian artery. He consequently has surgery to correct it.** You see Gareth four weeks after his surgery and he is pleased to inform you that his pain has now resolved. He also informs you that he has won the lawsuit.

References

Deyo RA, Weinstein JN. Low back pain. N Engl J Med. 2001;344:363–70.

Bogduk N. Clinical anatomy of the lumbar spine and sacrum. 3rd ed. Chapter 10. Fig. 10.13 Pg 143 In: Nerves of the lumbar spine. Churchill Livingstone; 1997.

Carette S, Phil M, Fehlings MG. Cervical radiculopathy. N Engl J Med. 2005;353:392–9.

Bogduk N, McGuirk B. Acute neck pain. In: Gebhart G, Basbaum A, Campbell J, Fitzgerald M, Flor H, Jensen TS, Linton SJ, McGrath PJ, McMahon SB, Porecca F, Portnoy R, Reeh PW, Turk DC, editors. Pain research and clinical management. Management of acute and chronic neck pain, an evidence based approach. 2006a, pp. 31–43, 79–90. Elsevier, Philadelphis, PA.

Bogduk N, McGuirk B. Chronic neck pain. In: Gebhart G, Basbaum A, Campbell J, Fitzgerald M, Flor H, Jensen TS, Linton SJ, McGrath PJ, McMahon SB, Porecca F, Portnoy R, Reeh PW, Turk DC, editors. Pain research and clinical management. Management of acute and chronic neck pain, an evidence based approach. 2006b, pp. 93–8, 115–21. Elsevier, Philadelphia, PA.

Bogduk N, McGuirk B. Mechanisms of whiplash. In: Gebhart G, Basbaum A, Campbell J, Fitzgerald M, Flor H, Jensen TS, Linton SJ, McGrath PJ, McMahon SB, Porecca F, Portnoy R, Reeh PW, Turk DC, editors. Pain research and clinical management. Management of acute and chronic neck pain, an evidence based approach. 2006c, pp. 125–136. Elsevier, Philadelphis, PA.

DaSilva AFM, Acquadro MA. Orofacial pain. Pain Manage Rounds 2005;2(1).

Chapter 27

Headache

Mani K.C. Vindhya, MD, Prasad Nidadavolu, MD, and Chris James, BA

Introduction

A headache is one of the common reasons for seeking medical attention. The term "headache" generally encompasses all aches and pains located in the head. It is plausible to ask: why so many pain symptoms are centered in the head? A reasonable explanation is that the face and scalp are richly supplied with pain receptors, more so than many other parts of the body (Zagami 1994). It is a well-designed mechanism that protects the precious contents of the skull (Fig. 27.1). When pain-sensitive structures, which reside in the skull, are attacked by disease or trauma, each structure has its own way of inducing pain (Headache Classification Committee of the International Headache Society 1998). This chapter is designed to give an introduction and overview to various types of headaches, their origin, presentation, pathophysiology, and treatment modalities.

In order to understand various types of headaches, it is essential to know the underlying pathophysiology of headaches. However, the pathogenesis of headaches is often unclear and multi-factorial. The most common underlying causes of headaches are:

- Vascular theory, which states that headache is the result of abnormal synthesis of vasoactive amines, such as nor-epinephrine, dopamine, and serotonin, which cause cerebral vasoconstriction followed by compensatory vasodilatation.
- Inflammatory theory, which states that substance P, a vasodilator released from trigeminal ganglia, causes neuro-inflammatory changes that stimulate pain-sensitive cranial arteries and subsequently cause pain.
- Genetics plays an important role in predisposing certain individuals to headaches.
- Physical abnormalities of the brain such as tumors, stroke, aneurysms.
- Psychological abnormalities such as anxiety, stress, and mood disorders, and
- Use of drugs.

Table 27.1 shows at least eight different types of headaches, general pathology, and presentation, and discusses each type in detail.

N. Vadivelu et al. (eds.), *Essentials of Pain Management*,
DOI 10.1007/978-0-387-87579-8_27, © Springer Science+Business Media, LLC 2011

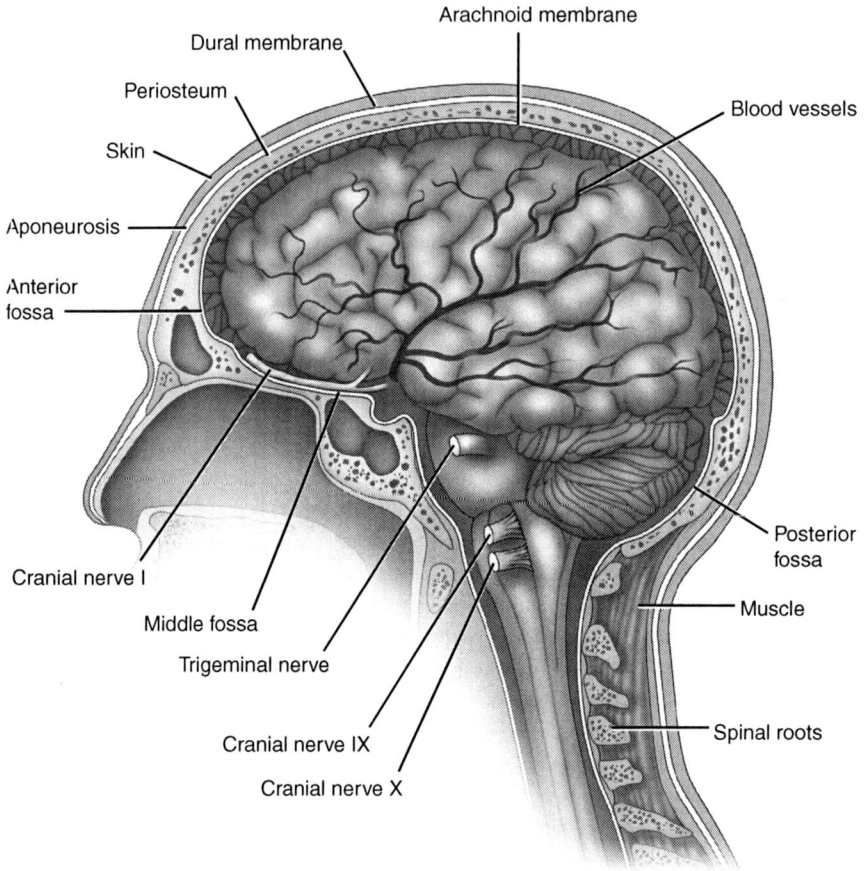

Figure 27.1   Major structures of the skull.

Migraine Headaches

Migraines are ubiquitous familial disorders commonly characterized by unilateral, periodic, often pulsatile pain that begins in the childhood, adolescence, or early adult life. It may recur with diminishing frequency during advancing years. Migraines can be further classified into two types:

- Migraine without aura
- Migraine with aura

Migraine Without Aura

An aura is a subjective sensation or motor phenomenon that precedes and marks the onset of an episode of a neurological condition, particularly an epileptic seizure or migraine. A

Table 27.1 Different types of headaches (general pathology, presentation, treatment).

	Types of headache	Pathology	Presentation	Treatment
1	**Migraine headache**	Vascular or inflammation, multi-factorial	May present with or without aura	Triptans, ergotamine, dihydroergotamine, NSAIDs, metoclopramide, phenothiazines, steroids, benzodiazepines, barbiturates, and opioids
2	**Cluster headache**	Exact mechanism is not known; neurovascular, histamine, ANS, or mast cell mediated	Severe unilateral headaches in temple and peri-orbital regions, occurring over a period of several weeks	Oxygen therapy, triptans, ergotamines, lidocaine, capsaicin, opioids, steroids
3	**Tension headache**	Multi-factorial, vascular, muscular, and psychogenic factors are suggested. Central sensitization at level of spinal dorsal horn/trigeminal nucleus leading to release of neurotransmitters that cause contraction of facial muscles, stress	Constant, tight band-like pressing pain in temporal, frontal, occipital, or parietal areas	Pharmacotherapy with NSAIDs, acetaminophen in combination with codeine or caffeine, anti depressants, tricyclics, non-pharmacological interventions like biofeedback, TENS, hot and cold applications, massage, and relaxation techniques
4	**Meningeal irritation**	Physical abnormalities like meningeal inflammation, aneurysms, hypertension	Fever, altered consciousness, nuchal rigidity, or perivenous hemorrhage of the fundus (subarachnoid hemorrhage secondary to hypertension)	Empiric antibacterial therapy for bacterial meningitis, antivirals for viral meningitis, acetaminophen, anti hypertensives, steroids
5	**Temporal arteritis**	Idiopathic autoimmune in etiology resulting in inflammatory reaction to the elastin component of the arteries	Usually unilateral, intense throbbing, or non-throbbing headache usually in the areas of affected cranial arteries	Steroids, immunosuppressant's like azathioprine, methotrexate, cyclophosphamide, etc.
6	**Posttraumatic headaches**	Headaches secondary to acute or chronic subdural hematomas	Dull, deep-seated unilateral pain often accompanied by confusion, drowsiness, and fluctuating hemiparesis	Management and treatment of the underlying traumatic brain injury. Antianxiety and antidepressant drugs
7	**Headaches of brain tumor**	Preexisting brain tumor	Deep non- throbbing, bursting like pain that may exacerbate with positional changes	Tumor irradiation, chemotherapy, and/or surgical resection
8	**Headaches of pseudo-tumor cerebri**	Idiopathic increase in intracranial pressure in patients with cerebral edema, increase in CSF leading to increased cranial pressure	Dull or pressure-like occipital or generalized headaches, sometimes associated with horizontal diplopia, transient visual obscurations, and vague dizziness	Acetazolamide, mannitol, digoxin, steroids , surgical procedures like lumbar punctures

NSAIDS=non-steroidal anti-inflammatory drugs; TENS=transcutaneous nerve stimulation; CSF=cerebrospinal fluid.

migraine without aura is also known as a "common" migraine. It usually presents as fronto-temporal headache. It is characterized by throbbing (pulsatile) pain, usually worse behind one eye or ear, which later becomes generalized with a dull ache and a sensitive scalp. It is common in adolescents and young to middle-aged adults and sometimes in children. It also occurs more commonly in women.

Diagnosis

Diagnosis of the common migraine can be made based on the following criteria:

- At least five headaches lasting 4–72 h each
- It has at least two of the following four characteristics:
  1. Pulsatile in nature
  2. Unilateral in location
  3. Moderate to severe in intensity (interferes with daily activities)
  4. Aggravation with physical activity (walking and routine daily activities)

At least one of the following symptoms can also occur: nausea, vomiting, photophobia (intolerance of visual light), and phonophobia (an irrational fear of sounds or of speaking loudly). Bright light, noise, tension, and alcohol worsen the symptoms (Spierings et al. 2001). These migraines are usually relieved by darkness and sleep.

It has been previously believed that migraines aura and headache were the result of the constriction and dilation of the cerebral and extracranial arteries, respectively. However, studies have shown a number of different mechanisms of the etiology of migraines (Lance 1993). One such theory states that substance P, a vasodilator released from trigeminal ganglia, causes neuro-inflammatory changes that stimulate pain-sensitive cranial arteries and subsequently cause pain associated with migraines. Vasoactive peptides such as serotonin and dopamine stimulate the inflammatory cascade causing release of platelets, mast cells, and cause vasodilatation. Studies have shown that platelets of migraine patients aggregate more readily than those of non-migraine patients. It is believed that platelets contain serotonin which can activate receptors that release nitric oxide, a vasodilator, subsequently causing migraines. Dopaminerigic activation is responsible for the hypersensitivity reactions such as nausea, vomiting, and irritability seen in association with migraines. Other causes such as stress, anxiety, and mood have also been linked to migraines. Twin studies reveal that almost all patients with migraines without aura have one or both parents who also suffer from the same migraines, thus suggesting a genetic predisposition to migraines.

Migraine with Aura

A migraine with aura is also known as a "classic" or a "neurologic" migraine. It has similar presentation to that of a migraine without aura, but shows a stronger familial inheritance. It is associated with a visual or sensory component such as scintillating lights and visual scotomas, which are areas of lost or depressed vision within the visual field surrounded by an area of less depressed or normal vision. It can also be associated with unilateral paresthesias, which are abnormal sensations such as burning, prickling sensations in the absence of stimuli), weakness, dysphasias (impaired speech), vertigo, and, rarely, confusion. The unilateral pulsating aspects of the migraine are its characteristic features in comparison to other headache types.

Diagnosis

Diagnosis of a classic migraine can be made if the patient suffers at least two attacks that satisfy three of the following four criteria:

- At least one aura symptom developing gradually (>4 min) or two or more symptoms occuring in succession.
- One or more reversible aura symptoms indicating focal cerebral cortical or brainstem dysfunction.
- No aura symptom lasts >60 min.
- Headache follows aura in < 1 h.

Treatment

Migraine treatments are usually individualized to meet the patient's needs (Lipton 2001). Analgesics like acetaminophen are usually used in uncomplicated, infrequent headaches. Combinations of acetaminophen with codeine or caffeine may be used for moderate to severe headaches. Non-steroidal anti-inflammatory drugs (NSAIDs) may be useful for the headaches mediated through the inflammatory process; however, they are less preferred in patients with hypersensitivity to aspirin, gastrointestinal ulcers, and undergoing anticoagulant therapy. Selective serotonin receptor agonists (5-HT1 agonists) such as triptans have significantly altered the treatment approach to the acute migraine attacks by selectively acting on the 5-HT1 receptors of the cranial arteries, causing vasoconstriction and suppressing the serotonin-mediated inflammation process. Table 27.2 shows the list of available triptans used for drug therapy. A new combination product Treximet (sumatriptan and naproxen) has been recently approved; it encompasses the benefits of both triptans and NSAIDs (Brandes et al. 2007). Ergot alkaloids like ergotamine and dihydroergotamine are direct vasoconstrictors of smooth muscles of cerebral arteries; they also alter the transmission at serotonergic, dopaminergic, and alpha-adrenergic junctions. Barbiturates have been used in combinations with acetaminophen and aspirin to relieve migraines; however, these are less preferred as they tend to cause rebound headaches and are addictive in nature. Barbiturates are more useful in

Table 27.2 List of available triptans used for drug therapy for migraine headache.

	Drug	Dosage	Maximum daily dose	Dosage forms
1	Almotriptan (Axert®; Ortho-McNeil-Janssen, Titusville, NJ)	12.5 mg q 2 h	25 mg	Tablets: 6.25, 12.5 mg
2	Sumatriptan (Imitrex®; Glaxo-Smith-Kline, Philadelphia, PA)	50–100 mg q 2 h	200 mg	Tablets: 25, 50, 100 mg Nasal: 5, 20 mg Injection: 6 mg/ml
3	Naratriptan (Amerge®; Glaxo-Smith-Kline, Philadelphia, PA)	1 or 2.5 mg q 4 h	5 mg	Tablets: 1, 2.5 mg
4	Zolmitriptan (Zomig®; Astra Zeneca, Wilmington, DE)	2.5 or 5 mg q 2 h	10 mg	Tablets/wafers: 2.5, 5 mg
5	Eletriptan (Relpax®; Pfizer, New York, NY)	20 mg q 2 h	80 mg	Tablets: 20, 40 mg
6	Rizatriptan (Maxalt®; Merck, Whitehouse Station, NJ)	5–10 mg q 2 h	30 mg	Tablets/wafers: 5, 10 mg
7	Frovatriptan (Frova®; Elan Pharmaceuticals, San Francisco, CA)	2.5 mg q 2 h	7.5 mg	Tablet: 2.5 mg

the treatment of tension headaches due to the ability to cause central nervous system (CNS) suppression, hence relieving stress and anxiety. Antiemetics like metoclopramide and phenothiazines have shown to block dopamine stimulation and hence are useful for symptoms of hypersensitivity in migraines with aura. Opioids are generally reserved for migraines that respond inadequately to all the other therapies due to their addictive properties. Steroids have shown some efficacy in treatment of migraines mediated by the inflammation; however, they are preferred only in acute treatment. Other methods such as relaxation techniques (meditation, acupuncture, hypnosis) have been shown to promote more restful sleep and reduce pain associated with migraines.

Migraine Prevention

Prophylaxis of migraine headaches is a critical part of the management of migraines. Several classes of drugs have shown to be effective in the prevention of acute attacks. Table 27.3 gives a list of selective classes of drugs used for prevention of migraine headaches.

Table 27.3 List of selective classes of drugs used for prevention of migraine headaches.

	Drug class	Drugs	Selected side effects
1	Antidepressants	Amytriptyline, fluoxetine	Drowsiness, headache, nausea, insomnia, nervousness
2	Beta-adrenergic receptor antagonists	Propranolol, metoprolol, nadolol, timolol	Reduced energy, tiredness, postural symptoms
3	Calcium channel blockers	Diltiazem, verapamil	Constipation, headache, cardiac conduction disturbances, edema
4	Anticonvulsants	Divalproex, gabapentin, topiramate	Drowsiness, weight gain, tremors, somnolence
5	Serotonin antagonists	Methysergide	Drowsiness, leg cramps, hair loss, retro peritoneal fibrosis

Other migraine variants include *basilar* migraine, *hemiplegic* migraines, and *ophthalmoplegic/retinal* migraines. Basilar migraines are relatively less common. They usually present with temporary cortical blindness associated with brainstem symptoms of vertigo, unsteady gait, limb ataxia (lack of muscle coordination), dysarthria (speech disorder due to loss of articulation), and tingling in hands, feet, and mouth followed by occipital headache. *Hemiplegic migraines* are headaches associated with paralysis of one side that may long outlast the headache. It is familial in inheritance. *Ophthalmoplegic or retinal migraines* are unilateral headaches associated with cranial nerve palsy, either third nerve palsy (presents as ptosis and ophthalmoplegia with or without pupil involvement) or sixth nerve palsy. Migraine may be a prominent feature in mitochondrial myopathy, encephalopathy, lactic acidosis, and stroke (MELAS), a mitochondrial disease common in children. It may also occur in a rare vasculopathy in adults called cerebral autosomal-dominant arteriopathy with subcortical infarcts and leukodystrophy (CADASIL).

Cluster Headache

Cluster headaches are also known as histamine headaches or migranous neuralgia. They commonly present as intense non-throbbing unilateral ocular pain associated with lacrimation (secretion of tears), rhinorrhea (discharge of a nasal mucus), conjunctival injection (blood-shot eyes), and ptosis (drooping of the upper eyelid). Diagnosis is based on symptoms. Cluster headaches are characterized by nightly recurrences usually occurring 1–2 h after falling asleep and are not associated with either aura or vomiting. These headaches recur with regularity for up to periods of 6–12 weeks, followed by symptom-free periods of months to years. Cluster headaches usually last for about 15–180 min. Same orbit is usually involved in recurring bouts. Cluster headaches are common in alcoholics, adolescents, and adult males.

Treatment

Treatment for cluster headaches may include oxygen therapy during earlier stage of acute attacks. Triptans such as sumatriptan can be used for treatment after the onset of the headache. Ergotamines are usually used as prophylactic agents. Capsaicin and lidocaine have shown to reduce intensity of cluster headaches when used intranasally. Steroids have shown to be beneficial by reducing the inflammatory modulators; however, they are only considered as short-term therapy. Opiates are used if inadequate relief is seen with the above agents. Tricyclic antidepressants and beta-blockers may be used prophylactically in treatment of chronic cluster headaches.

Tension Headache

Tension headache is the most common variety of headache (Bendtsen 2003). It usually occurs bilaterally with temporal occipitonuchal or frontal predominance. It can also diffuse and extend over the cranium. Diagnosis is made by symptoms. The pain is usually dull, aching, and may be associated with other sensations such as fullness, tightness, and pressure. Unlike the migraine headache, tension headache is not associated with throbbing pain, nausea, vomiting, photophobia, or phonophobia and usually does not interfere with day-to-day activities. Tension headache may persist for days, weeks, months, and years with mild fluctuations. It may be present throughout the day and is often associated with anxiety and depression. This headache is present when the patient awakens or may develop soon after awakening. Tension headaches occur most often in the middle-aged population and are often associated with anxiety, fatigue, and depression.

Treatment

Treatment is usually individualized with the recognition of underlying comorbid conditions such as anxiety, depression, and stress. Acetaminophen with or without codeine/caffeine and NSAIDs (aspirin, naproxen, ibuprofen, etc.) may be used for acute therapy, and antidepressants (amitriptyline), antianxiety drugs (buspirone), and calcium channel blockers may be used for the treatment of underlying comorbidities and as abortive therapy. Ergotamine and propranolol are not effective unless there is a migrainous component associated with the tension headache. Massage, hot and cold applications, transcutaneous nerve stimulation (TENS), meditation, and biofeedback mechanisms that cause relaxation may be useful.

Headaches Due to Meningeal Irritation

These headaches are usually due to a meningeal infection or rupture of an aneurysm. Meningitis and subarachnoid hemorrhage are the most common causes. Diagnosis is based on the patient's symptoms and imaging such as a computed tomography (CT) or a magnetic resonance imaging (MRI). The patient may present with a sudden onset of intense, deep pain, often worse in the neck, and evolving in minutes to hours. The pain can be generalized, bioccipital, or bifrontal. The patient may present with neck stiffness and have positive Kernig and Brudzinkis signs. Kernig's sign is indicative of meningitis; the patient feels pain when the knee and hip are bent, and is therefore asked to extend both the knee and the hip simultaneously. Brudzinki's sign is also indicative of meningitis; in this case, the patient will involuntarily lift his/her legs when their head is lifted while remaining in the supine position.

Treatment
Treatment of headaches due to meningitis usually involves treating the underlying comorbid condition. In the case of bacterial meningitis, empiric antibacterials are used, and viral meningitis is treated with antiviral agents. Acute therapy with steroids has shown to reduce the associated inflammation. Antihypertensives are used to prevent any rupture of brain aneurysms due to hypertension.

Headache of Temporal Arteritis
This headache is caused by inflammation of the cranial arteries and is usually seen in the elderly. It presents with increasingly intense throbbing or non-throbbing headaches. There is often a superimposed sharp, stabbing pain associated with thickened and tender arteries. The pain is usually unilateral, localized to the site of the affected arteries. However, it may also present as bilateral and explosive in nature in some patients. Pain may be present throughout the day and may be more severe at night. It may last for several months, if untreated. Diagnosis is often made based on the patient's age (>55 years of age), no previous history of symptoms, general malaise, weight loss, low-grade fever, and anemia. Erythrocyte sedimentation rate (ESR) may be elevated (>55 mm/h), and 50% of patients experience generalized aching of proximal limb muscles. A complication of temporal arteritis is blindness due to thrombosis of ophthalmic and posterior ciliary arteritis.

Treatment
Treatment consists of low-dose steroids which cause immunosuppression. High-dose steroids are usually reserved for ophthalmic and neurologic complications. Alternatively, other immunosuppressants like azathioprine, methotrexate, cyclophosphamide, and dapsone are used for their steroid-sparing effects.

Posttraumatic Headache
Headaches can occur secondary to acute or chronic subdural hematomas. It usually presents as a severe, chronic, continuous, or intermittent headache that may last several days or weeks. Patients with subdural hematomas may feel dull, deep-seated unilateral pain often accompanied by confusion, drowsiness, and fluctuating hemiparesis. Positional worsening of the symptoms is seen with acute hematomas. Eye pain is a common feature in tentorial hematomas, which is associated with the anatomical "tent" that covers the cerebellum. Diagnosis is established by CT and MRI imaging. Patients on anticoagulant therapy are at higher risk for hematomas. Either conservative treatment or surgical evacuation may be necessary.

Posttraumatic Nervous Instability

Posttraumatic nervous instability is a complex syndrome which involves giddiness, fatigue, nervousness, insomnia, irritability, trembling, tearfulness, lack of concentration, and a headache that resembles a tension headache. Mainstream treatment is supportive therapy, reassurances to the patient about benign nature of the symptoms, physical activity, and treatment with antianxiety and antidepressant drugs.

Headaches of Brain Tumor

Headache is a common symptom in two-thirds of patients with brain tumors. They are deep seated, usually non-throbbing (occasionally throbbing) and are often described as aching and "bursting." These headaches are non-specific in nature and are usually provoked by physical activity or changes in position.

Diagnosis can be made based on the presence of a preexisting brain tumor and signs/symptoms of increased intracranial pressure. These headaches are nearly always on the same side as the tumor and in later stages may be associated with projectile vomiting. Pain may last for hours and may recur many times during the day. These headaches are sometimes associated with vomiting, transient blindness, extremity weakness, and loss of consciousness which often show a high incidence of brain tumor.

Treatment

Treatment consists of correcting the underlying disease. It may involve tumor irradiation, chemotherapy, and/or surgical resection.

Headaches of Pseudo-tumor Cerebri (Idiopathic Intracranial Hypertension)

These headaches usually present as dull or pressure-like occipital or generalized headaches, sometimes associated with horizontal diplopia, transient visual obscurations, and vague dizziness. The most common etiology is idiopathic, but others include hypervitaminosis of vitamin-A, lead, and tetracyclines. Cerebral venous hypertensions, meningeal diseases, metabolic disturbances, gliomatosis cerebri are other causes. Diagnosis can be made if CSF pressure is found to be elevated to 250–450 mm H_2O and if there is papilledema with occasional cranial nerve palsy. A CT or an MRI may show normal or smaller ventricles.

Treatment

Treatment consists of osmotic agents like mannitol or carbonic anhydrase inhibitors like acetazolamide used to reduce intracranial pressure without any vision loss; digoxin has similar effects without severe adverse effects. In the case of severe symptoms like vision loss, high-dose steroids are used for short duration. Surgical treatment involves repeated lumbar punctures.

Secondary Causes of Headaches

Sometimes headache presents secondary to the underlying condition, such as cervical headaches, sinus headaches, psychogenic headaches, or drug-related headaches. The following briefly discusses these other causes.

Cervical Headache

Cervical headaches are usually due to a dysfunction in the cervical spine regions as a result of trauma to the cervical areas. It is one of the more difficult types of headache to diagnose due to its etiology. It is hypothesized that changes in the blood flow to the vertebral arteries due to cervical spine dysfunction are responsible for affecting the cranial blood flow, thus causing headaches. Treatment generally involves diagnosing the underlying cervical dysfunction and restoring the normal cranial blood flow.

Sinus Headache

Sinus headache is secondary to sinus infection or sinusitis. It usually manifests as headache with facial pain, fever, respiratory tract infections such as sore throat, nasal congestion, or ear infections. It may be due to bacterial or viral infection. Management of sinus headache is usually attained by reducing nasal congestion, as well as using antibiotics for the treatment of primary infection, decongestants such as pseudo-ephedrine or phenylephrine, and humidifiers.

Psychogenic Headache

Psychogenic headache is a new category of headache introduced by International Classification of Headache Disorders (ICHD) in 2004. It differs significantly from tension headache because its origin is attributed to underlying psychotic disorder. These headaches usually present with a psychotic disorder and resolve with the management of the disorder. The evidence for such headaches is currently limited, and is under investigation.

Headache Due to Cranial Neuralgia

Headaches due to cranial neuralgias are often associated with inflammation of nerves in the head or face. They usually manifest as throbbing pain in the head or face secondary to the inflamed nerve. They are often seen in association with conditions such as diabetes and multiple sclerosis.

Headache Due to Drugs

Certain drugs such as amphetamines, caffeine, acetaminophen, and ibuprofen can cause headache upon excessive use. Alcohol can cause a headache as one of its withdrawal symptoms. Nitrates and calcium channel blockers can cause a headache as side effect to their antihypertensive effect; niacin and propoxyphene overdose may also present headache as a symptom. Opioids and epileptic drugs are some of the most commonly seen drugs associated with headaches.

Case Scenario

Dr. Suneil Ramessur, MBBS, BSc (Hons), FRCA, DipHEP

Daisy is a 42-year-old female who is referred to your clinic by her PCP with complaints of facial pain. She has been getting intense periods of painful "electric shocks"

on the right side of her face. She has stopped applying makeup to her face for fear of triggering it and says that she is even scared to let her husband touch her face.

What is your diagnosis and how can you confirm it?
Take a full history and, as much as the patient will permit, perform a neurological examination. Her symptoms sound like typical trigeminal neuralgia (TGN). However, this patient is somewhat too young to present with this condition (the peak age at diagnosis is about 70 years), and therefore it is important to consider a latent demyelinating disease such as multiple sclerosis (MS). Some form of neurological imaging is important as 2% of patients presenting with typical TGN have a tumor – commonly a posterior fossa meningioma or a neuroma. MRI or MR topographic angiography (MRTA) will demonstrate the relationship between the nerve and blood vessels and can help identify nerve compression.

In her history, it is important to consider any recent dental work such as a root canal on the upper set of teeth which may have triggered her symptoms. Other conditions that can mimic TGN are

- Cluster headaches
- Short lasting unilateral neuralgiform headache with conjunctival injection and tearing (SUNCT)
- Chronic paroxysmal hemicrania (CPH)
- Jabs and jolts syndrome
- Cracked tooth syndrome
- Post-herpetic neuralgia
- Giant cell arteritis

Daisy did not have any facial weakness or sensory loss and nerve conduction studies were normal. The MRTA demonstrated compression in the nerve-pons junction. You explain there are pharmacological and non-pharmacological treatments available for her condition, and she prefers to avoid any procedural interventions at present.

What pharmacological treatment modalities are available to Daisy?
The anticonvulsants are the mainstay of treatment, in particular carbamazepine; dual therapy with gabapentin may be preferable to monotherapy with high-dose carbamazepine alone. A number of other pharmacological treatments have been used with varying degrees of success.

Daisy's symptoms have subsided slightly with the pharmacological regime on which you have placed her. However, 6 months later you receive a call asking you to urgently see her as an inpatient following a suicide attempt she has made, apparently due to an extreme exacerbation of her pain. You visit her and she tells you that, despite her fears, she is now ready to consider a surgical/procedural intervention.

What procedural treatments are available to Daisy?
The most established procedure is microvascular decompression (MVD). The initial reduction in symptoms is very high with over half still pain free 8–10 years later. Other possible procedures include:

Radiofrequency gangliolysis
Glycerol gangliolysis
Balloon decompression
Stereotactic radiotherapy
Peripheral neurectomy
Cryotherapy
Alcohol block

The patient should be advised to consult a neurosurgeon. The neurosurgeon's area of expertise and experience will generally dictate precisely which treatment will be best suited for your patient.

References

Bendtsen L. Central and peripheral sensitization in tension-type headache. Curr Pain Headache Rep. 2003;7:460.

Brandes JL, Kudrow D, Stark SR, O'Carroll CP, Adelman JU, O'Donnell FJ, et al. Sumatriptan-naproxen for acute treatment of migraine: a randomized trial. JAMA Apr 4 2007;297(13):1443–54. Medline

Headache Classification Committee of the International Headache Society. Classification and diagnostic criteria for headache disorders, cranial neuralgias and facial pain. Cephalagia 1998;8(suppl 7):1–96

Lance JW. Current concepts of migraine pathogenesis. Neurology Jun 1993;43(6 suppl 3): S11–5.

Lipton RB, Diamond S, Reed M, Diamond ML, Stewart WF. Migraine diagnosis and treatment: results from the American Migraine Study II. Headache 2001;41:638–45.

Spierings ELH, Ranke AH, Honkoop PC. Precipitating and aggravating factors of migraine versus tension-type headache. Headache 2001;41:554–8.

Zagami AS. Pathophysiology of migraine and tension type headaches. Curr Opin Neurol. 1994;7:272.

Chapter 28

Management of Cancer Pain

Joseph N. Atallah, MD

Epidemiology of Cancer Pain

Cancer is the second leading cause of death in the United States after heart diseases. Center of Disease Control estimated number of cancer deaths in 2005 to 559,312. Cancer constitutes 22.8% of the total death in the United States. Lung cancer is the most common fatal cancer in men (31%), followed by colon and rectum (10%), and prostate (9%). In women, lung (26%), breast (15%), and colon and rectum (10%) are the leading causes of cancer death. Most patients with cancer have pain. Cancer pain can develop from tumor invasion, musculoskeletal pain, visceral pain, radiation treatment effect, or neuropathy from chemotherapy. The incidence of pain in cancer patients receiving active treatment for early disease is about 20–25%. The incidence of pain in cancer patient with advanced disease is about 90%. More than 50% of patients with cancer pain have only one or two locations of pain. This fact usually gives the opportunity for interventional pain doctors to help patients with pain. Many cancer patients present with a combination of pain types such as visceral and somatic pain. Up to 90% of cancer pain patients respond well to medical treatment. A high percentage of the remaining individuals also respond well to interventional pain techniques (Portenoy 1989).

Barriers for Effective Pain Relief in Cancer Patients

There are several barriers for pain control in cancer patients. These barriers include family, patient him/herself and physician barriers. Family- and patient-related barriers consist of the fear of addiction from opioids, fear of other side effects from opioids, patient and family wrong belief that pain is inevitable with cancer and that opioids should be saved until they really need them (when the pain is intolerable. In addition, patients are afraid of being considered drug seekers or patient is afraid of distracting the physician from treating the main problem which is cancer. Physician and healthcare barriers are lack of education regarding pain treatment among physicians and healthcare workers, lack of knowledge by medical students and nursing staff on how to treat pain, fear from being prosecuted by state medical boards and other federal agencies for prescribing high doses of opioids, or unfamiliarity of physician and nursing staff with the fact that high opioid doses may be needed for cancer pain patients, especially in late stage of cancer. There is also a fear of side effects of opioids such as respiratory depression (Abram 1998, Benedetti 2000, Berland 2000).

N. Vadivelu et al. (eds.), *Essentials of Pain Management*,
DOI 10.1007/978-0-387-87579-8_28, © Springer Science+Business Media, LLC 2011

Assessment of Cancer Pain

Assessment of patients with cancer pain includes history of the pain, physical examination including a complete neurologic examination, diagnostic testing, and finally development of a management plan.

Obtaining History of Pain

A history of the pain includes information about its etiology, site(s) of pain, pattern and radiation, intensity of pain, description of pain and quality, factors exacerbating and relieving pain, previous forms of pain treatment, and pathophysiology of the pain (i.e., somatic, visceral, neuropathic). Somatic pain is described as dull or aching and is readily localized by the patient. Visceral pain is characterized as a deep, pressure-type sensation that is poorly localized; it may be diffuse and/or squeezing in nature. Neuropathic pain is described as a severe, burning, or a tingling sensation with a lancinating component.

Common forms of measurement include facial expression scale (see Chapter 5) or linear analog scale. Linear scale ranges from 0 to 10, in which 0 means no pain and 10 means the worst pain level imaginable (see Chapter 5). Scales may be verbal or written, and can be colors, numbers, or lines.

Other parts of patient history include past medical history such as information about comorbidity factors, current medications including all medications that the patient used for pain treatment in the past, social history including history of substance abuse, psychosocial evaluation including psychiatric history, patient distress, support systems, and patient/family attitudes about pain and its treatment.

It is important to repeat assessment of cancer pain on a regular basis to evaluate the treatment effectiveness and possible side effects. Repeat assessment can determine any change in the pain level or location (Burton et al. 2002, Burton et al. 2004b, Carr et al. 2000).

Physical Examination of Patient with Cancer Pain

Physical examination of the patient with cancer pain includes evaluation of patient weight including amount of weight loss, vital signs [temperature, heart rate (HR), blood pressure (BP), and respiratory rate (RR)]. Other aspects of evaluation should include: evaluation of pain as a fifth vital sign, general appearance of the patient, evaluation of gait, examination of heart and lungs and lymphatic system including examination of the blood flow to the extremities, and examination of the abdomen and pelvis. Complete neurological examination is essential which includes motor function of upper and lower extremities, deep tendon reflexes of the upper and lower extremities, sensory examination of the upper and lower extremities, and straight leg raising. Musculoskeletal examination including trigger point tenderness and evaluation of the possible sites of metastases is critical.

Diagnostic Testing of Cancer Pain Patients

Evaluation of the area of pain with diagnostic testing is essential. Diagnostic imaging modalities include plain films, computed tomography (CT) scan, positron emission tomography (PET) scan, and/or magnetic resonance imaging (MRI) of the affected area. Plain films are ideal for bone fractures. CT scan is helpful for bone metastasis, while MRI is helpful in soft tissue and bony metastatic disease. Bone scan is also useful in bone metastases. PET scan can detect soft tissue tumors and is also useful in detecting the response and/ or progress of cancer treatment.

Formulating a Plan of Care

Cancer pain can be changing based on the progress of disease and also based on the improvement in the size of the tumor. Formulating a plan of care is essential including a substitute plan in case of resistant pain. Discussing the whole plan with the patient is essential. Patient may need assurance that the first plan is not the only option available for them.

Pharmacologic Treatment of Cancer Pain

Analgesic Ladder

World Health Organization (WHO) developed guidelines for treatment of cancer pain (World Health Organization 1990, Zech 1995). It includes three-step "analgesic ladder" for pharmacologic management of cancer pain.

Application of the World Health Organization (WHO) analgesic ladder helps provide adequate analgesia in the majority of cases (Fig. 28.1) (Jacox et al. 1994, Miguel 2000, Patt 1993). The steps in the analgesic ladder are designed to treat mild, moderate and severe cancer pain:

- Mild pain: Non-opioid analgesics including non-steroidal anti-inflammatory drugs (NSAIDS; +/-) used in adjuvant therapy such as anticonvulsants and acetaminophen.
- Mild to moderate pain: Opioids and non-opioid analgesics and adjuvant therapy.
- Moderate to severe pain: Strong opioids such as long-acting opioids in addition to short-acting opioids and/or adjuvant therapy.

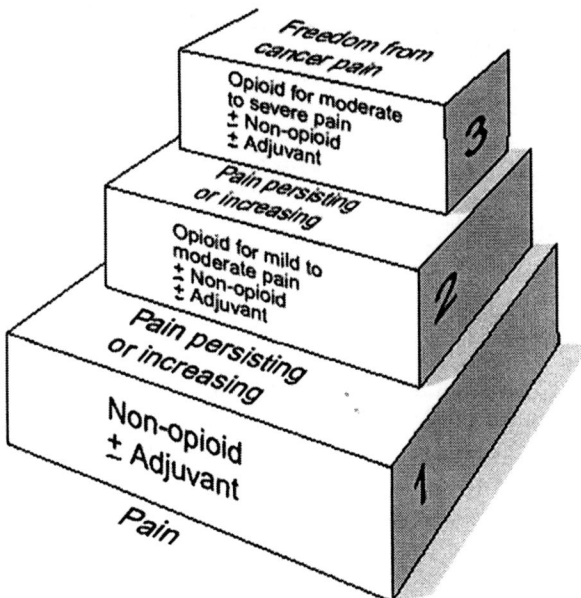

Figure 28.1 World Health Organization (WHO) Analgesic Ladder 1990.

Modified Analgesic Ladder

If the pain is persistent despite increasing doses of opioids, interventional treatment is warranted. Interventional procedures are demonstrated as Step 4 in the modified analgesic ladder below (Fig. 28.2). Interventional procedures are should be considered in cases of severe to intractable pain.

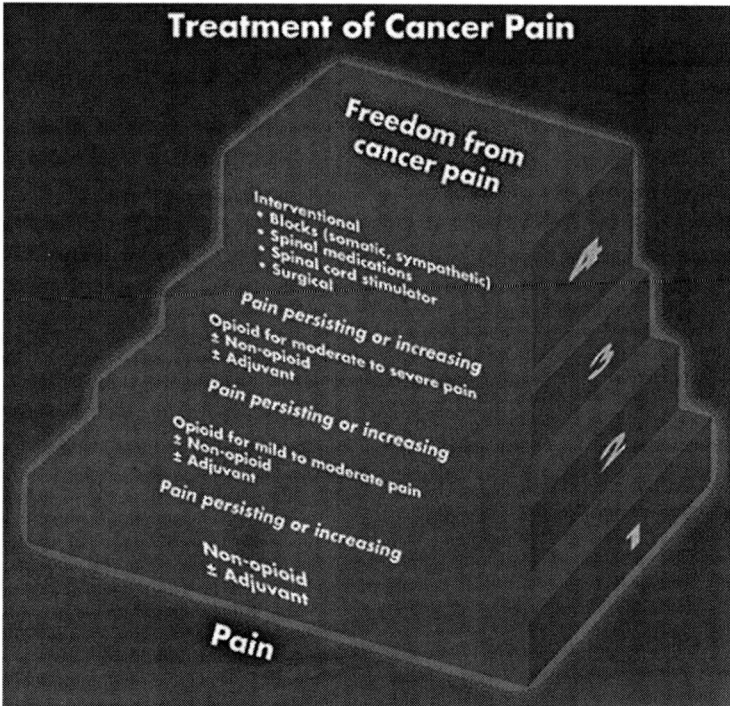

Figure 28.2 Modified World Health Organization (WHO) analgesic ladder for cancer pain, including interventional management. Adapted from Miguel (2000).

Non-opioid Analgesics

The first line of treatment includes non-opioid analgesics. Table 28.1 describes the commonly used non-opioid analgesics, their usual doses, route of administration, and possible side effects of each drug.

Opioid Therapy in the Treatment of Cancer Pain

When non-opioid analgesic fails to control the patient pain, opioid therapy plays an important role in treatment of cancer pain. Table 28.2 explains the difference in opioid peak onset based on route of administration (Fukshansky et al. 2005). Table 28.3 shows different opioids, available doses, route of administration, duration of action, and equi-analgesic doses (Burton 2004a). The characteristics of each drug, including side effects are discussed in different chapters in this book.

Combining short- and long-acting opioids in moderate to severe pain can be effective if the pain is not well-controlled and if the patient is already on PRN short-acting opioids.

Table 28.1 Commonly used non-opioid analgesics in cancer pain.

Drug	Usual dosage	Route of administration	Possible side effects	Other considerations
Acetaminophen	325–1500 mg	PO or suppository	Hepatotoxic on high dose	Do not exceed 4000 mg/day
Aspirin	81–325 mg/day	PO or suppository	Bleeding ulcers	
Ibuprofen	200–2400 mg/day	PO or suppository	Bleeding ulcers	Caution with renal patients
Ketorolac	10 mg PO q 4–6 h or 30 mg IV/IM q 6 h	Oral, IV, or IM	Bleeding ulcers	IV dose should not exceed 3–4 days
Naproxen	250–500 mg PO BID	Oral	Bleeding ulcers	Do not exceed a dose of 1000 mg/day for more than 6 months
Tramadol	50–100 mg PO q 6 h	Oral	Higher risk of seizures if used with antidepressants	Centrally acting non-opiate analgesic with low affinity for μ-opioid receptors
Tramadol-sustained release	100–300 mg/day	Oral	Same as above	Same as above

PO=per os.

Table 28.2 Opioid peak onset based on route of administration.

Route	Peak onset
Oral	60–90 min
Subcutaneous	30 min
Intravenous	15–20 min

In case of moderate to severe pain that is persistent throughout the 24-h period, combining long-acting opioids and short-acting opioids in cancer pain is often ideal. This can be done by adding a small dose of long-acting opioid to the already administered PRN short-acting opioid. Then, increase the dose of long-acting opioids gradually (every 1 to 2 weeks) until the dose of PRN short-acting opioids constitutes 15–20% of the total daily dose of patient's requirement of opioids. Figure 28.3 shows ideal treatment with long and short-acting opioids. It shows around the clock medication used long-acting opioids for persistent pain. Breakthrough pain is usually treated with breakthrough medication, which is a short-acting medication. Prescribing physician should be aware of the potential for overmedication, as shown in Fig. 28.3. If the patient is not using any short-acting or breakthrough medications, he/she may be approaching the overmedication line. Evaluation of the patient on a regular basis for signs of overmedication, such as sedation or drowsiness, is necessary.

Table 28.3 Routes and equianalgesic doses of selected opioids.

Drug	Available names and dosage	Duration of action	Equi-analgesic dose to 30 mg PO morphine per day		Route of administration
Morphine Sulfate instant release (MSIR)	• PO 15, 30 mg • Rectal 5, 10, 20, and 30 mg IV 1–10 mg dosage	3–4 h	30 mg PO is equivalent to 10 mg IV		PO, Rectal , IV, epidural, or intrathecal (only FDA approved opioid for intrathecal use in PF form)
Morphine sulfate-sustained release	MS contin ® 15, 30, 60, 100, 200 mg Ormamorph SR® 15, 30, 60, 100 mg Kadian® 20, 30, 50, 60, 100 mg Avinza® 30, 60, 90, 120 mg	8 h 12 h 24 h 24 h	30 mg PO morphine		Oral (tablet should not be broken or dissolved)
Hydromorphone (Dilaudid®)	Oral 2, 4, 8 mg Parenteral 1, 2, 4, 8 mg Suppository 3 mg	3 h	IV or suppository 2 mg	Oral 5 mg	Oral, IV, or suppository
Codeine	15, 30, 60 mg Oral	2–4 h	90 mg orally		Oral
Propoxyphene	Darvon 65 mg Darvon N 100 100 mg	3–4 h	200 mg orally		oral
Oxycodone	Oxycodone 5, 10 mg Oxy IR 5, 10, 15, and 30 mg Percocet 5/325, 7.5/500, and 10/650	3–4 h	20 mg orally		Oral or suspension
Oxycodone-sustained release	Oxycontin® 10, 20, 40, 80, 160 mg	12 h	20 mg		Oral (tablet should not be broken or dissolved)
Oxymorphone	Opana® 5, 10 mg 5, 10, 40 mg PO	4 h	20 mg		Oral tablets or suspension
Methadone		6–8 h	30 mg		
Fentanyl	• Transdermal patches (Duragesic®) 12, 25, 50, 75, or 100 mcgm/hr Q 48–72 h • Transbuccal lozenge (Actiq®) 200, 400, 600, 1200, or 1800 mcgm	72 h 2–4 h	100 mcgm		IV, transdermal, or transmucosal

FDA=Food and Drug Administration; IV=intravenous; PO=per os.

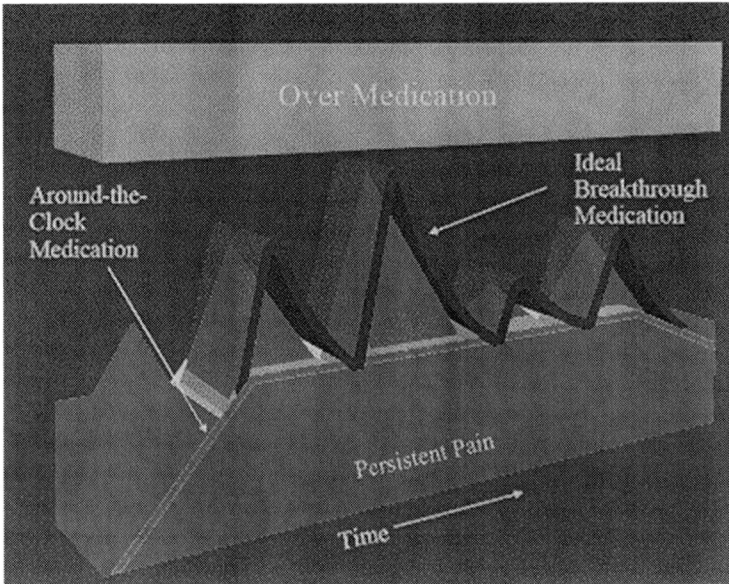

Figure 28.3 Ideal treatment of cancer pain with opioids using short- and long-acting agents. Long-acting opioids are used to help with the persistent pain, while short-acting opioids are used for the breakthrough pain. Please note the line for overmedication.

Patient-Controlled Analgesia in Cancer Pain

Patient with cancer pain who has intravenous (IV) access, unable to tolerate per os (PO) opioids, and prefers to have control over their pain management may benefit from patient-controlled analgesia (PCA). The patient can carry PCA machine in a backpack and deliver opioids through intermittent boluses controlled by the patient, and/or have a basal infusion of medications. Patient-controlled analgesia is described in detail in other chapters.

Interventional Management of Cancer Pain

If pain is not adequately controlled with pharmacologic treatments, consideration of alternative modalities is warranted. These modalities include antitumor therapy, neural blockade with or without neurolytic drugs, infusion therapy with opioids and/or local anesthesia with neuro-axial or peripheral nerves, central nervous system (CNS) opioid therapy, neurosurgery, or electrical stimulation. Table 28.4 shows examples of neurolytic blocks that can be helpful in alleviating cancer pain. Each block will be discussed separately in this chapter or indifferent chapters in this book. Table 28.5 shows different kinds of infusion therapy of opioids with or without local anesthesia either as neuro-axial analgesia or as regional anesthesia.

Surgical Treatment of Cancer Pain

Surgical treatment of cancer pain is rarely used now because of the development of intrathecal opioid infusions. These procedures include neurectomy, cordotomy, rhizotomy, or cingulotomy. These surgical options are beyond the scope of this text.

Table 28.4 Examples of Neurolytic Blocks for Cancer Pain.

Neurolytic blocks
- Celiac plexus
- Superior hypogastric plexus
- Ganglion impar
- Lumbar sympathetic chain
- Stellate ganglion
- Subarachnoid or epidural neurolysis
- Intercostal nerve
- Peripheral nerves

Table 28.5 Infusion therapy of opioids and/or local anesthesia.

Neuro-axial analgesia and/or anesthesia	Regional anesthesia
• Simple epidural infusion	• Brachial plexus (e.g., axillary, interscalene, supraclavicular, or infraclavicular infusion)
• Tunneled epidural infusion	• Lumbar plexus infusion
• Intrathecal programmable infusion	• Selective nerve infusion (e.g., sciatic or femoral nerve infusion)
• Implanted intrathecal programmable pumps	• Intrapleural catheter infusion
	• Paravertebral catheter infusion (e.g., thoracic or lumbar)

Radiation Treatment of Cancer Pain

Radiation therapy is used for pain relief if the tumor is invading bone or soft tissue. It is also used for decreasing the size of tumor mass. If bone metastases are limited to few sites, external beam radiation therapy may relieve pain and symptoms. In case of widely disseminated bone metastases, hemi-body irradiation has been utilized. This can produce complete pain relief in 20% of patients and partial pain relief in 75% of patients. Systemic radiopharmaceuticals have also been used in pain caused by various metastatic diseases. These agents are specific to each tumor. For example, one can provide pain relief in patients with well-differentiated thyroid cancer. Pain relief can occur within the first week of treatment and lasts for 2–4 months.

Neurolytic Visceral Sympathetic Blocks

Neurolytic sympathetic blocks can be very helpful in controlling pain that is visceral in origin. Visceral pain can occur when visceral structures are involved with cancer due to pressure, invasion, or stretching. Visceral pain can be dull, squeezing, and poorly localized. Referred pain can occur due to visceral pain. For example, patient can experience pain in the shoulder when the diaphragm is involved in the tumor. Sympathetic block can help visceral pain only. This means that other forms of pain that may be associated with the tumor cannot be affected and does not mean that the block is not successful. Visceral pain is transmitted along the

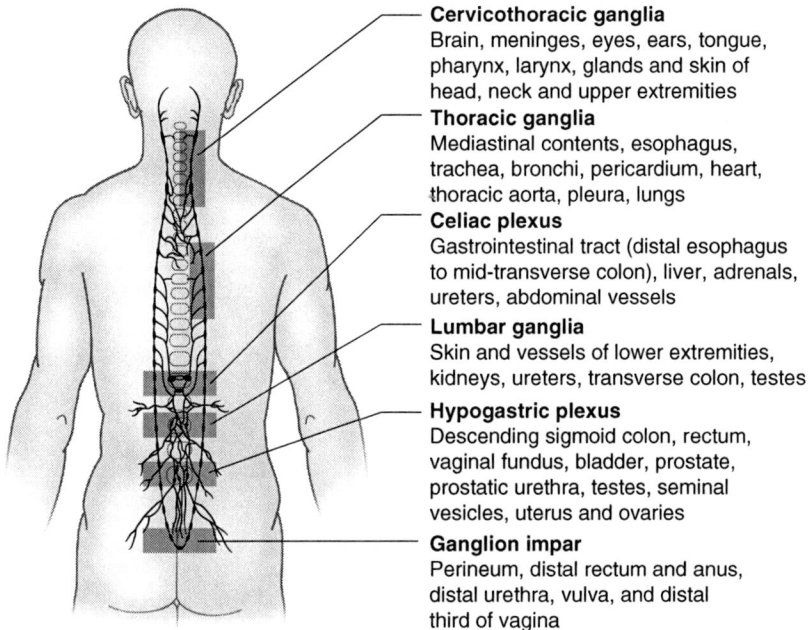

Cervicothoracic ganglia
Brain, meninges, eyes, ears, tongue, pharynx, larynx, glands and skin of head, neck and upper extremities

Thoracic ganglia
Mediastinal contents, esophagus, trachea, bronchi, pericardium, heart, thoracic aorta, pleura, lungs

Celiac plexus
Gastrointestinal tract (distal esophagus to mid-transverse colon), liver, adrenals, ureters, abdominal vessels

Lumbar ganglia
Skin and vessels of lower extremities, kidneys, ureters, transverse colon, testes

Hypogastric plexus
Descending sigmoid colon, rectum, vaginal fundus, bladder, prostate, prostatic urethra, testes, seminal vesicles, uterus and ovaries

Ganglion impar
Perineum, distal rectum and anus, distal urethra, vulva, and distal third of vagina

Figure 28.4 Schematic outline of the sympathetic nervous system with ganglia amenable to blockade highlighted.

sympathetic nervous system from the involved organ, relaying in para-vertebral ganglia that lie along the anterolateral portion of the vertebral column (Fig. 28.4). These ganglia are in perfect location for neurolytic destruction in case of cancer pain

Before performing any neurolytic block the physician should obtain pain history, and physical examination with identification of cancer as the main reason of pain. Neurological examination is mandatory before performing neurolytic blocks in order to identify any preexisting neurological deficit. The physician should perform examination of the site of the block to identify the presence of any infection and obtain coagulation profile including PT, INR, PTT, and platelet count because some of the cancer medications can affect platelets function and coagulation factors. The patient should have received appropriate trials of opioid and there should be a documentation of intolerance to opioids or ineffectiveness of opioids in relieving pain, despite increasing the dose. The physician should also obtain informed consent, explain in detail the procedure to the patient and also to the family if required, explain in detail and document all the risks and benefits of the blocks including the alternatives, the projected analgesic response, and the expected goals of therapy. Performance of local anesthetic block prior to neurolytic block is essential. This will enable the patient to be aware of the effect and possible side effects of the block, and also it will the patient and the healthcare providers to identify any neurologic deficits that may be intolerable to the patient. The most common neurolytic agents are alcohol or phenol. They both have equal effects. Table 28.6 shows the differences between alcohol and phenol as neurolytic agents.

Table 28.6 Differences between alcohol and phenol as neurolytic agents.

	Alcohol	Phenol
Concentration	50–100%	6–12%
Additives usually used	Local anesthetics (to relieve pain on injection)	Glycerin
Uses	Visceral ganglion neurolysis, subarachnoid injection, or peripheral nerve injection	Same
Patient response on injection	Pain (added local A. is helpful while keeping the concentration of alcohol above 50%)	Warm sensation. Usually no pain. It has local anesthesia. Property
Physical characters	Unstable at room temperature. Vials should open just prior to injection	Stable
Baricity	Hypobaric (i.e., will raise up in CSF)	Hyperbaric (i.e., will sink in CSF)
Effect	2–4 days	1–2 days
Duration of block	Long	Short
Neuronal generation	Possible	Possible

CSF=cerebrospinal fluid.

Celiac Plexus Block

Anatomy of the Celiac Plexus

The celiac plexus is the largest ganglia of the sympathetic nervous system located at prevertebral level of body of first lumbar vertebra. It innervates abdominal viscera and contains visceral afferent and efferent fibers. It also contains parasympathetic fibers from the vagus nerve. It does not contain any somatic fibers. Right-sided ganglion lies medial to inferior vena cava, while left-sided ganglia lies anterior to abdominal aorta (Waldman 2001, Wong and Brown 1997). Preganglionic axons from T5 through T12 leave the spinal cord with the ventral spinal routes to join the white communicating rami en route to the sympathetic chain. These axons do not synapse in the sympathetic chain but they pass through the chain to synapse at distal sites, including the celiac ganglia. Preganglionic nerves from T5 through T9 travel caudally from the sympathetic chain along the anterolateral aspects of the vertebral bodies. At the level of T9 and T10, the axons coalesce to form the greater splanchnic nerve. Sympathetic nerves from T10 through T11 and occasionally T12 combine to form the lesser splanchnic nerve. Their course parallels the greater splanchnic nerve in a posterolateral position and ends in either the celiac plexus or aorticorenal ganglion. The least splanchnic nerves arise from T12, parallel posteriorly the lesser splanchnic nerve, and synapse in the aorticorenal ganglion.

Indication of Celiac Plexus Block

The most common indication for celiac plexus block is malignancy in the gastrointestinal tract up to the transverse colon. The most common indication is cancer of the pancreas.

The following are some common indications for celiac plexus block:

1. Intra-abdominal visceral analgesia
2. Upper abdominal surgery combining intercostal block and celiac block
3. Intra-abdominal malignancy
4. Cancer of stomach

5. Pancreatic cancer
6. Gall bladder cancer
7. Adrenal mass
8. Common bile duct cancer
9. Chronic pancreatitis
10. Diagnostic neural blockade
11. Abdominal pain due to active intermittent porphyria

The efficacy of celiac plexus neurolytic block is related to the location and extends of cancer. It is overall considered as a good adjuvant to the pain management in cancer pain from the upper gastrointestinal tract. The main goal of this block is to eliminate the pain or decrease it, so oral opioids can control the pain without side effects.

Techniques

There are multiple techniques that can block visceral pain from the upper abdomen (Eisenberg et al. 1995).

These techniques include retrocrural posterior approach (behind diaphragm), transcrural posterior approach (through diaphragm), trans-aortic posterior approach, splanchnic nerve block, or an anterior approach which can be accomplished with either CT or ultrasound guidance. Table 28.7 and Figs. 28.5, 28.6, 28.7, and 28.8 compare the common techniques for posterior approach for celiac plexus block. Injection of dye is essential which shows good spread of the contrast at the anterolateral border of the corresponding vertebral body. If the patient has difficulty positioning prone, then anterior approach under CT guidance may be

Table 28.7 Comparison of the common techniques for posterior approach for celiac plexus block.

	Retrocrural (Fig. 28.5)	Transcrural (Fig. 28.6)	Trans-aortic (Fig. 28.7)	Splanchnic (Fig. 28.8)
Position	Prone	Prone	Prone or right lateral down position	Prone
Fluoroscopy use	Mandatory	Mandatory	Mandatory	Mandatory
Number of needles	Two	Two	One	Two
Type of needle	22G 5–7 in.	22G 5–7 in.	22G 7 in.	22G 5–7 in.
Level of needle insertion	first lumbar vertebrae 7 cm from midline bilaterally	first lumbar vertebrae 7 cm from midline bilaterally	first lumbar vertebrae 7 cm from midline on the left side	first lumbar vertebrae 7 cm from midline bilaterally
Direction of the needle	L1	L1	L1	T12
Final position of the left needle	Posterior to the aorta	Through the diaphragm and posterior to the aorta	Through the diaphragm and aorta. The needle tip just pass the wall of the aorta through continuous aspiration	Posterior to the aorta
Final position of the right needle	1 cm deeper than the left needle	Through the diaphragm	N/A	1 cm deeper than the left needle

N/A=not applicable.

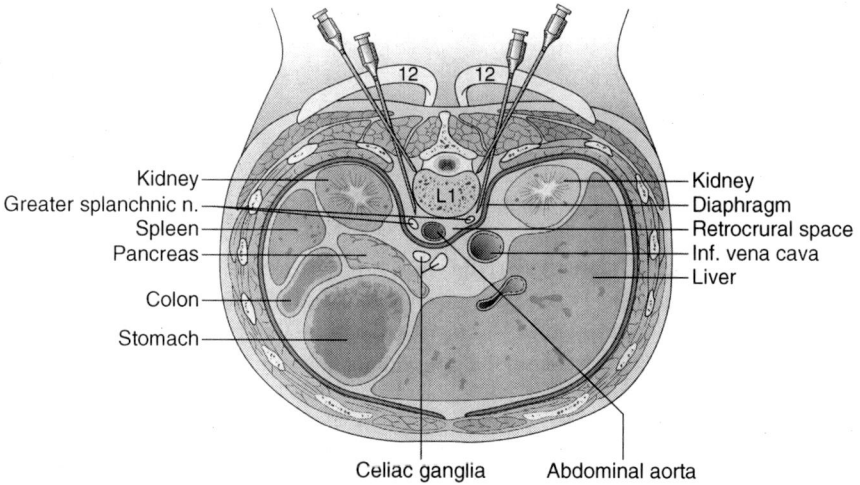

Figure 28.5   Retrocrural approach to the celiac plexus.

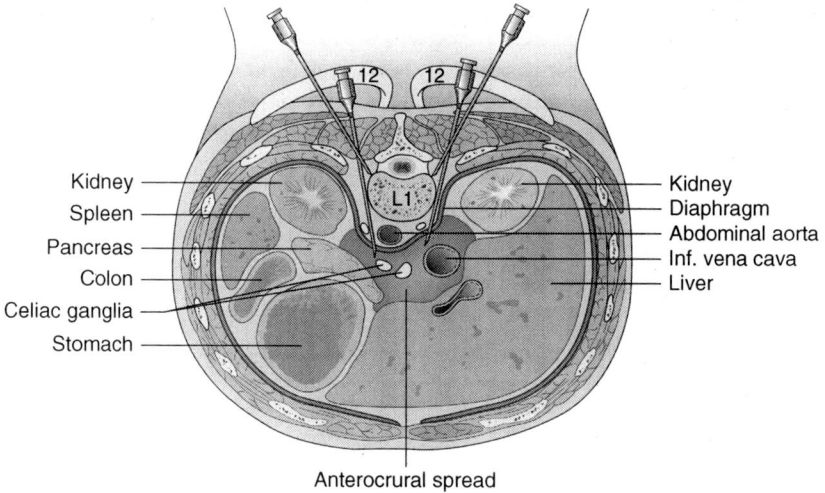

Figure 28.6   Transcrural approach to the celiac plexus.

appropriate. For a diagnostic block, 10 ml of bupivacaine 0.25–0.5% is injected on each side. For a neurolytic block, 15 ml of alcohol 100% mixed with 5 ml of lidocaine 2% (to avoid pain on injection) in each needle is injected. As an alternative, phenol 10% 10 ml can be injected in each needle without associated pain.

Complications

The most common side effect of celiac plexus block is orthostatic hypotension and is due to sympathetic block (Davies 1993, de Leon-Casasola 2000). It is usually transient and resolves

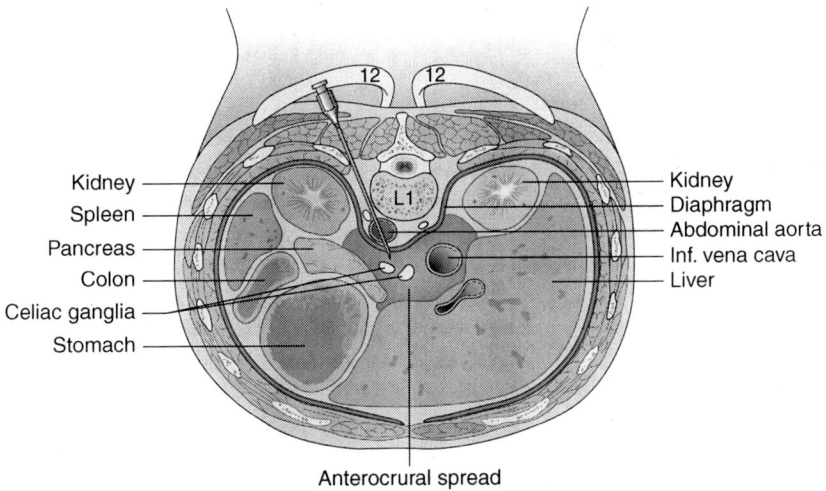

Figure 28.7   Transaortic approach to the celiac ganglia.

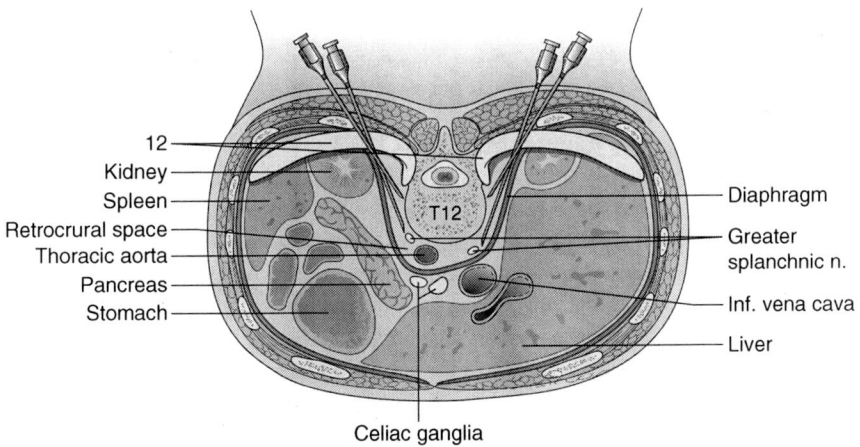

Figure 28.8   Splanchnic nerve block at the level of T12.

in 3–7 days. It is important to avoid sudden change in position in the first few days after the block. For the immediate effect after the procedure, we recommend a bolus of 500–1000 ml of normal saline before or during the procedure if the patient condition permits. Another common side effect is diarrhea, which is due to sympathetic block and usually is self-limited but should be treated with fluid resuscitation in debilitated or dehydrated patients. Paraplegia has been reported and has been attributed to injury or spasm of the lumbar segmental artery that supplies the spinal cord. This can be temporary or permanent. Another serious complication is retroperitoneal hematoma which can occur more frequently in patients who are on anticoagulation at the time of the procedure. The most common complaint after the procedure is back pain. A thorough patient history and physical examination will differentiate between back pain from needle placement and hematoma. CT scan is essential to rule out hematoma.

The Splanchnic Nerve Block

The indications for the splanchnic nerve block are similar to those for the celiac plexus block. It is indicated for patients with retroperitoneal pain and with upper abdominal pain not responding to the celiac plexus block because of the higher rate of complications associated with this block. The sympathetic supply for the abdominal viscera arises from the anterolateral horn of the spinal cord. Preganglionic fibers from T5 to T12 exit the spinal cord along with the ventral nerve roots and synapse in the celiac ganglia. Most of the preganglionic contribution to the celiac plexus is obtained from the greater, lesser, and least splanchnic nerves. The two needle retrocrural approach for the splanchnic nerve block is similar to that for the celiac plexus block, except that the needles are inserted in a more cephalad direction to rest on the anterolateral aspect of the T12 vertebral body (Shah et al. 2003).

Hypogastric Plexus Block

Hypogastric plexus block is located bilaterally in front of the anterolateral border of the lower 1/3 of L5 vertebral body. The ganglia are located in the retroperitoneum (Plancarte et al. 1997). Superior hypogastric plexus innervates the sympathetic structures of the lower abdominal and pelvic organs. Visceral pain is an important component in pelvic pain due to cancer. Pain relief from superior hypogastric plexus block is possible because afferent nerve fibers to the pelvic structures travel via sympathetic nerves and ganglia.

Indications for Superior Hypogastric Plexus Block

Hypogastric plexus block is useful in relieving visceral pain due to cancer from the descending colon, sigmoid colon, and rectum. It is also useful in pain originating from cancer of the bladder, prostatic urethra, prostate, seminal vesicles, and testicles. Pain from the cancer of the uterus, ovary, and vaginal fundus also can be treated with hypogastric plexus block. The efficacy of neurolytic block depends on the location and extent of the tumor. It is overall considered as a good adjuvant to pain management in cancer pain from the lower GI tract and pelvic organs. The goal is to eliminate the pain or decrease it, so that concomitant oral opioid administration can control the pain without significant side effects.

Technique

Hypogastric plexus is located at the lower 1/3 of L5 vertebral body in front of the anterolateral border of L5 on each side. Two needles are usually used to approach these ganglia. Table 28.8 describes the technique of this block. Figure 28.9 shows the final position of each needle. Injection of dye is essential to show good spread of the contrast at the anterolateral border of L5 vertebral body. For diagnostic block, 8–10 ml of bupivacaine 0.25–0.5% is injected on each side. For neurolytic block, 10 ml of alcohol 100% mixed with 5 ml of lidocaine 2% (to avoid pain on injection) in each needle is administered. As an alternative, phenol 10% 8–10 ml can be injected in each needle, usually with less associated pain.

Complications

One of the serious complications is retroperitoneal hematoma which occurs more frequently in patients who are on anticoagulation at the time of the procedure. The most common

Table 28.8   Technique of hypogastric plexus block.

Position	Prone with pillow under the abdomen
Fluoroscopy use	Mandatory
Number of needles	Two
Type of needle	22G 7 in.
Level of needle insertion	Lumbar vertebrae L4–5 interspace or L5 vertebral body 7 cm from midline bilaterally
Direction of the needle	Medial and caudal toward the lower 1/3 of L5
Final position of the left needle	Lower 1/3 of L5 vertebral body in front of the anterolateral border of L5
Final position of the right needle	Same

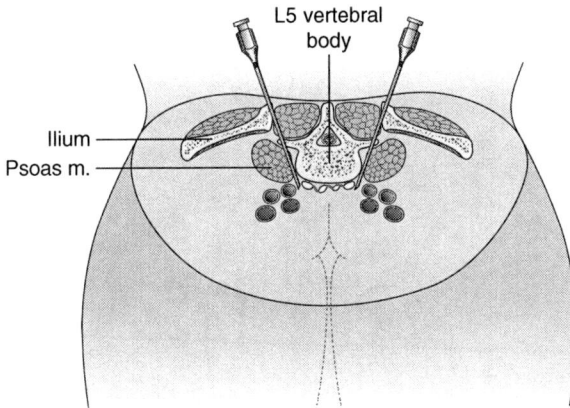

Figure 28.9   Hypogastric plexus block.

complaint after the procedure is back pain. A thorough patient history and physical examination will differentiate between back pain from needle placement or hematoma. CT scan is essential to rule out hematoma. Another common complaint is back pain which can be differentiated from back pain due to hematoma by the severity of pain and by performing serial exams. CT scan is diagnostic.

Ganglion Impar Block

The two sympathetic chains unite at the level of sacrococcygeal ligament. Ganglion impar is a solitary sympathetic ganglia at that level. Ganglion impar provides sympathetic supply to the perineum, distal rectum and anus, distal urethra, vulva, and distal third of vagina. This block can relieve cancer pain originating from the perineum, distal rectum and anus, distal urethra, vulva, and distal third of vagina.

Technique

Ganglion impar can be blocked at the level of the sacrococcygeal ligament. Needle should be bent at 45° angle to avoid injury to the anal canal or the rectum. Table 28.9 describes the technique of the block, and Fig. 28.10 shows the final position of the needle. Injection of dye is

Table 28.9 Technique of ganglion impar block.

Position	Prone, lithotomy, or lateral position
Fluoroscopy use	Mandatory
Number of needles	One
Type of needle	22G 3.5 in. bent 45° angle
Level of needle insertion	Anococcygeal ligament
Direction of the needle	Midline concavity posterior close to the sacrum
Final position of the needle	Level of the sacrococcygeal ligament

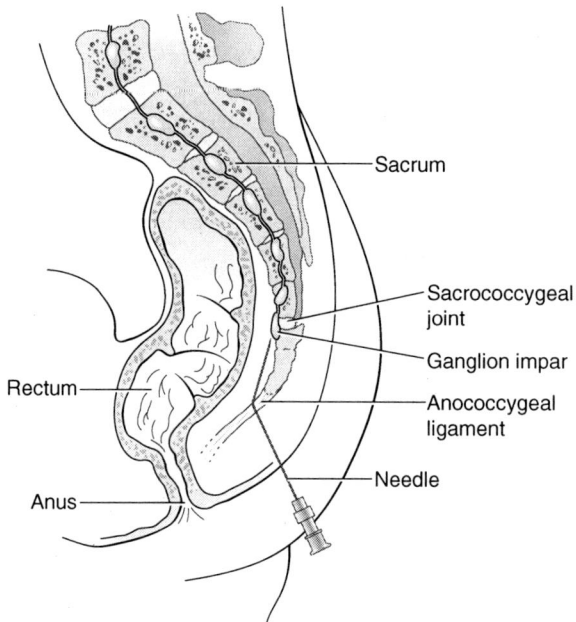

Figure 28.10   Ganglion impar block.

essential that shows good spread of the contrast in the retroperitoneal space and posterior to the rectum. For diagnostic block, 4–5 ml of bupivacaine 0.25–0.5% is injected. For neurolytic block, phenol 10% 4–5 ml can be injected.

Complications

Retroperitoneal hematoma can occur more frequently in patients who are on anticoagulation at the time of the procedure. The most common complaint after the procedure is back pain. As already discussed for other blocks, a good patient history and physical examination will help differentiate between back pain from needle placement and hematoma. CT scan is essential to rule out hematoma or bleeding. Another common complaint is back pain which can be differentiated from back pain due to hematoma by the severity of pain and by performing serial exams. CT scan is diagnostic. Perforation of the rectum or anus can occur. Another potential complication is injection of the neurolytic medication in the rectum or the sacrum. Injection of contrast dye before injection of neurolytic substances is therefore essential.

Stellate Ganglion Block

There are relatively few indications for cancer pain relief from stellate ganglion block. Cancer from head and neck and sympathetically mediated pain from the upper extremities are usually the main reasons for performing this block. The technique is the same as stellate ganglion block described elsewhere in the book, especially in relation to the management of the complex region pain syndrome (CRPS). Diagnostic block can be done by using 5 ml of bupivacaine 0.25–0.5%. Neurolytic block can be done using 6% phenol 3 ml and is used if diagnostic block is successful in controlling the pain on a temporary basis.

Complications

Common complications associated with neurolytic stellate ganglion block include prolonged Horner's syndrome, prolonged hoarseness of voice due to the effect on the recurrent pharyngeal nerve, permanent weakness or numbness of the upper extremity, possible injection of neurolytic medication in the epidural or intrathecal space which may cause permanent or temporary neurological deficits, and possible injection of neurolytic material in the vascular structures such as vertebral artery. Seizures or cerebral infarctions, sloughing of the skin or subcutaneous tissues and possible pneumothorax may occur.

Neurolytic Intercostal Nerve Block

Thoracic paravertebral nerve at each level gives anterior and posterior branches. The anterior branch is the intercostal nerve which gives lateral and anterior cutaneous branches. They provide motor supply to abdominal wall muscles via T7–T11 and muscles of the forearm and hand via T1. They provide sensory innervation of the skin of the chest and abdomen anterolaterally. The intercostal nerves travel in the inferior part of the ribs posterior to the intercostal artery. Subcostal nerve comes from the ventral ramus of T12 and is equivalent to the intercostal nerve at the above levels.

Technique

Neurolytic intercostal nerve block is indicated for cancer pain involving the chest wall and/or the ribs. It is also indicated in cancer pain involving the upper abdominal wall. Table 28.10 describes the technique of neurolytic intercostal nerve block for cancer pain. For diagnostic block, 1–2 ml of bupivacaine 0.25–0.5% is injected. Calculating the total milligrams of local anesthesia per body weight is important because of the potential local anesthesia toxicity. For neurolytic block, phenol 10% 4–5 ml can be injected. Alcohol should be avoided because of the risk of intercostal neuritis after the block. Most clinicians now favor the use of radiofrequency lesion of the intercostal nerves instead of injecting neurolytic medications because of the predictable lesion size of the radiofrequency probe. Radiofrequency lesion produces heat at the active tip of an insulated needle and causes destruction of the intercostal nerve.

Table 28.10 Technique of neurolytic intercostal nerve block.

	Neurolytic intercostal nerve block
Position	Prone with patient ipsilateral arm hanging off the procedure table
Fluoroscopy use	Mandatory
Number of needles	One or more based on how many levels
Type of needle	22G 3.5 in. or insulated 21 G with 5 mm active tip if using radiofrequency lesion (see below)
Level of needle insertion	Posterior axillary line needle advanced perpendicular to the skin until the rib is contacted
Direction of the needle	Needle withdrawn, then the skin and subcutaneous tissues are retracted inferiorly and the needle advanced again perpendicular to the skin until the needle pass 2 mm deeper than the level of the ribs. Fluoroscopy confirmation is essential
Final position of the needle	Needle just passed the inferior border of the rib and the needle is perpendicular to the skin in the costal groove.

Complications

Possible complication of intercostal nerve block include pneumothorax and intercostal local anesthetic toxicity, which can occur during the diagnostic block and also during the infiltration of local anesthesia before radiofrequency lesioning. Post-procedure intercostal neuropathy may occur, which can be treated with transcutaneous electrical nerve stimulation (TENS) unit, transdermal lidocaine patch, or antiseizure medications.

Subarachnoid Neurolytic Block

Relevant Anatomy

This procedure is suitable for patients who have significant cancer pain that is not responding to any other modalities. The pain should be localized into few sensory segments of the spinal cord. Sensory fibers arise from the dorsal aspect of the spinal cord while the motor fibers arise from the ventral aspect. The main goal of this block is to keep the neurolytic material around the sensory portion of the spinal cord (dorsal surface). This can be accomplished by a combination of positioning the patient in a way that the neurolytic materials (either hypo- or hyperbaric) remain localized in the dorsal surface of the spinal cord. Table 28.11 differentiates between the use of hypobaric and hyperbaric solution for neurolysis. The goal is selective destruction of the dorsal root ganglia. The physician should keep in mind that lower thoracic and lumbar nerves leave the spinal cord at a higher level when they exit the neural foramina. This is extremely important for the lower thoracic and lumbar neurolysis. For example, pain at the level of T9 nerve distribution requires neurolysis at T6, T7, and T8 levels. Volume to be injected is 0.6 ml within 80–90 s for each level with either agent. Diagnostic block using local anesthesia with the same baricity is essential prior to the actual block, to help evaluate the effects of the block, including any possible side effects. Complete neurological examination before and after the block is mandatory to evaluate for any neurological deficits. Extensive discussion with the patient and possibly family members about the risks and benefits of the block should take place, and possible side effects or complications should be explained at this time.

Table 28.11 Differences between hypobaric and hyperbaric solutions in subarachnoid neurolysis.

	Hypobaric neurolytic block	hyperbaric neurolytic block
Agent and concentration	Alcohol 100%	Phenol 6%
Additives usually used	None	Glycerin
Uses	Intractable unilateral cancer pain involving few dermatome	Same
Patient position	Lateral semi-prone position with area to be injected placed uppermost	Lateral semi-supine position with area to be injected lower most
Physical characters	Unstable at room temperature. Vials should opened just prior to injection	Stable
Baricity	Hypobaric (i.e., will raise up in CSF). Specific gravity of alcohol is 0.8 compared to 1.007 of CSF	Hyperbaric (i.e., will sink in CSF). Specific gravity of glycerin is 1.25 compared to 1.007 of CSF
Effect	2–4 days	1–2 days
Position after the block	Keep patient in the same position for 45 min after the procedure	Same
Fluoroscopy use	Mandatory	Same
Number of needles	Based on the level of pain	Same
Type of needle	22 or 25 G 3.5 or 5 in. based on the patient size	20–22 G needle (glycerin is very viscous and is harder to inject) 3.5 or 5 in. based on the patient size
Level of needle insertion	Based on the level of pain (see text)	Same
Final position of the needle	Free flow of clear CSF	Same

CSF=cerebrospinal fluid

Indications

Subarachnoid block may be suitable for unilateral intractable cancer pain not responding to conventional treatment, including treatment with opioids. The best location of pain for this block is unilateral cancer pain in the chest wall or abdominal wall, but it can be done for other locations such as lower and upper extremity pain. Pain should be somatic in nature. If the pain is visceral in nature, sympathetic block is advisable (see above).

Complications

The most common complication is motor weakness due to unintentional spread of neurolytic agents to the ventral surface of the spinal cord, and temporary or permanent weakness of the urinary or rectal sphincters. Post-dural puncture headache, especially in young patients, can occur.

Tunneled Epidural Catheter for Long-Term use for Cancer Pain

Anatomy

As mentioned in earlier chapters, the epidural space continues from foramen magnum superiorly to the sacrococcygeal membrane inferiorly. Epidural space contains fat, blood vessels, and connective tissues (Stoelting and Miller 2000). Epidural catheter can be placed at any level in the lumbar, thoracic, or cervical level. Infusion can be delivered at either level to help pain in cancer patients. Tunneled catheter is more advantageous than non-tunneled catheter because if infection occurs at the exit site, the infection will be far from the epidural

Table 28.12 Differences between simple one piece tunneled epidural catheter infusion and two pieces tunneled epidural catheter infusion.

	Simple one piece tunneled epidural catheter infusion	Tunneled two pieces epidural catheter infusion
Position	Prone or lateral based on the patient comfort level	Same
Fluoroscopy	Preferred	Preferred
Needles used	Tuohy needle # 17 or 18 × 2; one used for epidural space access and one for catheter tunneling	14 G, 7.6 cm Hustead needle
Site of needle position	Variable based on the pain level	Same
Needle insertion	Paramedian approach is preferable but midline approach can be used	Same
Catheter used	Radio opaque catheter is preferred	Radio opaque (proximal) catheter is included in the kit

space. Tunneled catheter is suitable for patients with cancer pain located anywhere from the neck to the lower extremities, and in patient with life expectancy of 3–6 months or less. Tunneled epidural catheter can be either simple epidural one piece catheter or tunneled epidural two-piece catheter with Dacron cuff and antibiotic cuff. The Dacron cuff is used to prevent slippage of the catheter out of the epidural space, and the antibiotic cuff is used to guard against infection. Infection is the most common complication of epidural catheter infusion. Table 28.12 describes the differences between the two types of epidural catheter. Figure 28.11a–f describes the implantation technique of a two-piece catheter.

Use and Maintenance Instructions (adopted with permission from Bard Access System manual)

General instructions:

- Postoperatively, the healthcare provider should observe incision sites for sepsis, inflammation, hematoma, seroma, and device erosion.
- Clamping is not necessary during either use or maintenance of the catheter. Toothed clamps, forceps, and scissors should not be used on or around the catheter.
- Routine catheter flushing is not required. If, however, the catheter is not used daily, it should be flushed once each week with 3 ml of sterile normal saline. Flush with saline (preservative free only), do not use any heparin-containing fluids.

Catheter dressing changes:

(1) Wash hands thoroughly with soap and water.
(2) Open dressing change supplies on a sterile field using sterile technique.
(3) Carefully remove the old dressing and wash hands again.
(4) Inspect catheter exit site closely for signs of infection or irritation.
(5) Clean any exudate from the exit site with hydrogen peroxide-soaked swaps.
(6) Using a povidone-iodine swab, apply gentle pressure and clean the exit site starting at the catheter and working outward in a circular motion. Never return to the catheter exit site with the same swab. Repeat the same procedure using two additional swabs.

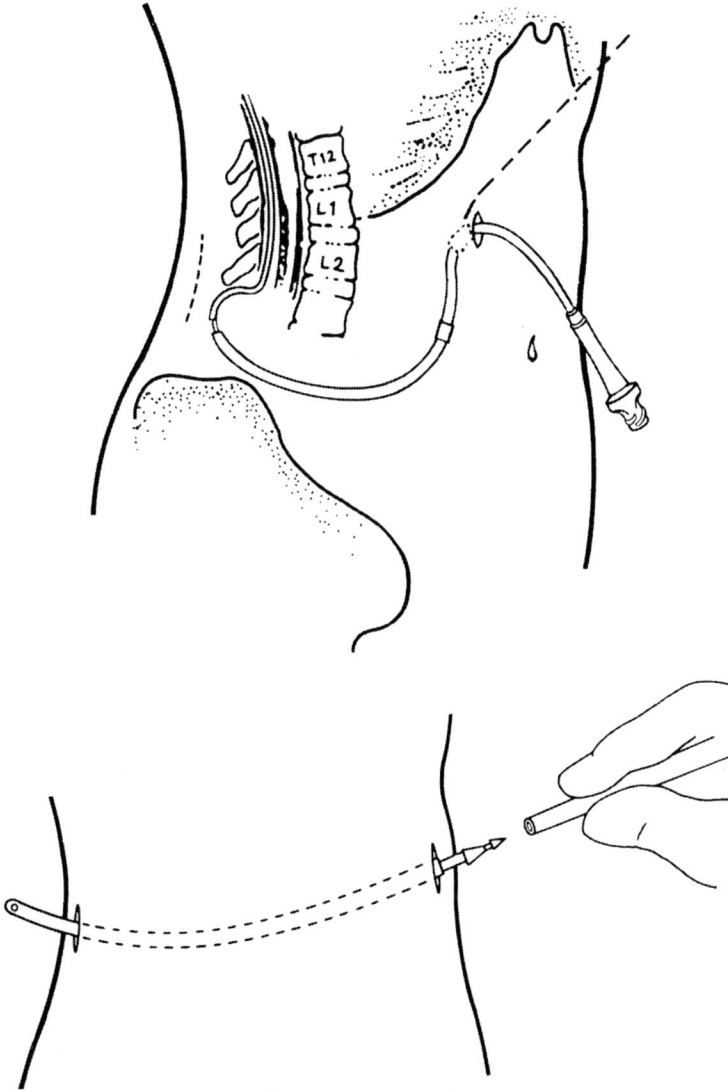

Figure 28.11 Technique of implantation of two-piece catheter. (a) Setup of implantable two-piece catheter including VitaCuff® Antimicrobial Cuff, ventral incision (exit site), distal catheter segment, SureCuff® Tissue Ingrowth Cuff, proximal catheter segment, paravertebral incision, connector. (b) 1. Tunnel simultaneously from ventral exit site. 2. Advance catheter over barbed area tunneler. 3. Draw tunneler and catheter through subcutaneous tunnel to paravertibral incision. (c) Trim tubing, eliminate any acute angles or bends. Advance to middle of the connector using non-toothed forcep and rubber shods. Detail of technique for advancing catheter over connector. Rubber shods to protect catheter. (d) Bridge ties. (e) Positioning of VitaCuff® including exit site, VitaCuff® Antimicrobial Cuff, and SureCuff® Tissue Ingrowth Cuff. (f) Securing suture provides strain relief while awaiting tissue ingrowth into the SureCuff® Tissue Ingrowth Cuff (with permission from Bard Access Systems, Salt Lake City, UT).

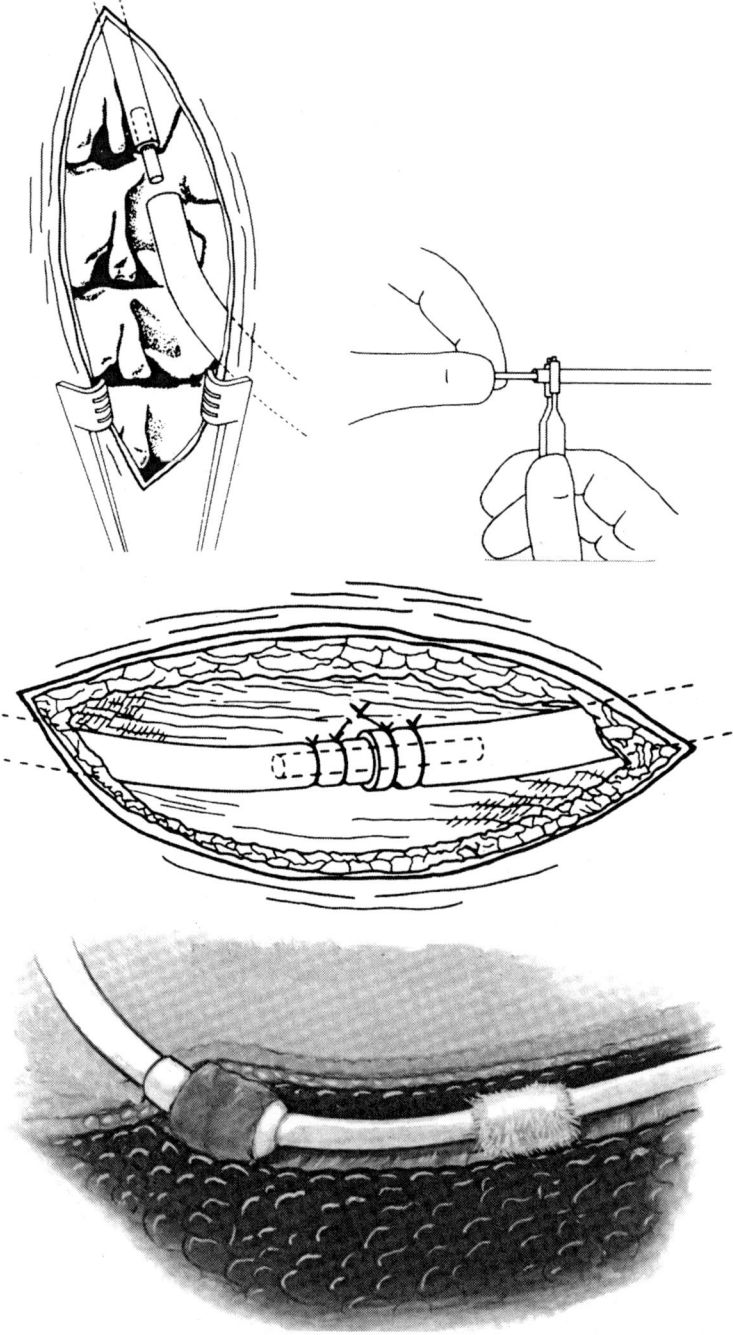

Figure 28.11 (Continued)

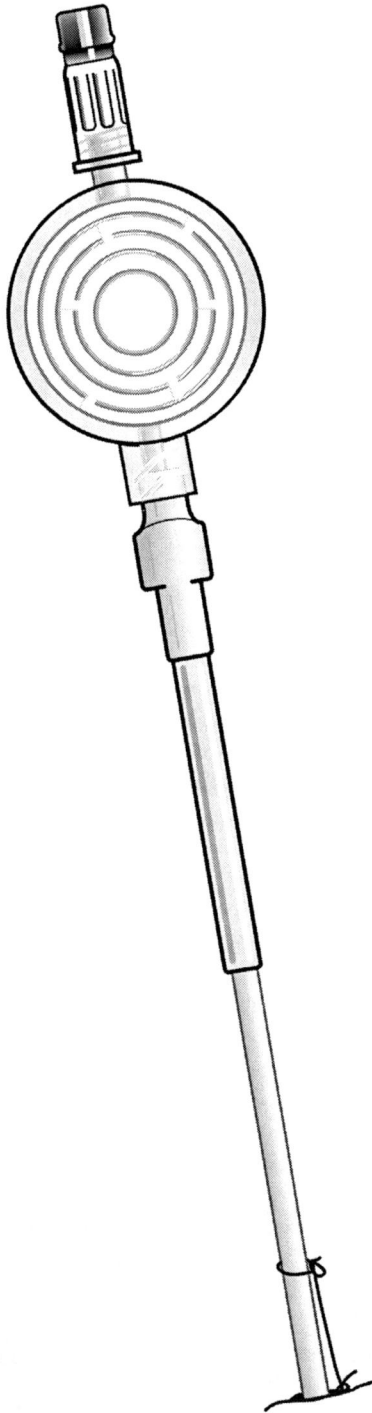

Figure 28.11 (Continued)

(7) Using another povidone-iodine swab, clean a 2 in. (5 cm) length of catheter extending from the exit site outward. Apply povidone-iodine ointment to the exit site and extending 1 in. from the exit site outward along the catheter.

(8) Apply a transparent dressing or sterile gauze dressing over the catheter exit site.

(9) Coil the catheter and secure it over dressing with tape.

(10) Date the dressing on the tape and document dressing change on patient's chart.

(11) If evidence of infection or incomplete wound healing such as redness, swelling, induration, pain, or exudate over the wound or at exit site is present, change dressing daily. If the wound site is completely healed, change dressing less frequently or in accordance with hospital policy. Exit site should be cleaned daily, however.

Filter and cap change:

(1) Wash hands thoroughly with soap and water.

(2) Open package containing special *Du Pen* epidural catheter filter with pre-attached injection cap #0602920. Cleanse junction of catheter connector and filter with a povidone-iodine swab. Allow to air dry for 2 min.

(3) Grasping old filter and catheter connector in opposite hands, gently twist counterclockwise to remove used filter.

(4) Remove shield from Luer fitting of new filter and attach securely to indwelling catheter Luer adapter by clockwise rotation.

(5) The filter and cap should be replaced every 48 h and anytime the filter is removed from the catheter. If any leaking at the septum or Luer connections is observed, the filter should be discarded and replaced immediately. 20 G × 1 in. (2.5 cm) needles, or smaller, are recommended for puncturing the injection cap.

(6) If a continuous epidural infusion is used, change tubing and filter daily.

Administration of medications:

(1) Wash hands thoroughly with soap and water.

(2) Draw up correct amount of morphine sulfate. If using a multidose vial, wipe top with povidone-iodine. Remove excess with sterile 2 in. × 2 in. (5 cm × 5 cm) gauze before puncturing vial top with needle.

(3) Wipe top of vial containing preservative-free sodium chloride with povidone-iodine. Remove excess with sterile 2 in. × 2 in. (5 cm × 5 cm) gauze before puncturing vial top with needle.

(4) Inject narcotic into vial of preservative-free sodium chloride to achieve desired dilution volume and gently mix by rocking the vial.

(5) Wipe top of preservative-free sodium chloride vial again with povidone-iodine. Remove excess with sterile 2 in. × 2 in. (5 cm × 5 cm) gauze.

(6) Aspirate morphine sulfate solution into a 12 cc syringe through a 1 in. (2.5 cm) 20 G needle.

(7) Wipe injection cap attached to catheter filter with povidone-iodine. Allow to air dry for 2 min. Remove excess with sterile 2 in. × 2 in. (5 cm × 5 cm) gauze.

(8) Insert needle into injection cap and slowly inject the morphine sulfate (1 cc/min or at a rate that is tolerated by the patient) using firm pressure. It is not necessary to flush the catheter after administering the medication.

Intrathecal Programmable Pumps

Intraspinal medication administration improves analgesia, while minimizing systemic side effects by delivery of the medication near the site of action in the dorsal horn (Erdine and Talu 1998). Intrathecal delivery of opioids into the CNS produces effective analgesia with doses lower than those used in oral or parenteral route. In general, the dose of morphine used for intrathecal administration is one to two hundredth that of an equivalent intravenous dose. Morphine is the only opioid approved for intrathecal use by the US Food and Drug Administration (FDA) for treatment of chronic and cancer pain. Other opioids have been used, such as hydromorphone, fentanyl, and sufentanil. Table 28.13 describes the differences between the properties of these drugs (Gilmer-Hill et al. 1999).

Table 28.13 Different properties of the commonly used drugs intrathecally.

	Morphine	Fentanyl	Sufentanyl
Lipid solubility (lipophilicity)	Low	High	High
Water solubility (hydrophilicity)	High	Low	Low
Onset	Slow	Fast	Fast
Duration	Prolonged	Short duration	Short duration
Ability to cross the dura	Yes because of it hydrophilic property	No because of its lipophilic property	No because of its lipophilic property
Rostral spread	Able to spread rostrally (can spread upward so the level of infusion of morphine does not have to be close to the level of pain)	Not able to spread rostrally (fentanyl should be administered at the spinal level of the pain)	Not able to spread rostrally (sufentanil should be administered at the spinal level of the pain)

Other drugs that are not opioids have also been used intrathecally in the treatment of cancer pain (Doggrell 2004, Eisenach et al. 1995). The most common drugs are clonidine, ziconotide, and bupivacaine. Usually one or more of these drugs are added to opioids in the intrathecal delivery system. Each patient should have individualized regimen plan based on the source of pain and opioid requirement prior to starting intrathecal infusion. Titration of the dose to effect is usually beneficial. Table 28.14 describes the properties of the commonly used non-opioids administered intrathecally.

Types of Intrathecal Implantable Pumps

Several manufacturers produce intrathecal pumps. Table 28.15 describes the differences between various kinds of intrathecal delivery systems.

Intrathecal delivery of opioids has been shown to reduce the level of pain in patients with intractable cancer pain (Bennett et al. 2000). A review of the literature by Gilmer-Hill and colleagues found that intrathecal delivery of morphine provided "good to excellent" pain

Table 28.14   Properties of commonly used non-opioids in the intrathecal pumps.

	Clonidine	Ziconotidine	Bupivacaine
Type	Alpha-2 adrenergic agonist	Calcium channel blocker	Local anesthetic
Mechanism of action	Alpha-2 receptors agonist on pre-synaptic primary afferents and on postsynaptic dorsal horn neurons of the spinal cord	Selectively blocks N-type calcium channels (prevents calcium influx and neurotransmitter release)	Sodium channel blocker (prevents the conduction of nerve impulses)
FDA approval	Approved for epidural use only	Approved for persistent chronic and cancer pain	Not approved for continuous intrathecal infusion
Advantage	Helpful in neuropathic pain	May be helpful in persistent cancer pain	Helpful in neuropathic and persistent pain
Disadvantage	Hypotension and sedation	Allergic reaction	Motor weakness on even small doses

Table 28.15   Different kinds of intrathecal drug delivery systems.

	Implantable fixed rate pump	Implantable programmable pumps
Approved by FDA	• Codman's model 400 (Raynham, Massachusetts) • Medtronic's Isomed (Minneapolis, Minnesota) • Arrow's M-3000 (Walpole, Massachusetts)	Medtronic's Synchromed II (Minneapolis, Minnesota)
Drug reservoir	Refillable	Refillable
Access side port (for CSF access without going through the drug reservoir for possible catheter integrity check)	Present	Present
Flow rate	Constant (0.5 or 1.0 ml/day)	The physician can change the daily rate (mg/day) including options of single bolus, timed-specific boluses, or a complex continuous delivery of drug
Change of dose	Change the drug concentration in the reservoir by aspirating the drug from the reservoir and re-injecting a higher or lower concentration to achieve the desired dose (mg/day)	Change the rate is easily accessible through a programmer including options of single bolus, timed-specific boluses, or a complex continuous delivery of drug. No need to access the drug reservoir
Advantage	Cheaper	More efficacious to patient needs on long-term basis
Disadvantage	Limited options of changing the dose (need to access the pump and change the concentration to change the daily dose	More expensive

FDA=Food and Drug Administration; CSF=cerebrospinal fluid.

relief. They also found that pain relief was associated with increased activity and improved quality of life in these patients. The technique of implanting intrathecal programmable pumps is as follows:

1. Prepare the patient using fluoroscopy to identify the appropriate intraspinous intervals. Make those intervals on the patient's skin, if desired.

2. Insert a Tuohy needle and place the catheter in the appropriate spinal location and corresponding to the patient's pain pattern. Verify the catheter placement using fluoroscopy.
3. Make an incision at the appropriate site. Withdraw the needle and guidewire.
4. Make an incision in the abdominal area and create a subcutaneous pocket for the pump.
5. Tunnel the catheter to the pump pocket and connect it to the pump.

Summary

Unrelieved pain associated with cancer can dramatically affect patients' quality of life. Intractable pain can be the main reason for poor functional status. It is essential for all healthcare providers to provide pain relief for cancer pain patients.

Case Scenario

Sreekumar Kunnumpurath, MBBS, MD, FCARCSI, FRCA, FFPMRCA

Nick is a 55-year-old insurance broker who has been recently diagnosed with multiple myeloma and is undergoing combined radiotherapy and chemotherapy in the hospital. Since admission, he has been complaining of pain in the back, right shoulder, and left groin. He has been evaluated thoroughly using MRI and bone scan, which have revealed wedge fractures of thoracic spine (T7 and T8) and osteolytic regions in the right humerus, ribs, and right femur. His medication regimen includes acetaminophen, tramadol, and morphine sulfate as needed. The attending hematologist is having problems with his pain control. As member of the palliative care team, you are requested to see him. As you go through his notes, you find that he is on antibiotics for left lower lobe pneumonia.

How are you going to assess him?
You need to obtain a detailed history of the pain and of his illness. Also, you need to perform a thorough physical examination, including a neurological assessment (this could be challenging when the patient is in a great amount of pain). During pain assessment, it is important to ascertain about sites, character, radiation, aggravating, and relieving factors. Individual pain scores should be recorded separately if possible, which will help to assess the pain and its progress. It is also important to understand the systemic impact of the pathological process. As you walk into the room, you notice that Nick looks unwell. He is on supplemental oxygen. He tells you that because of pain he is unable to take deep breaths or cough effectively. The physiotherapist who is with him says that Nick is unable to tolerate physiotherapy because of pain. His overall pain score at rest is a 6/10 and it worsens to 9/10 with movement.

What could be the cause of his respiratory infection?
Multiple myeloma itself can lead to increased susceptibility to infection and chemotherapy and radiotherapy are immunosuppressive. While strapping the chest to splint rib fractures may seem like a good idea, it impedes chest wall movement and prevents adequate inspiration and clearance of secretions. This can potentially lead to pulmonary atelectasis and pneumonia. Clearly, pain control here is not optimal, and it is important to note that the pain is getting worse with movement. Inadequate pain control has detrimental effects on various systems of the body and on the morale of the patient. An urgent review of his pain control is mandatory.

What are the different types of pain a cancer patient could experience?
Cancer patients can experience somatic, visceral, and neuropathic pain. Somatic pain is a constant, localized, aching pain that responds to opioids and non-steroidal anti-inflammatory drugs. Visceral pain is due to damage to viscera and is transmitted through the sympathetic system. This pain is hence poorly localized and may need sympathetic blockade to control it. Neuropathic pain in cancer could result from nerve damage secondary to tumor infiltration, chemotherapy, or radiotherapy. This type of pain can respond to anticonvulsants, antidepressants, or application of topical anesthetic agents.

You embark upon creating a pain management plan for Nick. You are now reviewing his pain medications. When you go through the laboratory reports you notice that his serum urea and creatinine levels are above the normal range. Nick mentions that he is afraid of taking too many painkillers, as he is worried about becoming addicted to morphine.

Describe your plan of care?
Nick is suffering from a continuous generalized pain and recurrent breakthrough pains exacerbated by movement. There are indications that he is developing complications secondary to inadequate pain relief. The first step is to stop ibuprofen immediately because of renal dysfunction. Nick needs baseline analgesia along with rescue medication. He also needs reassurance regarding his concern about opioid addiction, in order to improve compliance with treatment.

As a general rule, due consideration should be given to the WHO analgesic ladder. In the given clinical scenario the pain is severe. So the analgesic mainstay is opioids.

His analgesic plan may look like this:

Substitute morphine sulfate with oxycodone 5 mg every 4 h for continuous pain relief.

Oxycodone 5 mg PRN for breakthrough pain.

Oxycodone 5 mg 30 min before any planned activity (e.g., physiotherapy).

Acetaminophen 1 g every 6 h.

Nick needs to be seen on a regular basis, and physiotherapy and active mobilization need to be continued. Once satisfactory analgesia is achieved, the total dose of oxycodone can be administered as oxycontin in two divided doses 12 h apart. Oxycodone PRN dose should be retained for breakthrough pain.

Give reasons for not using long-acting opioid preparations to control breakthrough pain?
Increasing the dose of Oxycontin can result in unwanted side effects and toxicity.
The patient can get nausea and vomiting, constipation, urinary retention, respiratory depression, and so on. If the patient cannot take oral medication, then alternate routes such as transdermal, sublingual, subcutaneous, or intravenous should be considered.

Q Is there any role for interventional strategies?
Chemotherapy and radiotherapy are part of this approach to pain management. However, they do not provide immediate pain relief. On the other hand, epidural or intrathecal analgesics can provide excellent pain control. As a general rule, the intrathecal route is used if the patient is expected to survive for more than 3 months. If the expected survival time is less, then epidural drug delivery should be considered. The role of interventions such as neurolytic blocks is limited when there are multiple sites of pain. In cancer patients, the risk of complications arising from interventions is higher than in healthy population. Usually, these techniques are considered when pharmacotherapy fails.

Nick responds to the above regimen, his pain scores have come down, and he is able to cope very well with his regular physiotherapy and rehabilitation program. He is seen by the spine surgeons who recommend a dorso-lumbar spinal brace, and he is also scheduled for an assessment for a possible vertebroplasty. He completes his chemotherapy and radiotherapy, and he is able to manage his pain with acetaminophen, codeine, and occasional tramadol. Since multiple myeloma is not generally curable, he knows that he needs regular follow-ups and adjustments to his pharmacologic treatment.

References

Abram SE, ed. Pain management. In: Miller RD, editor. Atlas of anesthesia. Philadelphia, PA: Churchill Livingstone; 1998. Vol. 6.

Benedetti C, Brock C, Cleeland C, et al. NCCN practice guidelines for cancer pain. Oncology 2000;14:135–50.

Bennett G, Burchiel K, Buchser E, et al. Clinical guidelines for intraspinal infusion: report of an expert panel. J Pain Symptom Manage. 2000;20:S37–S43.

Berland D. Pain management in patients with advanced cancer. Ann Intern Med. 2000;132:593.

Burton AW, Driver LC, Mendoza TR, et al. Oral transmucosal fentanyl citrate in the outpatient management of severe cancer pain crises. Clin J Pain. 2004a;20:195–97.

Burton AW, Rajagopal A, Hassenbusch SJ, et al. Reduction in pain and oral opioid intake after intrathecal pump implantation. In: Program and abstracts of the International Association for the Study of Pain 10th World Congress on Pain, August 17–22, 2002, San Diego, CA.

Burton AW, Rajagopal A, Shah HN, et al. Epidural and intrathecal analgesia is effective in treating refractory cancer pain. Pain Med. 2004b;5:239–47.

Carr DB, Goudas LC, Balk EM, et al. Evidence report on the treatment of pain in cancer patients. J Nat Cancer Inst Monogri. 2004;32:23–31.

Cherny NI. The management of cancer pain. CA Cancer J Clin. 2000;50:70–116. Abstract

Davies DD. Incidence of major complications of neurolytic coeliac plexus block. J R Soc Med. 1993;86:264–266.

de Leon-Casasola OA. Critical evaluation of chemical neurolysis of the sympathetic axis for cancer pain. Cancer Control 2000;7:142–8.

Doggrell SA. Intrathecal ziconotide for refractory pain. Expert Opin Invest Drugs. 2004;13:875–77.

Eisenach JC, Du Pen S, Dubois M, et al. Epidural clonidine analgesia for intractable cancer pain. The Epidural Clonidine Study Group. Pain 1995;61:391–99.

Eisenberg E, Carr DB, Chalmers TC. Neurolytic celiac plexus block for treatment of cancer pain: a meta-analysis. Anesth Analg. 1995;80:290–5.

Erdine S, Talu GK. Cost effectiveness of implantable devices versus tunneled catheters. Curr Rev Pain. 1998;2:157–62.

Fukshansky M, Are M, Burton AW. The role of opioids in cancer pain management. Pain Pract. 2005;5:43–54.

Gilmer-Hill HS, Boggan JE, Smith KA, et al. Intrathecal morphine delivered via subcutaneous pump for intractable cancer pain: a review of the literature. Surg Neurol. 1999;51:12–5.

Jacox AK, Carr DB, Payne R, et al. Management of cancer pain: clinical practice guideline No. 9. Rockville, MD: Agency for Healthcare Policy and Research, US Department of Health and Human Services, Public Health Service; 1994: AHCPR Publication No. 94-0592.

Miguel R. Interventional treatment of cancer pain: the fourth step in the World Health Organization analgesic ladder? Cancer Control 2000;7:149–56.

Patt RB. Cancer pain. Philadelphia, PA: Lippincott; 1993.

Plancarte R, de Leon-Casasola OA, El-Helay M, et al. Neurolytic superior hypogastric plexus block for chronic pelvic pain associated with cancer. Reg Anesth. 1997;22:562–8.

Portenoy RK. Cancer pain: epidemiology and syndromes. Cancer 1989;63(11 suppl):2298–307.

Shah HN, Burton AW, Mendoza T, et al. Neurolytic blockade of the splanchnic nerves block relieves refractory pain associated with upper abdominal malignancy. In: Program and Abstracts of the Annual Meeting of the American Society of Anesthesiologists; October 11–15, 2003, San Francisco, CA; Abstract A1024.

Stoelting RK, Miller RD. Spinal and epidural anesthesia. In: Stoelting RK, Miller RD, editors. Basics of anesthesia. Philadelphia, PA: Churchill Livingstone; 2000. pp. 168–95.

Waldman SD. Interventional pain management. Phildelphia, PA: Saunders; 2001.

Wong GY, Brown DL. Celiac plexus block for cancer pain. In: Utney W, editor. Techniques in regional anesthesia and pain management. Vol. 1. Philadelphia, PA: W.B. Saunders; 1997.

World Health Organization. Cancer pain relief and palliative care: report of a WHO expert committee. WHO Tech Rep Ser. 1990;804:1–73.

Zech DFJ, Grond S, Lynch J, et al. Validation of World Health Organization Guidelines for cancer pain relief: a 10-year prospective study. Pain 1995;63:65–76.

Chapter 29

Ethics in Pain Management and End of Life Care

Jack M. Berger, MS, MD, PhD

Introduction

"Do the kind thing, and do it first," said William Osler as advice to physicians. But in 1904 there were limited things that physicians could do for their patients with chronic pain or who were in need of care at the end of life. In their article published in *Critical Care Medicine* in 1992, Cowley et al. concluded that "Despite the miraculous advances in medical theory and medical practice, the ethics surrounding medical care for the dying are more troubling today than they were in ancient Athens at the time of Plato. In classical antiquity, the primary concerns were for health and living well. The "Middle Ages" saw the emergence of the principle of sanctity of life. To these basic ideals, the "Renaissance" and the "Enlightenment" added the aspiration to prolong life. Finally, in the 20th century, modern science has rendered this aspiration a reality of unclear merit (Spiegel et al. 1998)."

According to Spiegel et al. (1998) here at the end of the 20th century, the old adage, to "cure rarely, relieve suffering often, and comfort always," has been rewritten. The doctor's job has become to "cure always, relieve suffering if one has the time, and leave the comforting to someone else." They further state that the acute disease model, which emphasizes diagnosis, definitive treatment, and cure, works in many situations, but the leading killers of Americans – heart disease, stroke, and cancer – are by and large chronic and progressive rather than acute and curable. Western medicine's success is also its weakness. The application of a curative model when disease management is all that can be given leaves doctors and patients dissatisfied.

Dotson (1997, 2000) stated that in the medical model of disease, "pain" is a symptom that would lead to the diagnosis of a disease and subsequently define appropriate treatment. This approach is clearly validated in such conditions as heart attack, appendicitis, and fractures of bones. However, culturally attached to this rational concept is the assumption that the physician's duty ends either when all conventional tests and examinations fail to find the cause of the pain, for example, in complex regional pain syndrome type I (CRPS I) or when the cause is found but does not respond to known specific treatments, for example, post-herpetic neuralgia.

Butler (1996a, b) and his associates and Dotson (1997, 2000) offer the opinion regarding both the scenarios given above that "the perception has been that nothing else can or should be done in these situations... despite the ancient and central professional taboo against abandonment of the patient." Dotson states that in the first situation the physician informs the patient that there is nothing really wrong, but that a psychiatric consultation might be helpful, the "it's all in your head" disposition.

Dotson further states that "in the second case, the patient is told that everything has been done, that the only thing left is narcotics, and we don't want to make you an addict" – the "learn to live with it" disposition.

In 1997, The American Society of Anesthesiology (ASA) Task Force defined the Purpose of Guidelines for Pain Management as the following:

- Optimize pain control, recognizing that a pain-free state may not be achievable
- Minimize adverse outcomes and costs
- Enhance functional abilities and physical and psychological well-being, and
- Enhance the quality of life for patients with chronic pain

Dotson (1997, 2003) defined this as a "Subject of Conscience." He asks, "Is not personal freedom the historical reason for the establishment of this nation [United States of America]? How does the endurance of pain fit into the pursuit of happiness? Is the individual the rightful owner of his/her own body (habeas corpus), or not? If there is no such thing as a truly objective 'pain meter,' – and there isn't! If the physician [or the HMO or Medicare] has been made the judge in our society of who gets what relief . . . and the physician has! How does the physician avoid being arbitrary and capricious in the exercise of such judgment? How does the physician avoid inflicting cruel and unusual punishment. . . . not upon the guilty, but upon the innocent? How does the physician hold the patient guilty (of malingering or drug abuse) until proven? And doesn't justice demand a burden of proof?"

Guiding Ethical Principles in Patient Care

In pain management and end of life care, there are four guiding ethical principles which govern our decision making and care of patients. These are the same principles that guide us in the conduct of medicine in general:

- Nonmaleficence: minimize harm (Hippocratic oath)
- Beneficence: do good if you can (St. Thomas Aquinas, 13th century)
- Patient autonomy: respect for the patient as a person, informed consent (Nuremberg trial of Nazi physicians who performed experiments on humans without consent is an example of violation of patient autonomy)
- Justice: fair use of available resources (not everyone is entitled to everything that medicine has to offer when resources are limited)

In implementing the above principles the physician has to balance three dichotomies:

- The potential benefits of treatment must be balanced against the potential burdens.
- Striving to preserve life but, when biologically futile, providing comfort in dying.
- Individual needs are balanced against those of society.

Eric J. Casssel, in his article regarding nature of suffering and the goals of medicine published in the *New England Journal of Medicine*, stated ". . .The relief of suffering and the cure of disease must be seen as twin obligations of a medical profession that is truly dedicated to care of the sick. Physicians' failure to understand the nature of suffering can result in medical intervention that (though technically adequate) not only fails to relieve suffering but also becomes a source of suffering itself."

In pain management as well as end of life care, providing pain relief can present a dilemma for physicians who operate under misconceptions of both the law and ethics. The Rule of Double Effect, which is the moral doctrine taken from the teachings of St. Thomas Aquinas of the 13th century, gives physicians the duty and obligation to relieve pain and suffering. Yet these philosophical arguments do not provide insight into the ambivalence that practitioners feel when they legitimately engage in these practices. Why should a physician feel ambivalent about doing the "right thing?"

The Rule of Double Effect states that an action having two effects, one good and one bad, is permissible if five conditions are fulfilled:

1. The act itself is good or at least morally neutral, e.g., giving morphine to relieve pain.
2. Only the good effect is intended (relieving pain) and not the bad effect (killing the patient).
3. The good effect is not achieved through the bad effect (pain relief does not depend on hastening death).
4. There is no alternative way to attain the good effect (pain relief).
5. There is a proportionately grave reason for running the risk, e.g., relief of intolerable pain.

Clearly, to justify use of this rule, the patient or surrogate decision maker would need to be informed of the risks and give valid consent. It is clear that any patient coming for surgery is expecting that his/her physician will attend to the pain which results from the surgery including the use of opioids. If other forms of pain relief are to be used such as epidural analgesia or peripheral nerve blockade, then additional consent discussions should be undertaken so that patients can make informed decisions about their pain management care.

According to the Rule of Double Effect it is clear in end of life care that there is ethical and legal sanctions for the use of whatever doses of opioids that are necessary so long as death is not directly intended. If the doses of the opioids necessary to relieve pain are large enough to produce deep sedation, this too would be permissible, if suffering can be relieved in no other way.

Thorn and Sykes (2000) studied 238 consecutive dying patients. In a retrospective study, they found that there was no difference in survival between those patients requiring escalating doses of opioids vs. those patients that were on stable doses of opioids. Because of this finding they concluded that the Rule of Double Effect was not even needed to justify the use of opioids for the control of pain at the end of life.

Much of inadequate pain management, particularly in end of life care, can be traced to lack of knowledge on the part of physicians. In a typical example, a physician stated, "We must wean off the morphine. We're killing him." This statement was in regard to an end-stage acquired immunodeficiency syndrome (AIDS) patient who had a do not resuscitate (DNR) status, documented pain scores of 5/10 and 6/10, and was currently receiving 3 mg/h IV morphine infusion. The physician wanted to give naloxone to reverse the effects of the morphine and then remedicate the patient with 25 mg meperidine IV q4h PRN for pain control. What is wrong with this scenario?

- 3 mg/h of IV morphine = 72 mg/day
- 1 mg morphine IV = 10 mg meperidine IV
- 72 mg morphine = 720 mg meperidine
- 25 mg meperidine q4h = 150 mg/day
- The patient was already in moderate to severe pain at the current dosage which was already inadequate, and the physician was reducing the dose by 80%. Further, by writing a PRN order, the physician was insuring that the patient would not even get the 25 mg of meperidine q4h.

This is a classic case of *"opiophobia"* – the unreasonable fear of opioid use, based on an inaccurate assessment of its dangers. It affects patients as well as physicians and may be one of the greatest barriers to the provision of effective pain medication. The 1993 California Medical Board Statement on the Prescribing of Controlled Substances stated that concerns about regulatory scrutiny should not make *physicians who follow appropriate guidelines* reluctant to prescribe or administer controlled substances, including schedule II drugs, for patients with a legitimate medical need for them.

Likewise, the Federal Controlled Substances Act (CSA) does *not* address medical treatment issues such as the selection or quantity of prescribed drugs. The CSA regulates drugs, not the practice of medicine. According to a Drug Enforcement Administration (DEA) policy, the practitioner's judgment, based upon training, medical specialty, and practice guidelines, determines what may be considered *legitimate medical purpose.* According to the Federal CSA, in order for a prescription to be valid, it must be issued for a legitimate medical purpose by an individual practitioner acting in the usual course of professional practice. A dentist, for example, cannot prescribe opioids for gynecological pain even though he/she has a DEA number.

Model Guidelines for the Use of Controlled Substances for the Treatment of Pain were developed jointly by the DEA and Federation of State Medical Boards of the United States and adopted on May 2, 1998. The purpose was (to) protect legitimate medical uses of controlled substances while preventing drug diversion and eliminating inappropriate prescribing practices. Simply put, you have a license to drive your car but you have to recognize stop signs and traffic lights.

Prescribing good faith requires an equally good faith history, physical examination, and documentation [of benefit]. One can always be sued by a patient claiming injury or becoming addicted to opioids. One can always be manipulated or deceived by individual patients seeking to abuse opioid medications. But careful monitoring, and particularly documentation of benefit, will reduce these risks to both the physician and the patient to a minimum.

The issue of the benefit of opioids in the treatment of chronic pain remains controversial. It is beyond this chapter to discuss the data supporting and not supporting opioids in chronic pain, but one issue should be considered. That is the issue of opioid contracts. Many pain management physicians feel that they should have a signed contract between them and their patients in which patients are required to agree to certain stipulations in order to continue treatment with opioids. However, contracts are legal documents which imply distrust between the parties; therefore, rules must be stipulated.

Therefore, a "contract" requirement establishes an "I don't trust you" relationship between the patient and the physician. Other physicians therefore call the "contract" an "agreement." This is a better term but it really does not convey the true intention of the document. The document is really an "informed consent agreement for treatment." The treatment of course is chronic opioid therapy, which carries with it certain risks, such as addiction, dependence, constipation, sedation, and confusion. It can also provide the benefit of pain relief.

These documents usually also contain conditions of treatment such as the patients can only obtain their prescriptions from one physician, they have a responsibility to keep track of their prescriptions such that they do not run out on weekends or holidays, and that they must refrain from using illicit drugs. The consequences of abnormal behavior are usually specified in the informed consent as well. But the document should be written in such a way that it is not threatening to the relationship between the doctor and the patient and to provide true informed consent to proceed with a treatment that does have risks as well as benefits associated with it, just like an invasive pain management procedure or a surgical procedure. The patient is also given information about the risks and benefits of alternatives to the opioid therapy to complete the process.

In providing symptom management and palliative care at the end of life, difficult decisions have to be made with respect to initiating therapeutic interventions or discontinuing interventions. It is interesting that there appears to be a great deal of discrepancy between what physicians state as to their biases for withdrawing life support measures and what they actually practice in real life. Asthenia, malnutrition, cachexia are common in dying patients with advanced cancer. They may in fact be adaptive mechanisms which do not require intervention.

Enteral feedings can lead to pneumonia from aspiration or diarrhea from poor absorption. Parenteral feeding requires intravenous access, and there is no evidence for improved survival, no evidence for improved tumor response to chemotherapy, and no evidence of decreased chemotherapy toxicity. The idea of decreased surgical complications with the use of total parenteral nutrition (TPN) is debatable. In animal studies there is evidence of actual enhanced tumor growth, but there is no evidence for enhanced quality of life or satisfaction of hunger.

In their study related to biases in how physicians choose to withdraw life support, Christakis and Asch (1993) reported that in order of preference, physicians find it easier to withdraw or withhold treatments in the following order: blood products, hemodialysis, intravenous vasopressors, total parenteral nutrition, antibiotics, mechanical ventilation, tube feedings, and finally intravenous fluids.

These therapies correlate with the preferences to withdraw forms of therapy supporting organs that failed for natural rather than iatrogenic reasons, to withdraw recently instituted rather than longstanding interventions, to withdraw forms of therapy resulting in immediate death rather than delayed death, and to withdraw forms of therapy resulting in delayed death when confronted with diagnostic uncertainty.

In their report on cancer patients receiving home TPN in 1997, Cozzaglio et al. (1997) retrospectively studied patients with metastatic cancer who were treated with home TPN. They note that the use of TPN in end-stage cancer patients varies from country to country. In the United States, Japan, and Italy, 40–60% of all patients getting home TPN have cancer, compared to only 18% in France and 5% in the UK. They further noted that the variance reflects a difference in cultural, ethical, social, and economic approaches to the problem, with a lack of a scientific basis resulting from the scarcity of specific literature.

They concluded that home TPN does not benefit cancer patients with a Karnofsky score of <50. In those patients who were treated for less than 3 months (Karnofsky < 50), there was no benefit in quality of life improvement.

Since dyspnea is a subjective experience similar to pain, it has a complicated pathophysiology that is affected by physical, psychological, social, and spiritual factors. The involvement of the entire interdisciplinary team is essential for treating dyspnea effectively, particularly in the terminal stages of disease.

Hydration is another area that presents ethical problems for physicians in the dying patient. Too much hydration in a patient who is unable to eliminate the fluid can lead to pulmonary congestion and dyspnea and edema around encapsulated tumors leading to pain.

In dealing with pain or end of life care, we must make every effort to control pain, being mindful of the risks of our interventions, but at the same time not be afraid to take action.

The late Primo Levi, an Italian journalist, said, "If we know that pain and suffering can be alleviated, and we do nothing about it, then we ourselves become the tormentors." However, according to another, unknown, author, "When men lack goals, they tend to engage in activity." Therefore, to reiterate the opening statement of this chapter, it is our job as compassionate and professional physicians to, "Do the right thing, and do it first" according to William Osler.

Case Scenario

Dr. Ganesh Kumar, MBBS, DA, MRCA and Sreekumar Kunnumpurath, MBBS, MD, FCARCSI, FRCA, FFPMRCA

Mariano is an 82-year-old millionaire industrialist who was diagnosed 2 months ago with advanced carcinoma of the pancreas. Though he has extensive bony metastasis, his main problem is severe, intolerable abdominal pain. His physician has requested that you, an interventional pain specialist, assess Mariano for a possible neurolytic celiac plexus block. He is doing so in order to keep the pain under control to enable the patient to be discharged and sent home. Mariano has expressed his desire to spend the last days of his life with his family.

Before meeting with Mariano, you decide to go through his medical records that show that his liver function tests are abnormal and his clotting is slightly deranged. His other medical problems include a 4 cm size aortic aneurysm, COPD, and hypertension. The MRI scan shows extensive degenerative changes of the spine and metastatic lesions on the lower thoracic vertebrae. A prior exploratory laparoscopy found the pancreatic tumor to be inoperable, and hence he had a course of palliative chemotherapy. You walk into Mariano's room and you notice that he is on PCA morphine and appears to be asleep with his son, Rocco, at his bedside. Rocco tells you that he does not want his father to be disturbed from his sleep and he asks you to discuss the procedure with him instead. Rocco says he is concerned that the morphine is making his father a "drug addict" and so he wants the celiac plexus block to be done so that the morphine can be stopped and his dad can make clear decisions about his estate and finances before he dies. Rocco requests you to proceed straight away and he says that presently his father cannot make any decisions for himself because of the morphine.

Do you agree with Rocco?

No necessarily. You always have to respect patient's autonomy. The other guiding principles in this situation include nonmaleficence, beneficence, and justice. So you have to reason with Rocco and tell him that first, you have to assess his dad in detail, including his mental capacity. "Capacity" is determined by the attending physician at the time of the interview with the patient that the patient is able to understand the therapeutic options and their inherent risks and benefits, can ask questions and process the answers, and make an informed decision about what he/she would like done or not done. This ability to have "capacity" to make health care decisions is not necessarily impaired by medications such as opioids; and does not require that the patient remember the conversation even 1 hour later. "Competency" on the other hand is the ability of the patient to make financial decisions about his/her will, and other socioeconomic decisions. This can be challenged by family members and is usually decided by a psychiatrist or a judge. If you are still in doubt about his ability to give a valid informed consent, then he will have to be assessed by a psychologist. You will also have to address Rocco's "Opiophobia." At this moment, Mariano wakes up and says, in a sleepy voice, "Hello doctor! Is my son is troubling you too? Do not listen to him. I am still the boss! You may ask me whatever you want to know."

What would you like to ask Mariano?

You need to assess whether Mariano is cognitively intact or not. If he is, then you can collect some detailed history, perform clinical examination, and complete your assessment. Mariano appears to be acting as if he is pretty much at his cognitive baseline. You discuss all of the pain management options with him in detail. Mariano asks you about the planned celiac plexus block and you explain potential risks and benefits. After the discussion, Mariano decides that he does not want to have the celiac plexus block as he wishes not to undergo any invasive procedures and he does not accept the risk of complications related to this block. He prefers to "die with dignity" at his home. He is very happy about the pain relief that he is receiving and would like to continue with current regimen. Impressed with your conduct, he requests you to take care of his pain from now on.

Would you accept his request?

There is no reason why you should not. However, in the given situation it is advisable to have an "opioid contract" signed between you and Mariano to avoid future litigations. Accepting his request would mean that you are not just an interventional pain management physician but that you would now be taking over the role of palliative care physician and you must have the resources to manage his care at home. It would be more appropriate to suggest home hospice care and that you would be able to participate in the management of the care provided by the hospice team. You should also explain that it would be better to try and convert him to oral long acting opioids such as methadone or sustained release morphine so that he would not have to have the intravenous medications and the intravenous access that the PCA requires. If he insists on having the PCA and since he has the financial resources, he can afford to pay for the extra costs, and he should have a more permanent intravenous access such as a chemo port inserted. Your decision to avoid the celiac plexus block might be challenged in a court of law and hence a consultation with the hospital legal department may be necessary.

References

Butler RN, Burt R, Foley KM, Morris J, Morrison RS. Palliative medicine: providing care when cure is not possible. A Roundtable discussion: Part 1. Geriatrics. 1996a May;51(5):33–6, 42–44.

Butler RN, Burt R, Foley KM, Morris J, Morrison RS. A peaceful death: how to manage pain and provide quality care. A Roundtable discussion. Part 2. Geriatrics 1996b Jun;51(6): 32–5, 39–40, 42.

Cassel EJ. Nature of suffering and the goals of medicine. NEJM 1982;306(11):639–45.

Christakis NA, Asch DA. Biases in how physicians choose to withdraw life support. Lancet 1993;342:642–6.

Cowley LT, Young E, and Raffin TA. Care of the dying: an ethical and historical perspective. Crit Care Med. 1992;20(10):1473–82.

Cozzaglio L, Palzola F, Cosantino F, et al. Outcome of cancer patients receiving home parenteral nutrition. Italian Society of Parenteral and Enteral Nutrition (S.I.N.P.E). J Parenter Enteral Nutr. 1997;1(6):339–42.

Dotson DA, Why not relief? Pain Physician 2000;3(1):65–68.

Dotson DA, Treat the disease or treat the patient? Am J Pain Manag 1997;7:130–132.

Doyle D, Hanks WC, MacDonald N, eds. Oxford textbook of palliative medicine. 2nd ed. New York, NY: Oxford University Press; 1998.

Practice guidelines for chronic pain management: a report by the American Society of Anesthesiology Task Force on Pain Management. Chronic Pain Section. Anesthesiology 1997;86:995–1004.

Saucier Lundy K, Janes S. The art of palliativge care – living with hope dying with dignity. Oncol Nurs Forum 1998;25(6):995–1004.

Spiegel D, Stroud P, Fyfe A. Complementary medicine. West J Med. 1998;168:241–7.

Thorns SA, Sykes N. Opioid use in the last week of life and implications for end of life decision making. Lancet 2000;356:398–9.

Section VIII

Additional Topics

Chapter 30

Pediatric Pain Management

Arlyne K. Thung, MD, Rae Ann Kingsley, APRN, and Brenda C. McClain, MD

Introduction

Over the years, significant advances have been made in the understanding and practice of pediatric pain management. Previous myths such as the inability of infants to experience pain or the inessential need to treat perioperative nociception or postoperative pain have been debunked by the evidence of mature nociceptive pathways by 30 weeks of gestation (Lowery et al. 2007) and the unquestionable benefits of treating noxious stimuli with analgesics (Anand et al. 1987, Anand and Hickey 1992).

Despite these important advances, pediatric pain management remains undertreated and challenging for the practitioner. In a study looking at the treatment of painful procedures in neonates in the intensive care unit, out of 42,413 painful procedures 79.2% were treated without specific analgesia (Carbajal et al. 2008). Furthermore compared to the pain assessment for adult and older pediatric patients, assessment of pain in nonverbal pediatric patients or patients with chronic diseases such as sickle cell is often more difficult for the practitioner. For the nonverbal infant, crying may not be due to pain but simple factors such as hunger or the stress of being in a strange hospital environment. For the sickle cell patient in acute crisis, the biophysical profile may not reflect typical changes seen in acute pain. Yet given the ever changing landscape of pediatric pain management with regard to newer assessment scales or pharmacological and non-pharmacological approaches, one basic principle remains clear. Communication among patient, parents, surgical, pediatric, and pain teams regarding assessment, treatment, potential treatment side effects, and treatment alternative is both an imperative and the foundation for a successful and sound pediatric pain management strategy.

Assessment

Pediatric pain assessment presents unique challenges to the medical practitioner not encountered with adult populations. Although infants and children experience pain through similar physiological processes as adults, their experiences cannot be measured with comparable assessment tools. The ability or willingness to communicate the child's experience of pain may often be limited by his/her age, developmental level, cognitive ability, previous pain experiences, and various ethnic/cultural influences. Furthermore, children may not know the meaning of "pain" and will often confuse fear and anxiety with pain which in turn may

N. Vadivelu et al. (eds.), *Essentials of Pain Management*,
DOI 10.1007/978-0-387-87579-8_30, © Springer Science+Business Media, LLC 2011

Table 30.1 Developmental Stages in the Pediatric Pain Patient.

Developmental stage	Abilities and attributes	Pain expressions
Infant	No verbal skills to describe pain Completely dependent on clinicians to assess and interpret behavioral exhibition of pain	Physical movements and responses: bodily arching, rigidity, thrashing, and drawing knees to chest Facial expressions: tightly closed eyes, furrowed brow, mouth open, and squarish Vocalization: intense, loud cry, and inconsolable Hypersensitivity/irritability Poor oral intake Poor sleep
Toddler/Preschooler	Minimal verbal skills Unable to abstract, quantify, or symbolize; literal, magical thinking Can report presence of pain, but unable to score and describe Does not understand cause and effect, may interpret pain as a punishment Vulnerable to secondary gains	Physical movements and responses: uncooperative, physical resistance, thrashing arms and legs, and guarding May be physically aggressive toward individual they believe to be responsible for the pain Vocalization: intense cry, verbally aggressive May regress or withdraw Poor oral intake Poor sleep Clingy to parent, caregiver, requests hugs, and kisses
School age	Can verbalize pain Able to localize and provide some description, cannot use adult assessment tools Beginning to understand abstract thought, not as literal, but not as sophisticated as adolescents and adults Understands rank and order Increase body awareness and fearful of bodily harm May exaggerate or provide inaccurate descriptions Influenced by ethnic culture	Physical movements and responses: muscle rigidity, body stiffness, and clenched fists Facial expressions: furrowed brow, closed eyes, and gritted teeth Poor sleep, nightmares Stalling behaviors
Adolescent	Appropriate primary source for information Able to use adult assessment tools Can abstract, quantify, qualify, and problem solve Lack of life experiences and maturity Influenced by ethnic culture	Muscle tension Deny pain in presence of peers Changes in activity, appetite, and sleep Regressive behavior

amplify the pain experience. Children may not cognitively understand that the pain can be treated. Given such obstacles, clinicians must have a keen awareness of the stages of pediatric growth and development to individualize pain assessment techniques and tools specific to each childhood stage (Table 30.1).

Components of a Pain History

A thorough pain assessment includes a comprehensive pain-focused history and physical examination. The QUESTT approach (Baker and Wong 1987) is commonly utilized as a global guide for pain assessment and evaluation:

Questt

Question the patient
Use a pain rating scale
Evaluate behavior and physiological signs
Secure the family's involvement
Take cause of pain into account
Take action and assess effectiveness

When obtaining the patient's history, the interview of both the child and the parents/caregivers is essential as children 5 years of age and older may be able to describe and portray their pain experience more accurately than their parents as parental perceptions, biases, and personal needs may be reflected in the parents' depiction of the pain history. The clinician should also be aware of the cultural beliefs surrounding the child's pain experience, the potential for secondary gains, and the overall family dynamic between the child and parent/caregiver when obtaining a complete history. The OLDCARTS mnemonic is often a useful guide when conducting a pain-specific history:

Oldcarts

Onset
Location
Duration
Character
Aggravating/associated factors
Relieving factors
Temporal factors
Severity

Onset:

- When did the pain begin?
- Was it sudden or insidious?
- Was it a result of injury or trauma?
- Is the pain acute or chronic?

Location:

- What is the point of origin?
- Is the pain localized or generalized?
- Is the pain superficial or deep?
- Does the pain follow the distribution of one of more nerve paths?
- Does the pain radiate or is it referred to areas other than the point of origin?
- Can the child identify or point to the painful body part or area?

Duration:

- How long has the pain lasted?
- If the pain is recurrent, how frequent and prolonged were the previous painful episodes?
- What is the typical progression and course of pain?

Character/quality:

- What descriptors or adjectives are used to describe the pain?
  - Bone – deep, aching, and boring
  - Muscle/fascia – dull, achy, sore, burning, and cramping
  - Nerve – sharp, knifelike, shooting, pins and needles, tingling, prickling, burning, and numb
  - Vascular – burning, stabbing, throbbing, tingling, and cold
  - Visceral – deep, cramping, and stabbing
- Is the pain constant or intermittent, dormant or progressive?

Aggravating/associated factors:

- How is the pain exacerbated?
- How has the pain impacted activity, appetite, sleep, concentration, mental and emotional status?
- Are there other symptoms resulting from the pain, i.e., nausea/vomiting, sweating, tremors, rigidity?

Relieving factors:

- How is the pain made better?
- Have any mediating activities been identified, i.e., prescription and non-prescription medications, dietary, vitamins, herbal supplements, complementary and alternative therapies
- What coping strategies have been helpful?

Temporal factors:

- What has been the chronological sequence of events?
- Is there a correlation to time of day, environmental conditions, specific events, or activities?
- Does anticipation intensify the pain?

Severity:

- How intense is the pain?
- What is the current, the highest, and the lowest pain level that is experienced?
- What is the acceptable level of pain?

Past Medical History/Family History/Social History

The next component of a thorough pain history is the past medical, family, and social history. The clinician should inquire about previous pain experiences and management strategies including pharmacological, non-pharmacological, and complimentary treatments, the presence of chronic pain conditions and any pertinent familial details. A thorough social history should recognize if the child's pain experience has impacted activities of daily living (i.e., sleep, work/school, mood, interactions with family and friends) and physical functioning.

Physical Examination

The physical examination should begin with the overall appearance of the child and recent physical vitals (blood pressure, heart rate, respiratory rate). When performing the actual physical examination, the clinician should take into consideration the child's level of discomfort and proceed from the areas causing the least to most pain.

Behavioral Signs of Pain

- Irritable crying
- Shallow breathing
- Splinting
- Changing facial expressions when touched or moved
- Resisting movement
- Rigid posture
- Difficulty sleeping
- Depressed mood

Physiologic Signs of Acute Pain

- Skin temperature changes
- Tachycardia
- Tachypnea
- Hypertension
- Sweating
- Decreased O_2 saturation

Physiologic Signs of Chronic Pain

- Involuntary muscle spasm
- Trigger points
- Decreased serotonin and endorphins
- Habituation of sympathetic response

Pain Measurement/Assessment Tools

The most accurate measure of pain is through patient self-report. The patient's description of the experience provides the clinician with the information needed to determine the location and severity of the pain. However, due to limitations in age or developmental level, the child may not be able to provide useful self-report. When a child is unable to provide self-report, clinicians must recognize certain physiological and or behavioral cues to determine treatment.

Observational assessment tools are indicated for children that are too young to understand the concept of self-report, too distressed to use self-report, or too restricted by cognitive or communicative impairments. Although pain assessment in this population can be achieved by using physiological and behavioral measures, the gathered information must be interpreted with caution. Physiological measures, such as heart rate, respiratory rate, and blood pressure, can provide clues to the presence of pain, but when viewed in isolation are not specific to pain.

Numerous pain assessment tools are available (Table 30.2) and the selection of the appropriate tool should be individualized to the child's age and developmental level.

Opioid Analgesics

Morphine

Morphine, the mainstay of pain therapy in the pediatric population, is the standard μ opioid analgesic to which all other opioids are compared (Table 30.3). Derived from the opium poppy, *Papaver somniferum*, morphine, along with codeine, is considered a naturally occurring opiate and is often the first-line agent for management of moderate to severe pain in the emergency room, operating room, ICU, and pediatric floor. Morphine can be given orally, intravenously, intramuscularly, neuraxially (via caudal, epidural, or intrathecal routes) but is often administered via intravenous patient-controlled analgesia (PCA) when used for hospitalized patients requiring acute or chronic pain management. Oral morphine is available in both immediate release and sustained release forms.

The hydrophilic nature of morphine allows a longer duration of analgesia when compared to more lipid soluble counterparts (e.g., fentanyl). Administration of intrathecal morphine may provide 12–24 h of analgesic effect due to the tendency to remain sequestered in the cerebrospinal fluid (CSF) with sustained interaction at the μ receptor in the substantia gelatinosa. Patients receiving neuraxial morphine (intrathecal or epidural) should be monitored for hypoxemia given the potential biphasic ventilatory depression caused by morphine (early respiratory depression at 1–2 h after neuraxial morphine administration and late depression up to 12 h after opioid injection).

The majority of morphine is metabolized by the liver to morphine-3-glucuronide (M3G) and morphine-6-glucuronide (M6G), with the latter being an active metabolite. Both M3G and M6G are water soluble and renally excreted. The ability to metabolize by glucuronidation, although immature, is present at birth and develops with age as morphine total body clearance may reach 80% of adult values by 6 months and 96% by 1 year of age (Bouweester 2004). In a review pooling the results of multiple pharmacological studies of pediatric patients receiving an intravenous (IV) morphine bolus and/or continuous IV infusions, Kart et al. (1997) noted the pooled half-life estimate for preterm neonates to be 9.0± 3.4 h, 6.5±2.8 h for term neonates, and 2.0±1.8 h for infants and children and clearance to be 2.2±0.7 ml/min^{-1}/kg^{-1} for preterm neonates, 8.1±3.2 ml/min^{-1}/kg^{-1} for term neonates, and 23.6±8.5 ml/min^{-1}/kg^{-1} for infants and children. As compared with adults,

Table 30.2 Pain assessment scales.

Pain assessment tool	Type of scale	Directions for use/scoring	Comments
Numeric Rating Scale (NRS)[a,b]	• Self-report • Administered either verbally or visually • Two scales: numbers or words	• Ask to give a verbal rating of pain using "0 = no pain to 10 = worst pain imaginable"	• Quick, simple, and easy to score • Easily translated to other languages • Decreased reliability with visual, auditory, or cognitive impairments and extremes in age
Visual Analog Scale (VAS)[c]	• Self-report • Administered visually	• Rate pain by making a mark on a 10-cm line	• Must understand concept of number and order • Quick and simple • Easily translated and available in multiple languages • Difficult for extremes in patient ages • High degree of sensitivity • Reliable tool for research
WongBaker FACES Rating Scale[d]	• Self-report • Administered visually • Three scales: faces, words, and numbers	• Ask the child to choose from the six cartoon faces the face that best describes your own pain • Smiling face represents "no hurt" to tearful face representing "hurts worst" • Do not use affected words	• Validated in children > 3 years of age • Simple, quick, and no gender influence • Emotion displayed on faces may reflect mood instead of pain • Available in multiple languages
Oucher[e]	• Self-report • Administered visually • Three scales: faces, words, and numbers	• Photographic scale • Child must seriate six geometric shapes; scored 0–5 • Ask the child to choose from the six the pictures "how much hurt you have right now" • Numeric scale if child can count to 100 by ones and identify the larger of two numbers. "no hurt" to the "biggest hurt you could ever have"	• Ages 3–13 years • Quick and simple • Available in three ethnic groups • May reflect mood instead of pain
Poker Chip[f]	• Self-report	• Four poker chips represent pieces of hurt • Ask how many pieces of hurt do you have right now	• Ages 3–7 years • Easy • Need some verbal skills
FLACC[g]	• Observational tool • Postoperative pain tool	• Five categories of pain behaviors: facial expression, leg movement, activity, cry, and consolability • Each scored 0–2	• Validated for scoring postoperative pain in infants and children • 2 months–7 years • (has been used 0–18 years) • Good evidence of reliability and validity
CHEOPS[h]	• Observational tool • Procedural pain	• Six behavioral items: cry, facial, child verbal, torso, touch, and legs • Scored 0–3; maximum score 13	• ages 1–17 years (has been used 4 months–17 years) • Good evidence of reliability and validity
Premature Infant Pain Profile (PIPP)[i]	• Observational tool	Scored <6 = minimal to no pain, 6–12 = mild to moderate pain, and >12 = moderate to severe pain	• <36 weeks of gestation
Neonatal Infant Pain Scale (NIPS)[j]	• Observational tool	• Six categories: facial expression, cry, breathing pattern, arms, legs, and state of arousal	• Use for children less than 1 year of age • Greater than 3 indicates pain

Table 30.2 Continued

Pain assessment tool	Type of scale	Directions for use/scoring	Comments
CRIES Pain Scale[k]	• Observational tool	• Five categories: crying, increased vital signs, expression (facial), and sleepless • Each scored 0–2	• Validated for neonates from 32 weeks of gestation to 6 months • Crying requires supplemental O_2 for saturation below 95% • Increased vital signs (arterial pressure and heart rate)
COMFORT Scale[l]	• Observational tool • Measures distress in unconscious or ventilated infants, children, and adolescents	• Eight items: alertness, calmness/agitation, respiratory response, physical movement, muscle tone, facial tension, blood pressure, and heart rate • Scored 1–5 • Scores range from 9 to 45; 17–26 generally indicate adequate sedation and pain control	• Newborn to 17 years • Requires unobtrusive observation for 2 min

[a] Downie et al. (1978).
[b] Jensen et al. (1986).
[c] Huskisson (1974).
[d] Wong et al. (2009).
[e] Beyer et al. (1992).
[f] Hester (1979).
[g] Merkel et al. (1997).
[h] McGrath et al. (1985).
[i] Stevens et al. (1996).
[j] Lawrence et al. (1993).
[k] Krechel and Bildner (1995).
[l] Ambuel et al. (1992).

these results showed age-related differences in half-life and clearance with half-life decreasing and clearance increasing with age.

Side effects of morphine include nausea/vomiting, pruritus, urinary retention, constipation, sedation, and confusion. Concomitant use of low-dose naloxone, an opioid receptor antagonist, has been shown in pediatric patients to decrease the untoward side effects of morphine without impacting its analgesic effect (Maxwell et al. 2005). Nevertheless, patients exhibiting side effects of morphine, other opioid analgesics, or epidural mixtures containing opioids should be thoroughly evaluated and treated appropriately (Table 30.4).

Fentanyl

Along with morphine, the synthetic opioid fentanyl is the most commonly used μ receptor agonist administered to pediatric patients by the anesthesiologist. The widespread use of fentanyl is marked by the multiple routes of administration (oral, intravenous, intramuscular, subcutaneous, transdermal, intranasal, epidural, and intrathecal). Pediatric uses of fentanyl include analgesia for intubated patients requiring mechanical ventilation, acute and chronic

Table 30.3 Systemic opioid analgesics.

Drug	Recommended dose	Interval	Comments
Codeine	1 mg/kg/dose Common elixir form: 12 mg codeine mixed w/ 120 mg acetaminophen	Q4 h PO	Ceiling effect with higher doses May show inter-individual variability
Oxycodone	0.1–0.15 mg/kg dose	Q4 h PO tab/elixir	Commonly used for postoperative analgesia
Morphine	50–100 mcg/kg	Q2–3 h IV	Histamine-related side effects
PCA dosing	30–50 mcg/kg	Load	
	15–20 mcg/kg	Bolus 6–10 min	
	15–20 mcg/kg/hr	Per hour infusion	
Morphine	0.2–0.5 mg/kg	Q4–6 PO	Immediate release
Fentanyl	1 mcg/kg/dose	Q1–2 h IV	Development of tolerance may occur with extended use
	1–4 mcg/kg/h	Per hour infusion	
Remifentanil	0.05–0.5 mcg/kg/min	Per hour infusion	Highly titratable Not suitable for patients requiring prolonged analgesia
Hydromorphone	10–15 mcg/kg	Q3–4 h IV	Minimal histamine-related side
PCA dosing	6–10 mcg/kg/dose	Load	
	3–4 mcg/kg/h	Per h infusion	
	75–100 mcg/kg/dose	Q3–4 h PO	
Methadone	0.1–0.4 mg/kg/dose	Q8–12 h PO	Prolonged half-life Multiple drug–drug interactions Unpredictable rates of metabolism

pain management, treatment of emergence delirium from general anesthesia, and preoperative anxiety. Compared with morphine, fentanyl is lipid soluble (accounting for its rapid onset and increased context sensitive half-life with prolonged infusion), 20–100 times more potent, has minimal histamine release even with high doses, and is more likely to cause opioid tolerance with extended use (Franck et al. 1998). Fentanyl is metabolized by the liver via the cytochrome P450 system with a small amount excreted unchanged by the kidneys. Age differences in fentanyl pharmacokinetics have been described with beta elimination half-life prolonged and clearance decreased the most in the preterm infant and neonate (Collins et al. 1985, Saarenmaa et al. 2000). However, results in pharmacokinetic studies with fentanyl have been largely variable making it difficult to demonstrate clear assessments in the pediatric population.

Additional side effects seen with fentanyl include chest wall rigidity, bradycardia, and laryngospasm (Baraka 1995), which may occur even with low doses.

Remifentanil

The high titratability and rapid metabolism of remifentanil distinguish it from other members of the opioid family and make remifentanil an analgesic alternative for patients undergoing both invasive and non-invasive procedures. Pediatric uses of remifentanil include sedation and analgesia for patients undergoing spinal surgery, plastic surgery procedures, magnetic

Table 30.4 Complications of opioid analgesia/postoperative epidural anesthesia and recommended intervention (Yaster et al. 1997, Dalens 1989).

Complication	Recommended intervention
Cardiovascular instability	1. Support airway, breathing, and circulation 2. Fluid bolus 10–20 ml/kg 3. Epinephrine 5–10 mcg/kg and then 0.1 mcg/kg/min titrated to effect 4. Discontinue epidural infusion if present
Severe respiratory depression (apnea, obtunded)	1. Support airway, supplemental o_2 2. Naloxone 5–10 mcg/kg IV $\pm$ infusion 5 mcg/kg/h 3. Stop all opioid containing infusions and boluses
Mild respiratory depression (slow respiratory rate, sedated)	1. Supplemental o_2 2. Naloxone 0.5 mcg/kg IV titrated to effect 3. Decrease epidural infusion rate 20–25%
Seizures	1. Support airway, breathing, and circulation 2. Discontinue infusion 3. Thiopental 2–3 mg/kg IV and midazolam 0.05–0.1 mg/kg IV
Motor blockade	1. Decrease concentration of local anesthetic in epidural mixture 2. Decrease epidural infusion rate 3. Withdraw epidural catheter 1 cm if one-sided block is present and reassess level
Pruritus	1. Nalbuphine 0.05–0.1 mg/kg q4–6 2. Naloxone 0.5–1.0 mcg/kg/IV $\pm$ infusion 0.25–1 mcg/kg/h 3. Diphenydramine 0.5 mg/kg/dose IV/PO q4–6 4. Decrease epidural rate by 10–20% if present; decrease/remove opioid
Nausea/vomiting	1. Ondansetron 0.05–0.1 mg/kg IV 2. Naloxone: see pruritus 3. Metoclopromide 0.1 mg/kg IV/PO q6
Urinary retention	1. Warm compresses and gentle bladder massage 2. Straight catheterization (q6 × 2); followed by indwelling catheter if necessary 3. Naloxone 0.5 mcg/kg IV
Signs of local infection	1. Remove catheter 2. Culture catheter tip 3. Careful follow-up
Leaking catheter	1. Carefully dry and redress catheter 2. Application of external pressure dressing

The authors' stress that these are only recommended interventions. Intervention should be based on and tailored to the needs of the patient and clinical situation.

resonance imaging (MRI), congenital heart surgery, cardiac catheterization, short oncological procedures (e.g., bone marrow aspiration), and short-term mechanical ventilation. Unlike other opioid analgesics, remifentanil is rapidly metabolized in the plasma by nonspecific esterases in the tissue and erythrocytes and does not accumulate with prolonged infusion. In looking at the pharmacokinetics of remifentanil in anesthetized pediatric patients, Ross et al. noted that age-related differences in clearance and volume of distribution were seen but not in half-life (3.4–5.7 min), with largest volume of distribution and rapid clearance noted in infants <2 months (Ross et al. 2001). As with other opioids, bradycardia and hypotension may occur, especially when giving boluses and large doses. Given its short duration of action, remifentanil is not a suitable option for patients requiring longer acting opioid therapy particularly in the postoperative period or for chronic pain management.

Codeine

Codeine, a naturally occurring opiate and weak μ opioid agonist, is typically given for the treatment of mild to moderate pain. It has one-tenth the potency of morphine and may be administered by oral, rectal, and intramuscular routes. Intravenous codeine is not a recommended route of delivery due to reports of profound hypotension seen in pediatric patients (Shanahan et al. 1983). Often given in combination with acetaminophen, codeine is a popular oral analgesic agent for children presenting for ambulatory surgery.

Following oral administration, codeine is quickly absorbed with peak plasma concentrations occurring within 1–2 h after ingestion. Codeine is metabolized in the liver in three ways, primarily by glucuronidation (75%), N-demethylation to norcodeine (15%), and 0-demethylation to morphine (10%) by the hepatic enzyme cytochrome P450 ED6 (CYP2DG6), a pathway that is hypothesized to be the major source of codeine's analgesic activity. Genetic polymorphism of CYP2DG6 is thought to account for the inter-individual variability in drug efficacy seen with codeine with 7% of Caucasians considered poor metabolizers of codeine (Alvan et al. 1990). Poor metabolizers will therefore generate little or no morphine from 0-demethylation, whereas extensive metabolizers may generate excessive amounts.

Side effects of codeine include nausea and vomiting, sedation, decreased gastric motility, pruritus/itching, and miosis, which may account for its ceiling effect when given in high doses (Williams et al. 2001).

Oxycodone

Oxycodone is an oral semi-synthetic μ opioid agonist that is 1.5–2 times more potent than oral morphine and typically used for moderate to severe pain. It may be given alone (available in immediate or sustained release form) or in combination with acetaminophen or acetylsalicylic acid. Oxycodone is metabolized by the liver to noroxycodone (major) and oxymorphone (minor). When given in immediate release form, peak plasma concentrations occur 1–2 h after oral administration with duration of action of approximately 4 h.

The pharmacokinetics of oxycodone has been described in the pediatric population. In a study looking at 18 children (2–10 years of age) who received intravenous oxycodone, terminal elimination half-life was approximately 100 min (less than observed adult values) and clearance was almost 50% higher in the pediatric population compared to adults (Olkkola et al. 1994). In infants less than 6 months who were given intravenous oxycodone, values for clearance and elimination half-life ($t^1/_2$) showed inter-individual variability (especially in patients <2 months) despite an overall assessment of clearance increasing and $t^1/_2$ decreasing with age (Pokela et al. 2005).

Hydromorphone

Due to its lack of associated active metabolite and histamine release, hydromorphone, a semi-synthetic morphine derivative, is a popular analgesic alternative to morphine for acute and chronic pediatric pain patients. It is commonly administered by intravenous, oral, and epidural routes and has a potency 5–7 times that of morphine. In addition, hydromorphone has similar drug onset to morphine and provides approximately 4–5 h of analgesia to the non-tolerant patient when given intravenously. The majority of hydromorphone is metabolized by the liver to the inactive metabolite hydromorphone-3-glucuronide which is then renally eliminated.

Methadone

Methadone is largely considered a second-line opioid for acute pain management due to its potential for drug to drug interactions, long half-life (18–24 h), and cases of serious side effects when patients were given large and frequent doses leading to gradual accumulation and toxic levels. However, methadone has been used safely in pediatric patients requiring relief for cancer pain (Miser and Miser 1985, Shir et al. 1998, Davies et al. 2008), burns (Williams et al. 1998), trauma (Shir et al. 1998), postoperative pain (Berde et al. 1991), and tapering for opioid dependency and withdrawal prevention (Tobias et al. 1990, Robertson et al. 2000, Siddappa et al. 2003). Methadone is a racemic mixture of L and D isomers, which acts both as a μ opioid agonist and as a N-methyl-D-aspartic acid (NMDA) antagonist. This latter property of methadone is of particular interest as the activation of NMDA receptors is noted to increase spinal neuron sensitivity to pain and reduce the activity of opioid agonists on neural opioid receptors. Methadone is metabolized by the hepatic cytochrome system which may show inter-individual variability. Therefore, patients who have received methadone should be closely monitored for potential drug–drug interactions and side effects of sedation and respiratory depression given its long half-life and potential unpredictable rates of metabolism.

Tramadol

A synthetic analog of codeine, tramadol has been increasingly used in the pediatric population. It has one-tenth the potency of morphine, is a weak μ opioid agonist, and a monoaminergic (serotonin and norepinephrine) reuptake inhibitor in the central nervous system (Bozkurt 2005). This latter activity of tramadol is thought to synergize with its μ opioid agonist property, thereby potentiating analgesia and perhaps minimizing side effects such as respiratory depression, nausea/vomiting, sedation, and constipation associated with the conventional μ opioid analgesics (Bosenberg and Ratcliffe 1998, Finkel et al. 2002, Chu 2006). To date, tramadol has been used for both acute and chronic pain management in the pediatric population and may be given by oral, intramuscular, intravenous, caudal/epidural routes or by local infiltration.

Patient-Controlled Analgesia

The patient-controlled analgesia (PCA) is the most common means of delivering intravenous opioids to the hospitalized pediatric patient for acute or chronic pain management. Long-acting analgesics such as morphine or hydromorphone are typically selected. PCA settings consist of a demand dose (drug delivered by pressing the PCA button when desired), basal hourly rate (drug dose delivered continuously during an hourly period), and lockout interval (time in minutes in which a patient is unable to have drug delivered). The use of PCA in younger patients less than 2 years of age is controversial. In younger pediatric patients who are unable to control the PCA, the demand dose may be given by nursing-controlled analgesia (NCA) or parent-controlled analgesia (PARCA). Pain management teams should always tailor the PCA settings to the needs of the patient either increasing the demand or basal dose if current settings are not adequately providing enough pain control or decreasing the demand or basal dose if the patient shows signs of being overdosed with opioids.

Non-opioid Analgesics

Acetaminophen

Acetaminophen (paracetamol) is a first-line anti-pyretic and analgesic for mild to moderate pain for pediatric patients of all ages. Its popularity is highlighted by its wide therapeutic window, over-the-counter accessibility, lack of systemic effects, safety profile when given in appropriate doses, and opioid sparing effect when given for pediatric ambulatory surgery (Korpela et al. 1999). Although the exact anti-nociceptive mechanisms of acetaminophen continue to be elucidated, proposed explanations have included interference with serotonergic descending pain pathways (Anderson 2008) and the central inhibition of the enzyme cyclo-oxygenase (COX), thereby preventing the production of prostaglandins from arachidonic acid. Prostaglandins are thought to play a role in nociceptive transmission by augmenting the release of excitatory neurotransmitters such as glutamate and substance P (Bjorkman et al. 1994, Choi et al. 2001) and blocking the release of inhibitory neurotransmitters (Ahmadi et al. 2002).

Acetaminophen may be given alone or in varying doses as a combination with codeine, oxycodone, or hydrocodone. When given alone, acetaminophen can be administered orally (multiple preparations), rectally or more recently, intravenously (mostly used outside the United States). Regardless of the route of administration, attention should be directed toward following acetaminophen dosing guidelines to avoid potential drug-induced toxicity (doses > 150 mg/kg or 10 times the recommended dose).

Following oral intake, acetaminophen plasma concentrations peak after 1–2 h with a reported half-life of 3–4 h. Recommended oral dose is 10–15 mg/kg q 4–6 h to a maximum dose of 50–75 mg/kg (Cranswick and Coghlan 2000). Rectal suppositories of acetaminophen, despite reported variability in absorption and pharmacokinetics (Anderson and Holford 1997), remain a popular means of drug delivery. Birmingham et al. (2001) recommended an initial dose of 40 mg/kg followed by 20 mg/kg doses every 6 h (Birmingham et al. 2001) based on a study age group of 3–12 years.

The use of intravenous acetaminophen in pediatric patients has increasingly garnered interest, with studies reporting predictable drug bioavailability (100%) and peak plasma concentrations occurring 1 h after injection (Anderson et al. 2005). However, given its relatively nascent and limited use in the United States, further studies are needed to clarify the role of IV acetaminophen in pediatric acute and chronic pain management.

Nonsteroidal Anti Inflammatory Drugs

Nonsteroidal anti inflammatory drugs (NSAIDs) are useful pharmacological agents for the treatment of mild to moderate pain and anti-pyrexia in the pediatric population. Their analgesic activity is thought to be due to the decrease in peripheral > central prostaglandin synthesis through the inhibition of the enzyme COX. Unlike acetaminophen which exhibits minimal peripheral side effects, prolonged NSAIDs use is associated with adverse complications including gastric wall thinning and ulceration, acute renal failure, and platelet dysfunction (Tobias 2000). Furthermore, the use of salicylates is thought to increase the risk of Reye's syndrome (characterized by acute hepatic failure and encephalopathy) and therefore not typically given for the treatment of fever or mild pain in pediatric patients exhibiting viral-like symptoms. NSAIDs may be administered orally, intravenously, intramuscularly, or rectally.

Ketamine

A phencyclidine derivative, ketamine, is well known for its dysphoria and dissociative anesthetic effects. Ketamine's analgesic properties are thought to be due to possible μ opioid activity (Finck and Ngai 1982, Smith et al. 1987) and NMDA receptor antagonism (Stubhaug et al. 1997, Stubhaug and Breivik 1997). Interest in ketamine has increased due to this latter activity as blockade of the NMDA receptor is thought to play a role in the development of central pain mechanisms such as "wind up" and hyperalgesia. Pediatric uses of ketamine include preoperative sedation, induction of general anesthesia, minimization of emergence delirium following general anesthesia, sedation/analgesia for invasive and non-invasive procedures (i.e., cardiac catheterization, wound dressing changes), and analgesic therapy for end-stage cancer pain (Abu-Shahwan and Chowdary 2007, Lois and De Kock 2008, Conway et al. 2009). Although ketamine causes minimal respiratory depression at sub-anesthetic doses, laryngospasm and hypersalivation are possible side effects (Green et al. 1998), with the latter effect being attenuated by the administration of an anti-cholinergic. Ketamine may be given intravenously, intramuscularly, or rectally.

Clonidine

Pediatric uses of clonidine (an α2-adrenergic agonist) include analgesic therapy (commonly as an adjunct to regional anesthesia) and treatment of preoperative anxiety (Mikawa et al. 1993, Ramesh et al. 1997, Bergendahl et al. 2004), postoperative nausea/vomiting (Handa and Fujii 2001), and emergence delirium (Kulka et al. 2001, Bock et al. 2002). Despite potential side effects of hypotension and bradycardia, clonidine is not associated with respiratory depression as seen with opioid analgesics. Clonidine may be administered by oral, rectal, or neuraxial (caudal, epidural) routes.

Regional Anesthesia

Regional anesthesia, whether performed alone or most commonly in conjunction with general anesthesia, provides an excellent and safe source of intra-operative and postoperative analgesia for pediatric acute pain management as well as analgesia for pediatric chronic pain management. The popularity of regional anesthesia is underscored by its ability to decrease intra-operative and postoperative requirement for opioids, intra-operative titration of volatile anesthetics, and to minimize side effects associated with opioid analgesia and volatile anesthesia such as sedation and nausea and vomiting. Techniques may include the neuraxial blocks (which encompass spinals, lumbar/thoracic epidurals, and caudals) and peripheral nerve blocks with and without the placement of catheters, although catheter placement is typical for the epidural technique. The decision to perform a regional anesthetic should be based on factors such as the patient (i.e., absence of coagulopathy or systemic infection), comfort level of the anesthesiologist, type of surgical procedure, location of the anticipated area of pain, parental consent, and patient cooperation (if performed awake).

Spinal Block

The placement of spinals (subarachnoid or intrathecal block) has been performed for over a century in pediatric patients as an alternative or adjunct to general anesthesia, particularly for abdominal or lower extremity procedures. Over the past 20 years, the use of spinal anesthesia has resurged particularly with neonates and infants undergoing inguinal hernia repair. Purported advantages include avoidance of endotracheal intubation and intra-operative hemodynamic stability. Disadvantages include finite spinal duration and potential inadequate level of surgical anesthesia.

Technique

When performed in the awake infant, routine anesthetic monitors (blood pressure cuff, EKG leads, and pulse oximetry) and supplemental oxygen (usually in the form of nasal cannula) should be placed and intravenous access should be obtained beforehand. Available assistance should be directed toward positioning the infant in the lateral or more commonly, sitting position while the anesthesiologist places the spinal at the L4-L5 interspace or below as the spinal cord may terminate at L3 in infants. Following sterile preparation, a 25–27 G spinal needle is carefully advanced until flow of CSF is noted and the syringe containing local anesthetic is quickly attached and slowly injected. The infant is then placed in the supine position. At the authors' institution, tetracaine (0.6–1 mg/kg) diluted with equal volume of 10% dextrose is the local of choice allowing for 60–90 min of surgical anesthesia time.

Complications

Complications associated with spinal placement in pediatric patients may occur but are infrequent. In a study looking at 1483 infants who successfully received spinal anesthesia (Williams et al. 2006), 56 infants (3.8%) had a sensory level that was higher than intended. Of these 56 infants 23 infants received supplemental oxygen while maintaining spontaneous ventilation while 10 infants showed airway compromise due to the high spinal level. These patients either received bag mask ventilation (five infants) or were intubated endotracheally (five infants). In the same study, bradycardia (as defined by <100 beats per minute) was another reported complication that occurred in 24 of the 1483 infants (1.6%). Fifteen infants received anti-cholinergics such as atropine or glycopyrrolate for bradycardia, while brady-cardia in three infants occurred in the setting of a high spinal. One of these infants required endotracheal intubation and chest compressions while the atropine circulated, but the infant was successfully extubated at the end of the surgical procedure without complication.

Epidural Block

Epidural anesthesia provides an effective form of analgesia for the pediatric patient intraoper-atively and postoperatively. In particular for pediatric patients undergoing upper abdominal or thoracic procedures such as for pectus excavatum, a working thoracic epidural provides an important component of pain management. Epidural placement may be achieved either with the patient awake or with the patient asleep after the induction of general anesthesia. An epidural infusion consisting of a local and opioid mixture is typically started during the surgical procedure and continued postoperatively for the duration of the epidural use.

Technique

The technique of epidural anesthesia is similar to adults although a shorter epidural nee-dle should be used when appropriate. The patient is either placed in a sitting (if awake) or lateral decubitus (awake or asleep) position following standard monitor application and IV access. Choice of epidural catheter placement (either lumbar or thoracic) should be deter-mined by the location of the surgical procedure (Table 30.5). If a lumbar epidural is chosen in

Table 30.5 Preferred levels of epidural catheter placement.

Upper abdominal or thoracic surgeries	T6-T10
Lower abdominal or pelvic surgeries	T10-L4
Lower extremity surgeries	L2-L5

infants, placement below L3 is recommended as the spinal cord in infants may terminate at L3. Following sterile preparation and drape, the epidural needle is carefully inserted until it is felt to engage the interspinous ligaments. The operator should be cautious when inserting the epidural needle as the epidural space is often more shallow than in their adult counterparts. After epidural needle engagement, the epidural needle is slowly advanced until the epidural space is identified with a loss of resistance technique. At the authors' institution, identification of the epidural space in pediatric patients is performed with a saline filled syringe to minimize the risk of air embolism. The epidural catheter is threaded and advanced in the epidural space anywhere between 1.5 and 5 cm depending on patient size and age and catheter desired tip location.

Complications

Possible complications associated with epidural anesthesia may include overadvancement of the epidural needle into the intrathecal space or "wet tap" and subsequent spinal headache and spinal anesthesia if local is inadvertently injected. Intravascular injection, epidural hematoma, and neurological injury are other possible risks of epidural anesthesia. Neurological injury following epidural catheterization is a potentially devastating but exceedingly rare complication whose incidence is difficult to quantify in the pediatric population although cases of spinal cord infarction following epidural placement and epidural steroid injection have been reported in the adult population (Ackerman et al. 1990, Bromage and Benumof 1998, Hobai et al. 2008, Ludwig and Burns 2005, Glaser and Falco 2005). In a 1-year prospective study by the French-Language Society of Pediatric Anesthesiologists (ADARPEF) designed to provide data regarding regional anesthesia epidemiology and complication incidence, the authors reported that out of 2396 lumbar epidurals, two patients experienced transient postoperative paresthesias (2 and 8 h) that resolved but could not be clearly attributed to the epidural placement versus nerve stretching from intra-operative positioning (Giaufre et al. 1996). In addition to complications from epidural technique, complications and side effects may arise from substances administered through the epidural, most often a mixture of opioid and local anesthetic (Table 30.6).

Caudal Block

Caudal anesthesia is the most common neuraxial block performed in the pediatric patient and is often an adjunct rather than alternative to general anesthesia. In the ADAPREF study looking at the epidemiology and complication incidence of regional anesthesia, out of 24,409 regional anesthetics 12,111 were caudals while epidurals and spinals accounted for 2396 and 506 regional blocks, respectively (Giaufre et al. 1996). Since the caudal space is contiguous

Table 30.6 Recommended solutions for epidural analgesia.

Solution	Rates (ml/kg/h)	Patients
Fentanyl 1 mcg/ml +Bupivacaine 1/16%	0.1–0.2	Neonates; <6 months
Fentanyl 2 mcg/ml +Bupivacaine 1/16%	0.1–0.4	>6 months
Hydromorphone 3 mcg/ml +Bupivacaine 1/16%	0.1–0.4	Neonates, infants, and toddlers
Hydromorphone 10 mcg/ml +Bupivacaine 1/32%	0.1–0.4	Toddler, school age children

with the epidural space, caudal blocks provide excellent analgesia for pediatric patients undergoing surgical procedures below the umbilicus. The popularity of caudal anesthesia is largely attributed to the low incidence of complications and relatively easy technique particularly in the pediatric patient. Little presacral fat seen in infants and children allows for the straightforward identification of bony anatomical landmarks. Caudal blocks may either be "single-shot" or continuous via caudal catheter for postoperative pain management.

Technique

The patient is placed in the lateral decubitus position and the sacral hiatus is identified following palpation of the sacral cornua, oftentimes located above the beginning of the gluteal cleft. Identification of the sacral hiatus may also be achieved through envisioning an imaginary equilateral triangle in which a line connecting the posterior iliac spines function as one side of the triangle with the remaining two sides joining at a point consistent with the location of the sacral hiatus. Following sterile preparation, an 18–22-g styleted beveled needle is directed at a 45° angle to the skin and advanced until a "pop" is felt when the needle pierces through the sacrococcygeal ligament. When using an intravenous catheter for the caudal needle, easy advancement of the catheter off the needle is indicative of penetration into the caudal canal. If the needle encounters bone before entering the sacral hiatus, the needle should be withdrawn and its angle should be decreased and readvanced until a "pop" is felt. Other reported methods confirming caudal placement include ultrasound imaging, nerve stimulation eliciting motor activity of the anal sphincter, and the "swoosh test" in which the injection of 2–3 ml of air through the caudal needle creates a "swoosh sound" with auscultation of the thoracolumbar spine. Of note, the "swoosh test" is not routinely performed due to the potential risk of air embolism. Following correct caudal needle placement, aspiration for CSF and blood and test dose (0.1 ml/kg) may be performed prior to full local anesthetic injection. At the authors' institution, 0.125–0.250% bupivacaine with 1:200,000 epinephrine at a dose of (0.8–1 ml/kg) (with 20 ml as the maximum allowable volume due to the risk of pressure-induced paresthesia) is the local of choice and is given incrementally, providing 4–8 h of analgesia. If a caudal catheter is planned, the catheter is threaded through the caudal needle to the desired thoracic or lumbar epidural space. Methods for confirming correct placement include the use of ultrasound (Chawathe et al. 2003), nerve stimulation (Tsui et al. 2004), and radiography with contrast (Valairucha et al. 2002).

Complications

Rare complications of caudal placement may include rectal perforation, intravascular injection, dural puncture, and neurological injury. If a caudal catheter is placed, fecal catheter contamination causing systemic infection is a potential but uncommon complication. In a study looking at bacterial colonization and infection rate in pediatric patients with continuous epidurals, similar rates of gram-positive colonization in caudal and lumbar epidural catheters (25% and 23%, respectively) were noted, while caudal catheters showed a higher percentage of gram-negative organisms (16%) versus lumbar epidurals (3%) (Kost-Byerly et al. 1998). Severe systemic infections did not occur in any of the studied patients. The practice at the authors' institution to minimize infection includes strict sterile technique with catheter placement, careful occlusive dressing of the catheter, and removal of the caudal catheter by postoperative days 2 or 3 when possible.

Peripheral Nerve Block

The use of peripheral nerve blocks is another means to provide analgesia for pediatric patients. Table 30.7 describes various peripheral blocks and potential pediatric uses. Benefits of peripheral nerve blocks include targeted deposition of local to specific nerves innervating the anticipated surgical or desired analgesic site and limited systemic effects as seen with neuraxial blocks (i.e., hypotension and respiratory depression from high spinal level). Peripheral block utilization in the pediatric population may range from the easily performed ilioinguinal/iliohypogastric and penile blocks for inguinal hernia and circumcision procedures to brachial plexus (interscalene, axillary) and lower extremity (femoral, sciatic, popliteal) blocks

Table 30.7 Peripheral blocks performed in pediatric patients.

Block	Pediatric Uses/Surgical Procedures
Intercostal	Thoracic procedures
Penile	Circumcision
Ilioinguinal/	Orchidopexy
Iliohypogastric	Inguinal hernia
	Miscellaneous groin procedures
Axillary	Arm/hand procedures
Interscalene	Shoulder procedures
Digital	Finger procedures
Femoral	Knee surgery
	Femoral Shaft Fractures
	Femoral Osteotomy
Sciatic	Foot/knee procedures
Popliteal	Leg/foot procedures
Auricular branch	Myringotomy/PE tube placement
Of Vagus (Nerve of	
Arnold)	
Infraorbital block	Cleft palate repair
Rectus sheath	Umbilical hernia repair
block	Epigastric hernia repair
	Nissen fundoplication
	Abdominal wall syndrome

Table 30.8 Maximum allowable single dosing for local anesthetics.

Local Anesthetic	Dose (mg/kg)
Bupivacaine	3
Ropivacaine	3
Lidocaine (plain)	5
Lidocaine with epinephrine	7

under the guidance of ultrasound and/or nerve stimulation to the application of novel blocks for common pediatric procedures such as myringotomy and PE (pressure equalizing) tube placement (Voronov et al. 2008). The practitioner should be cognizant of the maximal allowable local anesthetic dose to avoid systemic local toxicity when performing peripheral blocks (Table 30.8).

Hospital-Based Chronic and Recurrent Pain
Headaches
Children with chronic pain syndromes are often admitted for acute or abortive treatment of unbearable pain. Headaches and abdominal pain are among the most frequent reasons for pain-related admissions. Hospital admission for new-onset headache requires workup for organic disease. Occipital neuralgia with pain over the distribution of the lesser occipital nerve is common in children with achondroplasia secondary to stenosis of the foramen magnum (Kondev and Minster 2003). These acute pain episodes in the presence of chronic pain syndromes require knowledge of the chronic pain philosophies and treatment trends as well as the armamentarium to address the patient in pain extremis. One of the most frequent causes for hospital admission is headache such as in intractable migraine. Abortive migraine treatment includes oral preparations of NSAIDs, caffeine, and isometheptene. Nausea and vomiting may require administration of intravenous anti-emetics. The use of opioids or barbiturate compounds is acceptable as second-line therapy, but the trend is toward using the triptan preparations (Kondev and Minster 2003) instead of narcotics. The use of ergotamines and steroids is reserved for refractory cases.

Cystic fibrosis can be associated with headaches and facial pain due to sinusitis or coughing paroxysms (Marks and Kissner 1997, Stern et al. 1988). Migraine and tension headaches are the most common types of pediatric headaches. By age 15 years 5.3% of children have migraines and 15.7% have frequent non-migrainous headaches and 54% had infrequent non-migrainous headaches. More than 82% of children by late adolescence experience some type of headache (Lipton 1997).

Abdominal Pain
Abdominal pain is a frequent cause of hospital admission and missed school days. Abdominal pain is divided into two categories: functional and organic. Functional abdominal pain (FAP) encompasses a group of conditions characterized by chronic or recurrent symptoms that are not explained by biochemical, anatomical, or structural abnormalities (Saps and Di Lorenzo

2009). There is a higher incidence of symptoms of depression and anxiety in children with FAP. Prospective studies have shown that children of parents who have irritable bowel syndrome (IBS) where the most common presentation is chronic abdominal pain often report more gastrointestinal symptoms, have a higher rate of school absenteeism, and have more doctor's visits than children whose parents do not have IBS (Levy et al. 2004). Through the process known as "enabling" parents can inadvertently reinforce illness behaviors in their children when they attempt to be protective, compassionate, and nurturing (van Tilburg et al. 2009).

Abdominal pain due to organic disease accounts for less than 10% of the cases of recurrent abdominal pain (RAP). Genitourinary and gastrointestinal disorders are the most common organic causes of RAP. Recurrent urinary tract infection and hydronephrosis or obstructive uropathy can present with abdominal pain. Eventually, abnormal urinalysis and pyuria will focus attention to the underlying problem. Hemolytic uremic syndrome is the most common cause of renal failure in children (Jernigan and Waldo 1994).

Constipation is a common disorder and patients may experience crampy abdominal discomfort in association with the urge to defecate. A suggestive history and the demonstration on physical examination of bulky stool retained in the rectum should initiate a trial of appropriate treatment (Scott et al. 2000).

Particular aspects of the history that should alert suspicion of disease include significant recurrent pain in a child under the age of 3, consistent localization of pain away from the umbilicus, frequently awakening from sleep by pain, or repetitive vomiting. Pernicious or bilious vomiting that is accompanied by abdominal pain should always alert the clinician to the possibility of an intestinal obstruction. Malrotation or incomplete rotation of the mid-gut is a disorder that may present as a bowel obstruction and predisposes to the formation of intestinal volvulus (Scott et al. 2000). Vomiting, abdominal and flank pain, and ileus are the presenting signs for pancreatitis. Pancreatitis is uncommon in childhood and the etiology is diverse. The incidence of pancreatitis is unknown; however the disease occurs as a result of trauma then up to 50% of the cases will be complicated by the development of a pseudocyst (Hebra et al. 2008). There is a less than 2% prevalence of cholelithiasis in children although the number of cases is rising (Wesdorp et al. 2000).

Sickle Cell-Related Pain

Sickle cell disease was first described in 1910 by Herrick (1910) with the first molecular disease defined and described by Linus Pauling (1980). It was Sydenstricker who first used the word *crisis* to describe the abdominal pains and jaundice that occurs during the event. Ingram in 1956 examined the electrophoretic properties of normal and sickle hemoglobin and discovered the substitution of glutamic acid for valine at the sixth position of the hemoglobin chain which led to a change in ionic charge from neutral to phobic. Deoxygenation leads to crystal formation, tactoids, and stacking of red blood cells, such that sludging in the microvasculature occurs and results in ischemia and organ infarction. Hemolysis results in jaundice. The vaso-occlusive crisis of sickle cell disease is heralded by pain that may be localized or diffuse (Ballas 2002).

Over two million African-Americans and Hispanic-Americans are affected by sickle cell disease. Other people affected include those of Arab, Indian, and Asiatic descent or wherever there was malarial spread from equatorial Africa. Generally patients present with abdominal pain, back pain, or extremity pain, especially of the legs. Any one or combination of these regions may be affected during a vaso-occlusive crisis (VOC) (Wethers 2000, Serjeant and Serjeant 2004). Shapiro in the 1990s described the event as a *painful episode* to de-emphasize the emotional component in an effort to improve coping (Shapiro et al. 1995). Despite an attempt to control the behavioral facet by de-emphasizing the anxiety, it has been shown that many patients objectively test positive for anxiety and a sense of helplessness that may be a co-morbidity for this life-threatening disease. The unpredictability of onset and severity of pain coupled with the uncertainty of sequelae and shortened lifespan can be likened to living in a mine field.

Most patients with sickle cell disease have few crises that require hospitalization. Approximately 25% of all patients with sickle cell disease have frequent crises. Many VOC episodes are handled at home or in day hospitals which support the fact that early, effective intervention can curtail most uncomplicated crises (Benjamin et al. 2000). However, when a patient fails at home care, strong analgesics are indicated. Of patients who present to the emergency departments 50% do so for painful events. Approximately 30% present with febrile events and 20% for combined pain and fever (Frush et al. 1995). Patients often require large doses of opioids but obtain minimal relief due to the complex nature of the pain since rheological, inflammatory, and ischemic factors come into play. Elevated substance P levels appear to contribute to the acute episodes (Douglas 2008). Conversely, pain scores are not affected by the amount of opioid administration (Jacob et al. 2003). Since opioids do not have a ceiling effect of analgesia, increased doses are given in an effort to diminish the pain. Oftentimes, the sedation from the opioids can be severe, resulting in inadequate ventilation, hypoxia, and a worsening of the crisis pathophysiology. Acute chest syndrome, a complicated VOC presentation, has been associated with high-dose systemic exposure to morphine (Kopecky et al. 2004).

Cancer-Related Pain

A review by Docherty found that children and adolescents with cancer focused primarily on symptoms of pain and fatigue (Docherty 2003). Pain due to disease occurs in less than 50% of cases at the time of diagnosis in pediatric oncologic disease. However, children with cancer experience multiple types of pain during their course of care. Procedure-related pain due to venipunctures, bone marrow biopsies, and aspirates and lumbar punctures is common. Surgical resection of solid tumors and staged procedures requiring repeated operations, central intravascular access port placements, and subsequent removal are causes of procedure-related pain. Some chemotherapy regimens trigger the onset of neuropathic pain at a later time [e.g., granulopoiesis-stimulating factors (GSF) and vinca alkaloids] (Topp et al. 2000). Organic platinum compounds such as oxaliplatin can cause pain at the onset of infusion (Quasrhoff and Hartung 2002). Oral mucositis results from the cytotoxic effects of chemotherapy and radiation therapy. Apoptosis of the oral epithelium occurs and overgrowth of bacteria, fungi, and viruses in combination with the release of cytokines results in oral ulcers and a characteristic burning pain (Köstler et al. 2001). Resolution of the symptoms is temporally related to the restoration of the neutrophil count from the cytotoxic nadir (Lockhart and Sonis 1979).

Wolfe found that 89% of parents felt that their children experienced "a lot" or "a great deal" from at least one symptom at the end of life. Pain was the most common symptom, yet, only 27% of families found the symptom-specific interventions to be successful in managing the pain (Wolf et al. 2000). Parental distress can be great and is inversely proportional to the time elapsed since diagnosis (Boman et al. 2003).

Death distress is usually more profound in young patients and appears to be inversely correlated to spiritual "groundedness (Chibnall et al. 2002)." Differing spiritual beliefs between the caregiver and the adolescent patient can be a cause of worsening distress. Health professionals are encouraged to be familiar and non-judgmental of spiritual or religious beliefs of their patients (Lyon et al. 2001).

The Cancer Pain Relief Program of the World Health Organization (WHO) developed an analgesic ladder for the management of pain of increasing intensity (Jacox et al. 1994). For mild pain, the recommendations start with NSAIDs. This drug class must be used with caution in those patients receiving steroids as part of their oncologic management. NSAIDs are also contraindicated for patients who have renal insufficiency, intravascular volume depletion as seen with intractable vomiting, congestive heart failure, or peptic ulcer disease. A ceiling effect may occur and increasing doses will lead to side effects without additional benefits. Opioids have no ceiling effect. In the WHO ladder, moderate pain is treated with traditionally weak opioids. Agents such as codeine, oxycodone, hydrocodone, and meperidine are used. Mixed agonists–antagonists are incorrectly considered as protection against respiratory depression but may have greater side effects. These mixed agonists also have a ceiling effect. For severe pain, traditionally "strong" opioids are used. Unless contraindicated, morphine is generally considered the agent of choice. Other strong opioids include methadone, hydromorphone, levorphanol, and oxymorphone (Jacox et al. 1994).

Summary

The interpretation of "primum non nocere" or first do no harm does not translate into "do as little as possible." The practice of subtherapeutic dosing and erratic administration of analgesics predisposes the child to a prolonged pain experience. However, misconceptions and erroneous beliefs persist in the medical community despite advances in pediatric pain research. Walco has stated that assessment and treatment of pain in children are important parts of pediatric practice, and failure to provide adequate control of pain amounts to substandard and unethical medical practice (Walco 1994). Thus, the task of changing the culture of pain management for children is the charge of all healthcare professionals dedicated to the care of children.

Case Scenario

Dr. Suniel Ramessur, MBBS, BSc (Hons), FRCA, DipHEP

Justin is a 7-year-old boy who presents with severe abdominal pain and is now being assessed by the surgical team. You have been asked to see him in the emergency department to assist with his pain management.

What options can you consider to manage Justin's pain?
You will need to first assess Justin, which includes a medical history review and a physical examination. It is important to note the nature of his disease process and the pain pattern

– colicky pain may respond better to anti-spasmodics than to conventional analgesics. Note what, if any, analgesia he has already received. You will also need to assess the severity of his pain. While it is always prudent to begin at the bottom of the analgesic ladder, it is sometimes obvious that more than simple analgesics will be required.

Examine the child for signs of cardio-respiratory compromise as it may impact your analgesic regimen.

Acetaminophen would be a good background analgesic to use:

- Oral dose is 20 mg/kg (but be weary of using oral analgesics in this child as with an abdominal complaint, absorption may be variable and he may be vomiting).

A nonsteroidal can be considered but again remember the limitations of oral administration; rectal administration is likely to be distressing to a young child in pain and the IV route in a child may be controversial. It is also worth bearing in mind that the child may be dehydrated at this point and some argue that NSAIDs can predispose to intra-operative bleeding. For all these reasons it may be best to avoid a NSAID in the acute setting.

You may decide he requires IV morphine:

- IV dose is 50–100 mcg/kg in titrated doses while monitoring the SpO_2% and respiratory rate.

If giving opiates, then remember to prescribe an anti-emetic such as ondansetron 0.15 mg/kg.

Justin weighs 22 kg, and in addition to resuscitation fluids, you titrate 1.5 mg of morphine IV to settle his pain. He is more comfortable now and is having his SpO_2% monitored. The surgeons diagnose him with bowel intussusception and make arrangements for him to go to operating room.

What intra-operative analgesia strategies will you use?
In small children a caudal dose of local anesthetic can be very effective. It may be relatively contraindicated if he is septic or you suspect that he is still significantly hypovolemic. Many will use a rapid-onset and short-acting opiate such as fentanyl (1–3 mcg/kg) or alfentanil (10–20 mcg/kg). Depending on the situation, one could consider giving acetaminophen rectally before the end of the anesthetic. You can also ask the surgeon to place local anesthetics into the wound at the end of the case. Remember the following maximum doses:

- Lidocaine 5 mg/kg (plain)
- Bupivacaine 3 mg/kg

You decide to use fentanyl during the case and give a rectal dose of acetaminophen at the end of the case. The surgeons performed a laparotomy and resected some necrotic bowel. The plan is to extubate the child at the end of the case.

What postoperative analgesics do you think Justin will require?
In addition to background analgesia such as acetaminophen and the caudal, and in the absence of an epidural catheter, one will need to consider a long-acting opioid regimen. Depending on the age of the patient, patient- (or nurse) controlled analgesia should be considered (PCA/NCA). Each center will have its own protocol for setting up such an infusion. In case of significant respiratory depression, the dose of naloxone (0.01 mg/kg IV) should be administered.

References

Abu-Shahwan I, Chowdary K. Ketamine is effective in decreasing the incidence of emergence agitation in children undergoing dental repair under sevoflurane general anesthesia. Paediatr Anaesth. 2007;17(9):846–50.

Ackerman WE, Juneja MM, Knapp RK. Maternal paraparesis after epidural anesthesia and cesarean section. South Med J. 1990;83(6):695–7.

Ahmadi S, Lippross S, Neuhuber WL et al. PGE(2) selectively blocks inhibitory glycinergic neurotransmission onto rat superficial dorsal horn neurons. Nat Neurosci. 2002;5(1):34–40.

Alvan G, Bechtel P, Iselius L, et al. Hydroxylation polymorphisms of debrisoquine and mephenytoin in European populations. Eur J Clin Pharmacol. 1990;39(6):533–7.

Ambuel B, Hamlett K, Mrax C, Blumer J. Assessing distress in pediatric intensive care environments: the COMFORT scale. J Pediatr Psychol. 1992;17:95–109.

Anand KJ, Hickey PR. Halothane-morphine compared with high-dose sufentanil for anesthesia and postoperative analgesia in neonatal cardiac surgery. N Engl J Med. 1992;326(1):1–9.

Anand KJ, Sippell WG, Aynsley-Green A. Randomized trial of fentanyl anesthesia in preterm babies undergoing surgery: effects on the stress response. Lancet 1987;1:62–6.

Anderson BJ. Paracetamol (Acetaminophen): mechanisms of action. Pediatr Anesth. 2008;18(10):915–21.

Anderson BJ, Holford NHG. Rectal paracetamol dosing regimens: determination by computer simulations. Pediatr Anesth. 1997;7(6):451–5.

Anderson BJ, Pons G, Autret-Leca E, et al. Pediatric intravenous paracetamol (propacetamol) pharmacokinetics: a population analysis. Pediatr Anesth. 2005;15(4):282–92.

Baker CM, Wong DL. QUEST: a process of pain assessment in children. Orthoped Nurs. 1987;6(1):11–21.

Ballas SK. Sickle cell anaemia: progress in pathogenesis and treatment. Drugs 2002;62(8):1143–72.

Baraka A. Fentanyl-induced laryngospasm following tracheal extubation in a child. Anaesthesia 1995;50(4):375.

Benjamin LJ, Swinson GI, Nagel RL. Sickle cell anemia day hospital: an approach for the management of uncomplicated painful crises. Blood 2000;95(4):1130–6.

Berde CB, Beyer JE, Bournaki MC, et al. Comparison of morphine and methadone for prevention of postoperative pain in 3 to 7 year old children. J Pediatr. 1991;119(1):136–41.

Bergendahl HTG, Lonnqvist PA, Eksborg S, et al. Clonidine vs midazolam as premedication in children undergoing adeno-tonsillectomy: a prospective randomized controlled clinical trial. Acta Anaesthesiol Scand 2004;48(10):1292–300.

Beyer J, Denyes M, Villarruel A. The creation, validation, and continuing development of the Oucher: a measure of pain intensity in children. J Pediatr Nurs. 1992;7:335–46.

Birmingham PK, Tobias MJ, Fisher DM, et al. Initial and subsequent dosing of rectal acetaminophen in children: a 24-hour pharmacokinetic study of new dose recommendations. Anesthesiology 2001;94(3):385–9.

Bjorkman R, Hallman KM, Hedner J, et al. Acetaminophen blocks spinal hyperalgesia induced by NMDA and substance P. Pain 1994;57(3):259–64.

Bock M, Kunz P, Schreckenberger R, et al. Comparison of caudal and intravenous clonidine in the prevention of agitation after sevoflurane in children. Br J Anaesth. 2002;88(6):790–6.

Boman K, Lindahl A, Bjork O. Disease-related distress in parents of children with cancer at various stages after the time of diagnosis. Acta Oncologica 2003;42(2):137–46.

Bosenberg AT, Ratcliffe S. The respiratory effects of tramadol in children under halothane anesthesia. Anaesthesia 1998;53(10):960–4.

Bouwmeester NJ, Anderson BJ, Tibboel D, et al. Developmental Phamacokinetics of morphine and its metabolites in neonates, infants and young children. Br J Anaesth. 2004 Feb;92(2):208–17.

Bozkurt P. Use of tramadol in children. Pediatr Anesth. 2005;15(12):1041–7.

Bromage PR, Benumof JL. Paraplegia following intracord injection during attempted epidural anesthesia under general anesthesia. Reg Anesth Pain Med. 1998;23(1):104–7.

Carbajal R, Rousset A, Danan C, et al. Epidemiology and treatment of painful procedures in neonates in the intensive care units. JAMA 2008;300(1):60–70.

Chawathe MS, Jones RM, Gilersleve CD, et al. Detection of epidural catheters with ultrasound in children. Pediatr Anesth. 2003;13(8):681–4.

Chibnall JT, Videen SD, Duckro PN, et al. Psychosocial-spiritual correlates of death distress in patients with life-threatening medical conditions. Palliat Med. 2002;16(4):331–8.

Choi SS, Lee JK, Suh HW. Antinociceptive profiles of aspirin and acetaminophen in formalin, substance P and glutamate pain models. Brain Res. 2001;921(1–2):233–9.

Chu YC, Lin SM, Hsieh YC, et al. Intraoperative administration of tramadol for postoperative nurse-controlled analgesia resulted in earlier awakening and less sedation than morphine in children after cardiac surgery. Anesth Analg. 2006;102(6):1668–73.

Collins G, Koren G, Crean P, et al. Fentanyl pharmacokinetics and hemodynamic effects in preterm infants during ligation of patent ductus arteriosus. Anesth Analg. 1985;64(11)1078–80.

Conway M, White N, Jean CS, et al. Use of continuous intravenous ketamine for end-stage cancer pain in children. J Pediatr Oncol Nurs. 2009;26(2):100–6.

Cranswick N, Coghlan D. Paracetamol efficacy and safety in children: the first 40 years. Am J Ther. 2000;7(2):135–41.

Dalens B. Epidural anesthesia. In: Dalens B, editor. Pediatric regional anesthesia. Boca Raton, Florida; CRC Press; 1989. pp. 407–14.

Davies S, DeVlaming D, Haines C. Methadone analgesia for children with advanced cancer. Pediatr Blood Cancer 2008;51(3):393–7.

Docherty SL. Symptom experiences of children and adolescents with cancer. Ann Rev Nurs Res. 2003;21:123–49.

Douglas SD. Elevated plasma substance P in sickle cell disease and vaso-occlusive crisis. Med Hypoth 2008;70(6):1229.

Downie WW, Leatham PA, Rhind VM, et al. Studies with pain rating scales. Ann Rheum Dis 1978;37:378–81.

Finck AD, Ngai SH. Opiate Receptor mediation of ketamine analgesia. Anesthesiology 1982;56(4):291–7.

Finkel JC, Rose JB, Schmitz ML, et al. An evaluation of the efficacy and tolerability of oral tramadol hydrochloride tablets for the treatment of postsurgical pain in children. Anesth Anal. 2002;94(6):1469–73.

Franck LS, Vilardi J, Durand D, et al. Opioid withdrawal in neonates after continuous infusions of morphine or fentnayl during extracorporeal membrane oxygenation. Am J Crit Care 1998;7(5):364–9.

Frush K, Ware RE, Kinney TR. Emergency department visits by children with sickle hemoglobinopathies: factors associated with hospital admission. Pediatr Emerg Care 1995;11(1):9–12.

Giaufre E, Dalens B, Gombert A. Epidemiology and morbidity of regional anesthesia in children: a one-year prospective study of the French-Language society of Pediatric Anesthesiologists. Anesth Analg. 1996;83(5):904–12.

Glaser SE, Falco F. Paraplegia following a thoracolumbar transforaminal epidural steroid injection. Pain Phys. 2005;8(3):309–14.

Green SM, Rothrock SG, Lynch EL, et al. Intramuscular ketamine for pediatric sedation in the emergency department: safety profile in 1,022 cases. Ann Emerg Med. 1998;31:688–97.

Handa F, Fujii Y. The efficacy of oral clonidine premedication in the prevention of postoperative vomiting in children following strabismus surgery. Paediatr Anaesth. 2001;11(1):71–4.

Hebra A, Adams SD, Thomas PB. Pancreatitis and pancreatic pseudocyst. Available at http://.webmd.emedicine.com Sept 11, 2008. Accessed 10 August 2009.

Herrick JB. Peculiar elongated and sickle-shaped red blood corpuscles in a case of severe anemia. Arch Intern Med. 1910;6:517–21.

Hester N. The preoperational child's reaction to immunization. Nurs Res. 1979;28:250–4.

Hobai IA, Bittner EA, Grecu L. Perioperative spinal cord infarction in nonaortic surgery: report of three cases and review of the literature. J Clin Anesth. 2008;20(4):307–12.

Huskisson EC. Measurements of pain. Lancet 1974;2(7889):1127–31.

Jacob E, Miaskowski C, Savedra M, et al. Management of vaso-occlusive pain in children with sickle cell disease. J Pediatr Hematol/Oncol. 2003;25(4):307–11.

Jacox AK, Carr DB, et al. Management of cancer pain: clinical practice guideline. AHCPR Pub. No. 94-0592. Rockville, MD: Agency for Health Care Policy and Research, PHS, USDHHS, 1994.

Jensen MP, Karoly P, Braver S. The measurement of clinical pain intensity: a comparison of six methods. Pain 1986;27:117–26.

Jernigan SM, Waldo FB. Racial incidence of hemolytic uremic syndrome. Pediatr Nephrol. 1994;8:545–7.

Kart T, Christrup LL, Rasmussen M. Recommended use of morphine in neonates, infants and children based on a literature review: part 1-pharmacokinetics. Pediatr Anaesth. 1997;7(1): 5–11.

Kondev L, Minster A. Headache and facial pain in children and adolescents. Otolaryngol Clin N Am. 2003;(6):1153–70.

Kopecky EA, Jacobson S, Joshi P, et al. Systemic exposure to morphine and the risk of acute chest syndrome in sickle cell disease. Clin Pharmacol Ther. 2004;75(3):140–6.

Korpela R, Korvenoja P, Meretoja OA. Morphine-sparing effect of acetaminophen in pediatric day-case surgery. Anesthesiology 1999;91(2):442–7.

Kost-Byerly S, Tobin JR, Greenberg RS, et al. Bacterial colonization and infection rate of continuous epidural catheters in children. Anesth Analg. 1998;86(4):712–6.

Köstler WJ, Hejna M, Wenzel C, et al. Oral mucositis complicating chemotherapy and/or radiotherapy: options for prevention and treatment. CA Cancer J Clin. 2001;51:290–315.

Krechel SW, Bildner J. CRIES: a new neonatal postoperative pain measurement score – initial testing of validity and reliability. Paediatr Anaesth. 1995;5:53–61.

Kulka PJ, Bressem M, Tryba M. Clonidine prevents sevoflurane-induced agitation in children. Anesth Analg. 2001 93(2):335–8.

Lawrence J, Alcock D, McGrath P, Kay J, MacMurray S, Dulberg C. The development of a tool to assess neonatal pain. J Neonatal Nurs. 1993;12:59–66.

Levy RL, Whitehead WE, Walker LS, et al. Increased somatic complaints and health-care utilization in children: effects of parent IBS status and parent response to gastrointestinal symptoms. Am J Gastroenterol. 2004;99:2442–51.

Lipton RB. Diagnosis and epidemiology of pediatric migraine. Curr Opin Neurol. 1997;10:231.

Lockhart PB, Sonis ST. Relationship of oral complications to peripheral blood leukocyte and platelet counts in patients receiving cancer chemotherapy. Oral Surg Oral Med Oral Pathol. 1979;48:21–28.

Lois F, De Kock M. Something new about ketamine for pediatric anesthesia? Curr Opin Anesthesiol. 2008;23:340–44.

Lowery CL, Hardman MP, Manning N, et al. Neurodevelopmental changes of fetal pain. Semin Perinatol. 2007;31(5) 275–82.

Ludwig MA, Burns SP. Spinal cord infarction following cervical transforaminal epidural injection: a case report. Spine 2005;30(10):E266–8.

Lyon ME, Townsend-Akpan C, Thompson A. Spirituality and end-of-life care for an adolescent with AIDS. AIDS Patient Care Stds. 2001;15(11):555–60.

Marks SC, Kissner DG. Management of sinusitis in adult cystic fibrosis. Am J Rhinol. 1997;11(1):11–4.

Maxwell LG, Kaufmann SC, Bitzer S, et al. The effects of a small dose naloxone infusion on a opioid-induced side effects and analgesia in children and adolescents treated with intravenous patient-controlled analgesia: a double-blind, prospective, randomized, controlled study. Anesth Analg. 2005;100(4):953–8.

McGrath P, Johnson G, Goodman J, Schilinger J, Dunn J, Chapman J. CHEOPS: a behavioral scale for rating postoperative pain in children. In: Fields H, Dubner R, Cervero F, editors. Advances in pain research and therapy. New York, NY: Raven Press; 1985. pp. 395–402.

Merkel S, Voepel-Lewis T, Shayevits J, Malviya S. The FLACC: a behavioral scale for scoring postoperative pain in young children. Pediatr Nurs. 1997;23:293–297.

Mikawa K, Maekawa N, Nishina K, et al. Efficacy of oral clonidine premedication in children. Anesthesiology 1993;79(5):926–31.

Miser AW, Miser JS. The use of oral methadone to control moderate and severe pain in children and young adults with malignancy. Clin J Pain. 1985;1:243–248.

Olkkola KT, Hamunen K, Seppala T, et al. Pharmacokinetics and ventilatory effects of intravenous oxycodone in postoperative children. Br J Clin Pharmac. 1994;38:71–6.

Pauling L. The normal hemoglobins and the hemoglobinopathies: background. Tex Rep Biol Med. 1980–81;40:1–7.

Pokela M, Anttila E, Seppala T, et al. Marked variation in oxycodone pharmacokinetics in infants. Pediatr Anesth. 2005;15:560–5.

Quasrhoff S, Hartung HP. Chemotherapy-induced peripheral neuropathy. J Neurol. 2002;249:9–17.

Ramesh VJ, Bhardwaj N, Batra YK. Comparative study of oral clonidine and diazepam as premedicants in children. Int J Clin Pharmacol Ther. 1997;35(5):218–21.

Robertson RC, Darsey E, Fortenberry JD, et al. Evaluation of an opiate-weaning protocol using methadone in pediatric intensive care unit patients. Pediatr Crit Care Med. 2000;1(2):119–23.

Siddappa R, Fletcher JE, Heard AM, et al. Methadone dosage for prevention of opioid withdrawal in children. Paediatr Anaesth. 2003:13(9):805–10.

Ross AK, Davis PJ, Dear Gd GL, et al. Pharmacokinetics of remifentanil in anesthetized pediatric patients undergoing elective surgery or diagnostic procedures. Anesth Anal. 2001;93(6):1393–401.

Saarenmaa E, Neuvonen PJ, Fellman V. Gestational age and birth weight effects on plasma clearance of fentanyl in newborn infants. J Pediatr. 2000;136(6) 767-70.

Saps M, Di Lorenzo C. Pharmacotherapy for functional gastrointestinal disorders in children. J Pediatr Gastroenterol Nutr. 2009;48(suppl 2):S101-3.

Scott RB, Withers G, Morrison DJ, Zamora SA, Parsons HG, Butzner JP, Schreiber RA, Machida H, Martin SR. Manifestations of gastrointestinal disease in the child. In: Thomson ABR, Shaffer EA, editors. First principles of gastroenterology: the basis of disease and an approach to management; Canadian Association of Gastroenterology Staff; Canadian Association for the Study of the Liver Staff; Astra Zeneca Canada Inc Staff Thompson. 4th ed. Astra Zeneca Canada; 2000.

Serjeant GR, Serjeant BE. Sickle cell disease in Saudi Arabia: the Asian haplotype. Reflections on a meeting at Hofuf, September 2003. Ann Saudi Med. 2004;24(3):166-8.

Shanahan EC, Marshall AG, Garrett CP. Adverse reactions to intravenous codeine phosphate in children. A report of three cases. Anaesthesia 1983;38:40-3.

Shapiro BS, Dinges DF, Orne EC, et al. Home management of sickle cell-related pain in children and adolescents: natural history and impact on school attendance. Pain 1995;61(1):139-44.

Shir Y, Shenkman Z, Shavelson V, et al. Oral methadone for the treatment of severe pain in hospitalized children: A report of five cases. Clin J Pain 1998;14(4):350-3.

Smith DJ, Bouchal RL, deSanctis CA, et al. Properties of the interaction between ketamine and opiate binding sites in vivo and in vitro. Neuropharmacolgy 1987;26(9):1253-60.

Stern RC, Horowitz SJ, Doershuk CF. Neurologic symptoms during coughing paroxysms in cystic fibrosis. J Pediatr. 1988;112(6):909-12.

Stevens B, Johnston C, Petryshen P, Taddio A. Premature infant pain profile: development and initial validation. Clin J Pain. 1996;12:13-22.

Stubhaug A, Breivik H. Long-term treatment of chronic neuropathic pain with the NMDA receptor antagonist ketamine. Acta Anesthesiol Scand. 1997;41:329-31.

Stubhaug A, Brevik H, Eide PK. Mapping of punctuate hyperalgesia around a surgical incision demonstrates that ketamine is a powerful suppressor of central sensitization to pain following surgery. Acta Anaesthesiol Scand. 1997;41:1124-32.

Tobias JD, Schleien CL, Haun SE. Methadone as treatment for iatrogenic narcotic dependency in pediatric intensive care unit patients. Crit Care Med. 1990;18(11)1292-3.

Tobias JD. Weak analgesics and nonsteroidal anti-inflammatory agents in the management of children with acute pain. Pediatr Clin N Am. 2000;47(3):527-43.

Topp KS, Tanner KD, Levine JD. Damage to the cytoskeleton of large diameter sensory neurons and myelinated axons in vincristine-induced painful peripheral neuropathy in the rat. J Comp Neurol. 2000;424:563–76.

Tsui BC, Wagner A, Cave D, et al. Thoracic and lumbar epidural analgesia via a caudal approach using electrical stimulation guidance in pediatric patients: a review of 289 patients. Anesthesiology 2004;100(30):683–9.

Valairucha S, Seefelder C, Houck CS. Thoracic epidural catheters placed by the caudal route in infants: the importance of radiographic confirmation. Pediatr Anesth. 2002;12(5):424–8.

van Tilburg MA, Chitkara DK, Palsson OS, et al. Parental worries and beliefs about abdominal pain. J Pediatr Gastroenterol Nutr. 2009;48(3):311–7.

Voronov P, Tobin MJ, Billings K, et al. Postoperative pain relief in infants undergoing myringotomy and tube placement: comparison of a novel regional anesthetic block to intranasal fentanyl-a pilot analysis. Pediatr Anesth. 2008;18(12):1196–201.

Walco GA. Pain, hurt and harm—The ethics of pain control in infants and children. NEJM 1994;331(8):541–4.

Wesdorp I, Bosman D, de Graaff A, et al. Clinical presentations and predisposing factors of cholelithiasis and sludge in children. J Pediatr Gastroenterol Nutr. 2000;31(4):411–7.

Wethers DL. Sickle cell disease in childhood: Part I. Laboratory Diagnosis, pathophysiology and health maintenance. Am Fam Phys. 2000;62:1013–20.

Williams DG, Hatch DJ, Howard RF. Codeine phosphate in paediatric medicine. Br J Anaesth. 2001;86(3):413–21.

Williams PI, Sarginson RE, Ratcliffe JM. Use of methadone in the morphine-tolerant burned paediatric patient. Br J Anaesth. 1998;80:92–5.

Williams RK, Adams DC, Aladjem EV, et al. The safety and efficacy of spinal anesthesia for surgery in infants: the Vermont Infant Spinal Registry. Anesth Analg. 2006;102(1):67–71.

Wolfe J, Grier HE, Klar N, et al. Symptoms and suffering at the end of life in children with cancer. NEJM 2000;342(5):326–33.

Wong DL, Hockenberry-Eaton M, Wilson D, et al. Wong's essentials of pediatric nursing. 8th ed. St Louis, MO: Mosby; 2009.

Yaster M, Andresini J, Krane E. Epidural analgesia. In: Yaster M, Cote CJ, Krane EJ, Kaplan RF, Lappe DG, editors. Pediatric pain management and sedation handbook. St. Louis, MO: Mosby; 1997. pp. 113–46.

Chapter 31

Managing Pain in the Addicted Patient

Susan Dabu-Bondoc, MD, Robert Zhang, MD, and Nalini Vadivelu, MD

Approximately 20 million Americans have some form of substance abuse disorder, and about one-third of the US population has used illicit drugs (Substance Abuse and Mental Health Services Administration office of Applied Studies 2007). Substance abuse is known to occur in 10–16% of outpatients in general medical practice, 25–40% of hospital admissions, and 40–60% of major trauma patients (Manchikanti et al. 2003, Rosenblatt and Mekhail 2005). In chronic pain management settings, illicit drug use has been reported in 14–34% of patients (Manchikanti et al. 2006). Among the illicit drugs, use of marijuana is reported most common, followed by that of cocaine, hallucinogens, and methamphetamines. Such high prevalence of illicit use, along with concerns of drug abuse and addiction, and its association with life-threatening pathophysiological effects, often has a negative influence on pain treatment. Pain patients who have current or remote histories of drug abuse present a multitude of medical and psychosocial issues that hinder pain and symptom management. Physicians are often not well-versed with the conceptual or practical issues related to addiction, which causes difficulty in treating these patients effectively. In chronic pain patients, the high incidence of illicit drug use is intimately linked to opioid and prescription drug dependence, as well as to the psychosocial, cultural, and environmental factors that affect these individuals.

Diagnosing Substance Abuse and Addiction

Addiction is a primary, chronic, and neurobiologic disease with genetic, psychosocial, and environmental factors influencing its development and manifestations (Heit 2003). It is characterized by behaviors that include one or more of the following: impaired control over drug use, compulsive use, continued use despite harm, and craving for the drug (American Academy of Pain Medicine, American Pain Society, American Society of Addiction Medicine 2001, Rinaldi et al. 1988). This definition emphasizes that addiction is a psychological and a behavioral syndrome. *Physical dependence* is a state of neuroadaptation that is manifested by a drug class-specific withdrawal syndrome that can be produced by abrupt cessation, rapid dose reduction, decreasing blood level of the drug, and/or an administration of an antagonist. *Tolerance*, on the other hand, is a state of adaptation in which exposure to the drug induces changes that result in diminution of one or more of the drug's effects over time. Physical dependence and tolerance are neuropharmacological phenomena, while addiction is both a

N. Vadivelu et al. (eds.), *Essentials of Pain Management*,
DOI 10.1007/978-0-387-87579-8_31, © Springer Science+Business Media, LLC 2011

neuropharmacological and a behavioral phenomenon. Addiction may occur with or without physical dependence. *Pseudoaddiction*, a term coined by Weissman and Haddox in 1989 (Weissman and Haddox 1989), refers to behaviors that may mimic those commonly associated with opioid abuse but are instead indicative of unrelieved pain. The term is applied to an individual or a pain patient who seeks additional medications, whether appropriately or not, because of undertreatment of pain, and such inappropriate behavior ceases when pain is treated in the proper manner. Unlike addiction, this behavior resolves once the pain is under adequate control. *Pseudotolerance* is the need to increase medication (e.g., opioids for pain) when other factors, such as disease progression, new disease, increased physical activity, lack of compliance, change in medication, drug interaction, addiction, and/or deviant behavior, are present (Pappagallo 1998). *Abuse* is the use of medications outside the scope of usual medical practice or the use of illicit substances. Various definitions of abuse, which include the phenomena associated with physical dependence or tolerance, are often, however, not applicable to terminal pain patients (i.e., cancer patients) who receive potentially abusing drugs for legitimate medical indications (Passik et al. 1998, Passik and Portenoy 1998). *Diversion* is the use of legitimately prescribed medication for illicit, illegitimate purposes, with the intent to sell or distribute.

Evaluation of the drug-abusing patient must be comprehensive in all three key aspects of patient's problem: pain, addiction, and psychiatric component. Patients with a history of substance abuse or drug addiction can be classified into three categories: those who are actively involved in illicit drug use, those with a history of drug abuse, and those in methadone maintenance programs. Evaluation of addiction should include determination of the patient's history of which substances have been used over what time duration, history of prior substance abuse treatment, assessment of the severity of the patient's substance abuse problem and the extent of patient's involvement in treatment programs, what is the patient's level of motivation to change status, what is the duration of sobriety if in recovery, and how sobriety is maintained. In this population, it is not uncommon for pain, substance abuse, and psychiatric problems to act synergistically to lead to development of complex, difficult to manage syndromes. Consulting or involving substance abuse specialists such as psychiatry and/or addiction medicine professional may often be needed to clarify diagnosis and complete evaluation. Current or past history of a personality, anxiety, mood, or psychotic disorder warrants a psychiatric referral and evaluation. Careful chronology may reveal which component (pain versus psychologic versus addictive disorder) exacerbate or cause the other. Table 31.1 enumerates the various criteria used in diagnosing substance abuse and substance dependence as published in Diagnostic and Statistical Manual of Mental Disorders, 4th ed. (DSM-IV).

Assessing severity of abuse is, as established in DSM-IV criteria, based on the number of adverse consequences resulting from use. Not all the criteria in the DSM-IV, however, would be applicable in the chronic pain patient, and in fact some have been a source of confusion in diagnosing addiction. The form of addiction seen in the patient with pain is often not the same as the type seen in the street addict. The requirement in the DSM-IV criteria for substance dependence about giving up or decreasing social, occupational, or recreational activities because of substance abuse often is not found in the pain patient with dependence. Unlike the illicit addict, the pain patient does not usually compromise their lifestyle (e.g., drive long distances to seek drugs or involve himself in criminal activity or drug diversion).

Table 31.1 Diagnostic criteria of substance abuse and dependence in DSM-IV (American Psychiatric Association 1994).

A. Substance abuse
– maladaptive pattern of substance use leading to clinically significant impairment or distress, manifested by at least one of the following, occurring within a 12-month period, and symptoms have never met the criteria for substance dependence
1. Recurrent use resulting in failure to fulfill major role obligations at work, school, or home (examples: substance-related poor work performance, repeated absences, suspensions, expulsion from school, neglect of children, or household)
2. Recurrent use in physically hazardous situations such as driving a vehicle or operating a machine
3. Recurrent substance-related legal problems such as substance-related misconduct leading to arrests
4.Continued use despite substance use related persistent or recurrent social or interpersonal problems (examples: arguments with spouse about consequences of intoxication, physical fights)
B. Substance dependence
- a maladaptive pattern of substance use, leading to clinically significant impairment or distress, as manifested by three or more of the following, occurring at any time in the same 12-month period:
1. Tolerance – as defined by either of the following:
    a. need for markedly increased amounts of the substance to achieve intoxication or desired effect
    b. markedly diminished effect with continued use of the same amount of the substance
2. Withdrawal – as manifested by either of the following:
    a. the characteristic withdrawal syndrome for the substance
    b. the same or closely related substance is taken to relieve or avoid withdrawal symptoms
3. The substance is often taken in larger amounts or over a longer period than was intended
4. There is a persistent desire or unsuccessful effort to cut down or control substance abuse
5. A great deal of time is spent in activities necessary to obtain the substance (e.g., visiting multiple doctors or driving long distances), use the substance, or recover from its effects
6. Important social, occupational, or recreational activities are given up or reduced because of substance abuse
7. The substance use is continued despite knowledge or having a persistent or recurrent physical or psychological problem that is likely to have been caused or exacerbated by the substance (e.g., current cocaine use despite recognition of cocaine-induced depression)

Adapted From Diagnostic and Statistical Manual of Mental Disorders (1994).

Also, the classic sign of compulsive opioid use may not be apparent in the pain patient because opioid is prescribed and is readily available. The signs of prescription drug abuse, in contrast to that of illicit abuse, often are more subtle and may need a combination of multiple observations.

Toxicology screening can be a helpful clinical adjunct to identify aberrant behavior and to monitor problematic opioid use in addiction or diversion. Practitioners believe that all patients with chronic non-terminal pain who were treated with opioids should be subjected to random urine screening. This belief has been supported by survey studies demonstrating that about 40% of the patients with chronic non-cancer pain who were treated with opioids were found to be problematic, and about half of these problematic cases were identified through toxicology screening. The physician is, nevertheless, the ultimate responsible caregiver who determines the severity of the prescription drug abuse in his practice and to make the decision on whether toxicology would be utilized on a routine or an occasional basis.

The chapter covers a review of the most commonly encountered illicit drugs of abuse, their physicochemical characteristics and epidemiology, pathophysiological effects, and clinical manifestations. Management of pain in both the illicit and licit drug-abusing patient is then discussed focusing on the conceptual and practical issues associated with drug abuse in both the acute and chronic pain patient.

Illicit Drugs

Cocaine

In the United States, there are an estimated 2.4–5 million regular users of cocaine and among adults, approximately 30 million (15% of US population) have tried cocaine at least once (US Dept Health Human Services, Substance Abuse and Mental Health Services Administration, Office of Applied Studies 2006). Cocaine is an alkaloid extracted from the leaves of the shrub indigenous to South America, *Erythroxylon coca*. The drug was first introduced as a local anesthetic due to its topical numbing properties. It is commercially marketed in a hydrochloride form as powder, granules, or crystals, and is prepared by dissolving the alkaloid to form a water-soluble salt, cocaine hydrochloride. This can be converted back to its alkalinized (most popular) form by the addition of baking soda or ammonia plus water followed by heating, which is widely smoked and known as "crack," "rock," or free base. Crack cocaine can be 95% pure, is highly addictive and is ingested orally, smoked in a base pipe, snorted, or is injected. When smoked, it can provide an intense euphoria in less than 1 min, with duration of only 5–10 min (Perez-Reyes et al. 1982). Cocaine's low molecular weight and high lipid solubility allow easy diffusion across lipid membranes. The oral form is historically the oldest and was documented in reports of South American natives chewing coca leaves for recreational benefit. The bioavailability after oral ingestion is 30–40% and is about 80 or 90% after intranasal or inhalation route, respectively (Jeffcoat et al. 1989). While the onset of euphoric effects after the oral route is 10–20 min, peak plasma levels are obtained in less than 15 min via the intranasal route and in 3–5 min after intravenous administration. Patients with pseudocholinesterase deficiency are at increased risk of cocaine toxicity because cocaine is metabolized mainly by plasma and liver cholinesterases to water-soluble metabolites that are excreted in the urine.

As an indirect sympathomimetic agent, cocaine interferes with presynaptic reuptake of neurotransmitters norepinephrine, epinephrine, serotonin, and dopamine, thereby increasing their availability at adrenergic receptors (Carrera et al. 2004). Cocaine produces a dose-dependent increase in heart rate and blood pressure, heightens arousal, and improves performance on tasks of vigilance and alertness. The increase in dopaminergic activity in the cortico-limbic reward system of the brain contributes to cocaine's positive psychological effects such as euphoria, improved sense of self-confidence and well-being, and its abuse potential. As a local anesthetic, cocaine blocks the rapid increase in cell membrane permeability to sodium ions during depolarization and the propagation of the action potential leading to slowing or blocking of nerve conduction. Like other local anesthetics, cocaine's effects on Na channels also occur in cardiac myocytes causing negative chronotropic (e.g., prolonged QRS) and inotropic effects in severe overdose.

Cocaine toxicity can lead to sudden death. Severe reactions are characterized by their rapid onset and unpredictable effects, manifested as overwhelming stimulation of the central nervous, cardiovascular, and respiratory systems, culminating in seizures followed by profound depression and cardio-respiratory collapse (Mouhaffel et al. 1995). Alternatively, cardiac arrhythmias may occur and progress to ventricular fibrillation. Through vasoconstriction and vasospasm, cocaine compromises arterial blood flow to the heart and brain, leading to inadequate blood supply and oxygenation that may result into stroke, irreversible brain damage, myocardial depression, or myocardial infarction (MI) (Pitts et al. 1997, Feldman et al. 2000). Myocarditis, congestive heart failure, and dilated cardiomyopathy resulting from cocaine abuse have also been documented (Mouhaffel et al. 1995). Acute aortic dissection, although rare, may also occur due to abrupt, severe catecholamine release and hypertension (Hsue et al. 2002). The incidence of hemorrhagic strokes is also increased (Brust 1993). Pulmonary complications associated with cocaine use occur primarily in individuals who inhale crack and include chronic cough, asthma, hypersensitivity pneumonitis ("crack lung"), pulmonary edema, pneumo-pericardium, and pulmonary hemorrhage (Shanti and Lucas 2003, Albrecht et al. 2000). "Crack lung" or pneumonitis in a cocaine user is characterized by fevers, pulmonary infiltrates, and leukocytosis; it is treated with oral steroids but can be severe enough to cause acute respiratory failure and make patients ventilator dependent (Gatof and Albert 2002). Barotrauma resulting in pneu-mo-pericardium has been attributed to frequent Valsalva maneuvers performed by cocaine smokers or snorters.

Hyperthermia mediated by vasoconstriction and/or the hypermetabolic state of cocaine use may follow toxicity. This may be accompanied by rhabdomyolysis, acute renal failure, or convulsions (Marzuk et al. 1998). Other reported adverse effects of cocaine use include anxiety, restlessness, irritability, confusion, nasal septum infection or perforation, papillary dilatation, and seizures (Greydanus and Patel 2003). In the pediatric population, short- and long-term neurobehavioral problems have been associated with cocaine abuse. Multiple congenital anomalies, meconium staining, low birth weight, "withdrawal baby" syndrome (a constellation of symptoms including frequent sneezing, irritability, and diarrhea), increased incidence of sudden infant death syndrome (SIDS), and failure to thrive have all been associated with infants of cocaine-abusing mothers (Kain et al. 1993). Risk factors such as lack of prenatal care, history of preterm labor, and cigarette smoking should arouse suspicion of cocaine use in pregnancy. Because of its high lipid solubility, cocaine's rapid transplacental diffusion and consequent high fetal blood and tissue levels can result in reduced uteroplacental blood flow and hypoxia, uteroplacental insufficiency, acidosis, and fetal distress (Bhuvaneswar et al. 2008). In the third trimester, cocaine toxicity may cause preterm labor or delivery, premature rupture of membranes (PROMs), and abruptio placenta. Emergency abdominal delivery is fourfold higher in parturients; maternal seizures are commonly seen. While it is less clear if there is an increased risk of congenital anomalies in the fetus, chronic cocaine abuse has been known to produce permanent biochemical and functional changes affecting brain structures manifested as low IQ scores (Andres 1993). Cocaine in combination with benzodiazepines, at least in animal studies, increases the incidence of malformations such as hydronephrosis, cryptorchidism, and incomplete ossification of the skeleton (Mehanny et al. 1991). Other acute effects from cocaine intake in parturients include fetal tachycardia, hypertension, and intrauterine fetal death (IUFD).

Amphetamines and Related "Designer" Drugs

Also known as poor man's cocaine, this class of drug has a special feature of having a half-life that is said to be eight times as long as that of cocaine (Derlett et al. 1989). Amphetamines can be ingested orally, inhaled, or injected. Metabolism is variable and up to 30% can be excreted unchanged in the urine. Amphetamines and its metabolites can be detected in the urine for several days after ingestion and their plasma half-life is highly variable. Through central nervous system stimulation, they cause euphoria, increased alertness, aggression, and changes in personality. Both amphetamine and amphetamine "designer" drugs produce indirect sympathetic activation by releasing noradrenaline, dopamine, and serotonin from terminals in the central and autonomic nervous system (Christophersen 2000, Albertson et al. 1999).

The term "designer" drugs include a group of compounds that have been chemically altered from federally controlled substances to produce special effects and to bypass legal regulation. The largest group, and the most extensively studied, is the methylenedioxy derivatives of amphetamine and methamphetamine. The most known and widely used designer drug is 3,4-methylenedioxymethamphetamine (MDMA, or Ecstasy).

Ecstasy and Eve

MDMA or 3,4-methylenedioxyemethamphetamine, otherwise known as ecstasy (or the "love drug," Adam, Eve, X, E, XTC), is both a hallucinogen and a stimulant. It induces a state of euphoria and increased self-awareness (Milroy 1999). It was first synthesized as an appetite suppressant in 1914 but its euphoric and energizing qualities made it a popular street drug since the 1980s with a particular high prevalence of use in college campuses or "rave" (very large dance parties in abandoned warehouses) clubs (Greydanus and Patel 2003, Shulgin 1986, Boot 2000). It is readily absorbed through the gastrointestinal tract, is swallowed, used rectally, smoked/snorted, or injected. Its effects on mood are mediated by actions on dopamine and serotonin pathways, as well as on noradrenergic pathways. The drug has been found to have detrimental effects on serotonergic neurons in the CNS. As a result, memory and cognitive dysfunction as well as behavioral problems are common side effects. The most commonly seen reaction to toxic ingestion of MDMA is a syndrome of altered mental status, tachycardia, tachypnea, profuse sweating, and hyperthermia, which closely resembles that of acute amphetamine overdose (amphetamine is chemically similar to MDMA). Some of the more rare but serious side effects include malignant hyperthermia, rhabdomyolysis, kidney failure, heart failure, disseminated intravascular coagulation (DIC), fulminant liver failure, strokes, seizures, and death (Reneman et al. 2000, Rittoo and Rittoo 1992, Fiege 2003, Brauer 1997). The hallucinogenic and stimulant effects of the drug can last 3–6 h but can last up to several days. When taken in pregnancy, the risk of congenital effects, such as cardiac anomalies, cleft lip and palate, biliary atresia, fetal IUGR, IUFD, and cerebral hemorrhage, is increased (Eriksson et al. 2000).

Hallucinogens (Club Drugs)

Hallucinogens include lysergic acid (LSD), phencyclidine (PCP), mescaline, and psilocybin. These drugs are all ingested orally. They produce visual, auditory, and tactile hallucinations with distortions of body image, surroundings, and reality; as well as, anxiety, panic attacks, and a fear of going crazy (Abraham et al. 1996). Although mild and do not resemble the sympathetic discharge caused by cocaine, ecstasy, or amphetamines, hallucinogens cause hypertension and tachycardia, dilated pupils, and increased body temperature via activation of the sympathetic nervous system. Overdose can lead to respiratory depression, seizures, coma, or death. Hallucinogens are not associated with withdrawal symptoms and physical dependence but do cause psychological dependence and tolerance. In pregnancy, hallucinogen abuse leads to a higher risk of premature labor and delivery, fetal IUGR, meconium staining, and withdrawal syndrome.

Phencyclidine (PCP or "Angel Dust")

Discovered in 1926, phencyclidine is a hallucinogen that remained without significant utility until 30 years later when its potential to reduce or even eliminate pain was demonstrated in animal models. Briefly used as an analgesic–amnesic anesthetic, it was later abandoned due to high incidence of bizarre psychiatric effects such as delirium, agitation, disorientation, and hallucination (Abraham et al. 1996). Ketamine, a PCP derivative, is a well-known sedative, anesthetic, amnesic, and analgesic. PCP and similar compounds produce a dissociative phenomenon, in which the subject has an "out of body" experience. When taken orally, the effects develop in 1–2 h and last for about 10 h. Their mechanism of action is complex and includes agonist, partial agonist, and antagonist effects at various adrenergic, dopaminergic, and serotonin receptors (Abraham et al. 1996). Sympathetic activation, hallucination, delirium, amnesia, depression and, long-term memory and cognitive dysfunction are some of the common side effects. In high doses, respiratory arrest can occur. Alternatively, this class of drugs has the ability to antagonize N-methyl-D-aspartate (NMDA) receptors which has clinical implication in chronic pain. Activation of NMDA receptors causes the spinal cord neuron to become more responsive to all of its inputs, resulting in central sensitization. NMDA receptor activation not only increases the cell's response to pain stimuli but also decreases neuronal sensitivity to opioid receptor agonists.

Lysergic Acid Diethylamide

Lysergic acid diethylamide (LSD) is a semi-synthetic "psychedelic" drug, derived from morning glory seeds and ergot, a rye fungus. It is colorless, odorless, and tasteless. Its unusual psychological effects such as visuals of colored patterns behind the eyes, a sense of time distortion, and crawling geometric patterns has made it one of the most widely known psychedelic drugs. After its discovery in 1938 while investigating ergot compounds, LSD was used experimentally to treat neuroses, narcotic addiction, autism, alcoholism, and terminally ill cancer patients and to study the mechanisms of psychotic diseases like schizophrenia. Nearly 30 years after its discovery, manufacture, possession, sale, and use of LSD was restricted in the United States under the Drug Abuse Control Amendment of 1965. The central nervous system effects of LSD generally begin within an hour of intake and last for up to 12 h. Its mechanism of action is thought to involve an interaction with serotonin neurotransporters. The physical effects include loss of appetite, sleeplessness, pupil dilation, dry mouth, salivation, palpitations, perspiration, nausea, dizziness, blurred vision, as well as, increased body temperature, heartbeat, blood pressure, and blood sugar. The psychological effects include euphoria, dysphoria, visual hallucinations, as well as, intense changes in mood and emotion (Abraham and Aldridge 1993). LSD use is associated with two long-term effects: psychosis and hallucinogen persisting perception disorder (HPPD), also known as "flashbacks." LSD flashbacks may be exacerbated by use of drugs such as marijuana or serotonin reuptake inhibitors Prozac® (Eli Lily, Indianapolis, IN) and Zoloft® (Pfizer, New York, NY).

γ-Hydroxybutyrate (GHB)

γ-Hydroxybutyrate (GHB) is also known as "liquid ecstasy." It is a popular club drug which acts as a central nervous system (CNS) depressant, causes euphoria, and decreases inhibitions (Hernandez et al. 2005). Also one of the so-called designer drugs, it is often abused by placing it in party drinks to produce sedation and amnesia (Greydanus and Patel 2003). The effects of GHB occur within 10–20 min and can last up to 4 h. The drug is rapidly and completely metabolized in the body to carbon dioxide and water. Large overdoses may result in respiratory depression and death. Cessation from chronic use is associated with withdrawal. GHB was once used as an anesthetic but its usefulness declined as better anesthetic agents with lesser side effects were developed. There are no known antidotes for intoxication with rave or club drugs; treatment would be supportive if such case arises.

Marijuana

Marijuana is the most commonly used illicit substance in the United States. Also known as "pot," "grass," "weed," hash, or tetrahydrocannabinol (THC), it is a hallucinogenic agent prepared from the dried leaves of *Cannabis sativa*. Its primary psychoactive constituent is THC. The medical use of cannabis in the treatment of pain and other symptomatology has long been practiced. The first recorded use of medical cannabis dates back to 2700 BC; in the United States, medical marijuana was routinely used until 1942. However, because of growing concerns over its addictive potential, the medical and psychosocial side effects of its chronic use, US physicians had been prohibited by the federal government to prescribe these drugs. Other countries such as the Netherlands and Canada still routinely use medical marijuana in the treatment of pain and other disorders such as anorexia (Cohen 2008).

Marijuana is most commonly inhaled, i.e., smoked via cigarette, a water pipe, or a blunt (a hollow cigar filled with marijuana), but can also be taken orally (Hernandez et al. 2005). Users experience an intense feeling of relaxation and euphoria within minutes and its effects rarely last more than 2–3 h. However, due to its high lipid solubility cannabinoids may rapidly accumulate in adipose tissue which may in part account for the long elimination half-life of up to a week. While side effects include tachycardia, conjunctival congestion and anxiety, adverse reactions mostly include anxiety, depression, fear, delusions, hallucinations, and violent behavior. Chronic use may lead to cognitive impairment, shortened memory span, confusion, altered time perception, and dulled reflexes. Abstinence after chronic use can lead to a withdrawal syndrome characterized by troubled sleep and negative mood. When taken in combination, marijuana can augment the sedative effects of drugs such as alcohol and benzodiazepines or amplify the stimulatory actions of cocaine and amphetamines (Greydanus and Patel 2003). In recent years, there has been a renewed interest in both legalizing and legitimizing the use of marijuana especially in the treatment of chronic pain.

Heroin and Methadone

It is estimated that there are 980,000 long-term users of heroin in the United States, and in 1996 the cost of heroin addiction to society and the healthcare system was estimated at $5 billion and $22 billion, respectively (Mark et al. 2001). About 30% of adolescents who smoke heroin end up as heroin addicts; chance of relapse after discontinuation increases the younger and the greater number of years of addiction (Greydanus and Patel 2003).

Apparently, among opioid-dependent patients, only 12–15% are actively enrolled in methadone maintenance (Roundaville and Kosten 2000). This is unfortunate in the sense that methadone maintenance has been found to be effective in curtailing drug use, preventing overdose deaths, and the spread of infectious diseases, as well as reducing crime and enhancing social productivity (Strain et al. 1993).

Heroin was first synthesized in 1889 as a less addicting morphine substitute (Kain 2001). Also known as diacetylmorphine, it is constituted by a slight structural modification of morphine but is about three times as potent as morphine, penetrates the blood–brain barrier due to increased solubility, and produces an intense rush when smoked or injected (Porer 1999).

Opioid overdose is manifested by coma, circulatory collapse, pinpoint pupils, bradycardia, hypothermia, and severe respiratory depression. On the other hand, when symptoms of insomnia, dysphoria, restlessness, tachycardia, tachypnea, hypertension, and mydriasis occur, acute opioid withdrawal should be suspected and may initiate 4–6 h after the last opioid use and peaks about 48–72 h. Rhinorrhea, lacrimation, tremors, piloerection, and yawning are often signs of craving for the drug. Flu-like signs and symptoms such as anorexia, muscle aches, nausea, vomiting, hot and cold flashes, abdominal pain, and increased temperature are common. Heroin overdose can result to the development of pulmonary edema, myocardial involvement, or death.

Among pregnant women, heroin and methadone are the most commonly used opioids. Heroin use (smoked recreationally rather than injected, in formulations that are 1–98% pure) has increased in the past decade. Approximately 7000 opiate-exposed births occur annually (Luty et al. 2003), and there has been up to sixfold reported increase in obstetric complications associated with heroin use (Hulse et al. 1998). Opioid withdrawal syndrome can result in impaired fetal growth and neonatal abstinence syndrome characterized by tremulousness, irritability, wakefulness, temperature dysregulation, dysfunctional suck with subsequent failure to thrive, and seizures (Kusche 2007). It is a current standard of care to maintain opioid-dependent women on long-acting narcotics during pregnancy rather than having to resort to a withdrawal protocol in light of reported inferior fetal outcomes that were associated with withdrawal during pregnancy (Luty 2003).

Prescription Drugs

The concern for prescription drug abuse has recently overshadowed that of illicit drug abuse, as the non-medical use of scheduled medications prescribed for pain, pain-related symptoms, and psychiatric disorders began rising in the mid-1990s. Non-medical use of prescription drugs was previously estimated in about 0.7 million individuals, 0.5 million of which used prescription pain relievers such as codeine, meperidine, morphine, fentanyl, hydromorphone, hydrocodone, methadone, and oxycodone (Joranson et al. 2000). In 2003, the lifetime prevalence rates for non-medical use of opioids increased to about 3 million (Smith and Woody 2005). While opioid drug mentions decreased by 25% from 1990 to 1996, year 2000 and 2003 updates showed a significant increase in oxycodone mentions (Joranson et al. 2000, Office of Applied Studies, Substance Abuse and Mental Health Services Administration 2003). The prevalence of opioid abuse is now similar to that of cocaine and only second to that of marijuana. Consequent to this, the government has become more involved in trying to curb the growing menace of prescription drug abuse. But beyond regulatory oversight, the intrinsic difficulties of treating pain especially in individuals with history of substance abuse and in those with prescription drug abuse pose special dilemmas even for experienced practitioners. Non-medical users of prescription drugs have been described to be more likely Caucasian, use alcohol, cocaine, or heroin, or use needles to inject drugs compared to those who reported using illicit drugs only. Youths and young adults who used prescription drugs non-medically have a higher rate of other illicit drug use as well.

Use of opioids often leads to rapid tolerance and eventually to physical and psychosocial dependence. Physical dependence and withdrawal due to opioid use results from upregulation of the cyclic aminophosphorase (cAMP) pathway at the locus coeruleus (Kasser et al. 1998). Unlike addiction which is a pathologic process, physical dependence is a natural expected physiologic response that can occur with use not only of opioids but also of benzodiazepines, alcohol, antidepressants, corticosteroids, diabetic agents, cardiac medications, and many other medications used in clinical medicine (Pastermark 2001). Tolerance is also a normal expected physiologic response that can occur with exposure to not only opioids but also certain class of drugs or substance like alcohol. Pain tolerance develops presumably as a result of decreased endogenous opioid release leading to the individual experiencing exaggerated pain. Administering the drug daily in increasing doses makes addiction to opioids occur more rapidly. Abrupt cessation or rapid dose reduction resulting in decreasing blood level of the drug and/or administration of an antagonist to the drug can produce a withdrawal syndrome that includes, but is not limited to, diaphoresis, nausea, vomiting, abdominal cramps, convulsions, or death (Nestler 2001). Chronic opioid use leads to cross tolerance to anesthetic and other depressant drugs as a result of chronic receptor stimulation. Opioids known to have been abused include codeine, meperidine, oxydocone, fentanyl, morphine, methadone, heroin, pentazocine, and propoxyphene. It is important to note, however, that most of these medications mentioned, though capable of producing physical dependence, are not associated with the disease of addiction (Portenoy 2007). A heroin addict, for example, is both physically dependent and addicted to the narcotic, while the pain patient taking opioids is physically dependent, but not necessarily addicted (Heit 2003, Pastermark 2001). Both will experience withdrawal if the drug is abruptly stopped, and both can exhibit tolerance to the drug.

Abuse and Addiction in Pain Patients

Opioid abuse is found in 9–41% of chronic pain patients, while illicit drug abuse is found in 14–34% (Heit 2003, Schnoll and Weaver 2003). Illicit drug use is reported more commonly in patients younger than 45 years, after a motor vehicle injury, in patients with involvement of multiple (three or more) regions in the body, and in patients with past history of illicit drug use. Most studies suggest that addiction per se is not common in acute, chronic, and cancer pain treatment (Portenoy and Savage 2007, Schnoll and Weaver 2003, Ballantyne and LaForge 2007). The prevalence of addiction varies from 0 to 50% in chronic non-malignant pain patients and from 0 to 7.7% in cancer patients depending on the subpopulation studied and the criteria used (Hojsted and Sjogren 2007). Few problems evolve when treating chronic non-malignant pain with opioid and dose escalations do not develop. In cancer patients, the diagnosis and treatment of chronic pain in an individual with substance abuse have been deemed complex and challenging because one is known to complicate the other.

Although the increase in availability of prescription opioids may have led to an increase in their diversion into the illicit market, it has been noted that the increased medical use of opioid analgesics to treat pain does not appear to contribute to increase in the health consequences of opioid analgesic abuse (Joranson et al. 2000). In addition, pain itself does not appear to be an independent factor for abuse of pain medications, and that majority of legitimate pain patients do not abuse their analgesic medication (Compton and Volkow 2006).

Treating Pain in Patients with Addictive Disorder

A patient with addictive disorder is a tremendous challenge in pain management. Some of the major dilemmas the clinician has in treating pain in a patient with history of substance use or abuse include the potential consequences of not achieving the proper balance between undertreating or overtreating pain, the risks of precipitating worsening addictive behaviors with the utilization of opiates, and the medicolegal implications that may be associated with opioid use. In the next sections, treatment of pain in this population according to whether pain is acute or chronic is discussed.

Acute Pain

Pain is considered acute when it is self-limited. It is usually associated or caused by disease or acute medical condition, trauma, inflammatory process, surgery, or a physiological process such as labor. In acute pain, the nervous system is usually intact, and a variety of autonomic changes which may potentially be harmful are identifiable. These include tachycardia, hypertension, sweating or vasoconstriction, increased rate and decreased depth of respiration, increased gastrointestinal secretions, decreased intestinal motility, skeletal muscle spasm and immobility, increased sphincter tone, venous stasis, or urinary retention. Other potential harmful effects include thrombosis or pulmonary embolism, anxiety, confusion, or delirium. Acute pain usually decreases or ceases as wound or injury heals or as medical condition improves.

Acute and chronic pain may, in some instances, overlap. Certain severe and prolonged acute pain may progressively become more like chronic pain. Patients with chronic pain may have superimposed acute pain such as when they develop bone fracture secondary to metastatic malignancy or when they require surgery. In such cases, the nervous system may not be intact and they may have significant pre-existing psychological problems, opioid tolerance, and other complicating conditions.

Opioids are the mainstay for treatment of severe acute pain in the addicted patient. Because pharmacologic tolerance to opiates is common in these individuals, the doses required are usually higher than in the non-addicted patient. Concerns of abuse of opiates in these individuals having been documented escalating, a collaborative effort by the clinician, the psychiatrist, and the addiction medicine should be attempted.

Guidelines for successful management of acute pain in the known or suspected opiate addict have been published by Portenoy and Payne (1992). The recommended first step is to define the pain syndrome and provide treatment for the underlying disorder. As mentioned in the prior sections, it is important to distinguish the patient with a remote history of drug abuse from one who is actively abusing drugs and one who is receiving methadone maintenance. This is followed by appropriate pharmacologic principles of opioid use. Opioids are used in adequate doses, dosing intervals, and appropriate route of administration. The use of concomitant nonopioid therapies such as nonopioid analgesics and nonpharmacologic therapies when appropriate are encouraged. Specific drug abuse behaviors need to be recognized. Excessive negotiation over specific drugs and doses is discouraged. Early consultation to appropriate services such as psychiatry and substance abuse services, and if available, pain service is advocated. If outpatient treatment is required, problems associated with opioid prescription renewals should be anticipated.

In surgical pain, other therapeutic options include alternative route of administration of either opioid, local anesthetic, or both. The use of regional analgesia (e.g., intrathecal or epidural techniques) and/or peripheral nerve blockade is used to increase control of pain in addicted patients. In certain cases, pain treatment may require extensive and sympathetic blockade to relieve acute pain such as during major surgery or in profoundly severe acute pains refractory to other modalities of treatment. Patient-controlled analgesia (PCA) modality is often withheld from these individuals because of the concern that self-administered analgesic delivery may reinforce drug-seeking behavior (Sinatra 1998), and neural blockade or epidural analgesic techniques are substituted. More recent thinking allows selected patients presenting with cocaine and alcohol abuse to use PCA in well-supervised settings. Patients with a history of chronic pain and significant opioid tolerance require increased amounts of drug to compensate for both baseline requirements, as well as that needed to control pain following surgery. In general, health providers tend to limit opioid administration to patients who have a history of substance abuse despite the fact that perioperative patients with history of substance abuse or tolerance experience the same intensity of postsurgical discomfort. Physicians fear that pain medications may mask status changes and risk patient addiction. It appears, however, that iatrogenic addiction may not be a concern of significant magnitude as one would expect (Sinatra 1998). In a survey of over 10,000 patients from 151 burn centers, for example, no cases of iatrogenic opioid addiction were reported (Perry and Heidrich 1982). In the patient with history of addiction the chronic use of opiates poses a significant risk of exacerbating a substance abuse problem.

Management should be centered in recognizing and accepting the addiction problem and on providing structured, consistent care, preferably with input from addiction or psychiatric specialists. Multimodal, team-oriented approach to treatment, although cumbersome and impractical, may well be cost-effective for this complex type of patient. The incidence of addiction in the opioid-treated population ranges from 3 to 19%. Incorrectly assuming that patients with addictive illness will develop addiction plays a negative role in effectively treating pain.

Chronic Pain

Chronic pain, as has been agreed arbitrarily, is pain which persists for more than 3 months or which persists past the time of healing (Merskey and Bogduk 1994). After severe trauma, major surgery, or painful diseases such as pancreatitis, severe acute pain can persist more than 10–14 days and become essentially chronic (Bonica 1985). Chronic pain progressively leads to limitation of physical, mental, and social activities, and it is not uncommon for it to cause anger, depression, and family and socioeconomic perturbation (Siddall and Cousins 1998). In chronic pain, sympathoadrenal responses are not apparent and are seemingly habituated or exhausted, and vegetative responses such as irritability, loss of appetite, sleep disruption, depression, or attenuation of motor activity emerge. Patients may be sad, subdued, or sleepy secondary to excessive consumption of medications. Such affect may mask the presence of pain. Psychological disturbances may result from severe refractory chronic pain. Such various components of chronic pain syndromes must be recognized and addressed when treating this type of pain.

About one-third of the American population experiences chronic pain. Billions of dollars are lost yearly due to health care expenses and missed workdays for chronic pain. Addictive illness has been rapidly evolving in the social, medical, and legal/regulatory environment. Like that of acute pain, there is a consensus that patients involved with substance abuse are generally undertreated by clinicians for their chronic pain due to biases, misconceptions, and systems issues.

The goal of management in chronic pain is to increase function and decrease pain while monitoring for side effects of the prescribed medication.

A history of substance abuse has been previously considered a contraindication to opioid therapy for chronic pain. It appears that individuals with a prior history of recent substance abuse are more likely to have abuse recurrence than individuals with a distant polysubstance abuse or isolated alcohol abuse. Currently, opioid therapy in patients with a recent history of substance abuse is controversial. Existing studies report mixed results. Preventing or detecting addiction recurrence is key.

Although patients with chronic pain may be at increased risk for addiction, clinical research shows that the general population has demonstrated similar addiction rates. Indeed, it has been noted that addiction does not occur in the majority of chronic pain patients who are properly evaluated and treated with opioids. Individuals receiving opioids, whether it is for appropriate reasons or for the disease of addiction, are expected to experience physical dependence and tolerance when taking opioids regularly (Nestler et al. 2001). One must always ask if the patient is being undertreated for the pain syndrome. Constant reevaluation of pain treatment is key to prevent undertreatment. A variety of assessment and treatment approaches have been formulated to make managing pain abusers more effective.

There has been an unequivocal support for the notion that pain medication should not be withheld from pain patients, even in the presence of addiction. Individuals with substance abuse or dependence can be effectively treated for pain provided their substance abuse disorder is addressed immediately and treatment of substance dependence be included in the management plan (Passik and Kirsh 2005, Weaver and Schnoll 2002, Coluzzi and Pappagallo 2005, Savage 2002, Compton and Athanasos 2003). It is recommended that monitoring should be increased, more frequent visits initiated, and the amount of medication available at one time limited. To detect the presence of illicit drugs or substances not prescribed for pain management and to verify that the patient is taking the prescribed opioid instead of selling it, random urine drug tests are utilized. Certified substance abuse treatment provider should be consulted, appropriate medication-assisted treatment initiated, and participation in 12-step programs encouraged. With the patient's permission, it is prudent to consult and coordinate with the designated substance abuse treatment provider on an ongoing basis. When warranted, opioid treatment must be discontinued (e.g., prescription forgery, opioid diversion, continued inappropriate opioid use). Providing opioid analgesia to patients who are psychologically dependent does not necessarily worsen their dependence, nor will withholding opioids increase their likelihood of recovery; however, unrelieved pain can trigger relapse (Compton and Athanasos 2003, Alford 2006, Gourlay 2005). Below are some of the recommended strategies to have higher chances of successful outcome when dealing with this patient population.

How to talk to patients with pain about substance use problems (Weaver and Schnoll 2002):

1. Be nonjudgmental – patients are more likely to be forthcoming.
2. Avoid yes/no questions that do not allow patients to express their feelings.
3. Start with sweeping questions (e.g., "How helpful have your medications been for you?") rather than begin with questions about medication misuse.
4. Listen to what patients say about how and why they take their medications.
5. Use existing tools for screening.
6. Ask questions about warning signs (e.g., "Have you ever taken your pain medication for other reasons?").
7. Inquire about their willingness to try alternative, nonopioid forms of therapy.

In Table 31.2, guidelines for prescribing drug with abuse liability in pain patients with history of addiction are outlined. Physicians should set clear rules and expectations for them and the patient and have both sign an agreement. Based on current evidence, physicians assume that patients adhering to controlled substance agreements and without obvious dependency behavior do not abuse either illicit or licit drugs. The dose of the medication should be set at the appropriate level to treat the condition and titrate as necessary. Using feedback from patient to set dose is often helpful. To prevent undertreatment of pain or treatment gaps, physician should give enough medication plus rescue doses. Patients should be asked to bring in all original medication bottles with or without medication including the date they are filled, the prescribing physician and the dispensing pharmacy, the number of pills dispensed, and the number of remaining pills. Physicians should monitor for lost or stolen prescriptions and obtain random urine screens, as well as, obtaining knowledge of

Table 31.2 Guidelines for prescribing drug with abuse liability in pain patients with history of addiction.

1. Set clear rules and expectations for you and the patient, have both sign an agreement
2. Set the dose of the medication at the appropriate level to treat the condition, and titrate as necessary
3. Use feedback from patient to set dose
4. Give enough medication plus rescue doses
5. Ask patient to bring in all original medication bottles with or without medication: date filled, pharmacy, prescribing physician, number of pills dispensed, and number of remaining pills
6. Monitor for lost or stolen prescriptions
7. Obtain random urine screens
8. Know the drugs for which the laboratory screens
9. Use adjunctive medications as necessary
10. Document, document, document
11. See the patient as frequently as needed
12. Work with significant others or closed family members
13. Know how to withdraw the patient from the medication
14. Know the pharmacology, duration of action, and parenteral to oral conversion ratio of the drugs being prescribed
15. Bring patient in for unscheduled visits
16. Obtain release to contact other health care providers
17. Limit p.r.n. medications since this promotes drug-seeking behavior
18. Adequately treat the condition and trust the patient to avoid problems of pseudoaddiction

Adapted from: Schnoll and Weaver (2003).

the drugs for which the laboratory screens. Adjunctive medications are often prudent to use as necessary to avoid unnecessary escalation of opiate doses. Documentation is key to prevent confusion and overprescription. Good practice dictates seeing the patient as frequently as needed, working with significant others or any closed family member. Knowing how to withdraw the patient from the medication is important, as well as, bringing patient in for unscheduled visits. PRN medications need to be limited to prevent drug-seeking behavior. And last, to avoid problems of pseudoaddiction, trust the patient and adequately treat the condition.

No known modality is appropriate as a single intervention for all types of pain. Multimodality, multidisciplinary approaches appear to hold the most promise. Constant reassessment and adjustment to the treatment plan are essential. Opioid analgesics may be an integral part of the treatment plan for many patients, but long-term efficacy, i.e., improved analgesia, improved functional levels and quality of life, and minimized side effects is essential. Few pain specialists have cross-training in managing addictive illness and, similarly, few addiction specialists have cross-training in pain management. Developing collaborative treatment and monitoring plans between the specialties is essential to successful outcomes. The medical and social complexity of treating pain patients with addictive behavior certainly calls for a systematic, structured, and multidisciplinary approach to achieve better outcome, but to date such strategies, however, have not been tested through research.

Considerable experience exists with the use of non-opiate pain medications for chronic pain. There has been widespread success with the use of anti-inflammatory medications, antidepressants, and antiepileptics.

Opioids have long been used to treat moderate to severe chronic pain. When opioids are used to treat moderate to severe pain, physical dependence and tolerance occur, but the disease of addiction occurs only in some patients. The clinician can use either a short-acting opioid such as morphine, hydromorphone, or oxycodone; a short-acting opioid in a controlled-release delivery system such as Oxycontin® (Purdue Pharma, Cranberry, NJ) or Duragesic® TTS patch (Ortho-McNeil-Janssen, Titusville, NJ); or a long-acting opioid such as methadone or levorphanol. While physical dependence is inevitable with opioid therapy, clinicians should work to minimize tolerance and abuse. By definition, an increased opioid requirement is considered "tolerance" only when all other conditions are stable, i.e., there is no disease progression, new disease, excessive physical activity that exacerbates pain, skipped analgesic doses, drug interaction, etc., that would lower analgesic effectiveness. Evidence suggests that the use of a long-acting opioid medication such as methadone and controlled-release opioids are less likely to induce tolerance and abuse than that of a short-acting opioid (Garrido and Troconiz 1999, Brookoff 1993). The short-acting opioids usually should be reserved for breakthrough or incidental pain. Dose increase and opioid rotation are rational responses to inadequate pain relief, but again, reasons for a diminution in analgesic effect must be investigated to rule out other reasons, i.e., progression of the disease or psychosocial factors that may aggravate the pain experience. For most mu-receptor agonists, there is no pharmacological ceiling dose – the dose beyond which no additional analgesic effect will be achieved in an opioid-responsive condition (Chang et al. 2007, Rich 2007).

During pregnancy, the clinician has several options recommended for managing opioid abuse. One is methadone maintenance, which has been the standard of care since the early 1970s. Another is the use of buprenorphine and naltrexone. Although not yet established, buprenorphine and naltrexone appear equally safe. While limited clinical trials exist, opioid detoxification preferably during the second trimester is considered another option. When used for maintenance in pregnancy, the dose of methadone should be adjusted according to their current withdrawal signs and symptoms caused by methadone's increased metabolism (via the effect of increased progesterone on liver cytochrome P450 enzymes) and decreased plasma protein binding (Wolff et al. 2005). Patients already on methadone maintenance should be continued on their outpatient dose (McCarthy et al. 2005). To have fewer withdrawal cycles, heroin and fentanyl users are converted to using methadone during pregnancy. Conversion has been associated with fewer spontaneous abortions and a reduced risk of intravenously transmitted infections (McCarthy et al. 2005). The rate of spontaneous abortion with methadone (3–4%) has been found to be lower (Kashiwagi et al. 2005) compared with that of pregnant individuals who continue to use heroin (10–20%). This was attributed to fetal stress secondary to fluctuating levels of opiates. The recommended starting dose of methadone for conversion often ranges from 1 to 20 mg; patients are then dosed on an as needed basis every 6 h depending upon signs and symptoms of opiate withdrawal including subjective cravings. Most patients reach a stable dose after 48–72 h (Kashiwagi et al. 2005).

Methadone Therapy

Methadone administration historically has been the responsibility of both the Food and Drug Administration (FDA) and the Drug Enforcement Agency (DEA). This organizational structure's policies has historically isolated methadone therapy from the medical mainstream and limited the development of physician expertise. However, the Drug Addiction Treatment Act of 2000 expanded the avenues for the treatment of opioid dependence in the United States from specially licensed methadone facilities to physicians' private offices, where Schedule III–V drugs can be prescribed (Fiellin and O'Connor 2002). Opioid substitution treatment has now been monitored by the Substance Abuse and Mental health Administration and has allowed the expansion of treatment to private practice, which supposedly will create opportunities to provide comprehensive care for addicted patients. It was aimed to reduce stigma associated with the use of opioids, bring addiction treatment into the mainstream of health care, and treatment become similar to that of other chronically ill patients. In addition, it was also hoped such expansion could perhaps provide public health benefits such as reducing heroin demand.

Buprenorphine Therapy

The approval by DEA and FDA of the office-based use of methadone, as well as buprenorphine, to treat opioid addiction expanded treatment options for opioid addiction (Resnick 2003). Pain management physicians now prescribe buprenorphine in the treatment of pain in patients with a history (documented or otherwise) of addiction, assuming that the etiology of the pain is well documented and the patient is not drug seeking in an attempt to maintain a habit. Pain management specialists will therefore likely encounter buprenorphine either as a current medication in patients who are maintained on the drug or in those patients who paradoxically deteriorate despite being on escalating doses of traditional narcotic pain medication. The utility of this drug in controlling chronic pain in those suffering with chemical dependencies, however, still warrants further exploration.

If a history of addiction exists, or an occult dependency is suspected, it is important for physicians treating chronic pain to understand the unique pharmacology of buprenorphine. This can be accomplished by close communication with addiction medicine physicians or via patient referrals to physicians trained in addiction medicine who, by virtue of that training and certification, have special knowledge and privilege in relationship to the drug, or with psychiatrists with special certification in addictions who have received special training and a special DEA number allowing them to prescribe buprenorphine in a maintenance fashion. Buprenorphine both structurally and clinically provides an elegant alternative to treating legitimate chronic pain in the patient with predilection to addiction (Bickel et al. 1988, Amass et al. 2000, Giacomuzzi et al. 2006). Buprenorphine's clinical efficacy results from its unique molecular structure: it is a partial mu-opioid agonist and a weak antagonist. It has a high affinity for the mu receptor, with slow dissociation resulting in a long duration of action and an analgesic potency 25–40 times greater than morphine. The main reason the drug is considered in populations with addictive predisposition is its safety profile. At higher doses, its agonist effects plateau while its antagonist effects predominate, limiting the drug's desirability as a substance of abuse and decreasing the potential for respiratory depression. As with other narcotics, withdrawal symptoms and abstinence syndromes, although mild, also do occur.

In France since February 1996, general practitioners have also been allowed to prescribe buprenorphine in high dosage for maintenance treatment of major opioid drug addiction. A prospective cohort study (Duburcq et al. 2000) of 919 major opioid addicts was performed to assess patient outcomes with a follow-up of up to 2 years. High dosage of buprenorphine was prescribed by general practitioners for 3 months to opioid addicts who had a long serious history of drug addiction, parallel consumption of cocaine, and other illicit drugs. In 2 years, about two-thirds of the patients remained in follow-up by two general practitioners; there was a reduction in drug-related harm such as seroconversions for hepatitis B, hepatitis C, and HIV; substitution treatment rate was 84%; duration of prescription and dispensing increased; heroin intake fell by 25%; and declaration of drug intake fell by about 30% (Duburcq et al. 2000).

Buprenorphine as an alternative to methadone in pregnancy has been validated by several naturalistic studies in France, where outpatient physicians can treat with buprenorphine without specialized training; up to 70,000 patients annually have received the medication on an outpatient basis since the 1996 liberalization of policies (Auriacombe et al. 2004). Despite positive findings for buprenorphine in pregnancy by several French and some American studies (Fischer et al. 2006, Auriacombe et al. 1999), one Finnish study described greater severity of the neonatal abstinence syndrome and higher rates of SIDS (Kahila et al. 2007). Naltrexone is thought to possibly play a role in relapse prevention, and it has been utilized for maintenance after an initial taper with buprenorphine. Naltrexone was used, in one small Australian study, for a detoxification protocol during pregnancy and showed favorable results. Naltrexone implant is currently being studied and initial results seem promising.

Oxymorphone (Opana)

Oxymorphone or 14-hydroxydihydromorphinone is a semi-synthetic opioid analgesic that is derived from thebaine and is approximately six to eight times more potent than morphine. It is a powerful opioid agonist that specifically binds to mu-opioid receptor, is marketed in oral form (Opana, Opana ER) in 5, 10, 20, and 40 mg tablets, as a suppository (Numorphan) in

5 mg, and as an injectable hydrochloride salt in 1 mg doses. Until its removal from the US market in the early 1970s, oxymorphone (popularly known as "blues") was one of the most sought-after opioids by the intravenous drug using population. Containing very few insoluble binders which made them easy to inject, the extended release blue-colored tablets were profoundly potent when used intravenously. These tablets were known to be extremely euphoric which is comparable to or better than heroin. As with other opioids, oxymorphone can cause physical dependency and has the potential for abuse. Being especially potent, oxymorphone can be used to alleviate dyspnea in patients with left ventricular failure.

Having been shown by placebo-controlled trials to be effective in alleviating moderate to severe pain associated with osteoarthritis (Matsumoto et al. 2005, McIlwain and Ahdieh 2005), cancer (Sloan et al. 2005), orthopedic surgery (Ahdieh et al. 2004), and chronic low back pain (Hale et al. 2005, Gammaitoni et al. 2007), oxymorphone may be a new treatment option for use in the illicit or licit substance-abusing patient and for use during opioid rotation. For patients with addictive disorder, it is an option for the relief of moderate to severe pain, as a preoperative medication to alleviate apprehension, maintain anesthesia, and as an obstetric analgesic. At least in chronic low back pain patients, oxymorphone is found equally effective in both opioid-naive and opioid-experienced patients. It may be given in 0.5 mg increments up to a total of 2 mg especially in patients who have required at least 4 mg of hydromorphone. The extended release formulation is designed to continuously release drug during the 12-h period and its pharmacokinetic properties are consistent with its use for around the clock therapy. A steady state is usually achieved within 3 days with a relatively stable plasma concentration (Adams and Ahdieh 2004). Having both the extended- and immediate-release formulations provide flexibility in dosing that is useful when converting patients from different opioids (Adams and Ahdieh 2004, Adams and Ahdieh 2005).

Management of Patients Taking Suboxone

Suboxone is a mixed opioid agonist/antagonist, with buprenorphine as its active ingredient. Suboxone has a high affinity for the opiate receptor which can block the effect of other narcotics if taken in conjunction with it. It provides analgesia and euphoria but its primary indication is for the treatment of narcotic addiction. When patients with narcotic addiction let their narcotic level fall below their threshold, they begin to experience profound withdrawal syndrome producing sweats, cramps, diarrhea, mood swings, and agitation. Although suboxone can be displaced by higher doses of narcotics, it generally holds patients at a level which curbs withdrawal and craving, while it keeps them from moving up their narcotic level when they take perioperative opioids. Suboxone is typically given between one and three tablets sublingually daily. The other unique feature of suboxone is its having a peak ceiling effect; therefore, patients will not step up their narcotic level even if they take more than the recommended daily dose. This is another great advantage of the drug in deterring its abuse potential. The naloxone in suboxone is not bioavailable sublingually and its main role is to deter inappropriate use of the medication.

There is no gold standard for treating patients taking suboxone before elective surgery. Careful titration of perioperative narcotics with appropriate monitoring for side effects remains the mainstay of treatment. Typically, specalists recommend that suboxone be stopped for 2–3 days before elective surgery to make traditional opiates be more effective as its level falls. Patients are prescribed short-acting narcotics such as percocet for a couple of days to ward off withdrawal as they stop taking suboxone in anticipation of elective surgery. In the operating room, narcotics should be continuously titrated to effect, may use regional anesthesia techniques and field blocks, and consider using non-narcotic analgesics where indicated. In the recovery room, traditional narcotics should be used when patients are in pain. Postoperative narcotics need to be titrated gently and appropriately, as respiratory depression is the principal side effect that merits extreme vigilance. Alternatively, other clinical providers continue patient's baseline suboxone dose into the operative period and titrate additional short-acting opioids as necessary to control perioperative pain. There is no consensus regarding the discharge of patients in suboxone. The risk of restarting the patient's narcotic addiction needs to be considered. Patients should be transitioned back to their suboxone around the time patients are moved-off their post op narcotics. To avoid withdrawal symptoms, patients need to be in their prior narcotic level when they start suboxone.

Case Scenario

Sreekumar Kunnumpurath, MBBS, MD, FCARCSI, FRCA, FFPMRCA

You are requested by the surgical team to see Gregory, a 30-year-old actor. He is due to have arthroscopic reconstruction of the cruciate ligament of his knee next week.

Gregory is worried about the anesthesia and the surgery itself. He mentions that his pain tolerance is very low and that he had a terrible experience during previous knee surgery. He reluctantly reveals that he had been using heroin during the time of his previous surgery, but had not mentioned this to the anesthesiologist. He mentions that during the postoperative period he went "cold turkey."

What further information do you require for managing Gregory's anesthetic and pain management?
Your first task is to get a detailed history of his substance abuse. Gregory might be suffering from addiction, physical dependence, or tolerance. The suggestion of withdrawal symptoms could have been due to pseudoaddiction. You will need to know about his current drug use, and possibly seek the help of a psychologist and/or addiction services. It is worth looking at the medical records from the first surgery to have a better understanding of what happened.

A detailed assessment reveals Gregory has been using heroin for about 3 years, and he has been in a rehabilitation program for the last 6 months. He is currently taking 60 mg of methadone a day. He admits to occasional cocaine and cannabis use, which he claims to be a "professional hazard." His medical records reveal that the previous episode of inadequate pain relief followed a closed reduction of a fractured ankle. At the time he had been prescribed only non-steroidal analgesics, and developed withdrawal symptoms in the afternoon following the operation. He required large doses of morphine and was placed on morphine PCA for 3 days. He was later referred to the psychologist for further management of his drug addiction.

Enumerate key components of Gregory's preoperative evaluation with regards to management of his pain?

You have to assess his (anticipated) pain and addiction status. Although he states that he is in rehabilitation and has been "clean" for a while, bear in mind that Gregory may still withhold key information. It is advisable to gather information about Gregory's compliance directly from the rehabilitation program. You will also need to know whether he is taking any prescription medications, and you may have to confirm this with his PCP. His surgery is scheduled for tomorrow morning and you are seeing Gregory to discuss the anesthetic plan.

Outline your analgesic plan for Gregory?

A detailed plan must be outlined with Gregory's consent. You use a multimodal analgesic regimen utilizing simple analgesics, opioids plus or minus a regional technique. A collaborative approach involving the clinician, the psychiatrist, and the addictions unit should be attempted. Excessive negotiation over specific drugs should be discouraged, and the use of morphine or hydromorphone PCA should be done in a well-supervised setting. Consider a toxicology screen of a urine sample on the day of surgery, since it could be valuable given the history of multiple substance abuse.

Gregory agrees to undergo the operation under general anesthesia combined with a sciatic and femoral nerve block. You advise Gregory to continue to take methadone on top of other analgesics, which include acetaminophen, ibuprofen, and buprenorphine as needed. The operation is successful and Gregory recovers uneventfully. He is discharged home on the third postoperative day and advised to continue methadone, acetaminophen, and ibuprofen.

A day later, you receive a call from the hospital requesting you to evaluate Gregory because he has returned to the hospital with severe pain in his operated knee. When you see Gregory he is screaming with pain and is verbally abusive. He is sweating profusely and looking very pale.

How will you manage Gregory?

The possibilities are that Gregory is in real pain (pseudoaddiction), withdrawing, drug seeking, or intoxicated with other illicit drugs. Your management depends on your assessment, which would be based on the history, physical examination, and laboratory investigations. You take a quick but thorough history (Gregory is in no mood to talk to you) and he tells you that his operated knee is "killing" him and he is demanding morphine. He swears that he has not touched any illicit drugs other than what you had prescribed. On examination, Gregory's knee is swollen and angry, and it is tender and warm to touch. The cause of Gregory's pain appears to be an infected knee. You prescribe morphine IV for pain. Further investigations show a fluid collection inside the knee joint. An orthopedic surgeon is consulted and he aspirates pus from the knee. Then, Gregory undergoes an urgent arthrotomy. You see Gregory in the recovery, and he is awake and cheerful. "An actor and a junky: a bad combination to convince people the pain is real," he laughs.

References

Abraham H, Aldridge A, Gogia P. The psychopharmacology of hallucinogens. Neuropsychopharma 1996;14:285–98.

Abraham H, Aldridge A. Adverse consequences of lysergic acid diethylamine. Addiction 1993;88:1327–34.

Adams MP, Ahdieh H. Pharmacokinetics and dose-proportionality of oxymorphone extended release and its metabolites: results of a randomized crossover study. Pharmacotherapy 2004;24:468–76.

Adams MP, Ahdieh H. Single- and multiple-dose pharmacokinetic and dose-proportionality study of oxymorphone immediate-release tablets. Drugs R D 2005;6:91–9.

Ahdieh H, Ma T, et al. Efficacy of oxymorphone extended release in postsurgical pain: A randomized clinical trial in knee arthroplasty. J Clin Pharmacol. 2004;44:767–76.

Albertson TE, Derlet RW, Van Hoozen BE. Methamphetamine and the expanding complications of amphetamines. West J Med. 1999;170:214–9.

Albrecht CA, Jafri A, Linville, L, et al. Cocaine-induce penumopericardium. Circulation 2000;102:2792–4.

Alford DP, Compton P, Samet JH. Acute pain management for patients receiving maintenance methadone or buprenorphine therapy. Ann Intern Med. 2006;144(2):127–34.

Amass L, Kamien JB, Mikulich SK. Efficacy of daily and alternate-day dosing regimens with the combination buprenorphine-naloxone tablet. Drug Alcohol Depen. 2000;58:143–52.

American Academy of Pain Medicine. American Pain Society, American Society of Addiction Medicine. Definitions related to the use opioids for the treatment of pain [consensus document]. Glenview, IL, American Academy of Pain Medicine; 2001.

American Psychiatric Association. Diagnostic and statistical manual of mental disorders. 4th ed. Washington, DC: Author; 1994.

Andres RL. Social and illicit drug use in pregnancy. In: Resnik RR, Ceasy R, editors. Maternal-fetal medicine. Philadelphia, PA: WB Saunders; 1993. pp. 145–64.

Auriacombe M, Affelou S, Lavignasse P, et al. Pregnancy, abortion and delivery in a cohort of heroin dependent patients treated with drug substitution (methadone and buprenorphine) in Aquitaine. Presse Med. 1999;28:177.

Auriacombe M, Fatseas M, Dubernet J, et al. French field experience with buprenorphine. Am J Addict. 2004;13(suppl 1):S17–S28.

Ballantyne JC, LaForge KS. Opioid dependence and addiction during opioid treatment of chronic pain. Pain 2007;129(3):235–55.

Bhuvaneswar CG, Chang G, Epstein LA, Theodore SA. Cocaine and opioid use during pregnancy: prevalence and management. Prim Care Companion J Clin Psychiatry. 2008;10(1):59–65.

Bickel WK, Slitzer ML, et al. A clinical trial of buprenorphine: Comparison with methadone in the detoxification of heroin addicts. Clin Pharmacol Ther. 1988;43:72–8.

Bonica JJ. Biology, pathophysiology, and treatment of acute pain. In: Lipton S, Miles J, editors. Persistent pain. Orlando, FL: Grune & Stratton; 1985. vol. 5. pp. 1–32.

Boot BP, McGregor IS, Hall W. MDMA (Ecstasy) neurotoxicity: assessing and communicating the risks. Lancet 2000;355:1818–21.

Brauer RB, Heidecke CD, Nathrath W, et al. Liver transplantation for the treatment of fulminant hepatic failure induced by the ingestion of ecstasy. Transpl Int. 1997;10:229–33.

Brookoff D. Abuse potential of various opioid medications. J Gen Intern Med. 1993;8:688–90.

Brust JC. Clinical, radiological, and pathological aspects of cerebrovascular disease associated with drug abuse. Stroke 1993;24:1129–33.

Carrera MR, Meijler MM, Janda KD. Cocaine pharmacology and current pharmacotherapies for its abuse. Bioorg Med Chem. 2004;12:5019–30.

Chang G, et al. Opioid tolerance and hyperalgesia. Med Clin North Am. 2007;91(2): 199–211.

Christophersen AS. Amphetamine designer drugs: an overview and epidemiology. Toxicol Lett. 2000;112:127–31.

Cohen S. Cannabinoids for chronic pain. BMJ 2008 Jan;336:167–8.

Coluzzi F, Pappagallo M. Opioid therapy for chronic noncancer pain: Practice guidelines for initiation and maintenance of therapy. Minerva Anestesiol 2005;71(7–8):425–33.

Compton P, Athanasos P. Chronic pain, substance abuse and addiction. Nurs Clin North Am. 2003;38(3):525–37.

Compton WM, Volkow ND. Abuse of prescription drugs and the risk of addiction. Drug Alcohol Depend. 2006 Jun;83(suppl 1):S4–7.

Derlett RW, Rice P, Horowitz BZ, Lord RV. Amphetamine toxicity: experience with 127 cases. J Emergency Med. 1989;7:157–61.

Duburcq A, Charpak Y, et al. Two years follow-up of a heroin users cohort treated with high dosage buprenorphine. Results of the SPESUB study (pharmacoepidemiologic follow-up of general practice Subutex). Rev Epidemiol Sante Publique. 2000;48(4):363–73.

Eriksson M, Jonsson B, Zetterstrom R. Children of mothers abusing amphetamines: head circumference during infancy and psychosocial development until 14 years of age. Acta Paediatr. 2000;89:1474–8.

Feldman JA, Fish SS, Beshansky JR, et al. Acute cardiac ischemia in patients with cocaine associated complaints: results of a multicenter trial. Ann Emerg Med. 2000;36:469–76.

Fiege M, Wappler F, Weisshorn R, et al. Induction of malignant hyperthermia in susceptible swine by 3,4-methylenedioxymethamphetamine ("ecstasy"). Anesthesiology 2003;99: 1132–6.

Fiellin DA, O'Connor PG. Clinical practice: office-based treatment of opioid-dependent patients. N Engl J Med. 2002;347:817–23.

Fischer G, Ortner R, Rohrmeister K, et al. Methadone versus buprenorphine in pregnant addicts: a double blind, double dummy comparison study. Addiction 2006;101:275–81.

Gammaitoni E, Gould H, Ahdieh T. Opana ER improves pain quality measures in opioid-experienced patients with chronic low back pain. J Pain 2007;8(4 suppl):S44.

Gatof D, Albert RK. Bilateral thumb burns leading to the diagnosis of crack lung. Chest 2002;121:289–91.

Giacomuzzi S, Kemmler G, Ertl M, Riemer Y. Opioid addicts at admission vs. slow-release oral morphine, methadone, and sublingual buprenorphine maintenance treatment participants. Subst Use Misuse 2006;41(2):223–44.

Gourlay DL, Heit HA, Almahrezi A. Universal precautions in pain medicine: A rationale approach to the treatment of chronic pain. Pain Med. 2005;6(2):107–12.

Garrido MJ, Troconiz IF. Methadone: a review of its pharmaco-kinetic/pharmacodynamic properties. J Pharmacol Toxicol Methods 1999;42:61–6.

Greydanus DE, Patel DR. Substance abuse in adolescents: a complex conundrum for the clinician. Pediatr Clin North Am. 2003;50:1179–223.

Hale ME, Dvergsten C, Gimbel J. Efficacy and safety of oxymorphone extended release in chronic low back pain: Results of a randomized, double-blind, placebo- and active-controlled phase III study. J Pain. 2005;6:21–8.

Heit HA. Addiction, physical dependence, and tolerance: precise definitions to help clinicians evaluate and treat chronic pain patients. J Pain Palliat Care Pharmacother. 2003;17(1): 15–29.

Hernandez M, Birnbach D, Zundert A. Anesthetic management of the illicit-substance using patient. Curr Opin Anaesthesiol. 2005;18:315–24.

Hojsted J, Sjogren P. Addiction to opioids in chronic pain patients: A literature review. Eur J Pain. 2007;11(5):490–518.

Hsue PY, Salinas, CL, Bolger AF, et al. Acute aortic dissection related to crack cocaine. Circulation 2002;105:1592–95.

Hulse GK, Milne E, English DR, et al. Assessing the relationship between maternal opiate use and neonatal mortality. Addiction 1998;93:1033–42.

Jeffcoat AR, Perez-Reyes M, Hill JM, Sadler BM, Cook CE. Cocaine disposition in humans after intravenous injection, nasal insufflation (snorting), or smoking. Drug Metab Dispos. 1989 Mar–Apr;17(2):153–9.

Joranson DE, Ryan KM, Gilson AM, Dahl JL. Trends in medical use and abuse of opioid analgesics JAMA 2000;283(13):1710–4.

Kahila H. Saisto T, Kivitie-Kallio S, et al. A prospective study on buprenorphine use during pregnancy: effects on maternal and neonatal outcome. Acta Obstet Gyncol Scand. 2007;86:185–90.

Kain ZN, Barash PG. Anesthetic implications of drug abuse. ASA refresher course lectures. Ed: Alan Jay Schwartz vol 29.

Kain ZN, Rimar S, Barash PG. Cocaine abuse in the parturient and effects on the fetus and neonate. Anesth Analg. 1993;77:835–45.

Kashiwagi M, Arlettaz R, Lauper U, et al. Methadone maintenance program in a Swiss perinatal center, 1: management and outcome of 89 pregnancies. Acta Obstet Gynecol Scand. 2005;84:140–4.

Kasser CL, Geller A, Howell E, Wartenberg A. Principles of detoxification. In: Graham AW, Schultz, editors. Principles of addiction medicine. 2nd ed. Chevy Chase, MD: American Society of Addiction Medicine; 1998. pp. 423–30.

Kusche C. Managing drug withdrawal in the newborn infant. Semin Fetal Neonatal Med. 2007;12:127–33.

Luty J, Nikolau V, Beam J. Is opiate detoxification unsafe in pregnancy? J Subs Abuse Treat. 2003;24:363–7.

Manchikanti L, Cash KA, Damron KS, Manchukonda R, Pampati V, McManus CD. Controlled substance abuse and illicit drug use in chronic pain patients: An evaluation of multiple variables. Pain Phys. 2006;9:215–25.

Manchikanti L, Pampati V, et al. Prevalence of illicit drug use in patients without controlled substance abuse in interventional pain management. Pain Phys. 2003;6(2):173–8.

Mark TL, Woody GE, Juday T, et al. The economic costs of heroin addiction in the United States. Drug Alcohol Depend. 2001;61:195–206.

Marzuk PM, Tardiff K, Leon AC, et al. Ambient temperature and mortality form unintentional cocaine overdose. JAMA 1998;279:1795–800.

Matsumoto AK, Babul N, Ahdieh H. Oxymorphone extended-release tablets relieve moderate to severe pain and improve physical function in osteoarthritis: results of a randomized, double-blind, placebo- and active-controlled phase III trial. Pain Med. 2005;6:357–66.

McCarthy JJ, Leamon MH, Parr MS, et al. High dose methadone maintenance in pregnancy: maternal and neonatal outcomes. Am J Obstet Gyncol. 2005;193:606–10.

McIlwain H, Ahdieh H. Safety, tolerability, and effectiveness of oxymorphone extended release for moderate to severe osteoarthritis pain: a one-year study. Am J Ther. 2005;12:106–12.

Mehanny SZ, Abdel-Rahman MS, Ahmed YY. Teratogenic effect of cocaine and diazepam in CF1 mice. Teratology 1991;43:11–7.

Merskey H, Bogduk N. Classification of chronic pain: descriptions of chronic pain syndromes and definitions of pain terms. 2nd ed. Seattle, WA: IASP Press; 1994.

Milroy CM. Ten years of "ecstasy". J R Soc Med. 1999;9268–71.

Mouhaffel AH, Madu EC, Satmary WA, et al. Cardiovascular complications of cocaine. Chest 1995;107:1426–34.

Nestler EJ, Hyman SE, Malenka RC. Reinforcement and addictive disorders. In molecular neuropharmacology: a foundation for clinical neuroscience. New York, NY: McGraw-Hill; 2001.

Office of Applied Studies. Substance abuse and mental health services administration. The DAWN Report, January 2003.

Pappagallo M. The concept of pseudotolerance to opioids. J Pharm Care Pain Symp Control. 1998;6:95–8.

Passik SD, Kirsh KL. Managing pain in patients with aberrant drug-taking behaviors. J Support Oncol. 2005;3(1):83–6.

Passik SD, Portenoy RK, Ricketts PL. Substance abuse issues in cancer patients part 1: prevalence and diagnosis. Oncology 1998;12(4):517–21.

Passik SD, Portenoy RK. Substance Issues in palliative care. In: Berger A, et al, editors. Principles and practice of supportive oncology. Philadephia, PA: Lippincott-Raven; 1998. pp. 513–24.

Pastermark GW. The pharmacology of mu analgesics: from patients to genes. Neuroscientist 2001;7(3):220–31.

Perez-Reyes M, Di Guiseppi S, Ondrusek G, et al. Free-base cocaine smoking. Clin Pharmacol Ther. 1982;32:459–65.

Perry S. Heidrich G. Management of pain during debridement: a survey of U.S. burn units. Pain 1982;13:267.

Pitts W, Lange R, Cigarroa J, et al. Cocaine-induced myocardial ischemia and infarction: physiology, pathology, recognition, and management. Prog Cardiovasc Dis. 1997;40:65–76.

Porer K. Acute heroin overdose: update. Ann Intern Med. 1999;130:584–90.

Portenoy RK, Payne R. Acute and chronic pain, In: Lowinson J, Ruiz P, Millman RB, et al, editors. Substance abuse: a comprehensive textbook. 2nd ed. Baltimore, MD: Williams & Wilkins; 1992. pp. 691–721.

Portenoy RK, Savage SR. Clinical realities and economic considerations: special therapeutic issues in intrathecal therapy-tolerance and addiction. J Pain Symptom Manage. 2007;14(3):S27–S35.

Reneman L, Habraken JB, Mojoie CB, et al. MDMA ("ecstasy") and its association with cerebrovascular accidents: preliminary findings. Am J Neuroradiol. 2000;21:1001–07.

Resnick RB. Food and drug administration approval of buprenorphine-naloxone for office treatment of addiction [letter]. Ann Intern Med. 2003;138:360.

Rich BA. A Chronic pain patient's perspective on opioid tolerance. J Pain Palliat Care Pharmacother 2007;21(1):43.

Rinaldi RC, Steindler EM, Wilford BB, Goodwin D. Clarification and standardization of substance abuse terminology. JAMA 1988;259:555–7.

Rittoo DB, Rittoo D. Complications of "ecstasy" misuse. Lancet 1992;340:725–6.

Rosenblatt AB, Mekhail NA. Management of pain in addicted/illicit and legal substance abusing patient. Pain Pract. 2005;5(1):2–10.

Roundaville BJ, Kosten TR. Treatment for opioid dependence: quality and access. JAMA 2000;283:1337–9.

Strain EC, Stitzer ML, et al. Methadone and treatment outcome. Drug Alcohol Depend. 1993;33(2): 105–17.

Savage SR. Assessment of addiction in pain-treatment settings. Clin J Pain. 2002;18(4 suppl):S28–S38.

Schnoll SH, Weaver MF. Addiction and pain. Am J Addict. 2003;12(suppl 2):S27–35.

Shanti CM, Lucas CE. Cocaine and the critical care challenge. Crit Care Med. 2003;31: 1851–9.

Shulgin A. The background and chemistry of MDMA. J Psychoact Drugs 1986;18:291–304.

Siddall PJ, Cousins MJ. Introduction to pain mechanisms. Implications for neural blockade. In: Cousins MJ, Bridenbaugh PO, editors. Neural blockade in clinical anesthesia and management of pain. 3rd ed. Philadelphia, PA: Lippincot-Raven; 1998. pp. 692–3.

Sinatra RS. Acute pain management and acute pain services. In: Cousins MJ, Bridenbaugh PO, editors. Neural blockade in clinical anesthesia and management of pain. 3rd ed. Philadelphia, PA: Lippincot-Raven; 1998. p. 802.

Sloan P, Slatkin N, Ahdieh H. Effectiveness and safety of oral extended-release oxymorphone for the treatment of cancer pain: a pilot study. Support Care Cancer 2005;13:57–65.

Smith MY, Woody G. Nonmedical use and abuse of scheduled medications prescribed for pain, pain-related symptoms, and psychiatric disorders: patterns, user characteristics, and management options. Curr Psychiatry Rep. 2005;7(5):337–43.

Substance Abuse and Mental Health Services Administration office of Applied Studies. National Survey on Drug Use and Health, Results 2007. Washington DC: US Department of Health and Human Services;2007.

US Department of Health Human Services, Substance Abuse and Mental Health Services Administration, Office of Applied Studies. Results from the 2005 National Survey on Drug Use and Health: National Findings. Rockville, Md: US Dept Health Human Services; 2006.

Weaver MF, Schnoll SH. Opioid treatment of chronic pain in patients with addiction. J Pain Palliat Care Pharmacother 2002;16(3):5–26.

Weissman DE, Haddox JD. Opioid pseudoaddiction—an iatrogenic syndrome. Pain 1989;36(3):363–6.

Wolff K, Boys A, Rostami-Hodjegan A, et al. Changes to methadone clearance during pregnancy. Eur J Clin Pharmacol. 2005;61:763–8.

Chapter 32

Pain Management in Elderly Patients

Shamsuddin Akhtar, MBBS, Roberto Rappa, MD, and M. Khurrum Ghori, MD

Introduction

The aging process leads to progressive physiological changes. Individuals are more vulnerable to injury at both extremes of age. This chapter will emphasize the changes that one experiences with aging. Chronological age refers to age according to birth date, whereas biological age is the estimated age based on the degree of physiological degeneration or loss of physiologic reserve (Lee 2003). Physiologic changes do not necessarily parallel that of chronological age. Furthermore, specific physiological processes may age at different rates in the same individual. In addition to normal physiologic changes that occur with aging, coexisting medical conditions are also more prevalent in the elderly. The normal physiological changes associated with aging are distinct from changes brought on by disease. The pharmacokinetic, pharmacodynamic, neurologic, and cognitive changes in the elderly are affected as much by normal physiology as they are by disease.

Elderly patients become more sensitive to the therapeutic and toxic effects of many drugs (Vuyk 2003). The increased sensitivity has been studied for a variety of agents in a variety of settings. In general, it is important to recognize that differential sensitivity to drugs in the elderly population is a result of complex age-related changes in normal physiology, pharmacokinetics, pharmacodynamics, and organ system pathology. The rapidity and degree of these changes are influenced largely by the same factors that contribute to pathology, namely, genetics, environmental exposures, and diet. The following chapter will describe some of the more fundamental physiological changes to occur in the elderly population and how those changes affect basic pharmacokinetic and pharmacodynamic parameters. It will conclude with a brief discussion on the neurobiology of pain, pain assessment in the elderly, and its management.

Physiological Changes in the Elderly

Body Composition

Body composition changes quite significantly with aging. There is an overall reduction in lean muscle mass with an incremental increase in total body fat. These changes cause a corresponding reduction in total body water. It has been estimated that body fat increases by approximately 20–40% and body water decreases by 10–15% in old age (McLean and

N. Vadivelu et al. (eds.), *Essentials of Pain Management*,
DOI 10.1007/978-0-387-87579-8_32, © Springer Science+Business Media, LLC 2011

Couteur 2004). These changes have far reaching consequences on the bioavailability and volumes of distribution of commonly administered drugs (see below).

Cardiovascular System

The cardiac manifestations of aging are a direct result of complex biophysical, biochemical, molecular, ionic, and structural changes that occur at the level of the myocyte. There is a global reduction in the number of cardiac myocytes with aging (Vuyk 2003). Additional changes in the structural components [extracellular matrix (i.e., collagen)] result in a natural degree of "stiffening" of the myocardium and the vasculature.

The stiffened myocardium and vasculature become gradually less compliant to changes in fluid volume. This means that at similar filling volumes, the cardiovascular system operates at a higher pressure (mean arterial pressure, MAP). Increases in the MAP consequently cause a steady increase in left ventricular afterload, resulting in decreased stroke volume. Compensatory changes in the left ventricle (concentric hypertrophy) attempt to restore stroke volume (SV) at the expense of further reductions in myocardial compliance. This results in increased diastolic dysfunction and reduced left ventricular end diastolic volume (EDV). Preload is therefore reduced, causing further reductions in stroke volume and cardiac output. Though CO appears to be maintained in well-conditioned healthy elderly individuals, compensatory responses of CO to "stress" can be decreased (Mangoni and Jackson 2004, Morgan 2007).

In addition to changes at the cardiac myocyte level there are accompanying changes in the autonomic nervous system. There is an overall dampening of autonomic and baroreceptor activity with aging (Vuyk 2003, Mangoni and Jackson 2004, Prough 2005). This results in a decreased resting heart rate (HR). In addition, there is a decreased ability to increase cardiac output by changes in HR. As compared to younger patients, increases in CO are facilitated by increasing EDV, as opposed to increasing HR. This results in an increased reliance on atrial filling for maintenance of CO. As a result, dysrhythmias in the elderly can significantly affect their hemodynamic integrity. Overall, the hemodynamic response to physiological stress is diminished with aging.

Respiratory

Complex physiologic changes occur in the respiratory system with aging (Morgan et al. 2007, Leung 2007, Sadean and Glass 2003, Stoelting and Miller 2007). Respiratory mechanics is altered due to changes in the lung parenchyma, the thorax, and the medullary respiratory centers. These changes account for the increased degree of ventilation/perfusion (V/Q) mismatching and intrapulmonary shunting that is observed with normal aging. In addition, resting arterial oxygen tension, compensatory responses to hypoxia and hypercarbia, protective upper airway reflexes, and the work of breathing are all affected with age (Morgan et al. 2007, Leung 2007). It is estimated that arterial oxygen tension decreases by an average rate of 0.35 mm Hg per year (Morgan et al. 2007). However, because the arterial partial pressure of carbon dioxide ($PaCO_2$) does not change much with age, there is a compensatory increase in minute ventilation (Sadean and Glass 2003).

In addition to changes in pulmonary architecture, there are corresponding changes in the medullary respiratory centers of the central nervous system. This results in impaired ventilatory responses to hypoxia and hypercarbia with increasing age (Morgan et al. 2007,

Leung 2007). This phenomenon partially accounts for the exaggerated respiratory effects of benzodiazepines and opioids in this patient population. There is a higher incidence of transient apnea and episodic breathing in the elderly after exposure to central nervous system depressants (Stoelting and Miller 2007).

Protective airway reflexes (laryngeal, pharyngeal, and cough) are also impaired with increasing age, which can contribute to a higher incidence of pulmonary aspiration and postoperative respiratory morbidity and mortality in this population (Stoelting and Miller 2007).

Finally, the work of breathing in the elderly population is increased as compared to younger patients. This is attributed to the gradual stiffening and calcification of the costochondral joints of the thorax, resulting in a less compliant chest wall. This, in conjunction with the increased incidence of smaller airway closure, makes breathing more laborious in the elderly. Elderly patients are more predisposed to acute postoperative respiratory failure than their younger counterparts.

Gastrointestinal

With advancing age there is a general decline in hepatocyte mass, with a proportional reduction in hepatic blood flow. Blood flow to the liver, and its corresponding mass, decreases by approximately 40% with increasing age (McLean and Couteur 2004). Although oxidative drug metabolic processes may become less efficient with aging, studies demonstrate that phase I and phase II enzymatic reactions appear to be well preserved with increasing age (McLean and Couteur 2004). Serum albumin concentration decreases by approximately 10% in older patients (McLean and Couteur 2004).

Renal

Overall, renal mass, renal blood flow, tubular function, and glomerular filtration rate (GFR) are all reduced with age. The mass of the kidney decreases by 20–25% between the age of 30 and 80 years (McLean and Couteur 2004). There is a gradual increase in blood urea nitrogen by approximately 0.2 mg/dl per year. Interestingly, despite these changes, serum creatinine concentration remains largely unchanged. This is attributed to the proportional decrease in lean body mass and creatinine production in the elderly population (Prough 2005).

GFR declines by less than 1 ml/min/yr after middle age. As old age is also associated with increased rates of hypertension, vascular disease, and diabetes, it is difficult to accurately predict to what extent decrease in GFR is purely related to age. Additional changes include a blunted renin–angiotensin–aldosterone system (RAAS) response, increased antidiuretic hormone (ADH) levels, and increased atrial natiuretic peptide (ANP) release, especially in the perioperative period (Morgan et al. 2007, Prough 2005).

Central Nervous System (CNS)

There is a reduction in cortical neuronal density with accompanying changes in cerebral blood flow with aging (Morgan et al. 2007, Prough 2005, Sadean and Glass 2003). Cerebral blood flow decreases by 10–20% in proportion to neuronal losses. This is largely attributed to increased apoptotic activity of cerebral neurons, particularly in the cerebral cortex and frontal lobes. Additionally, deranged cellular calcium homeostatic mechanisms cause altered

synaptic activity and signal transduction. The number of synapses and their corresponding receptors are reduced [i.e., decreased serotonergic, adrenergic, and gamma-aminobutyric
acid (GABA) binding sites]. There is also a reduction in neuronal regenerative capacity (Vuyk
2003). Additionally, N-methyl-D-acetate (NMDA) receptor-binding sites have been reported
to decrease by 50% in aged animals (Vuyk 2003).

Pharmacokinetic Changes in the Elderly

Pharmacokinetics is the study of drug movement throughout the body and it is described
by four basic parameters: drug absorption, distribution, metabolism, and excretion. All
parameters are affected by aging to a varying extent.

Changes in body composition with aging have profound influence on the distribution of
drugs and their resultant steady-state plasma concentrations. With increases in total body
fat and concomitant decreases in total body water, the elderly experience alterations in their
volumes of distribution (Vd) to many pharmacological agents. This has far reaching implications in the peak plasma concentrations of drugs, the time course of their action, and the
degree to which they exert their therapeutic and adverse effects (Sadean and Glass 2003).

Highly water soluble drugs (i.e., acetylsalicylic acid), as well as their hydrophilic metabolites, would be expected to achieve higher overall plasma concentrations in the setting of
decreased total body water. Similarly, lipophilic drugs (i.e., diazepam) would be expected to
achieve a lower overall plasma concentration, as they are taken up more avidly and stored
by the increased adipose tissue. This results in an increased Vd and a prolonged elimination
half-life for lipid-soluble agents (Sadean and Glass 2003).

Changes in cardiovascular physiology also have a profound impact on the distribution
of drugs. As expected, decreases in cardiac output that accompany the normal aging process
result in reduced tissue perfusion. This results in increased circulatory times, a delay of drug
transfer from their sites of administration to their sites of action, and a delay to peak drug
effects. Furthermore, decreased perfusion to excretory organs, such as the liver and kidneys,
results in an overall increase in the duration of action of many commonly administered drugs.

In addition to reduced perfusion, reductions in hepatic and renal mass are expected to
result in a reduced clearance of many drugs. As described above, reductions in hepatocyte
mass, along with reduced hepatic perfusion, are expected to slow metabolic processes in the
liver. This is particularly important for those drugs that are highly extracted by the liver or
for drugs that undergo extensive first-pass metabolism. These agents depend on hepatic blood
flow for their overall elimination (i.e., morphine sulfate), and in the setting of reduced hepatic
perfusion, their clearance can be reduced by as much as 30–40% (McLean and Couteur 2004).
As a result, one should reduce maintenance dosing for those particular agents in the elderly.

Age-related changes in serum albumin concentration can also affect the Vd of many commonly administered medications in the elderly. There is an apparent 10% increase in the
unbound fraction of many pharmacologic agents in the elderly, mirroring the decrease in
serum albumin (McLean and Couteur 2004). The effects of decreased protein binding are
more pronounced for drugs that are highly extracted by the liver, extensively protein bound,
and administered intravenously. This includes agents such as fentanyl, haloperidol, lidocaine,
and midazolam. As a result, dosage readjustments are often necessary to avoid excessive
toxicity associated with the increased bioavailability of those particular agents (McLean and
Couteur 2004, Sadean and Glass 2003).

Similarly, reduced renal mass, renal blood flow, and glomerular filtration is expected to slow drug excretion from the body, particularly for those agents that rely heavily on renal elimination pathways [i.e., nonsteroidal anti-inflammatory drugs (NSAIDs)] (McLean and Couteur 2004). These two processes operate in tandem and have profound influences on drug elimination in this population. As a result, initial dosing and maintenance dosing should be adjusted, as many circumstances call for dose reductions of 10–25% in the elderly.

Pharmacodynamics

Pharmacodynamics is the study of the biochemical and physiologic effects of drugs and the molecular mechanisms by which those effects are produced. Age-related changes in pharmacodynamics are complex and variable for different agents. In order to establish clear pharmacodynamic distinctions, studies of differential drug sensitivity require measurements of serum drug concentrations. Because age-related pharmacokinetic changes will often result in differences in drug bioavailability, conclusions about pharmacodynamic relationships are often difficult to ascertain. Most of our understanding of the pharmacodynamic changes in the elderly, is therefore, derived from the study of specific agents. The following section describes some of the more established pharmacodynamic changes associated with aging.

Elderly patients are more sensitive to the therapeutic effects and more vulnerable to the adverse effects of neuroleptics and benzodiazepines (McLean and Couteur 2004). Extrapyramidal side effects, postural hypotension, acute delirium, and arrhythmias are more frequent in this patient population at lower antipsychotic doses (Mangoni et al. 2004). Similarly, sedation is often induced at lower serum drug concentrations of benzodiazepines than in younger patients. For example, the effective concentration for sedation in 50% of patients (EC50) after intravenous midazolam is reduced by approximately 50% in older patients, despite similar pharmacokinetic profiles (McLean and Couteur 2004). These differences may be attributed to upregulated GABA receptor activity in the central nervous system (CNS) (see below) and possibly account for the association of benzodiazepines with falls and hip fractures in older people.

Elderly patients also demonstrate increased sensitivity to opioid analgesics. It has been consistently demonstrated that older patients experience enhanced sedation, analgesia, and adverse effects from opioid administration. This may be attributed to the differential expression of opioid receptors in the elderly population (Vuyk 2003, Sadean and Glass 2003, Berger 2007, Mann 2003). The dose requirement for fentanyl significantly decreased with advancing age (a 50% decrease between the ages of 20 and 89 years), despite little differences in pharmacokinetic parameters (Scott and Stanski 1987).

Neurobiology of Pain

There often exists the pretense that age dulls the sense of pain. Along with this sentiment, there is the belief that old people are less sensitive to the effects of pain. There have been many studies conducted examining the pain threshold responses of the elderly to a variety of noxious stimuli (Gibson and Helme 2001). The results have provided interesting insights on the neurobiology of pain evolution in the aging population.

Psychophysical studies of heat pain thresholds in young and older adults have revealed age-related increases in thermal pain threshold. A 20% increase in radiant pain threshold has been observed for most elderly patients, particularly those greater than 70 years of age.

Additionally, studies have revealed modest increases in pressure and sharp pain thresholds, 15 and 20%, respectively (Gibson and Helme 2001).

Visceral pain thresholds have also been studied in the elderly. There is a significant age-related increase in pressure pain threshold of visceral tissue (Gibson and Helme 2001). For example, gastric and esophageal distension studies (with an inflatable balloon) have shown a 50% increase in reported visceral pain among older individuals (Gibson and Helme 2001). This may partially explain the diminished and atypical pain presentations for common organ system pathology (i.e., myocardial infarction) in this patient population.

Descending neuro-inhibitory pathways have also been studied in the elderly population. Studies directed at activating these endogenous analgesic systems (i.e., repeated ice water immersion) have revealed that post-exposure analgesic responses (measured by post-exposure pain threshold responses) are markedly reduced in persons of advanced age. For example, elderly patients were found to have only a 40% increase in pain threshold after repeated ice water immersion as compared to a 150% increase as seen in younger adults (Gibson and Helme 2001). This may explain some of the age variations in reported pain tolerance levels and the ability to cope with severe or chronic persistent pain.

Studies in the elderly have demonstrated clear associations between pain perception and mood disorders. Patients who are anxious or depressed voice more localized and intense pain than do their non-anxious/non-depressed counterparts (Berger 2007). Given the fact that mood disorders are increasingly prevalent in the elderly population (i.e., prevalence of major depressive disorder 1–2% in community-dwelling elderly and 5–6% in older patients in the primary care setting), it is especially important to recognize co-morbid psychiatric disease in this patient population. Sometimes adequate pain control can be achieved from simple psychological or psychiatric interventions.

Pain Assessment in the Elderly

The assessment of pain requires time and patience. Thorough history and physical examination are a crucial part of the assessment. First interview should focus on vital signs, state of hydration, and conversation style of the patient. If these patients are confused or show memory deficit or incoherent speech, then bedside psychological tests should be done to diagnose cognitive deficit. Elderly patients who have difficulty communicating with clinicians are at particular risk of under treatment (Bernabei et al. 1998, Pargeon and Hailey 1999, Fineberg 2006). Detailed chronological history may be collected from the patient, previous medical records or if patient shows memory difficulties or uncooperative behavior, direct interview of family members or caregivers residing with the patient. Systematic physical examination of body should be part of the pain assessment protocol. As most elderly patients suffering from pain are on multiple medications, adverse drug interactions should be kept in mind. Just as a routine physical exam includes inspection, palpation, percussion, and auscultation, same system is used for physical exam of pain patients with some modifications. While performing clinical examination of elderly, the description of pain with movement is noted. Changes in gait with reference to gravity, supportive aids used, dragging or pulling of upper or lower extremities should be recorded in the initial and subsequent notes.

Tools to assess pain in the elderly are the same as in any other adult patient. However, they are impractical in acute delirium or of minimal value in patients with dementia or cognitive dysfunction. Furthermore, the first-hand information regarding injury, type of injury, damage to organs, and baseline function of the patient may not be available and would have to be obtained from the caregivers. All these factors can make the assessment of pain in the elderly quite challenging. For the purpose of assessment, pain in elderly can be categorized into acute and chronic entities. Acute pain is either caused by perioperative injury or non-operative trauma or disease. Typical expected duration of acute pain may range from 1 to 6 months. Any condition in which pain duration is more than usually expected time or lasts more than 6 months is called chronic pain.

Acute pain can be assessed using Visual Analog Pain Scale (VAS). In cooperative patients it is a sensitive test, correlates well with verbal pain score, and should be recorded on each visit to assess the severity of pain. In patients who are demented and cognitively challenged, physical cues like moaning, grimacing, restlessness, and agitation may represent pain behavior. Chronic pain can be assessed using McGill Pain Questionnaire (MPQ), Illness Behavior Questionnaire (IBQ), and Minnesota Multiphasic Personality Inventory (MMPI). They are not recommended for patients with cognitive impairment and dementia (Ferrell et al. 1995, Hurley and Volicer 2001).

When geriatric patients cannot explain their symptoms due to memory or neurological insufficiency, or history and physical examination are insufficient to diagnose a pain symptom, diagnostic tests become more important and may help clarify the ambiguity. Painful conditions in old age are difficult to separate from one another. For example, lower extremity pain may come from a variety of pain conditions, like spinal stenosis, diabetic neuropathy, nerve entrapment by disc herniation or osteophyte formation or intermittent claudication due to vascular insufficiency or other causes. To separate each condition various diagnostic tests are used. Sequence of testing typically starts with plain X-rays of the affected region or organ followed by more advanced imaging techniques (CT scan, MRI) followed by specialized diagnostic modalities (electrophysiological studies, electromyography, nerve conduction velocities, discography, myelography, etc.) (Manchikanti et al. 2008, Boswell 2007).

Management of Pain in the Elderly

Management of pain in the elderly involves a multi-modal approach. It is dependent on the etiology of pain, duration of pain, and the associated co-morbidities in a particular individual. Pain secondary to acute insult can be intense, however, potentially easier to control with analgesics (opioid and non-opioid medications) and/or neuraxial blocks or peripheral nerve blocks. The management of chronic pain on the other hand can be very challenging. It frequently involves the use of analgesics, adjuvant medications, and advanced invasive interventions. Furthermore, psychological support, rehabilitation, psychological and physiatrist support play an important role in the management of chronic pain. In the elderly, with significant incidence of co-morbidities and terminal conditions, palliative and hospice care also contribute to the overall management of pain.

Pharmacological Interventions

Pharmacological interventions are the mainstay of pain management strategies in any group. Pain medications should be used in stepwise approach as recommended by World Health Organization (WHO) (Boswell 2007). NSAIDs and non-opioid analgesics are recommended as first-line medications. If the pain persists or increases, opioids can be added to manage mild-to-moderate pain. Stronger opioids are recommended for moderate to severe pain as part of multimodal therapy. Adjuvant medications (anti-depressants, anti-psychotics, and anticonvulsants) which help modulate pain can be added at each step to complement therapy. Furthermore corticosteroids, local anesthetics, and muscle relaxants can also be used for short period of time to complement pain management.

Prostaglandin Inhibitors

These drugs inhibit central and peripheral prostaglandin formation, thus inhibiting pain transmission. They are broadly classified into two groups: non-specific cyclo-oxygenase (COX) inhibitors (ibuprofen, naproxen, aspirin, acetaminophen, ketorolac, and diclofenac) and specific COX-2 inhibitors (celecoxib, rofecoxib, valdecoxib, and parecoxib). These drugs are effective for bone-related pain and are frequently used to treat mild to moderate acute pain, chronic pain, cancer-related pain, arthritic pain, inflammatory pain, and fever. Side effects of these medications limit their use in the elderly. Ibuprofen and naproxen can prolong prothrombin time in patients on warfarin which can lead to excessive bleeding (Schulman and Henriksson 1989, Dijk et al. 2004, Visser et al. 2005). They should be used with caution in patients with gastrointestinal ulcers, renal insufficiency, and hepatic sufficiency. Ketoralac is an intravenous analgesic and effective for orthopedic and somatic pain. However it has nephrotoxic effects and may precipitate renal failure in elderly and dehydrated patients (Schoch et al. 1992, Haragsim et al. 1994). Diflunisal is another antiarthritic medications that can increase the levels of indomethacin if taken concomitantly and the combination can lead to significant gastrointestinal bleeding (Mano 2006, Verbeeck 1990). Acetaminophen effects are thought to be due to inhibition of brain prostaglandin synthetase. Acetaminophen neither interferes with platelet function nor causes gastric irritation; however, it should be used with caution in elderly patients with anemia or hepatic disease. Since malnutrition, thrombocytopenia, and alcoholic liver disease is more prevalent in the elderly, chronic ingestion of acetaminophen may cause neutropenia, pancytopenia, leukopenia, and thrombocytopenic purpura (Barker et al. 1977, Lane 2002).

Opioid Analgesics

Opioid analgesics stimulate the endogenous opioid receptors. They can be administered orally, subcutaneously, intravenously, neuro-axially, transdermally, rectally, or through the oral mucosa. However, opioids can cause significant sedation, confusion, respiratory depression, urinary retention, constipation, nausea, and vomiting. Opioids should be used with caution and their dose should be reduced in the elderly, especially those patients with significant co-morbidities. Patients with history of chronic obstructive pulmonary disease, asthma, emphysema, central or obstructive sleep apnea, obesity, renal failure, and hepatic failure are especially prone to the side effects of opioids.

Opioids differ in potency and hence different agents can be used for varying intensity of pain. Codeine is used for mild to moderate pain. Hydrocodone is commonly using in the elderly for acute or chronic pain. Morphine is the most commonly prescribed pain medication in elderly patients. Oxycodone is used for moderate to severe acute or chronic pain. It should be used cautiously in the post-operative elderly patients to avoid serious respiratory depression. Meperidine can cause seizures, myoclonus, and agitation in elderly patients and should be avoided in elderly patients with low ejection fraction and impaired renal function (Szeto 1977, Danziger et al. 1994, Clark et al. 1995). Hydromorphone has been used safely, especially in those patients in the elderly for the management of acute and chronic pain.

It is five times more potent than morphine, has no active metabolite, and can be administered orally, epidurally, and intravenously. Methadone is a synthetic opioid with prolonged half-life. Its effects on QT interval have recently raised questions about its use in elderly pain patients (Pearson and Woosley 2005, Sticherling et al. 2005, Krantz 2003). Fentanyl is a fast-acting narcotic analgesic. Typically fentanyl is administered intravenously. However, it can also be administered transdermally for the management of cancer or chronic pain. Transdermal fentanyl can take 24–72 h to reach steady-state level and another 15–21 h for the effect to dissipate after it is discontinued. Additional narcotics should be administered cautiously in elderly patients who are receiving transdermal fentanyl.

Adjuvants and Other Analgesics

Adjuvant drugs include anti-depressant drugs, traditional anticonvulsant medications, or psychotropic medications. Systemic administration of alpha-2 agonists and NMDA antagonists can help control moderate to severe pain. Many of these medications have significant cardio-respiratory and central effects. Due caution should be exercised in prescribing these medications to the elderly with especial attention given to drug–drug interaction and drug–disease interactions (Jano and Aparasu 2007).

Non-pharmacological Interventions

Anesthetic Techniques

Severity of pain, systemic side effects of narcotics, or concomitant co-morbidities may preclude the use of high doses of narcotics to control moderate-to-severe pain. Reversibly inhibiting the transmission of pain pathways at the level of the spinal cord or nerve, by neuraxial or peripheral nerve blocks, respectively, would alleviate pain. Neuro-axial administration of opioids, low dose local anesthetics and in combinations with systemic administration of alpha-2 agonists, NMDA antagonists can effectively control moderate to severe pain. In the elderly, these techniques and medications can be used to reduce the systemic doses of opioids and other analgesic medications. Spinal and epidural blocks can be very effective in relieving perioperative pain. However, elderly patients are more prone to hypotension produced by the concomitant sympathetic block when neuraxial local anesthetics are used (Meyhoff et al. 2007). Seemingly normal adult doses of opioids, benzodiazepines can cause respiratory depression and mental status changes in elderly debilitated patients. Smaller doses of local anesthetics and opioids are recommended in the elderly.

Advanced Interventional Techniques

Multiple intervention modalities can be used to control pain, when pharmacological pain control is suboptimal. Some of these include transcutaneous electrical nerve stimulation (TENS) unit patch, trigger point injections, epidural pumps, acupuncture, intrathecal pump placement for morphine, clonidine and other medications, intradiscal electrothermal therapy (IDET), nerve ablation therapy, facet joint injections, cryoablation, radiofrequency nerve ablation, peripheral nerve blocking catheters, fluoroscopic guided nerve blocks for cancer pain, and ganglion blocks for chronic regional pain syndrome (CRPS). Use of a particular technique in a patient, is guided by etiology of pain, concomitant co-morbidities, and the patient's current clinical status, than by age. Cancer is most prevalent in the elderly and is the third leading cause of death in the geriatric population. Celiac plexus block, hypo-gastric block, individual sympathetic nerve, and ganglion blocks are examples of blocks used to relieve chronic pain. Interventional radiologists, pain specialists, and neurosurgical specialists use such techniques in cancer-related or sympathetically mediated or debilitating chronic pain conditions. As with any invasive technique, it is important to exclude contraindications to the technique. Cardio-respiratory illnesses, cognitive dysfunction, and coagulopathy (secondary to anti-platelet or anti-coagulant therapies) may preclude certain interventions in the elderly (Boswell et al. 2007).

Rehabilitation

Injury due to fall is the most common cause of fracture-related morbidity in elderly population (Berry and Miller 2008, Gibson et al. 2008). Injuries may range from fracture of hip joint to intracranial hematomas. Medications used to treat these patients may significantly limit the activity of an elderly individual. Many elderly patients are already dependent on social support system for exercise and activity. Furthermore, Alzheimer and other cognitive disorders may cause low compliance to rehabilitation activities causing worsening pain and quality of life. This lack of activity increases chances of delayed healing, deep vein thrombosis, and pulmonary embolism (Labropoulos et al. 2009, Yablon et al. 2004). The best way to avoid this situation is to involve elderly pain patients in healthy exercise activities, use proper pain medications for physiotherapy needs, and improve range of motion of joints with the help of physiatrists and rehabilitation teams.

Psychological Interventions

Psychological problems can frequently present as physical complaints. Most common finding in such patients is that pain symptoms are inconsistent with the anatomical distribution of pain fibers (Stone et al. 2005). Depression is commonly found with chronic pain in elderly patients. For this reason psychological evaluation of the elderly patient in pain is considered standard protocol in the majority of pain clinics. However psychological evaluation can be challenging, as confused, demented, and delirious patients may not be able to express their symptoms and can lead to inappropriate therapy for their painful condition. In patients with diagnosis or signs of psychiatric disorder, primary treatment of disorder is an integral part of their therapy. Social support is also an important aspect of treatment of chronic pain in elderly patients.

Hospice and Palliative Care

Unrelieved pain is the most important symptom to be addressed, when providing support and comfort to an elderly, at the end of life stage. This requires special skills in pain management at the end of life. A survey of hospice nursing home patients showed that 85% patients suffered from moderate to severe pain at the end of life (Bernabei et al. 1998, Pargeon et al. 1999, Fineberg et al. 2006). For this reason a balanced technique of social support, pain control with fewer side effects while keeping patients wishes, is a priority. Optimum pain control with narcotic analgesics, nerve blocks, rhizotomy, implantable devices, and palliative sedation are various ways to alleviate painful dying process. When dealing with an elderly patient for palliative care, patient's wishes, social support of family, friends, or hospice care nurses need to be collaborated in a multi disciplinary pain management protocol.

Summary

There are many physiological changes that occur with aging. Many of these changes have a significant impact on pharmacokinetic and pharmacodynamic of analgesic medications. Elderly patients are much more prone to sideeffects and drug dosages should be reduced in this population. The elderly also have significant co-morbid diseases that include dementia, Alzheimer's disease, cardio-respiratory dysfunction, renal dysfunction, and musculoskeletal disorders. These concomitant disorders may not only limit the administration of medications, but also may preclude certain invasive, pain interventions for pain relief. They also make pain assessment challenging and pain management difficult in the elderly. Psychiatric conditions and/or psychological impact of pain and chronic primary conditions, e.g., cancer, needs to be taken into account when managing elderly patients with pain. A management strategy for chronic pain typically involves many disciplines, including chronic pain specialist, social worker, physiatrist, rehabilitation physician, and potentially a psychiatrist. Furthermore, social, cultural, and ethical issues should also be kept in mind when managing pain in an elderly patient.

Case Scenario

Shamsuddin Akhtar, MBBS, Roberto Rappa, MD, and Ghori Mohammed, MD

A 76-year-old male, Patrick, presents for a total right hip replacement. The patient has a history of osteoarthritis, chronic atrial fibrillation, hypertension, chronic obstructive pulmonary disease, and type 2 diabetes mellitus. He denies significant cardio-respiratory symptoms, his recent stress test was negative for ischemia, and ejection fraction was reported as 56%. His medications include lisinopril, coumadin, glipizide, and naproxen. He occasionally takes tramadol for moderate-to-severe pain. You are asked to see Patrick and discuss the anesthetic plan. Patrick's wife had a similar surgery under general anesthesia with an epidural for postoperative pain control. She was extremely pleased with this choice because she did not feel any pain at all after the operation. She attributes the success of the operation to the anesthetic she had. Patrick is keen to have a similar anesthetic.

Can spinal or epidural anesthesia be used for this patient?
Since the patient is on coumadin, neuraxial blockade may be contraindicated.

Spinal or epidural anesthesia is contraindicated in patients with coagulopathy. ASRA (American Society of Regional Anesthesia) guidelines generally state that the coagulation studies need to be within the normal range before elective placement of the neuraxial block. If spinal anesthesia is used for surgery, long-duration preservative-free morphine (Astramorph) can be administered intrathecally with the local anesthetic (beware of respiratory depression). Intrathecal opioids can provide pain relief for many hours after surgery. If epidural anesthesia was used, the patient could receive an initial dose of dilute local anesthetic solution with opioids and subsequently a continuous infusion of local anesthetic plus an opioid. Since the patient's INR comes back at 1.5, he undergoes the surgery under general anesthesia without spinal or epidural.

Patrick recovers from the anesthetic, but he is still not fully awake. He is maintaining his airway, breathing at a rate of 14 breaths per minute, and his saturation is 98% on oxygen. You leave him in recovery under the care of nursing staff. Half an hour later, your are urgently requested to see Patrick as he is agitated and thrashing about in bed.

What could be the reason for this?
The assessment in this situation should follow the ABCDs (airway, breathing circulation, and disability). Elderly patients are more sensitive to the depressant effects of anesthetics, sedatives, and opioid analgesics. Airway and breathing, if compromised can lead to hypoxia with accompanying cerebral hypoxia, resulting in agitation, anxiety, and confusion. Circulatory depression can lead to the same clinical picture in addition to clammy skin, sweating, and reduced capillary refill time. Postoperative cognitive dysfunction is an entity on its own in elderly population, the cause of which is still unclear. A full bladder or inadequate analgesia can also present in a similar way. On review, you find that the cause of his agitation is likely postoperative pain.

How would you manage his postoperative pain?
Pain can typically be controlled with intravenous opioids in combination with regular acetaminophen. Patient-controlled analgesia (PCA) is used if the patient is cooperative. If patient is not cooperative, IV opioids may have to be administered on as needed basis.

Hydromorphone PCA was chosen as it is more potent, has a shorter duration of action, and no active metabolites compared to morphine. As soon as the patient was able to tolerate food orally, he was started on oral pain medication. Percocet, which is the combination of oxycodone and acetaminophen is commonly prescribed after surgery. Excessive sedation can occur with opioid medication in the elderly. Hence, they should be started on lower doses and medication should be carefully titrated. He tolerated the medication and was discharged home on postoperative day #4.

However, on his postoperative visit, he is still complaining of significant pain at the operative site. His activity is limited due to pain. How will you work up this patient? What medications will you prescribe?
The persistent postoperative pain is unusual. General approach to pain is to examine the patient and confirm the diagnosis. Appropriate investigations such as radiological imaging may be needed.

Physical exam revealed limited range of motion with no apparent signs of infection. Patient underwent hip X-rays that showed a possible collection of fluid at the operative site, which was further characterized by CT scan of the hip. The fluid collection was drained, which released pressure and decreased the intensity of pain. Regular physiotherapy is very important in order to reestablish the range of movement after many orthopedic surgeries. Failure to do so can lead to contractures and worsening pain syndromes. Patrick underwent regular physiotherapy that helped the recovery process and decreased pain considerably.

References

Barker JD, Jr, de Carle DJ, Anuras S. Chronic excessive acetaminophen use and liver damage. Ann Intern Med. 1977;87:299–301.

Berger JM. Pain management. In: Silverstein JH, Rooke GA, Reves JG, editors. Geriatric anesthesiology. 2nd ed. New York, NY: Springer; 2007. pp. 308–21.

Bernabei R, Gambassi G, Lapane K, Landi F, Gatsonis C, Dunlop R, Lipsitz L, Steel K, Mor V. Management of pain in elderly patients with cancer. SAGE Study Group. Systematic Assessment of Geriatric Drug Use via Epidemiology. JAMA 1998;279:1877–82.

Berry SD, Miller RR. Falls: epidemiology, pathophysiology, and relationship to fracture. Curr Osteoporos Rep. 2008;6:149–54.

Boswell MV, Trescot AM, Datta S, Schultz DM, Hansen HC, Abdi S, Sehgal N, Shah RV, Singh V, Benyamin RM, Patel VB, Buenaventura RM, Colson JD, Cordner HJ, Epter RS, Jasper JF, Dunbar EE, Atluri SL, Bowman RC, Deer TR, Swicegood JR, Staats PS, Smith HS, Burton AW, Kloth DS, Giordano J, Manchikanti L. Interventional techniques: evidence-based practice guidelines in the management of chronic spinal pain. Pain Phys. 2007;10:7–111.

Clark RF, Wei EM, Anderson PO. Meperidine: therapeutic use and toxicity. J Emerg Med. 1995;13:797–802.

Danziger LH, Martin SJ, Blum RA. Central nervous system toxicity associated with meperidine use in hepatic disease. Pharmacotherapy 1994;14:235–8.

Ferrell BA, Ferrell BR, Rivera L. Pain in cognitively impaired nursing home patients. J Pain Symptom Manage. 1995;10:591–8.

Fineberg IC, Wenger NS, Brown-Saltzman K. Unrestricted opiate administration for pain and suffering at the end of life: knowledge and attitudes as barriers to care. J Palliat Med. 2006;9:873–83.

Gibson RE, Harden M, Byles J, Ward J. Incidence of falls and fall-related outcomes among people in aged-care facilities in the Lower Hunter region, NSW. N S W Public Health Bull. 2008;19:166–9.

Gibson SJ, Helme RD. Age-related differences in pain perception and report. Clin Geriatr Med. 2001;17:433–56, v–vi.

Haragsim L, Dalal R, Bagga H, Bastani B. Ketorolac-induced acute renal failure and hyperkalemia: report of three cases. Am J Kidney Dis. 1994;24:578–80.

Hurley AC, Volicer L. Evaluation of pain in cognitively impaired individuals. J Am Geriatr Soc. 2001;49:1397–8.

Jano E, Aparasu RR. Healthcare outcomes associated with beers' criteria: a systematic review. Ann Pharmacother. 2007;41:438–47.

Krantz MJ, Kutinsky IB, Robertson AD, Mehler PS. Dose-related effects of methadone on QT prolongation in a series of patients with torsade de pointes. Pharmacotherapy 2003; 23:802–5.

Labropoulos N, Gasparis AP, Pefanis D, Leon LR, Jr, Tassiopoulos AK. Secondary chronic venous disease progresses faster than primary. J Vasc Surg. 2009;49:704–10.

Lane JE, Belson MG, Brown DK, Scheetz A. Chronic acetaminophen toxicity: a case report and review of the literature. J Emerg Med. 2002;23:253–6.

Lee CY. Manual of anaesthesia. New York, NY: McGraw-Hill; 2006.

Leung JM. Elderly patient. In: Stoelting RK, Miller RD, editors. Basics of anesthesia Philadelphia, PA: Churchill Livingstone Elsevier; 2007. pp. 518–29.

Manchikanti L, Singh V, Derby R, Schultz DM, Benyamin RM, Prager JP, Hirsch JA. Reassessment of evidence synthesis of occupational medicine practice guidelines for inter-ventional pain management. Pain Phys. 2008;11:393–482.

Mangoni AA, Jackson SH. Age-related changes in pharmacokinetics and pharmacodynamics: basic principles and practical applications. Br J Clin Pharmacol. 2004;57:6–14.

Mann C, Pouzeratte Y, Eledjam JJ. Postoperative patient-controlled analgesia in the elderly: risks and benefits of epidural versus intravenous administration. Drugs Aging 2003;20: 337–45.

Mano Y, Usui T, Kamimura H. In vitro drug interaction between diflunisal and indomethacin via glucuronidation in humans. Biopharm Drug Dispos. 2006;27:267–73.

McLean AJ, Le Couteur DG. Aging biology and geriatric clinical pharmacology. Pharmacol Rev. 2004;56:163–84.

Meyhoff CS, Hesselbjerg L, Koscielniak-Nielsen Z, Rasmussen LS. Biphasic cardiac out-put changes during onset of spinal anaesthesia in elderly patients. Eur J Anaesthesiol. 2007;24:770–5.

Morgan GE, Mikhail MS, Murray MJ. Clinical anesthesiology. 4th ed. New York, NY: McGraw-Hill; 2007.

Pargeon KL, Hailey BJ. Barriers to effective cancer pain management: a review of the literature. J Pain Symptom Manage. 1999;18:358–68.

Pearson EC, Woosley RL. QT prolongation and torsades de pointes among methadone users: reports to the FDA spontaneous reporting system. Pharmacoepidemiol Drug Saf. 2005;14:747–53.

Prough DS. Anesthetic pitfalls in the elderly patient. J Am Coll Surg. 2005;200:784–94.

Sadean MR, Glass PS. Pharmacokinetics in the elderly. Best Pract Res Clin Anaesthesiol. 2003;17:191–205.

Schoch PH, Ranno A, North DS. Acute renal failure in an elderly woman following intramuscular ketorolac administration. Ann Pharmacother 1992;26:1233–6.

Schulman S, Henriksson K. Interaction of ibuprofen and warfarin on primary haemostasis. Br J Rheumatol. 1989;28:46–9.

Scott JC, Stanski DR. Decreased fentanyl and alfentanil dose requirements with age. A simultaneous pharmacokinetic and pharmacodynamic evaluation. J Pharmacol Exp Ther. 1987;240:159–66.

Sticherling C, Schaer BA, Ammann P, Maeder M, Osswald S. Methadone-induced Torsade de pointes tachycardias. Swiss Med Wkly. 2005;135:282–5.

Stoelting RK, Miller R. Basics of anesthesia. 5th ed. Philadelphia, PA: Churchill Livingston; 2007.

Stone J, Smyth R, Carson A, Lewis S, Prescott R, Warlow C, Sharpe M. Systematic review of misdiagnosis of conversion symptoms and "hysteria". BMJ 2005;331:989.

Szeto HH, Inturrisi CE, Houde R, Saal S, Cheigh J, Reidenberg MM. Accumulation of normeperidine, an active metabolite of meperidine, in patients with renal failure of cancer. Ann Intern Med. 1977;86:738–41.

van Dijk KN, Plat AW, van Dijk AA, Piersma-Wichers M, de Vries-Bots AM, Slomp J, de Jong-van den Berg LT, Brouwers JR. Potential interaction between acenocoumarol and diclofenac, naproxen and ibuprofen and role of CYP2C9 genotype. Thromb Haemost. 2004;91:95–101.

Verbeeck RK. Pharmacokinetic drug interactions with nonsteroidal anti-inflammatory drugs. Clin Pharmacokinet 1990;19:44–66.

Visser LE, van Schaik RH, van Vliet M, Trienekens PH, De Smet PA, Vulto AG, Hofman A, van Duijn CM, Stricker BH. Allelic variants of cytochrome P450 2C9 modify the interaction between nonsteroidal anti-inflammatory drugs and coumarin anticoagulants. Clin Pharmacol Ther. 2005;77:479–85.

Vuyk J. Pharmacodynamics in the elderly. Best Pract Res Clin Anaesthesiol. 2003;17:207–18.

Yablon SA, Rock WA, Jr, Nick TG, Sherer M, McGrath CM, Goodson KH. Deep vein thrombosis: prevalence and risk factors in rehabilitation admissions with brain injury. Neurology 2004;63:485–91.

Chapter 33

Management of Oro-dental Pain

Amarender Vadivelu, BDS, MDS

Pain arising in the oral tissues can cause considerable discomfort and interfere with oral function. The teeth are primarily important for mastication of food, and the mouth is the first part of the gastrointestinal tract to initiate digestion process. Other functions of the teeth include facilitating speech, swallowing, and contributing to aesthetics which in turn instills a sense of self-esteem and confidence.

Oro-dental pain as a specific modality (Clark 2006) and a cardinal sign occurs as a result of inflammation and traumatic injuries or as a complication of elective oral and maxillofacial surgery. Toothache has been compared with earache and labor pain for its intensity and propensity for acute discomfort.

Common diseases affecting the oral structures are dental caries and gum disease, oral ulcers, and dentine hypersensitivity. The need for regular oral care by the patient and preventive visits to the dental office cannot be overemphasized since the above disorders can lead to a host of complications, which can include intractable pain.

Dental caries is known to be the highest incidence of any disease that besets mankind. Orson had called this the "triple tragic triangle of tooth decay" and had implicated fermentable carbohydrates, oral bacteria, and susceptibility of the individual. Tooth decay can progress by a burrowing effect, ultimately destroying the dentin, and reaches the nerve center of the tooth which constitutes the dental pulp. The dentin plays a vital role by acting as a thermal insulator and helping withstand the extremes of temperature, like having an ice cream or a hot cup of tea.

The concept of remaining dentine thickness (RDT) is of paramount importance in preventing hypersensitivity and pain. Dental caries reduces the dentin thickness and hence the protection afforded against extremes of temperature variations is hampered. Needless to say that dental caries is an infection with organisms like *Streptococcus mutans* and *Lactobacillus acidophilus*. Dental caries, if unattended, is progressive and can lead to irreversible damage of the pulp and its attendant complications.

The periphery of the pulp is lined by odontoblasts which send their protoplasmic processes into the dentin. Cavities placed closer to the pulp could injure underlying odontoblasts (Murray et al. 2002).

There is a subodontoblastic nerve plexus in the dental pulp called the plexus of Raschkow. The density of free nerve endings in the dental pulp is very high compared to other parts of the body, and this accounts for the severe pain felt during tooth infection. Each tooth can be innervated by about 1000 afferent sensory nociceptive neurons which branch extensively.

The tooth dentine has A-beta fibers and A-delta fibers which modulate tactile and pain sensation. The pulp has A-delta and C fibers. The C fibers are polymodal and can respond to mechanical stimulation, cooling, heating, and chemical stimuli in the form of pain.

Conditions affecting the dental pulp as a sequelae to dental caries are pulp hyperemia, acute pulpitis, chronic pulpitis, and acute periapical abscess.

Diseases Affecting the Pulp

Clinical insults such as dental caries, dental trauma, and dental operative procedures can cause pulp tissue breakdown and painful symptoms in dental pulp (Bergenholtz 1990).

Pulp Hyperemia

A very typical acute pain is felt due to cold or hot stimulus which is transient and the pain subsides after removal of the stimulus. This condition is reversible if promptly treated.

Acute Pulpitis

Acute pulpitis results in a throbbing pain in the tooth, and the pain is severe on application of hot or cold stimulus. The condition is called irreversible pulpitis when the dental pulp undergoes degeneration and necrosis. This requires investigation like dental x-rays to visualize the extent of damage and determine the need for root canal treatment and restorative care. The pain increases in the supine position.

Acute Periapical Abscess

Once periapical pathology sets in, the tissues surrounding the tooth (including the alveolar bone) are affected, culminating in liquefaction necrosis and formation of a tooth abscess. The abscess can present as a dental emergency with varying degrees of cellulitis and fascial space infection.

The tooth in question is tender to touch and there is increase in local temperature. The patient may present with pyrexia and regional lymphadenitis with inability to chew on the affected side. Infection with periorbital edema due to an upper premolar or molar infection needs urgent attention for infection and pain control.

The root apices of the lower second molar are anatomically located in the bone more caudal than the mylohyoid muscle, also known as the oral diaphragm. An infected lower second molar has the propensity to trigger a space infection called Ludwig's angina.

Ludwig's angina is an emergency and presents with boardlike rigidity of the floor of the mouth, with elevation of the tongue and respiratory embarrassment, pyrexia, pain, and swelling of the face. The condition requires hospitalization and management by a maxillofacial surgeon.

Miscellaneous Dental Conditions Causing Pain
Trauma from Occlusion

The teeth undergo physiological wear with age, and the surface of the grinders, namely the premolars and molars undergoes uneven wear. This can lead to pernicious wear facets which produce lateral forces termed parafunctional forces. These parafunctional forces affect the attachment apparatus of the tooth. The suspensory ligament of the tooth, the periodontal ligament, undergoes varying degrees of damage. Forces greater than 100 pounds per square inch can be generated in the interdigitating molar areas. A high filling or a foreign body encountered during chewing can also cause trauma from occlusion. The tooth is tender with inability to chew on the affected side. The condition is generally reversible unless simultaneously affected by progressive inflammatory gum disease.

Wasting Diseases of the Teeth

These are grouped as attrition, abrasion, and erosion and can be a source of pain.

Loss of tooth substance reduces the RDT giving rise to persistent pain and sensitivity in the affected teeth. Tooth brush abrasion can cause the gum margin to recede and expose the root surface, causing gingival recession. Incorrect brushing technique is the culprit. Gingival recession can lead to cervical hypersensitivity and cosmetic insult. Sensitivity at the necks of the teeth can be persistent and annoying.

Hyperemesis gravidarum in the first trimester of pregnancy can cause the acidic vomitus to erode the lingual surfaces of the upper front teeth, leading to sensitivity and dental erosion. Soft drinks can also be a cause of erosion. Another cause for attrition is audible bruxism. Bruxers generally grind their teeth at night and wear out the occlusal surfaces, which leads to increased sensitivity. Bruxism is a parafunctional oral habit, which has a psychosomatic etiology. The patient requires multidisciplinary management to address psychological stress and dental management. It is generally the partner who hears the grinding sound and this input could be valuable in diagnosis.

Pathological Painful Lesions Affecting Oral Soft Tissues

Oral Ulcers

Ulcers in the mouth can be a cause of severe recurrent pain. The various ulcers can be grouped as recurrent oral aphthae, acute herpetic gingival stomatitis, acute candidiasis, and acute necrotizing ulcerative gingivitis. Aphthous ulcer is recurrent, stress induced, and painful. Diagnosis is clinical. A large aphthous ulcer is designated a major aphthous and heals by scarring.

Viral infection due to herpes simplex virus I occurs in children and presents with vesicles which rupture and cause ulcers. These are painful during the course of the disease. Affected children are prone to dehydration, and hence prompt attention to monitor the child during the acute phase is necessary.

Radiation-Induced Mucositis

Radiation treatment for oral cancer can cause dryness of the mouth due to reduced salivary secretion. The normal lubrication function of the saliva is compromised, leading to pain and inflammation. Osteoradionecrosis is due to radiation for oral cancer treatment and can induce endarteritis. Any minor trauma leads to infection with debilitating consequences.

Autoimmune Diseases

Diseases such as oral lichen planus pemphigus and cicatricial pemphigoid can all cause oral ulcers which are painful and affect the quality of life.

Acute Pericoronitis

This is a relatively common condition and is defined as the inflammation of the soft tissues around an erupting tooth. The patient may present with pain and trismus. Fascial space infection and peritonsillar abscess are potential complications. This condition is often associated with an impacted tooth.

Oral Conditions Affecting Hard and Soft Tissues

Periodontal Diseases

Gum disease is a chronic disease which can manifest with potential ulcerated pus pockets. This is a chronic inflammatory disease initiated by oral bacteria and sustained by the host immune response. Chronic gum disease is characterized by the absence of acute pain as a warning signal, and this in turn could lead to destruction of periodontal tissues by the disease process without the patient being aware of it. However, exacerbation of a chronic lesion can produce varying degrees of pain. Hence the need for preventive checkup to detect disease is important.

The bacterial plaque on the teeth surface functions as a biofilm, which is firmly adhering and has an organized structure which ultimately causes a recalcitrant anaerobic infection.

Dental plaque, being a complex mixture of antigens, elicits an immune response and causes the host cells to secrete enzymes and toxins which destroy the tooth-supporting bone. The teeth become loose and there is discomfort in chewing; eventually the patient risks losing his/her teeth. The major risk factors for periodontal disease are male gender, smoking, stress, and poor oral hygiene.

Dry Socket

This is a painful condition which occurs following dental extraction. The clot is lost due to inadvertent forceful rinsing, leading to osteitis.

Oral Conditions and Remote Systemic Effects

Periodontal Disease, Preterm Low Birth Weight, and Cardiac Disease

The emergence of a new discipline of periodontal medicine toward the end of the last millennium has driven researchers to explore the propensity of chronic inflammatory gum disease in modulating preterm births, still births, and intrauterine growth restriction.

Needless to say that acute periodontal abscesses can cause rapid destruction of alveolar jaw bone and cause pain and oral disability. Epidemiological data show a trend that mothers with poor periodontal health are at risk of producing preterm babies.

Paquette et al. (1999) have shown that cord blood from pregnant mothers with gum disease shows a higher titer of IgM antibodies to specific oral bacteria than do periodontally healthy mothers. It is of interest to note that chronic gingivitis is reversible if treated, but periodontitis which involves tooth socket bone loss is chronic and essentially irreversible. The latter condition has a prevalence of between 8 and 20% in different populations. Studies by Beck et al. (2002) revealed an association between gum disease and heart disease. Periodontal disease causes an elevation of C reactive proteins in the blood.

Notwithstanding the multifactorial nature of cardiac disease and preterm anomalies, chronic inflammatory gum disease can induce a "bandwagon effect" in susceptible patients and hamper the quality of life and have an influence on longevity as well.

However, robust research evidence is needed to implicate periodontal disease as a major culprit. Preventive oral health and dental pain management have become a priority in these special groups of patients as an integral part of antenatal care and cardiac rehabilitation programs.

Musculoskeletal Pains

Temporomandibular Joint Pain

The mandible is the movable member of the stomatognathic system and articulates with the skull with the help of the temporomandibular joint. Joint pathologies can cause pain, clicking, dislocation, and subluxation which can interfere with optimal function.

Intractable Pain

Burning Mouth Syndrome

This occurs mainly in female patients after menopause. A neuropathic relationship has been suggested (Forssell et al. 2002). This may be accompanied with glossodynia or glossopyrosis.

Neuralgias

Trigeminal neuralgia can present as pain in the teeth, often described as cutting or stabbing in nature. This can often be confused with atypical facial pain (Türp and Gobetti 2002).

Atypical Odontalgia

Phantom toothache occurs in an area where the tooth is extracted. This occurs in women and is termed atypical odontalgia. Emotionally labile women are more prone to this condition.

Diagnosis

Pain as a modality has the perceptual component, the visceral component, the emotional component, and the referral component. A careful history of pain, its duration, frequency, character, intensity, radiation, and exacerbating factors are significant inputs to decide on the strategy of pain control. Ulcers due to autoimmune diseases can be diagnosed by incisional biopsy which aids in microscopic and immunological evaluation. X-rays with intraoral films, panoramic views of the jaws, magnetic resonance imaging of the temporomandibular joints, and cone beam computerized tomograms are used to aid in diagnosis. These aids help in delineating the extent of bony pathology giving rise to the plethora of symptoms which includes pain.

Electromyography is used to study the activity of the masticatory muscles. Electric pulp tester is used to monitor the sensitivity of the pulp. Hemograms aid in planning surgical procedures for the gums. A local anesthetic can clinch the diagnosis of pain on the affected side if administering it abolishes the sensation of pain at that point in time.

Management of Oro-Dental Pain

Dental Hypersensitivity

Periodic 6-monthly preventive visits to the dentist go a long way in preventive pain management. Dentine hypersensitivity is treated by in-office application of unfilled resin and photopolymerization and fluoride application with 2% sodium fluoride. Commercially available fluoride varnishes such as Duraphat® can be used in the office. Over-the-counter pastes such as Sensoform® and Sensodyne® are available. Trowbridge and Silver (1990) have recommended the use of cavity varnishes, calcium hydroxide, potassium oxalate, fluoride compounds, and restorative resins for desensitization among other agents.

Avoiding cross-brushing will prevent gingival recession and protect the thin cementum at the neck of the teeth. Acute toothache can be treated with local anesthetic block injections for temporary relief. Local anesthesia can be administered with 2% lidocaine hydrochloride with 1:80,000 epinephrine. Non-steroidal anti-inflammatory agents such as ibuprofen and ketorolac can be used to control pain. Standard dosages should be reduced when used in children and the geriatric population. It is important to take timely medication for pain control to maintain the therapeutic blood level.

Control of Pain in the Dental Operating Suite

Preanesthetic medication is medication administered prior to the induction of local anesthesia. The main rationale is to anxiety. A benzodiazepine such as diazepam 5 mg (adult patients) is administered orally 1 h before the procedure. Atropine 0.3 mg may be given intramuscularly in case of excessive salivary secretion. Ambulatory patients must be advised not to drive after a dental procedure if sedating premedication was used. Nitrous oxide–oxygen conscious sedation may be employed. Indications for conscious sedation are mild pain, fear and anxiety, excessive gag reflex, and prolonged treatment time (Paarman and Royer 2008).

Treatment of Acute Pulpitis

Tooth abscesses are drained by making an opening in the tooth under local anesthesia. Root canal treatment is done with an inert material – gutta percha, which seals the pulp canal space. Special injections called periodontal ligament injections can be employed for individual tooth anesthesia.

Management of Ulcers

Viral infections with herpes can be managed with oral Acyclovir 200 mg five times daily for 5 days along with oral non-opioid analgesics. Fungal infections such as angular cheilitis can be managed with Mycostatin ointment, while denture sore mouth can be managed with nystatin oral solution.

Aphthous ulcers can be treated with triamcinolone acetonide in an 0.1% orabase-topical application. Alternative stress reduction strategies such as meditation and yoga can be employed. Vitamin B complex is often prescribed to forestall micronutrient deficiencies. Bruxism can be managed with night bite guards and dental crowns.

Management of Temporomandibular Joint Pain

Improper occlusion of the teeth can precipitate pain in the jaw joints. Ultrasound is useful for the alleviation of pain arising from a temporomandibular disorder (TMD). Occlusal splints can give relief for jaw joint pain, and resisted jaw exercises can help strengthen the joints. Tricyclic antidepressants (amitriptyline) have been reported to have analgesic effects in the management of TMD by blocking reuptake of noradrenaline and serotonin. A second mechanism attributed is the antagonistic effects on NMDA receptors (Feinmann 1985).

Management of Oral Ulcers in Autoimmune Disease

A dermatological referral to assess the lesion is often necessary. The oral lesion could be a stand-alone lesion or be a part of chronic dermatosis. Topical application of fluocinonide 0.05% and oral steroids in the appropriately titrated dosages is the mainstay of treatment. Appropriate dosages of steroids are started and gradually decreased in a step-down manner. Pain control can be done by application of orabase (carboxymethyl cellulose) and mouth rinse containing diphenhydramine. Side effects of systemic steroids warrant that the steroid regimen should be monitored by a dermatologist.

Radiation Mucositis

Radiation mucositis can be treated with topical application of carboxymethyl cellulose and topical application of benzocaine 20%.

Management of Osteoradionecrosis

All infected teeth in the line of radiation are extracted prior to commencement of radiation therapy. At least 2 months are given for extraction sockets to heal. Prevention of radiation caries is effected by application of topical fluoride to the teeth.

Management of Neuropathic Pain

Pain caused by a lesion of the peripheral or central nervous system is commonly termed neuropathic pain. This could be a source of pain in the teeth along the course of the nerve which innervates the teeth on the ipsilateral side of the jaw. Fractures of jaw bones can cause injury to the nerves. This can result in neuropraxia or neurotmesis leading to paresthesia, resulting in patient biting on the tongue and causing traumatic ulcers.

Trigeminal neuralgia responds to treatment with carbamazepine. Monitoring of plasma concentrations is important to prevent unwanted side effects. Mental nerve avulsion under local anesthesia gives pain relief for variable periods of time. Phenytoin sodium has also been used for pain relief in trigeminal neuralgia as a second line of treatment. However, supplementation with folic acid is important.

Management of Acute Pericoronitis

The offending impacted tooth has to be extracted. Trismus is treated with methocarbamol, and metronidazole can be given to treat an infection. Gentle debridement is carried out under the operculum to clear food debris.

Management of Dry Socket

The socket is irrigated with saline and any slough removed. Whiteheads varnish may be helpful, and non-steroidal anti-inflammatory drugs could be used for pain relief.

Management of Burning Mouth Syndrome

This is a difficult condition to treat, and reassurance is important. Possible causes implicated are chronic infections, reflux of stomach acid, hormone imbalances, and medication side effects (Gorsky et al. 1991).

Management of Periodontal Disease

Gum disease is managed by good preventive care such as brushing, flossing, use of oral irriga-
tor, and regular scale and polish. It is imperative to schedule an appointment with the dentist.
Pain due to periodontal surgery can be managed by non-steroidal anti-inflammatory agents.
Regular use of essential oil mouth washes and diet containing citrus fruits and vegetables
helps reducing halitosis. The tongue is the principal site for the collection of volatile sulphur
compounds. Hence tongue cleaning should be an integral part of any oral hygiene regimen
to reduce the bacterial count.

Summary

This chapter has reviewed the causes of oro-dental pain and its management. The key to
successful pain control is early diagnosis so that carious cavities are filled and incipient gum
disease is treated before it becomes chronic. The loss of tooth substance as a major cause of
hypersensitivity is emphasized. Early treatment of painful conditions helps prevent the phenomenon of peripheral and central sensitization (Greene 2009). Regular dental screening as
an integral part of antenatal check for pregnant mothers would be an effective strategy for
preventive pain management (Paarmann and Royer 2008). Qualitative research across pain
clinic settings needs to be carried out to collect data and set strategies for optimal pain management pertaining to outcomes in quality-of-life parameters (Sessle et al. 2008). Table 33.1
reviews the therapeutic management of oral pain.

Table 33.1 Therapeutic management of oral pain.

Clinical manifestation	Class of drug	Name of drug	Dose	Route of administration
Dental caries prevention	Topical fluorides	Neutral sodium fluoride gel 1.0%	In-office procedure	Topical
Xerostomia	Saliva stimulants	Pilocarpine hydrochloride 5-mg tablets	1 tablet t.i.d.	Oral
Radiation mucositis	Topical anesthetic	Dyclonine HCL 0.5 %	1 teaspoonful rinse three times and expel	Topical
	Alkaline saline (salt bicarbonate)	Half teaspoonful salt and baking soda in water	Rinse four times a day with copious amount	Topical
Autoimmune disease – erosive lichen planus pemphigus	Topical steroids	Dexamethasone elixir 0.5 mg/5 ml	15 ml q.i.d. rinse and swallow 3 days; gradual step down till asymptomatic	Topical/oral
	Systemic steroids	Dexamethasone phosphate	4 mg/ml inject 1 ml around lesion after LA twice a week	Injectable Intralesional for severe oral lesions
Gingival enlargement	Vitamins oral rinse	Folic acid oral rinse	1 mg/ml rinse l teaspoonful b.i.d. and expel	Topical
Burning mouth syndrome	Antihistamine	Diphenhydramine elixir 12.5 mg/5 ml	Rinse 1 teaspoonful 2 min three times/swallow	Oral/topical
	Antidepressants	Amitriptyline tablet 25 mg	one tablet h.s. for 1 week increase to 3 tablets – maintain	Oral

Case Scenario

Dr. Suresh Menon, MBBS, DA, FRCA and Sreekumar Kunnumpurath, MBBS, MD, FCARCSI, FRCA, FFPMRCA

Melinda is a 19-year-old university student who is suffering from left-sided facial pain. The pain began a week ago and was of gradual onset. She initially felt it on the side of her face, in front of her left ear. Her primary care physician noted that there was a slight tenderness over the front of her left ear. Her external auditory meatus appeared normal and during the examination of her ear when traction was applied on the pinna, she jumped from pain. She had an elevated white cell count and a diagnosis of otitis externa was made. She was sent home with advice to take acetaminophen for pain and antibiotics to control infection.

A few days later she returns to her PCP complaining that the pain is worse and she cannot open her mouth. The PCP immediately decides to refer the patient to you, a dental surgeon. On arrival to your clinic you examine her and note that she is febrile and has visible swelling on the left side of her cheek.

What is the possible diagnosis?
Melinda could be suffering from a dental abscess or she could have an impacted wisdom tooth. In order to arrive at a diagnosis, you need to obtain a detailed history, perform a physical examination, and then order appropriate investigations.

Melinda tells you that she cannot open her mouth because of pain. You examine Melinda in the dental chair. In spite of pain, she is able to cooperate with your dental examination. You manage to visualize the oral cavity and note that her gums are swollen. You can see that she has an infected lower molar tooth. Furthermore, the pus extruding from the margins of the gum is visible.

How would you confirm the diagnosis?
Confirmation of diagnosis can be done by taking a dental x-ray. It also helps to assess the extent of the disease process and help with treatment planning. You decide that the abscess needs to be drained immediately to avoid the spread of inflammation.

Describe your perioperative pain management?
Immediate dental pain control can be achieved with simple analgesics such as acetaminophen, ibuprofen, or ketorolac (intravenous). Ketorolac has the advantage of parenteral administration. In severe cases when the above medications fail to control pain, you can consider prescribing an opioid such as vicodin or percocet. Once the acute pain has subsided, drainage of the abscess can be undertaken in the dental chair or in an operating room with appropriate antibiotic coverage. In the dental chair, Entonox (nitrous oxide-oxygen mix) or a dental nerve block using local anesthetic can be employed for the treatment. The local anesthetic technique can provide variable duration of postoperative pain relief, depending on the agents used. If Melinda prefers a general anesthetic then the procedure may need to be undertaken in an operating room. Drainage of the abscess itself would reduce the postoperative analgesic requirement, and this could be often achieved with simple analgesics such as acetaminophen or NSAIDs.

To prevent dental pain from recurring, the dental specialist may have to carry out definitive procedures such as filling the caries, root canal treatment, or extraction of non-salvageable teeth. The importance of oral hygiene in preventing dental and oral disease should be emphasized.

References

Beck J, Elter J, Heiss G, Couper D, Mauriello S, Offenbacher S. Relationship of periodontal disease to carotid artery intima-media wall thickness: the atherosclerosis risk in communities (ARIC) study. Arterioscler Thromb Vasc Biol. 2001 Nov;21(11):1816–22.

Bergenholtz G. Pathogenic mechanisms in pulpal disease. J Endod. 1990 Feb;16(2):98–101.

Clark G. Persistent orodental pain, atypical odontalgia, and phantom tooth pain: when are they neuropathic disorders? J Calif Dent Assoc. 2006 Aug;34(8):599–609.

Feinmann C. Pain relief by antidepressants: possible modes of action. Pain 1985 Sep;23(1): 1–8.

Forssell H, Jääskeläinen S, Tenovuo O, Hinkka S. Sensory dysfunction in burning mouth syndrome. Pain 2002 Sep;99(1–2):41–7.

Gorsky M, Silverman SJ, Chinn H. Clinical characteristics and management outcome in the burning mouth syndrome. An open study of 130 patients. Oral Surg Oral Med Oral Pathol. 1991 Aug;72(2):192–5.

Greene C. Neuroplasticity and sensitization. J Am Dent Assoc. 2009 Jun;140(6):676–8.

Murray P, About I, Lumley P, Franquin J, Remusat M, Smith A. Cavity remaining dentin thickness and pulpal activity. Am J Dent. 2002 Feb;15(1):41–6.

Paarman C, Royer R. Pain control for dental practitioners. In: Paarman C, Royer R, editors. An interactive approach. Lippincott Williams and Wilkins, Baltimore, MD, 2008.

Paquette D, Madianos P, Offenbacher S, Beck J, Williams R. The concept of "risk" and the emerging discipline of periodontal medicine. J Contemp Dent Pract. 1999 Nov;1(1):1–8.

Sessle BJ, Lavigne GJ, Lund JP, Dubner R. eds. Orofacial pain-from basic science to clinical management: the transfer of knowledge in pain research to education. Quintessence Publishing Co Inc, Hanover Park, IL; 2008.

Trowbridge H, Silver D. A review of current approaches to in-office management of tooth hypersensitivity. Dent Clin North Am. 1990 Jul;34(3):561–81.

Türp J, Gobetti J. Trigeminal neuralgia – an update. Compend Contin Educ Dent. 2000 Apr;21(4):279–82, 84, 87–8 passim; quiz 92.

Chapter 34

Drug Formulary for Pain Management

Anita Hickey, MD and Ian Laughlin, MD

Opioids

The use of opioids as the most effective treatment for moderate to severe acute pain and cancer pain is well established. This is in part due to their predictable dose-dependent response, lack of ceiling effect, and predictable production of profound analgesia with progressive dose escalation. Long-term use of opioids does not result in organ toxicity with the exception of methadone and toxic metabolites of meperidine, morphine, and proproxyphene. Escalation of dose is associated with side effects which increase proportionately in the acute pain setting. The side effects may differ according to the opioid administered, due to mediation of both analgesia, and adverse side effects by the mu opioid receptor (Intrurrisi and Lipman 2009).

The choice to administer opioids in chronic benign pain remains controversial. Opioids have been shown to significantly reduce pain as well as improve mood and function in chronic nonmalignant pain, including neuropathic, nociceptive, and mixed pain. However, no quality long-term studies greater than 16 weeks have been performed (Gallagher and Rosenthal 2008).

Iatrogenic addiction of individuals is reported to vary between 0.05 and 32% depending on the medical setting, the patient population served, and the presence of risk factors such as a history of addiction or drug abuse. Long-term opioid use can be effective and safe when established opioid guidelines are followed (Gallagher and Rosenthal 2008).

It is clinically useful to classify opioids as weak or strong depending on their relative efficacy. Weak opioids are used for moderate or less severe pain, and their efficacy is limited by an increased incidence of side effects at higher doses [e.g., nausea and constipation with codeine, and central nervous system (CNS) excitation with propoxyphene].

Some opioids have analgesic actions limited to the mu, kappa, and delta opioid receptors. For purposes of acute pain management, the mu opioid agonist agents are the primary drugs of choice. Opioids that are more useful in chronic pain and neuropathic pain have analgesic effects not only at the mu opioid receptor but are also enhanced by actions as N-methyl-D-acetate (NMDA) receptor antagonists, and by central neuromodulating effects through inhibition of reuptake of serotonin and norepinephrine similar to many antidepressants. Some opioids have all three properties (e.g., methadone). The common opioids used in practice are divided as to their mu opioids actions vs. NMDA receptor antagonism and hormonal reuptake inhibitory actions, and are listed in Table 34.1. The strong mu agonists

N. Vadivelu et al. (eds.), *Essentials of Pain Management,*
DOI 10.1007/978-0-387-87579-8_34, © Springer Science+Business Media, LLC 2011

Table 34.1 Broad spectrum versus narrow spectrum opioid analgesics.

Broad-Spectrum opioids with NMDA receptor blocking action	Broad-spectrum opioids which inhibit reuptake of serotonin and norepinephrine	Narrow-Spectrum opioids with analgesic action limited as mu opioid agonist
Methadone	Methadone	Morphine
Ketobemidone	Levorphanol	Hydromorphone
Dextroproxyphene	Dextromethorphan	Codeine
Dextromethorphan	D-Propoxyphene	Etorphine
Meperidine (pethidine)	Tramadol	Fentanyl
	Meperidine (pethidine)	Sufentanyl
		Oxycodone
		Hydrocodone
		Buprenorphine

NMDA= N-methyl-D-acetate.
With permission from Morley (1999).

and mixed agonist–antagonist opioids are listed together with important characteristics and properties in Table 34.2. Patient-controlled analgesia (PCA) dosing for opioids commonly used for acute postoperative pain control is listed in Table 34.3.

Many of the common oral opioids are used in fixed dose combinations with nonopioid analgesics. The efficacy of these agents is limited by the maximal safe dose for the acetaminophen, aspirin, or nonsteroidal anti-inflammatory drugs (NSAIDs) component. The most common preparations of the combination opioids are listed in Table 34.4 emphasizing the maximum dosage based on the adjuvant medication. If the patient requires a higher dose of opioids than would be allowed in the combination drug, it would be better to prescribe a pure opioid and permit the patient to supplement with NSAIDs or acetaminophen in appropriate doses at regular intervals. Even standard dosing of NSAID medications may result in toxicity in patients with impaired renal and hepatic function, with greater than moderate chronic alcohol use, and in malnourished or dehydrated children (Mazer and Perrone 2008, Chun et al. 2009, Amar and Schiff 2007). NSAID dosage information, classification by mechanism, and important characteristics are listed in Table 34.5.

Opioid conversion

The following formula is used to convert one opioid to another using the conversion factor.

$$\frac{\text{Dose of current medication}}{\text{Conversion factor of current medication}} = \frac{\text{Dose of new medication}}{\text{Conversion factor of new medication}}$$

For example, patient has used 42 mg of IV morphine in the last 24 h. To convert to oral morphine equivalent:

$$\frac{42\,\text{mg IV morphine}}{10\,\text{mg IV morphine}} = \frac{?\,\text{dose of PO morphine}}{30\,\text{mg PO morphine}}$$

Table 34.2 Strong mu Opioids, Agonist-Antagonist Opioids, and Partial u Agonists with Morphine Dosing Equivalents and Important Characteristics.

Opioid analgesics commonly used for severe pain

Name	Equianalgesic Parenteral Dose (mg)	Parenteral/oral Potency (mg) (Conversion Factor)	Starting oral Dose range (mg)	Plasma Half-Life (h)	Epidural Conversion Factor	Intrathecal Conversion Factor	Comments	Precautions
Morphine	10	30	30–60/24 h in divided doses	2–4	1 mg	0.1 mg	Standard of comparison for opioid analgesics. Extended-release preparations available	Those with impaired ventilation, bronchial asthma, increased intracranial pressure, and liver and renal failure. Lower doses for elderly
Hydromorphone	2	8	4–8	2–3	0.4 mg	0.08 mg	Slightly shorter acting. High-potency parenteral dosage form for tolerant patients	Like morphine
Methadone	1		5–10	13–50	–	–	Good oral potency. Long but variable plasma half-life. Rotation dose depends on prior opioid dosage. May prolong QT interval in non-dose-dependent manner in susceptible individuals	Like morphine. May accumulate with repetitive dosing causing excessive sedation. For conversion in morphine equivalents for chronic use, use 6:1 ratio, (morphine to methadone equivalents) with baseline and postdosing ECGs
Propoxyphene	–	200	32–65	3.5	–	–	"Weak" opioid; often used in combination with nonopioid analgesics	Cumulative with repeated doses; convulsions with overdose
Levorphanol	2	4	2–4	12–16	–	–	Like methadone	Like methadone
Oxycodone	–	20	5–20	2–4	–	–	Immediate release and extended release oral dosage forms. Also available as rectal suppository	Like morphine
Meperidine	100	300	Not recommended	3–4	–	–	Slightly shorter acting than morphine. Used orally for less severe pain	Normeperidine metabolite can cause CNS excitation and seizures with repeated dosing for longer than 24 h. Avoid in renal insufficiency and those taking MAOIs
Codeine	75	130	30–60	3	–	–	Used orally in combination with nonopioids for less severe pain	Like morphine
Hydrocodone	–	30	2.5–10	3.5–4.5	–	–	Used orally in combination with nonopioids for less severe pain	Like morphine

Table 34.2 (Continued)

Opioid analgesics commonly used for severe pain

Name	Equianalgesic Parenteral Dose (mg)	Parenteral/oral Potency (mg) (Conversion Factor)	Starting oral Dose range (mg)	Plasma Half-Life (h)	Epidural Conversion Factor	Intrathecal Conversion Factor	Comments	Precautions
Mixed agonist–antagonists								
Pentazocine	60	3	See comments	2–3	–	–	Used orally for less severe pain. A mixed agonist–antagonist	May cause psychomimetic effects. May precipitate withdrawal in opioid-dependent patients. Not for myocardial infarction patients
Nalbuphine	10	See comments	See comments	5	–	–	Not available orally. Like parenteral pentazocine but not scheduled drug	Incidence of psychomimetic effects lower than with pentazocine
Butorphanol	2	See comments	See comments	2.5–3.5	–	–	Not available orally. Like parenteral nalbuphine	Like nalbuphine
Partial mu agonists								
Buprenorphine	0.3	See comments	See comments	3–5	–	–	Not available orally. Only parenteral form approved in the United States for pain. Does not produce psychomimetic effects	May precipitate withdrawal in opioid-dependent patients. Not readily reversed by naloxone. Avoid in labor
Novel synthetic dual-action opioids								
Tapentadol (Nucynta)®	See comments	See comments	50–100 mg Q4–6 h maximum 600 mg daily	4	–	–	Centrally acting analgesic. Dual mode of action with agonist activity at μ-opioid receptor and norepinephrine reuptake inhibitor activity. Considered to have potency between tramadol and morphine	Use caution in patients with decreased liver function, (starting dose of 50 mg PO limited to 50 mg PO TID)
Tramadol (Ultram)®	See comments	See comments	50–100 mg Q 6 h maximum 400 mg daily		–	–	Weak μ-opioid agonist and norepinephrine and serotonin reuptake inhibitor action. In animal models, M1 metabolite up to six times more potent than tramadol in producing analgesia and 200 times more potent in μ-opioid binding	Increased risk of seizures and serotonin syndrome at doses over 400 mg daily and in combination with TCA, SSRI, and MAOI medications

SSRI = selective serotonin reuptake inhibitors; MAOIs = monoamine oxidase inhibitors; TCA = tricyclic antidepressants; CNS = central nervous system; ECG = electrocardiogram.
Adapted from Bonica's management of pain. 4th ed. Ch. 78, pp. 1174–9.

Table 34.3 Intravenous Patient-Controlled Analgesia (PCA) Regimens for Acute Pain.

Medication	Pharmacodynamics	Bolus	Lockout interval (min)
Morphine	Mu opioid receptor agonist	0.5–2.5 mg	5–10
Fentanyl	Mu opioid receptor agonist	10–20 mcg	5–10
Hydromorphone	Mu opioid receptor agonist	0.25–0.5 mg	5–10
Alfentanil	Mu opioid receptor agonist	0.1–0.2 mg	5–8
Methadone	Mu opioid receptor agonist; NMDA receptor antagonist	0.5–2.5 mg	8–20
Meperidine	Mu opioid receptor agonist	5–25 mg	5–10
Oxymorphone	Mu opioid receptor agonist	0.2–0.4 mg	8–10
Buprenorphine	Mu opioid receptor partial agonist; kappa opioid receptor antagonist	0.03–0.1 mg	8–20
Nalbuphine	mu opioid receptor antagonist; kappa opioid receptor agonist	1–5 mg	5–15
Pentazocine	Mu opioid receptor antagonist; kappa opioid receptor agonist	5–15 mg	5–15

All doses are for adult patients. The anesthesiologist should proceed with titrated intravenous loading doses if necessary to establish initial analgesia. Individual patient's requirements vary widely, with smaller doses typically given for elderly or compromised patients. Continuous infusions are not initially recommended for opioid-naive adult patients.
Adapted from Bonica's management of pain. 4th ed. Ch. 51, p. 706.

Table 34.4 Combination opioids available for oral administration.

Trade name	Opioid component	Dose of opioid (mg)	Adjuvant drug	Dose of adjuvant (mg)	Tablets/capsules per day
Advil®	–	–	Ibuprofen	200	12
E.S. Tylenol®	–	–	Acetaminophen	500	8
Tylenol-3®	Codeine	30	Acetaminophen	300	13
Tylenol-4®	Codeine	60	Acetaminophen	300	13
Darvon®	Propoxyphene	65	–	–	No limit
Darvocet®	Propoxyphene	65	Acetaminophen	325	13
Darvocet N-100®	Propoxyphene	100	Acetaminophen	325	13
Vicodin®	Hydrocodone	5	Acetaminophen	500	8
Vicodin ES®	Hydrocodone	7.5	Acetaminophen	750	5
Lortab Elix®	Hydrocodone	7.5	Acetaminophen	500	8
Lorcet 10/650®	Hydrocodone	10	Acetaminophen	650	6
Norco®	Hydrocodone	10	Acetaminophen	325	13
Vicoprofen®	Hydrocodone	7.5	Ibuprofen	200	12
Percodan®	Oxycodone	5	Aspirin	325	6
Percocet®	Oxycodone	5 or 10	Acetaminophen	325	13
Tylox®	Oxycodone	5	Acetaminophen	500	8
Oxycodone®	Oxycodone	5	–	–	No limit
Ultram®	Tramadol	50	–	–	8
Ultracet®	Tramadol	37.5	Acetaminophen	325	10

With the exception of tramadol containing products, the dose is limited by the adjuvant, not the opioid component. The maximum doses should be reduced in the elderly or in the presence of liver or renal insufficiency. Notice that the oral equivalent for 10 mg of intravenous morphine is 30 mg of oral hydrocodone. But when hydrocodone is combined with acetaminophen, the ratio is such that a toxic dose of acetaminophen would be taken with the hydrocodone. It is better to convert to a pure immediate release opioid agonist until such time that it is established that a reasonable dose of combination medication can be given safely.

Table 34.5   NSAID Classification and dosing.

Acetaminophen and nonsteroidal anti-inflammatory drugs (NSAIDs) available in the United States

Medication	Proprietary (Trade) name	Half-Life (h)	% Protein bound	Usual 24-h adult dose range	Adult daily dose and frequency		Usual Daily pediatric dose mg/kg/per 24 h
					Dosage	Schedule	
Para-Aminophenol derivative							
Acetaminophen	Tylenol, others	2	20–50	2–4 g	325–650 mg / 650 mg–1 g	q4h / QID	Dose varies with body weight and age
Salicylates							
Aspirin	Multiple	2–3	~90	2.4–6 g	600–1,500 mg	QID	80–100 mg/kg/24 h
Choline	Trilisate	2–3	90	1.5–3 g	500–1,000 mg	TID	50–65 mg/kg/24 h
magnesium trisalicylate	Tricosal				750–1,500	BID	
Diflunisal	Dolobid	8–12	99	1–1.5 g	500–750 mg	BID	NA
Salsalate	Disalcid	1	90	1.5–3 g	750–1,500 mg	BID	NA
Propionic acid derivatives							
Fenoprofen	Nalfon	2	99	1.2–2.4 g	300–600 mg	QID	900 mg–1.8 g per body surface area (m²)
Flurbiprofen	Ansaid	2	99	200 mg	100 mg	BID	NA
Ibuprofen	Motrin, Advil, others	6	99	1.2–2.4 g (pain) 2.4–3.2 g (inflammation)	OTC: 200–400 mg Rx: 400, 600, 800 mg	QID	30–40 mg/kg/day as 3–4 doses
Ketoprofen	Orudis	2–4	99	225 mg	75 mg	TID	NA
Naproxen	Naprosyn, others	14	99	750 mg–1 g	250, 375, 500 mg	BID	10–20 mg/kg/24 h as two doses
Oxaprozin	Daypro	40–60	99	1.2 g	1.2 g	Once daily	10–20 mg/kg/24 h

Table 34.5 (Continued)

Acetaminophen and nonsteroidal anti-inflammatory drugs (NSAIDs) available in the United States

Medication	Proprietary (Trade) name	Half-Life (h)	% Protein bound	Usual 24-h adult dose range	Dosage	Schedule	Usual Daily pediatric dose mg/kg/per 24 h
Fenamates							
Meclofenamate	Meclomen	2–3	99	150–400 mg	50–100 mg	TID, QID	NA
Diclofenac	Voltaren, in Arthrotec	1–2	99	150–200 mg	50 mg / 75 mg	TID / BID	2–3 mg/kg/24 h
Tolmetin	Tolectin	5	99	800–2,400 mg	400, 600, 800 mg	TID, QID	20–30 mg/kg/24 h as 3–4 doses
Ketorolac	Toradol	4–6	99	Oral: not >60 mg/day; Parenteral 30–60 mg, then 15–30 mg	Oral: 10 mg q6h for not >5 days total	QID	IV: 0.5 mg/kg/day single dose only; IM: 1 mg/kg/day single dose only
Mefenamic acid	Ponstel	3–4	99	1.0–4.0 g	250 mg	QID	NA
Enolic acid derivatives (Oxicams)							
Meloxicam	Mobic	15–20	99	7.5–15 mg	7.5 mg (OA); 15 mg (RA)	Once daily / Once daily	NA
Piroxicam	Feldene	40–50	99	20 mg	10, 20 mg	Once daily	NA
Nabumetone	Relafen	24	99	1.0–1.5 g	500–750 mg	BID	NA
Acetic acid derivatives							
Etodolac	Lodine	7	99	400–1,200 mg	200–300 mg maximum: 1,200 mg	BID, TID, QID	15–20 mg/kg/24 h
Indomethacin	Indocin, Indocin SR, others	4.5	90	<200 mg	25–50 mg; SR: 75 mg; rarely >150 mg	TID or QID BID	2–4 mg/kg/24 h
Sulindac	Clinoril	8–16	99	400 mg	150, 200 mg	BID to TID	NA
COX-2 selective NSAID (Coxib)							
Celecoxib	Celebrex	6–12	97	200 mg	100–200 mg; 400 mg acute pain	1–2 times daily	3 mg/kg BID

Adapted from Bonica's management of pain. 4th ed. Ch. 77, p. 1159.

$$\frac{30\,\text{mg PO morphine} \times 42\,\text{mg IV morphine}}{10\,\text{mg IV morphine}} = 126\,\text{mg PO morphine}$$

Morphine

Morphine is the prototypical strong mu agonist opioid and is still the most commonly used opioid worldwide. Orally administered morphine is available in both immediate acting and extended release formulations. A combination of both immediate acting and extended release morphine is typically used in chronic pain management. Morphine metabolites include *morphine-3-glucuronide* (hyperalgesia, agitation, myoclonus; can accumulate in renal insufficiency or prolonged high doses), *morphine-6-glucuronide* (more potent than morphine; can accumulate in renal insufficiency or prolonged high doses), and *normorphine* (allodynia, myoclonus).

Many opioids are available orally in extended release preparations. The most common are given below.

Extended-Release Morphine

MS Contin® 10, 30, 60, 100, 200 mg tablets dosing is q8h or q12h (often has end-of-dose failure with q12h dosing). Tablet cannot be broken, chewed, dissolved, or crushed. Absorption: single peak with T_{max} occurring at 2–3 h. Patients can take it in fasting or fed state.

Kadian® 10, 20, 30, 50, 60, 80, 100, and 200 mg capsules dosing is q24h (often has end-of-dose failure at 18 h). Capsule can be opened and administered in food or as slurry down a G-tube. Absorption: single peak with T_{max} occurring at approximately 8 h. Alcohol will not affect absorption.

Avinza® 30, 45, 60, 75, 90, 120 mg capsules dosing is q24h (often has end-of-dose failure at 18 h). Capsule can also be opened and administered in food. Avoid coadministration with alcohol (ingestion of alcohol will result in rapid absorption of total dose). Fumaric acid is an inactive ingredient and can cause renal toxicity in high doses; thus, daily dose of Avinza® must not exceed a max of 1,600 mg/day. Absorption: contains both immediate release and extended release beads of morphine sulfate for fast onset with sustained effect. T_{max} occurs in approximately 1.5 h with a more even plateau than Kadian. Can be taken in fasting or fed state.

Oramorph®SR 15, 30, 60, 100 mg tablets dosing is q8h or q12h. Tablet cannot be broken, chewed, dissolved, or crushed. Absorption: single peak T_{max} occurring at 3.5–4 h.

Sustained Release Oxymorphone

Opana®ER 5, 7.5, 10, 15, 20, 30, 40 mg tablets dosing is q12h. Tablet cannot be broken, chewed, dissolved, or crushed. Should be dosed at least 1 h prior to or 2 h after eating. Avoid coadministration with alcohol. Absorption: single peak with T_{max} occurring at approximately 3 h.

Sustained Release Oxycodone

OxyContin® 10, 15, 20, 30, 40, 60, 80, 160 mg tablets, dosing is q12h (rarely necessary to dose q8h, approximately 20% absorption in first hour, then steady absorption of the rest). Tablet cannot be broken, chewed, dissolved, or crushed. OxyContin exhibits a biphasic absorption pattern with two apparent absorption half-lives of 0.6 and 6.9 h.

Sustained Release Tramadol

Ultram®ER 100, 200, 300 mg tablets, dosing q24h (max 300 mg/day). Tablet cannot be broken, chewed, dissolved, or crushed. Absorption: single peak with T_{max} occurring at approximately 12 h. Risk for seizures and serotonin syndrome when taken with other serotonergic medications.

Transdermal Fentanyl Patch

Duragesic® 25 μg/h, 50 μg/h, 75 μg/h, 100 μg/h. Delivers a continuous dose per hour of fentanyl transcutaneously. Normally a patch is adequate for continuous dosing over 72 h. They require about 12–18 h to reach steady-state absorption, and 12 h to clear when patch is removed. Not affected by obesity or cachexia except in time elapsed to reach steady state. Heat (i.e., heating pads) or fever associated with peripheral vasodilation can *significantly* increase absorption rate. Approximately 60 mg/day of intravenous morphine or 180 mg/day of oral morphine will be equivalent to a 100 μg/h fentanyl patch.

Transbuccal Fentanyl

Actiq® (fentanyl lollipop) 200 μg, 400 μg, 800 μg, 1,200 μg. Lozenge should be held against the inside of the cheek. Approximately 25% of the dose is absorbed directly through the buccal mucosa, the rest is swallowed and another 25% of the total dose is then slowly absorbed from the stomach. T_{max} occurs in 20–40 min. Patient can remove the lozenge from the mouth if pain relief is obtained prior to full dissolution, discarding the rest of the lozenge. The lozenges contain sugar and can cause tooth decay if used frequently in the same area.

Fentora® (fentanyl buccal tablet) 100, 200, 300, 400, 600, 800 mcg dosing q4h. Dissolves rapidly. Following buccal administration of Fentora®, fentanyl is readily absorbed with an absolute bioavailability of 65% (50% absorbed transmucosally, 15% absorbed through the gastrointestinal tract). T_{max} occurs in approximately 45 min. Due to higher bioavailability, dosing *is not* equivalent from Actiq to Fentora® – transition patients from Actiq per guidelines in Fentora package insert.

Stool Softeners and Laxatives

Since opioids can cause constipation, either a stool softener, or a laxative, or a combination should be used. Other than lactulose, none of the stool softeners, laxatives, or combinations requires a prescription. Colace, Surfak, Peri-Colace, Senokot and Senokot-S can all be given as one or two capsules at bed-time.

Colace® (docusate sodium) 100 mg – softener (this product is a sodium salt)
Surfak® (docusate calcium) 240 mg – softener (this product is a calcium salt)
Peri-Colace® (docusate + sennosides) – combination laxative and softener
Senokot® (senna) – stimulant laxative
Senokot-S® (docusate + senna) – combination laxative and softener
Milk of Magnesia® (magnesium hydroxide) – osmotic laxative
Miralax® (polyethylene glycol) – osmotic laxative
Magnesium Citrate® osmotic laxative (generally not used for opioid constipation)
Lactulose® osmotic laxative (synthetic disaccharide; requires a prescription)

Anticonvulsants

Actions of Anticonvulsants in Pain Therapy

Similarities between the pathophysiological phenomena observed in some epilepsy models and in neuropathic pain models justify the rational use of anticonvulsant drugs in the symptomatic management of neuropathic pain disorders. The availability of newer anticonvulsants tested in higher quality clinical trials has marked a new era in the treatment of neuropathic pain.

Today, gabapentin (Neurontin®) and pregabalin (Lyrica®) have become the first-line anticonvulsants used in pain management. Considerable research has defined the mechanisms by which these agents produce antinociception. The drugs bind to the A-2D subunit of the presynaptic voltage-gated calcium channel on C-nociceptor fibers entering the spinal cord, preventing calcium entry into the cell, thus preventing the fusion of the neurotransmitter releasing vesicles to the cell membrane which is necessary for the release of the neurotransmitters into the synapse. Side effects include weight gain, peripheral edema, and short-term memory loss. Package insert specifies dosing for renal failure.

Gabapentin (Neurontin®): 100, 300, 400, 600, 800 mg tablets; 100, 300, 400 mg capsules. Functions as an A-2D subunit blocker on voltage-gated calcium channels in the spinal cord as well as a tetrodotoxin-resistant sodium channel (TTXr) blocker. Considered first-line therapy for neuropathic pain. Daily dose 900–4,000 mg/day in TID or QID dosing. Elderly may only tolerate 100 mg QD-TID.

Pregabalin (Lyrica®): 25, 50, 75, 100, 150, 200, 225, 300 mg capsules. Functions as an A-2D subunit blocker on voltage-gated calcium channels in the spinal cord. Approved for use in the treatment of postherpetic neuralgia (PHN), diabetic neuropathy, and fibromyalgia, but is used in many neuropathic pain syndromes. Start 50–75 mg dosing TID or QID titrated up to 400 mg/day.

Topiramate (Topamax®): 25, 50, 100, 200 mg tablets; 15, 25 mg capsules. Blocks voltage-dependent sodium channels, augments gamma aminobutyric acid (GABA) at some subtypes of the GABA-A receptor, antagonizes the AMPA/kainate subtype of the glutamate receptor, and inhibits the carbonic anhydrase enzyme. Dosing 75–600 mg QD or BID, Food and Drug Administration (FDA) approved for use in migraine prophylaxis. Does not cause weight gain (may cause mild to moderate weight loss – thought to be due to carbonic anhydrase appetite suppression) and is often used as a substitute in women with neuropathic pain who are concerned about weight gain. Inhibition of carbonic anhydrase can also result in nephrolithiasis ($CaPO_4$ stones). May cause closed-angle glaucoma in susceptible individuals – discontinue if blurred vision and eye pain develop.

Lamotrigine (Lamictal®): Na^+ channel blocker, 50–400 mg QD or in divided doses. Need to monitor for side effects (liver function). Found to be effective in central poststroke pain syndrome.

Carbamazepine (Tegretol®): Older agent, only proven effectiveness is in trigeminal neuralgia. Functions as a Na^+ channel blocker. Many side effects, including potential hepatic and/or bone marrow damage. Need to monitor liver function and blood count. Particular caution must be taken in patients with bone marrow depression. Can result in hyponatremia so serum Na^+ must be monitored when titrating. Dosing is usually initiated at 100 mg BID as tolerated. Effective dose range for pain control varies from 200 to 1,200 mg/day.

Oxcarbazepine (Trileptal®): A structural derivative of carbamazepine, with a ketone substitution on the dibenzazepine ring. Reduced impact on the liver with metabolism. Avoids the risk of anemia or agranulocytosis occasionally associated with carbamazepine. Can result in hyponatremia so serum Na^+ must be monitored when titrating. Dosing is usually initiated at 300 mg BID as tolerated. Recommended daily dose is 1,200 mg/day.

Phenytoin (Dilantin®): older agent, first-generation sodium channel blocking anticonvulsant. Used for neuropathic pain (PO dose 100 mg TID). Need to monitor therapeutic level. Major precautions: porphyria, liver disease, myocardial insufficiency, cardiac arrhythmias, hypotension. Intravenous (IV) phenytoin 15 mg/kg infused over 2 h can provide up to 7 days of pain reduction in a crisis (McCleane 1999). Gingival hyperplasia can be disturbing to patients.

Next Generation Anticonvulsants (GABA Enhancers)

Vigabatrin (Sabril®) – newly approved (2009) antiepileptic drug indicated for refractory complex partial seizures in adults. Vigabatrin inhibits the breakdown of GABA by irreversibly inhibiting GABA transaminase. It is an analog of GABA, but it is not a receptor agonist. Shown to cause irreversible bilateral concentric visual field constriction in 30% of patients – baseline vision testing and eye exams q3mo. *Not likely to find common use in pain medicine due to high incidence of vision loss.*

Tiagabine (Gabitril®): An antiepilepsy drug available in 2, 4, 12, 16 mg tablets. Binds to recognition sites associated with the GABA uptake carrier. It is thought that tiagabine blocks GABA uptake into presynaptic neurons, permitting more GABA to be available for receptor binding on the surfaces of postsynaptic cells. Approved in 1997, FDA required revised package insert in 2005 secondary to reports showing an association with new onset seizures and status epilepticus in patients without epilepsy. In most cases, patients were using concomitant medications that lower the seizure threshold. *Off-label use of Gabitril [bipolar, neuropathy, depression, posttraumatic stress disorders (PTSD)] is now strongly discouraged by the FDA.*

Ganaxolone (INN, also known as CCD-1042): a neurosteroid related to pregnanolone which has sedative, anxiolytic, and anticonvulsant effects. It is a potent and selective positive allosteric modulator of GABA-A receptors.

Phase 2b studies of ganaxolone are ongoing to study and evaluate safety, tolerability, and efficacy in adults with complex partial seizures. Any effect on neuropathic pain has yet to be formally studied.

Retigabine: Acts on potassium ion channels and effects GABA neurotransmission by action at the GABA-A receptor. Retigabine is a psychoactive drug and research chemical under development as a novel anticonvulsant agent. Its acts as a neuronal KCNQ/Kv7 potassium channel opener, a mechanism of action completely different from those of presently marketed antiepileptics. Retigabine is currently in phase III clinical trials as an adjunctive treatment for partial-onset seizures in adult patients with refractory epilepsy. GlaxoSmithKline (GSK) and Valeant Pharmaceuticals International (VRX) announced on October 30, 2009 that they filed a New Drug Application with the US Food and Drug Administration (FDA) for retigabine, used as adjunctive therapy to treat adult epilepsy patients with partial-onset seizures. Preliminary animal models have shown effectiveness in diminishing neuropathic pain (Blackburn-Munro and Jensen 2003).

Antidepressants

A major depressive episode (Diagnostic and Statistical Manual of Mental Disorders, 4th ed.; DSM-IV) implies a prominent and relatively persistent (nearly every day for at least 2 weeks) depressed or dysphoric mood that usually interferes with daily functioning, and includes at least five of the following nine symptoms: depressed mood, loss of interest in usual activities, significant change in weight and/or appetite, insomnia or hypersomnia, psychomotor agitation or retardation, increased fatigue, feelings of guilt or worthlessness, slowed thinking or impaired concentration, and a suicide attempt or suicidal ideation.

Tricyclic Antidepressants

Tricyclic antidepressants are used for depression and neuropathic pain. They are inhibitors of reuptake of norepinephrine and serotonin in the descending projections from the brain to the dorsal horn of the spinal cord resulting in modulation of the incoming nociceptive signals. Norepinephrine seems to be more important for analgesia whereas serotonin is more important for antidepressant effects. The sedating effects may be helpful with sleep. Usually these agents are initiated as an evening dose, escalating every 3–5 days. Beneficial effects may not be noticed, however, for 1–3 weeks. There are common side effects of all of the tricyclic antidepressants, although to varying degrees. Dry mouth, blurred vision, urinary retention, constipation and reflux (anticholinergic), weakness, lethargy, and fatigue can occur. Secondary amines tend to be better tolerated than the tertiary amines. A comparison of the most common TCAs can be found in Table 34.6. Caution must be taken with these agents to evaluate for exacerbation of psychiatric symptoms, postural hypotension, benign prostate hypertrophy, urinary retention, and closed-angle glaucoma. Cardiac dysrhythmias are more common than with the specific serotonin reuptake inhibitors (SSRIs).

Table 34.6 Tricyclic Antidepressants with Dosing and Common Side Effect Profiles.

Tricyclic antidepressants					
Name	Anticholinergic	Sedation	Comments	Initial dose	Max dose
Tertiary amines					
Imipramine (Tofranil®)	+++	+++	• First TCA introduced (1957)	10–25 mg qhs	300 mg/day
Clomipramine (Anafranil®)	++++	+++	• Especially effective for OCD • Most serotonergic TCA	10–25 mg qhs	300 mg/day
Amitriptyline (Elavil®)	+++++	+++++	• 10–30 mg qhs for sleep disorders and chronic pain	10–25 mg qhs	300 mg/day
Doxepin (Sinequan®)	+++	++++	• Most histamine block	10–25 mg qhs	300 mg/day
Secondary amines					
Nortriptyline (Aventyl®)	+	+	• Less hypotension • Lower maximum dose compared to other TCAs	10 mg qhs	150 mg/day
Desipramine (Norpramin®)	+	+	• Most NE activity • Least anticholinergic TCA	10–25 mg qhs	300 mg/day

Serotonin and Norepinephrine Reuptake Inhibitors (SNRIs)

Venlafaxine (Effexor®) =150 mg for norepinephrine. Start at 37.5 mg QD advancing every 3–5 days. Must reach =150 mg/day to obtain the norepinephrine reuptake inhibition effect. Differs from other agents in that it lacks anticholinergic, antiadrenergic, and antihistaminergic side effects.

Duloxetine (Cymbalta®) 30 mg/day advancing to 60–120 mg/day. Approved for use in diabetic neuropathy and postherpetic neuralgia but is commonly used in neuropathic pain syndromes associated with situational depression as an adjunct to the anticonvulsants and opioids. It has the advantage of limited anticholinergic effects, and the onset of analgesia occurs within a few days instead of several weeks.

Bupropion (Wellbutrin®SR, Zyban®) 150–300 mg/day. Wellbutrin SR is given BID (Wellbutrin XL is given QD). Bupropion is an atypical antidepressant that acts as a norepinephrine and dopamine reuptake inhibitor, and nicotinic antagonist. Bupropion lowers seizure threshold in higher doses. However, at the recommended dose the risk of seizures is comparable to that observed for other antidepressants. Bupropion is an effective antidepressant on its own but it is particularly popular as an add-on medication in the cases of incomplete response to the first-line SSRI antidepressant. It also seems to be effective in patients who have a history of alcohol or substance abuse who require long-term opioid therapy for chronic pain.

Trazadone (Desyrel®) 50–300 mg/day (avoid in men due to risk of priapism). A favorable response in association with other adjunctive drugs and again particularly useful to restore evening sleep given at night.

Selective Serotonin Reuptake Inhibitors

These agents are primarily effective for the treatment of depression associated with chronic pain syndromes. Although there are sporadic reports of the effectiveness of certain SSRIs in pain treatment, they are for the most part adjuncts to the other nonopioid analgesics. Care must be used in combination with other serotonergic medications as serotonin toxicity (serotonin syndrome) can occur. The combination of SSRIs and monoamine oxidase inhibitors (MAOIs) pose a particularly severe risk of a life-threatening serotonin syndrome. Clinical features of serotonin toxicity are included in Table 34.7.

Table 34.7 Clinical signs and symptoms of serotonin toxicity.

Autonomic effects	Somatic effects	Cognitive effects
• Hyper/hypotension	• Tremors	• Confusion
• Tachycardia	• Myoclonus	• Agitation
• Hyperthermia	• Hyperreflexia	• Hallucinations
• Diarrhea		• Central nervous system hyperactivity
• Nausea/vomiting		

Fluoxetine (Prozac®) 10–80 mg/day (10, 20, 40 mg capsules)
Sertraline (Zoloft®) 50–200 mg/day (25, 50, 100 mg tablets)
Paroxetine (Paxil®) 10–50 mg/day (10, 20, 30, 40 mg tablets) Best for anxiety-related disorders.

Aripiprazole (Abilify®) maximum dose 30 mg/day (2, 5, 10, 15, 20, 30 mg tablets, 1 mg/ml oral solution). Best for add-on adjunct to other antidepressants, or for bipolar disease or schizophrenia.

Olanzapine (Zyprexa®) usual dose range 10–15 mg/day, safety of doses greater than 20 mg/day have not been established (2.5, 5, 7.5, 10, 15, 20 mg tablets, and disintegrating tablets of 5, 10, 15, 20 mg). Bipolar disorder and schizophrenia.

Citalopram (Celexa®) 20–40 mg/day (10, 20, 40 mg tablets and 2 mg/ml solution).

Escitalopram (Lexapro®) 10–20 mg/day (5, 10, 20 mg tablets; oral solution 1 mg/ml). S-stereoisomer of citalopram. More rapid onset of antidepressant effects with less side effects.

Monoamine Oxidase Inhibitors

Monoamine oxidase inhibitors work by binding to the enzyme monoamine oxidase, thus inhibiting the breakdown of monoamines at the synaptic junction which increases the concentration of the neurotransmitters epinephrine, norepinephrine, and dopamine at various sites in the central nervous system (CNS) and sympathetic storage sites. Therapeutic effect takes 2–4 weeks. Patients prescribed these agents should avoid foods high in tyramine such as cheeses, yeast supplements, and red wines. Meperidine (Demerol®) must be avoided because of risk of serotonin syndrome and malignant hyperpyrexia.

Isocarboxacid (Marplan®): 30–50 mg/day (10 mg tablets)
Phenelzine (Nardil®): 45–90 mg/day (15 mg tablets)
Tranylcypromine (Parnate®): 20–60 mg/day (10 mg tablets)

Neuroleptics (Antipsychotics)

Traditional Neuroleptics

These drugs function as antipsychotics by antidopaminergic effects particularly at the D2 receptors in the brain. They have major side effects to include movement disorders.

Phenothiazine (Thorazine®): 10, 25, 50, 100, 200 mg tablets
Thioridazine (Mellaril®): 10, 25, 50, 100 mg tablets
Fluphenazine (Prolixin®): 1, 2.5, 5, 10 mg tablets
Trifluoperazine (Stelazine®): 1, 2, 5, 10 mg tablets
Haloperidol (Haldol®): 0.5, 1, 2, 5 mg tablets

Atypical Neuroleptics

These agents have lesser D2 antagonism but also block serotonin-2 receptors and to a variable degree D4 receptors. They may be more effective than typical neuroleptics but have less psychotic effects.

Risperidone (Risperdal®): 0.5, 1, 2, 3, 4 mg tablets
Clozapine (Clozaril®): 25, 100 mg tablets
Olanzapine (Zyprexa®): 2.5, 5, 10 mg tablets

Mood Stabilizers
Mood Stabilizers for Bipolar Depressive Disorders
Lithium
Lithium is the most frequently used agent for bipolar disease but it has a very narrow therapeutic index. Lithium is formulated as a chemical salt, of which lithium carbonate is the most commonly prescribed (citrate, sulfate, orotate are alternatives). Dosing is BID or TID. Therapeutic trough levels are typically 1.0–1.5 mEq/l for acute mania and 0.6–1.2 mEq/l for chronic maintenance. Regular serum lithium level testing is necessary. Important to monitor renal and thyroid function. Can be used in the treatment of cluster headache syndromes.

Valproic acid (Depakote®): GABA transaminase inhibitor as well as inhibitor of voltage-gated sodium channels and T-type calcium channels. Valproate is a known folate antagonist, which can cause neural tube defects, so avoid in pregnancy if possible.

Carbamazepine (Tegretol®): previously discussed under "Anticonvulsants."
Lamotrigine (Lamictal®): previously discussed under "Anticonvulsants."

Anxiolytics
Anxiety is a very common concomitant condition in patients with chronic pain, presenting as panic, PTSD, obsessive/compulsive disorder (OCD), etc. Although *anxiolytics do not possess intrinsic analgesic activity*, anxiety is often accompanied by somatic complaints of chest pain, GI upset, or neurologic symptoms such as dysesthesias, headache, which may be relieved by anxiolysis. Benzodiazepines are also a mainstay in the treatment of restless legs syndrome (RLS). Although most RLS studies were conducted with clonazepam, current recommendations focus on shorter acting benzodiazepines such as triazolam (Silber et al. 2004).

Benzodiazepines
Benzodiazepines are the most common class of agents for anxiety.

Clonazepam (Klonopin®): 0.5, 1, 2 mg tablets. Considered both as a psychotropic agent (anxiolysis) as well as an adjunct in the treatment of neuropathic pain (lancinating pain).

Buspirone (Buspar®): 5, 10, 15, 30 mg tablets. Acts as a 5-HT-1A agonist and can potentiate the effects of the SSRIs. It is titrated at 5 mg TID to start increasing to 10 mg TID as tolerated, if necessary.

Alprazolam (Xanax®): 0.25, 0.5, 1, 2 mg tablets. (Xanax®XR): 0.5, 1, 2, 3 mg tablets.
Chlordiazepoxide (Librium®): 5, 10, 25 mg capsules.
Flurazepam (Dalmane®): 15, 30 mg capsules.
Diazepam (Valium®): 2, 5, 10 mg tablets. Injectable solution 5 mg/ml. Oral solution 5 mg/ml.
Lorazepam (Ativan®): 0.5, 1, 2 mg tablets. Injectable solution 2, 4 mg/ml. Oral solution 0.5 mg/5 ml. Can be administered intravenously.

Midazolam (Versed®): Injectable solution 1, 5 mg/ml. Oral solution 2 mg/ml. Used primarily as an intravenous agent for antianxiety and amnesia in surgical procedures as a premedication. Can be administered orally in children as an anxiolytic for surgery.

Oxazepam (Serax®): 10, 15, 30 mg capsules.
Temazepam (Restoril®): 7.5, 15, 22.5, 30 mg capsules.
Triazolam (Halcion®): 0.125, 0.25 mg tablets.

Nonbenzodiazepine Anxiolytics

Buspirone (Buspar®): 5, 10, 15, 30 mg tablets. Acts as a 5-HT-1A agonist and can potentiate the effects of the SSRIs. Start at 5 mg TID and slowly titrate to effective dose (max 60 mg daily). Mechanism of action is unrelated to benzodiazepines and will not prevent or shorten benzodiazepine withdrawal.

Psychostimulants

Agents which are used in patients with attention deficit disorder, parkinsonism, narcolepsy, workshift sedation, and treatment-resistant depression to augment antidepressants, to counter iatrogenic sedation from opioids and other adjunctive medications, and to treat fatigue or sedation in terminal illness. The majority of psychostimulants are amphetamine based and can cause dopamine release in increasing doses, which can result in behavioral changes. Care must be taken with these drugs since significant abuse potential can occur.

Dextroamphetamine (Dexedrine®): 5–60 mg/day
Methylphenidate (Ritalin®): 10–30 mg/day
Magnesium pemoline (Cylert®): 37.5–112.5 mg/day

Amphetamine/Dextroamphetamine (Adderall®): Extended release action; 10–40 mg/day, used for adult attention deficit disorder if patient had favorable response to Ritalin®.

Nonamphetamine Stimulants

Modafinil (Provigil®): 100, 200 mg tablets. The mechanism of action of modafinil is unknown.
Armodafinil (Nuvigil®): 50, 100, 150, 200, 250 mg tablets. Armodafinil is the active R-enantiomer of modafinil. The mechanism of action of armodafinil is unknown.
Caffeine: 100 mg tablets. Functions as an adenosine receptor antagonist in the CNS.

Local Anesthetics

Lidocaine

Lidocaine is a membrane stabilizer and a Na^+ channel blocker. Intravenous lidocaine can be effective as a diagnostic or therapeutic treatment for neuropathic pain. Lidocaine (1–5 mg/kg) is dissolved in 50–100 ml saline and infused over 15–30 min. The key to this test or treatment is that the patient must reach an adequate blood level of lidocaine to feel some toxicity such as slurring of speech, ringing in the ear, circumoral numbness, or difficulty completing a sentence. When any of these occurs, the infusion rate is stopped or slowed down until the symptoms begin to resolve and then the infusion is restarted. Significant pain relief is diagnostic for neuropathic pain. As a therapeutic procedure, ketorolac 15–30 mg, magnesium sulfate 1 g, and Decadron® 4–6 mg can be added to the lidocaine to treat "total body pain syndromes" such as fibromyalgia. During the time of the infusion, positive reinforcement suggestions for healing can be given to the patient since the infusion produces a light trance state with the patient in a receptive state. Lidocaine may also be used as a nasal spray or gel for intractable cluster headaches.

Mexilitine (Mexitil®): Sodium channel blocker, antiarrhythmic and antineuropathic pain adjunct. Based on effective intravenous Lidocaine trial, Mexilitine can be started at 100–150 mg qhs advancing as tolerated to 900 mg/day in divided TID or QID dosing. Nausea and vomiting can occur but heartburn is especially common for approximately 15 min after ingestion which is not relieved by antacids but is also not damaging to the gastric mucosa.

Tocainide (Tonocard®): another oral local anesthetic antiarrhythmic, sodium channel blocker neuropathic pain adjunctive medication. Rarely employed today. Tonocard is no longer available in the United States secondary to the risk of severe lung and blood disorders as a result of its use.

LidoDerm® 5% Lidocaine patches: approved for use in postherpetic neuralgia (PHN) as a transdermal topical analgesic. The single dosage patch is applied for 12 h/day to the painful area. The lesions of the acute phase of herpes zoster must be healed however, as the patch can only be applied to intact skin. While FDA approval is specific for PHN, physicians are using these patches for other conditions such as low back pain, painful scars, and myofascial pain with some success.

Local anesthetics such as bupivacaine are also used in continuous intrathecal administration therapy through in-dwelling spinal catheters and pumps in concentrations as high as 40 mg/ml of bupivacaine mixed with other agents such as opioids, baclofen, clonidine, or ziconotide.

NMDA Antagonists

Ketamine

Ketamine is a phencyclidine analog, usually administered intravenously during anesthesia but can be given orally for chronic pain. However, the therapeutic window between the disphoric and hallucinogenic doses and analgesic doses is very small and many patients do not tolerate this agent orally. Newer prospective studies have shown efficacy in the treatment of complex regional pain syndrome (CRPS) (Sigtermans et al. 2009).

Dextromethorphan: (100 mg QID) found in cough syrup usually at 30 mg/tablespoon. Can be compounded by a pharmacist in any dose capsule. Recommended starting dose is 30 mg PO TID.

Alpha-2 Agonists

These agents have been shown to be effective in the management of acute postoperative pain and in chronic pain states, (including disorders involving spasticity or myofascial pain, neuropathic pain, and chronic daily headaches).

Clonidine (Catapres®, Duraclon®): 0.1, 0.2, 0.3 mg tablets; 0.1, 0.5 mg/ml injectable solution. A centrally acting, direct α-adrenergic receptor agonist (α2 > α1) which can be given PO, IV, epidural injection, and intrathecal injection. The analgesic effect of clonidine is felt to occur at presynaptic and postjunctional α2-adrenergic receptors in the spinal cord.

Dexmedetomidine (Precedex®): 100 mcg/ml injectable solution. Dexmedetomidine is a relatively selective α2-adrenergic agonist. It is currently approved by the FDA for ICU sedation (continuous infusion not to exceed 24 h) and sedation of nonintubated patients prior to and during surgical procedures. New studies have shown that dexmedetomidine has significant opioid sparing effects and can be effective when included in PCA formulations containing opioids (Lin et al. 2009).

Tizanidine (Zanaflex®): α2-adrenergic agonist often used as an antispasmodic agent. Initial dose may have to be as low as 0.25 mg because of potential significant sedation. Titrate up to 2–4 mg every 6–8 h until relief or excessive side effects occur; hypotension, sedation, asthenia, and dry mouth (dose related) are frequent; need to monitor for elevated liver function enzyme levels and hepatotoxicity. Maximum dose recommended is 36 mg/day. Zanaflex has 1/10 to 1/50 the potency of clonidine in lowering blood pressure. Concomitant use of tizanidine with fluvoxamine or with ciprofloxacin (potent inhibitors of CYP1A2) is contraindicated.

Antispasmodic Agents (Muscle Relaxants)

Baclofen (Lioresal®): GABA receptor antagonist, descending pain modulation best for pain associated with spasticity through central pain modulating mechanisms. Oral tablets of 5 and 10 mg dosed TID; may titrate every 3 days to effect with maximum dose: 80 mg/day. Can cause sedation, dizziness, weakness, hypotension, nausea, respiratory depression, constipation; discontinue by slow taper; withdrawal syndrome consists of hallucinations, seizures; need to monitor liver function since it may increase alkaline phosphatase and AST levels; dose adjustment is necessary in patients with renal impairment. Baclofen is available for intrathecal administration to control severe spasticity. Initial intrathecal trial of 50–100 µg to measure reduction in spasticity. Must be done in a monitored setting with resuscitation equipment available. Pyridostigmine (Antilirium®) 1 mg IV is the antidote.

Dantrolene: Oral administration is 25 mg QD × 7 days, then 25 mg TID × 7 days, then 50 mg TID × 7 days, then 100 mg TID. Blackbox warning about symptomatic fatal or nonfatal hepatitis; discontinue drug if no benefit is observed after 45 days.

Diazepam (Valium®): Adults: 2–10 mg TID-QID, elimination half-life 100 h: avoid in elderly, avoid in patients with renal or hepatic impairment. It has a significant abuse potential; dizziness, drowsiness, confusion; children >6 months: 1–2.5 mg half-life 20–50 h; active metabolites extend half-life up to 100 h. It must be withdrawn slowly from high doses to avoid seizures (4–6 weeks).

Tizanidine (Zanaflex®): α2-Adrenergic agonist, initial dose may have to be as low as 0.25 mg because of potential significant sedation. Titrate up to 2–4 mg every 6–8 h until relief or excessive side effects occur; hypotension, sedation, asthenia, and dry mouth (dose related) are frequent; need to monitor for elevated liver function enzyme levels and hepatotoxicity. Maximum dose recommended 36 mg/day.

Cyclobenzaprine (Flexeril®), 5 mg TID; may increase to 10 mg TID; elimination half-life ~18 h in young subjects, ~33 h in elderly, and ~46 h in patients with hepatic impairment.

Anticholinergic effects (drowsiness, urinary retention, dry mouth): avoid in elderly; QT prolongation: avoid in patients with arrhythmias, cardiac conduction disturbances, heart block, heart failure, or recent myocardial infraction; may raise intraocular pressure: avoid in patients with glaucoma.

Carisoprodol (Soma®) 350 mg tablets; maximum recommended dose is TID or QID. Not recommended in children <12 years; drowsiness; can cause psychological and physical dependence (metabolized to meprobamate, a barbiturate tranquilizer), withdrawal symptoms can therefore occur with discontinuation; excessive use, overdose, or withdrawal may precipitate seizures; reports describe idiosyncratic or allergy-type reactions after first dose (mental status changes, transient quadriplegia, fever, angioneurotic edema, asthmatic episodes).

Chlorzoxazone (Parafon forte); Adults: 250–750 mg TID-QID. Dizziness and drowsiness may occur with rare cases of hepatotoxicity, gastrointestinal irritation, and rare cases of gastrointestinal bleeding; it may also cause red or orange urine; should be avoided in patients with liver impairment. Children: 125–500 mg TID-QID or 20 mg/kg/day in three or four divided doses; same side effects and toxicities can occur as in adults.

Metaxalone (Skelaxin®): 800 mg TID-QID. Not recommended in children <12 years; do not use in patients with renal or hepatic failure or a history of anemia; dizziness or drowsiness; rare cases of leukopenia or hemolytic anemia may occur. Reported to be less sedating than other muscle relaxants.

Methocarbamol (Robaxin®): 1,500 mg QID for the first 2–3 days, then 750 mg QID. Available orally in 500, 750, and 1,000 mg tablets. Robaxin is also available as an injectable. Do not use injection in patients with renal failure; may cause brown-to-black or green discoloration of urine; may impair mental status; may exacerbate symptoms of myasthenia gravis.

Orphenadrine (Norflex®): (available generic only) 100 mg BID; orally, combination products are given TID-QID: it should be avoided in the elderly; it may raise intraocular pressure and should therefore be avoided in patients with glaucoma; it can be associated with gastrointestinal disturbances; elimination half-life 13–20 h which may be extended when use is prolonged; it should be avoided in patients with cardiospasm or myasthenia gravis; and it is contraindicated in duodenal or pyloric obstruction or stenosing peptic ulcers. The anticholinergic effects (drowsiness, urinary retention, dry mouth) can be prominent.

Headache Medication

Migraine Headache

The mainstay of chronic migraine treatment is abortive therapy with NSAIDs, Triptans, and Ergot derivatives (Table 34.8). Migraine prophylaxis is typically reserved for patients with frequent headaches that are nonresponsive to abortive therapy. Prophylaxis can include beta-blockers, anticonvulsants such as Topiramate, and supplements such as magnesium and riboflavin (Table 34.9).

Cluster Headache

Acute treatment for cluster headaches can include triptans, Ergot derivatives, and even intranasal lidocaine. Prophylactic treatment includes verapamil, glucocorticoids, topiramate, and lithium.

Table 34.8 Oral acute migraine treatments.

Nonspecific treatments	Specific treatments
Acetaminophen (1,000 mg)	Triptans
Aspirin (900 mg)	Sumatriptan (Imitrex®) 50 or 100 mg
	Naratriptan (Amerge®) 2.5 mg
Antiemetics/prokinetics	Rizatriptan (Maxalt®) 10 mg
Promethazine (Phenergan®) 25 mg	Zolmitriptan (Zomig®) 2.5 or 5 mg
Metoclopramide (Reglan®) 10 mg	Eletriptan (Relpax®) 40 or 80 mg
	Almotriptan (Axert®) 12.5 mg
NSAIDs	Frovatriptan (Frova®) 2.5 mg
Naproxen (500–1,000 mg)	
Ibuprofen (400–800 mg)	Ergot derivatives
	Ergotamine (1–2 mg)

NSAIDs = nonsteroidal anti-inflammatory drugs.
Adapted from Bonica's management of pain. 4th ed. Ch. 61, p. 866.

Table 34.9 Preventative treatments in migraine.

Drug	Dose	Selected side effects
Pizotifen	0.5–2 mg QD	Weight gain, drowsiness
β-Blockers		
Propranolol	40–120 mg BID	Reduced energy, tiredness, postural symptoms, contraindicated in asthma
Tricyclics		
Amitriptyline	25–75 mg	Drowsiness
Desipramine	qhs	(note: some patients are very sensitive and may only need a total dose of 10 mg,
Nortriptyline		although generally 1–1.5 mg/kg body weight is required)
Anticonvulsants		
Valproate	400–600 mg BID	Hair loss, drowsiness, weight gain, fetal abnormalities, hematological or liver abnormalities, pancreatitis
Topiramate	50–200 mg QD	Tremor, weight loss, care with a family history of glaucoma, nephrolithiasis, dizziness, sedation, paresthesia
Gabapentin	900–3,600 mg QD	Cognitive dysfunction, vertigo, weight gain, fluid retention, blurred vision, adjust dose in patients with renal insufficiency
Methysergide	1–6 mg QD	Drowsiness, leg cramps, hair loss, retroperitoneal fibrosis (1 month drug holiday is required every 6 months)
Flunarizine	5–15 mg QD	Drowsiness, weight gain, depression, parkinsonism
Nutraceuticals		
Riboflavin	400 mg QD	Gastrointestinal upset
Coenzyme Q10	100 mg TID	

Adapted from Bonica's management of pain. 4th ed. Ch. 61, p. 865.

Tension Headache

Acute treatment typically involves NSAIDs or acetaminophen. Prophylactic treatment can include TCAs, SNRIs, SSRIs, anticonvulsants such as topiramate and gabapentin, and trigger point injection with botulinum toxin.

Corticosteroids

Methylprednisolone acetate (Depo Medrol®): strength 40 or 80 mg/ml, supplied in 1, 5, or 10 ml vials. High potency with high glucocorticoid effect and low mineralocorticoid effect.

Triamcinolone acetonide (Kenalog®): strength 40 mg/ml, supplied in 5 ml vials. High potency with high glucocorticoid effect and low mineralocorticoid effect. Triamcinolone acetonide does not contain polyethylene glycol.

Triamcinalone diacetate (Aristocort®): strength 10 or 20 mg/ml, supplied in 1 and 5 ml vials. High potency with high glucocorticoid and low mineralocorticoid effect. Other drugs include:

Betamethasone (Celestone®): 6 mg/ml, 5 ml vials (highest glucocorticoid potency).
Dexamethasone (Decadron®): 4 mg/ml, 5 ml vials (next highest glucocorticoid potency).

Sedative Hypnotics (Sleep Aids)

Benzodiazepine Sedative Hypnotics

Benzodiazepine sedative hypnotics have an associated dependency risk and a higher incidence of next day sedation. All have risk of "sleep driving" and other complex, hypnotic behaviors.

Estazolam (ProSom®): 1, 2 mg tablets. Dose is 1–2 mg qhs (generic available)
Flurazepam (Dalmane®): 15, 30 mg capsules. Dose is 15–30 mg qhs (generic available)
Quazepam (Doral®): 7.5, 15 mg tablets. Dose is 7.5–15 mg qhs
Temazepam (Restoril®): 7.5, 15, 22.5, 30 mg capsules. Dose is 7.5–30 mg qhs (generic available)
Triazolam (Halcion®): 0.125, 0.25 mg tablets. Dose is 0.125–0.25 mg qhs (generic available)

Nonbenzodiazepine Sedative Hypnotic

It includes medications (Lunesta and Ambien CR) that have been studied for up to 6 months and are FDA approved for long-term use in adults. Lower incidence of next day sedation compared to benzodiazepines.

Eszopiclone (Lunesta®): 1, 2, 3 mg tablets. Dose is 1–3 mg qhs. Approved for long-term use.
Zalepon (Sonata®): 5, 10 mg capsules.
Zolpidem (Ambien®): 5, 10 mg tablets. (Ambien®CR): 6.25, 12.5 mg tablets. Approved for long-term use.

Melatonin Receptor Agonist Hypnotic

Ramelteon (Rozerem®): 8 mg tablets. Melatonin receptor agonist hypnotic which selectively binds to MT1 and MT2 receptors. Approved by the FDA in 2005. Dose is one tablet within

30 min of bedtime. Angioedema and anaphylaxis have been reported. Patients should not take in conjunction with fluvoxamine (Luvox®). Approved for long-term use.

References

Amar PJ, Schiff ER. Acetaminophen safety and hepatototoxicity—where do we go from here? Expert Opin Drug Saf. 2007 Jul;6(4):341–55.

Blackburn-Munro G, Jensen BS. The anticonvulsant retigabine attenuates nociceptive behaviours in rat models of persistent and neuropathic pain. Eur J Pharmacol. 2003;460: 109–16.

Gallagher RM, Rosenthal LJ. Chronic pain and opiates: balancing pain control and risks in long-term opioid treatment. Arch Phys Med Rehabil. March 2008;89(suppl 1):577–82.

Intrurrisi CE, Lipman AG. Opioid analgesics, In: Fishman SM, Ballentyne JC, Rathmell JP, editors. Bonica's management of pain. 4th ed. Philadelphia, PA: Lippincott Williams& Wilkins; 2009. pp. 1172–4.

Lin TF, Yeh YC, et al. Effect of combining dexmedetomidine and morphine for intravenous patient-controlled analgesia. Br J Anesth. 2009;102(1):117–22.

Mazer M, Perrone J. Acetaminophen-induced nephrotoxicity: pathophysiology, clinical manifestations, and management. J Med Toxicol. 2008 Mar;4(1):2–6.

Chun LJ, Tong MJ, Busuttil R, Hiatt JR. Acetaminophen hepatotoxicity and acute liver failure. J Clin Gastroenterol. Apr. 2009;43(4):342–9.

McCleane GJ. Intravenous infusion of phenytoin relieves neuropathic pain: a randomized, double-blinded, placebo-controlled, crossover study. Anesth Analg. 1999;89:985–8.

Morley J. New perspectives in our use of opioids. Pain Forum 1999;8(4):200–5.

Scanzello CR, Moskowitz NK, Gibofsky JD. The post-NSAID era: what to use now for the pharmacologic treatment of pain and inflammation in osteoarthritis. Curr Pain Headache Rep. 2007;11:415–22.

Sigtermans MJ, et al. Ketamine produces effective and long-term pain relief in patients with complex regional pain syndrome type 1. Pain 2009;145:304–11.

Silber MH, et al. An algorithm for the management of restless legs syndrome. Mayo Clin Proc. 2004;79(7):916–22.

Appendix

Multiple Choice Questions

Sreekumar Kunnumpurath, MBBS, MD, FCARCSI, FRCA, FFPMRCA

Choose the Single Best Answer for Each of the Following Questions

Chapter 1: Introduction to Pain Management, Historical Perspectives, and Careers in Pain Management

1. The "fifth vital sign" is
   A. Hear rate
   B. Oxygen saturation
   C. Pain
   D. Urine output

2. The concept of "four humors" was applied to medicine by
   A. Aristotle
   B. Hippocrates
   C. Huang Di Nei Jing
   D. Socrates

3. All of the following treatments are based on the gate control theory of pain EXCEPT
   A. TENS
   B. Spinal cord stimulation
   C. Deep brain stimulation
   D. Radio frequency ablation

Answers

1. The answer is C.
2. The answer is B. Hippocrates described the humors as related to one of the four constitutions, each of which was also correlated with the changing seasons and representative natural elements.
3. The answer is D. Radiofrequency ablation destroys the nerve fiber by heating it and thereby producing analgesia.

N. Vadivelu et al. (eds.), *Essentials of Pain Management*,
DOI 10.1007/978-0-387-87579-8, © Springer Science+Business Media, LLC 2011

Chapter 2: Multidisciplinary Approach to Pain Management

1. **The following is true of chronic pain:**
   A. Analgesics have no role in the multidisciplinary management of chronic pain
   B. Perpetuating factors may be remote from the originating cause
   C. It can be effectively managed in a primary care setting
   D. Immobilization of the affected part helps in the healing process

2. **Ann is 35-year-old woman who has been suffering from a headache for the last 6 months. She is on various medications and the side effects of these are affecting her work and daily activities. During assessment for the MPC (Multidisciplinary Pain Center) program she mentions that she recently has suffered two episodes of jerky movements of the right arm which made her wake up from sleep. Which of the following would be appropriate?**
   A. Conduct a detailed psychological assessment to rule out a somatization disorder
   B. Advise her to reduce or stop her current medications
   C. Ask her to increase the dose of diazepam that she is taking at bedtime
   D. Refer to a physician for further clinical evaluation and investigations

3. **Which of the following is part of a multidisciplinary approach to pain management?**
   A. Emphasize active patient participation and responsibility
   B. Provide education and training in the use of specific skills
   C. Help the patient re-conceptualize pain and associated problems from uncontrollable to manageable
   D. All of the above

4. **Which of the following statements regarding the role of medications in pain management program is *not* true?**
   A. Analgesics are given on a time-contingent basis
   B. Patients in an MPC program do not generally derive adequate pain relief from analgesic medication
   C. Pain cocktail technique involves mixing various opioids and NSAIDs in a masking vehicle
   D. Long-term use of other medications is discouraged both because of their potential side effects and the philosophy that the patient must learn to control his or her pain

5. **Success of a pain management program can be measured by all EXCEPT**
   A. Utilization of health care system following treatment
   B. Elimination or reduction of opioid medication
   C. Pain reduction
   D. Oswestry Disability Index (ODI)

Answers

1. The answer is B. Pain persisting after the healing process is complete does not serve any meaningful purpose. On the other hand, acute pain serves to protect the affected body part and it actually helps the healing process. Multidisciplinary management, though it encourages the patient to reduce analgesics, has a role in during acute exacerbations.

2. The answer is D. One of the aims of assessment for MPC is to rule out those patients who have a medical or psychological contraindication to such a program. Ann could be having a focal seizure and this needs to be investigated.
3. The answer is D. In patients suffering from chronic pain, complete freedom from pain is often impossible to achieve. Programs usually emphasize physical conditioning, medication management, acquisition of coping and vocational skills, and gaining knowledge about pain so that the pain becomes manageable.
4. The answer is C. The pain cocktail technique is a method of converting all opioids to an equivalent dose of sustained acting opioids or methadone and delivered with a masking vehicle. The dose is then tapered over the period of treatment. Most of the medications except antidepressants are finally stopped.
5. The answer is D. ODI is used to assess disability due to pain.

Chapter 3: Anatomic and Physiologic Principles

1. **The following statement regarding nociceptors is true:**
   A. visceral structures respond to pain induced by ischemia, spasm, inflammation, and mechanical stimulation
   B. Both cornea and tooth are innervated by A-β, A-δ, and C fibers
   C. Pain from ischemic bowel is well localized around the umbilicus
   D. Nociceptors are abundant in the brain

2. **Regarding pain hypersensitivity,**
   A. It is purely due to peripheral mechanisms
   B. Allodynia is persistent pain after the removal of the painful stimulus
   C. Hyperalgesia is when a noxious stimulus produces an exaggerated response
   D. Hyperpathia is pain produced by cold

3. **Which of the following regarding A-delta fibers is true?**
   A. They are unmyelinated
   B. They are associated with sharp localized pain
   C. They do not respond to mechanical stimulus
   D. They are are fast conducting at a speed of 40 m/sec

4. **Regarding spinal cord, which of the following statements is FALSE?**
   A. A-δ and the C fibers give branches to innervate neurons in Rexed's laminae I and II
   B. Axons of the second-order neurons in laminae IV–VI cross the midline and ascend into the brainstem
   C. Laminae are composed of white matter
   D. The spinal cord is divided into 10 laminae

5. **The beneficial effects of cognitive-behavioral therapy in chronic pain are mediated by**
   A. Augmenting descending inhibitory pathways
   B. Blocking transmission of pain in the spinothalamic tract
   C. By releasing acetylcholine from parasympathetic nerve endings
   D. None of the above

Answers

1. The answer is A. Cornea is devoid of C fibers. Visceral pain is poorly localized and brain is insensitive to pain.
2. The answer is C. Both central and peripheral mechanisms are implicated in pain hypersensitivity. Allodynia is when pain is produced by stimuli which are not normally painful (e.g., touch) and hyperpathia is when repetitive stimuli produces the sensation of pain.
3. The answer is B. A-delta fibers are myelinated and fast conducting at 20 m/sec. They do respond to mechanical stimulus which is above a specific threshold.
4. The answer is C. The spinal gray matter is divided into 10 laminae depending on the histological appearance.
5. The answer is A. Outflow of descending inhibitory impulses from frontal cortex, cingulate gyrus and hypothalamus are influenced by the patient's psychological and emotional state. Psychological support, including imagery, biofeedback, and music therapy can reduce pain intensity by either facilitating descending pathways or inhibiting cortical perception.

Chapter 4: Acute and Chronic Mechanisms of Pain

1. **Evan is a 45-year-old man who had undergone lumbar discectomy for back pain and leg pain about 3 weeks ago. He is now complaining of constant dull ache in his lower back along with sharp shooting pain down his right leg. He is also complaining of occasional burning sensation in the anterior aspect of his right thigh. Evan is likely suffering from**
   A. Neuropathic pain
   B. Nociceptive pain
   C. Mixed pain
   D. Physiologic pain

2. **Ionic basis of activation of nociceptors involves all EXCEPT**
   A. An inward sodium current
   B. A depolarizing calcium current
   C. Activation of nerve endings by potassium and hydrogen ions
   D. Hyperpolarization of cell membrane

3. **Action potentials through the sensitized nociceptors release the following peptides in and around the site of injury EXCEPT**
   A. Prostaglandin α
   B. Calcitonin gene-related peptide
   C. Cholecystokinin
   D. Substance P

4. **The correct sequence of the noxious stimulus from the periphery to the sensory cortex is**
   A. Aδ/C fibers→dorsal ganglia→spinothalamic tract→hypothalamus→thalamus→sensory cortex
   B. Aδ/C fibers → dorsal ganglia→spinothalamic tract→medulla→thalamus→sensory cortex

C. Aδ/C fibers → spinothalamic tract→ dorsal
ganglia→medulla→thalamus→sensory cortex

D. Aδ/C fibers → spinothalamic
tract→ dorsal ganglia→medulla→hypothalamus→sensory cortex

5. **The correct statement regarding NMDA receptor is**
   A. It is a 4-subunit, voltage-gated ligand-specific ion channel
   B. Glutamate binding to NMDA receptors sustains an outward Ca^{2+} flux
   C. Are responsible for producing analgesia
   D. Ketamine acts as an NMDA agonist

Answers

1. The answer is C. This pain has feature of both neuropathic and nociceptive pain. It has radiation that is indicative of nerve damage either pre-existing or secondary to surgery. Assessing qualitative aspect of pain is important in diagnosis and management.
2. The answer is D. Transduction is the process by which the noxious stimulus at the nerve ending converted to electrical activity. Activation of nociceptor triggers a generator potential mediated by calcium ion which in turn activates an inward sodium current resulting in propagation of action potential along the axon. Potassium and hydrogen ions are involved in activation of the nerve endings. Hyperpolarization makes the cell membrane less excitable.
3. The answer is A. Prostaglandin α is not a peptide but an eicosanoid.
4. The answer is B.
5. The answer is A. The effect of glutamate on NMDA receptor is sustained Ca^{2+} influx and it amplifies pain. Ketamine is NMDA receptor antagonist.

Chapter 5: Assessment of Pain: Complete Patient Evaluation

1. **Somatic and visceral pain could be distinguished by the following:**
   A. Somatic pain is likely to be sharp, burning, and poorly localized
   B. Visceral pain is likely to be dull, diffuse, and well localized
   C. Referred pain is suggestive of its visceral origin
   D. Autonomic disturbances are characteristic of somatic pain

2. **A 48-year-old bus driver is complaining of acute left buttock pain moving down the back of thigh and leg to the heel. On examination, he has grade 4 flexion of the knee and 1+ ankle reflex on the left. He has reduced sensation to light touch over the same area. He is likely to have**
   A. S2 radiculopathy
   B. Left sacro-iliac joint pain
   C. Fracture of the left femur
   D. Lumbar facet joint arthropathy

3. **Which of the following statement is FALSE regarding cranial nerve testing?**
   A. Conjugate gaze testing assesses the functions of cranial nerves II, III, and VI
   B. Trigeminal nerve has both sensory and motor functions
   C. Gag reflex assesses the function of vagus nerve
   D. Facial nerve has only motor function

4. **Which of the following is true regarding psychological evaluation using Mini-Mental examination?**
   A. Testing of orientation, registration, language, attention and calculation
   B. A maximum score is 30, and any score less than 23 is considered abnormal
   C. It provides information about the potential source of a patient's mental deficit
   D. Level of education has no effect on the result

5. **Choose the correctly matched pair:**
   A. Fact G questionnaire – Cancer pain
   B. SF-36 – lower scores indicating better health
   C. Brief Pain Inventory – Single-dimension survey
   D. VAS and VRS – Multi dimension Survey

Answers

1. The answer is C. Somatic pain is well localized where as visceral pain is poorly localized with associated autonomic disturbances such as sweating bradycardia and hypotension.
2. The answer is A. He is suffering from S2 nerve root pain. Nerve root pain follows this distribution. It could be a result of disc prolapse, infection, or tumor.
3. The answer is A. Conjugate gaze testing assesses cranial nerves III, IV, and VI. The tests for II nerve are visual acuity and visual field testing. Trigeminal nerve controls the muscles of mastication.
4. The answer is B. It involves testing five areas of mental status: orientation, registration, attention and calculation, recall, and language. In the case of the last two responses, the opposites are true.
5. The answer is A. In SF-36, higher scores indicate better health. VAS and VRS are single-dimension surveys, whereas BPI is a multi-dimensional survey.

Chapter 6: Diagnostic Imaging in Pain Management

1. **A patient has developed low back pain after straining from lifting a heavy piece of furniture. He has localized back pain for the first time, no radicular symptoms, and a normal neurologic exam. Next step in the evaluation should be**
   A. Order an MRI of the spine with contrast
   B. Order an MRI of the spine without contrast
   C. Obtain X-rays of the spine
   D. Defer imaging for now and provide conservative therapy

2. **Intrathecal pumps are a contraindication to performing an MRI**
   A. True
   B. False

3. **For the evaluation of which of the following conditions is the triple-phase bone scan is most useful?**
   A. Complex Regional Pain Syndrome (CRPS)
   B. Prosthetic loosening without infection
   C. Osteomyelitis
   D. Cancer metastases

4. **The only imaging modality that provides real-time imaging is**
   A. MRI
   B. CT Scan
   C. Ultrasound
   D. Plain Radiograph

5. **Complications following myelography include:**
   A. Headache
   B. Arachnoiditis
   C. Meningitis
   D. All of the above

Answers

1. The answer is D. Without radicular or neurologic signs, conservative management is the initial management of simple low back pain. With radicular signs or altered neurologic exam, an MRI is the test of choice.
2. The answer is B. A presence of an implanted intrathecal pumps used for pain, such as the Medtronic SynchroMed^{TM} pump, is not an absolute contraindication to MRI. The pump itself may stop functioning during the MRI exposure, but will resume thereafter. It is recommended that the pump programming be checked immediately after the MRI to verify that it has not been altered.
3. The answer is C. Although classically advocated for use in identifying Complex Regional Pain Syndrome, a regular single-phase bone scan is equally effective for the diagnosis of this condition. Triple-phase bone scan is an imaging modality that is more useful for osteomyelitis. A triple-phase bone scan, as its name implies, has three phases: a dynamic phase (performed immediately after radiotracer injection), a blood pool phase (performed 3–5 min after injection), and a delayed bone phase (performed 2–6 h after injection). In this scan, both blood flow and bone turnover are also evaluated as opposed to evaluation of only bone turnover in a plain bone scan. In the dynamic phase, the general amount of blood flow to an area is determined; in the blood pool phase, the amount of extravasation of tracer into the surrounding tissue is detected. In the delayed phase, bone uptake is measured. Because infections lead to increased blood flow in the area of infection as well as leaky tissue (osteomyel-"*itis*"), the two initial phases of a three-phase bone scan are useful in their diagnosis. The final phase, the delayed bone scan phase, localizes this infection to the bone ("*osteo*"-myelitis) by demonstrating increased bone turnover. Fractures and metastases as well as infections may cause hyperperfusion and hyperemia resulting in positive three-phase bone scans. When diagnostic doubt exists and greater specificity is needed, a subsequent scan using indium-111-tagged leukocytes will be positive for infection but not the other conditions. In this scan, leukocytes are withdrawn from a patient, labeled with indium-111, and re-injected. Detection is performed 24 h later with the hope that these labeled leukocytes will concentrate at an area of infection.
4. The answer is C. Ultrasound uses high-intensity sound waves in the range of 2–20 MHz to generate images of internal structures. It is attractive in that it is portable, and images can be achieved in real time. Furthermore, this modality does

not employ ionizing radiation or contrast agents, thus minimizing side effects and damage.
5. The answer is D.

Chapter 7: Opioids: Pharmacokinetics and Pharmacodynamics

1. **The following statement regarding μ receptors is FALSE:**
   A. Therapeutically useful receptor is μ1
   B. μ2 activation leads to side effects
   C. These receptors are proteins
   D. κ receptor mediates visceral and spinal analgesia

2. **Biotransformation of opioids primarily occurs in the liver by**
   A. Phase I reaction, mostly hydroxylation
   B. Cytochrome P450, which has a major role in opioid metabolism
   C. Phase II reaction involving conjugation with glucuronide
   D. All of the above

3. **Administration of morphine by oral route is very effective in controlling pain. Bioavailability by this route is**
   A. 75%
   B. 25%
   C. 50%
   D. 90%

4. **The advantages of the use transdermal opioids include the following EXCEPT**
   A. Noninvasive
   B. Effective
   C. Uses a small electric charge to propel the drug across the skin
   D. Avoids gastrointestinal side effects

5. **The most concerning side effect of intrathecal opioid delivery is**
   A. Itching
   B. Delayed respiratory depression
   C. Urinary retention
   D. Nausea and vomiting

Answers

1. The answer is C. Opioid receptors are glycoproteins. μ1 and receptor activation produces analgesia, while that of μ2 leads to the observed side effects such as respiratory depression, nausea, vomiting, euphoria, decreased gastrointestinal motility, urinary retention, tolerance, dependence, histamine release, miosis, and/or anorexia.
2. The answer is D. Phase I reaction produces more water-soluble and less active metabolite. Phase II reaction yields a large molecular weight compound which is usually inactive and is more easily excreted.
3. The answer is B. Despite significant first-pass metabolism, oral administration is made effective by proper scheduling and dosing adjustments.

4. The answer is C. The medication is delivered through passive diffusion. Iontophoresis uses electric charge for drug delivery.
5. The answer is B. Intrathecal opioids can spread rostrally producing delayed respiratory depression at a time when patient is least monitored. This is a real concern in the case of hydrophilic opioid like morphine.

Chapter 8: Opioids: Basic Concepts in Clinical Practice

1. **The following is NOT a therapeutic indication for opioids:**
   A. Constipation
   B. Diarrhea
   C. Pain
   D. Cough

2. **Patients on long-term therapy with opioids do NOT develop tolerance to**
   A. Pain
   B. Nausea and vomiting
   C. Constipation
   D. Respiratory depression

3. **A 65-year-old woman undergoes knee arthroscopy, and in recovery she complaints of severe postoperative pain despite have been given substantial dose of intravenous morphine. Review of her past medical records reveals that she has been taking dihydrocodeine for the past year for arthritis. She is likely suffering from**
   A. Addiction
   B. Pseudo addiction
   C. Cross-tolerance
   D. Physical dependence

4. **Opioid rotation is indicated when**
   A. There is decreasing analgesic efficiency
   B. There are persistent side effects
   C. Patient requests it
   D. All of the above

5. **Which of the following opioids can potentially cause convulsions secondary to a metabolite?**
   A. Fentanyl
   B. Diacetylmorphine
   C. Meperidine
   D. Sufentanil

Answers

1. The answer is A. Opioids can be used for symptomatic relief of diarrhea. Opioids also have antitussive properties.
2. The answer is C.
3. The answer is C. She has developed tolerance to morphine secondary to the long-term use of dihydrocodeine.

4. The answer is D. It also may be indicated when the patient cannot take oral medication.
5. The answer is C. Normeperidine is a metabolic byproduct of meperidine. Normeperidine has less analgesic potency than meperidine, but has the pharmacological property of decreasing seizure threshold and inducing central nervous system hyperexcitability and seizures.

Chapter 9: Nonopioid Analgesics in Pain Management

1. **The following is an undesirable effect of combined administration of an NSAID and acetaminophen:**
   A. Increased incidence of gastrointestinal bleeding
   B. Decreased analgesic effect
   C. Renal failure
   D. Reduced antipyretic activity

2. **The analgesic potency of 30 mg of ketorolac is equivalent to**
   A. 30 mg of morphine
   B. 5 mg of morphine
   C. 3 mg of morphine
   D. 10 mg of morphine

3. **Methyl prednisolone acetate used for interventional pain procedures**
   A. Has high mineralcorticoid and low glucocorticoid effect
   B. Has significant systemic effect due to rapid absorption
   C. Can produce chemical arachnoiditis
   D. Can be safely used for cervical transforaminal epidural steroid injections

4. **Which of the following is true regarding the treatment of neuropathic pain?**
   A. Carbamazepine alleviates pain by decreasing conductance in Na^+ channels
   B. Gabapentin acts by enhancing calcium entry into the cell
   C. Bioavailability of Gabapentin is more than pregabalin
   D. Convulsion is a side effect of Gabapentin

5. **Which of the following benzodiazepines is used in the treatment of trigeminal neuralgia?**
   A. Temazepam
   B. Diazepam
   C. Clonazepam
   D. Nitrazepam

Answers

1. The answer is A. The combination can produce GI bleeding even in the presence of proton pump inhibitors (PPIs).
2. The answer is D. Ketorolac has been shown to have opioid-sparing action when used for postoperative pain relief. However, it is not potent enough to be used as a sole analgesic after major surgery.
3. The answer is C. Methyl prednisolone acetate has high glucocorticoid and low mineralcorticoid activity. It is slowly absorbed from the site of injection and can lead to vascular occlusion, which is blamed for neurological damage following nerve root injections.

4. The answer is A. Gabapentin and pregabalin both have anticonvulsant properties and the latter has more bioavailability and hence the lower dose requirement. They block calcium entry into the cell, preventing the release of neurotransmitters.
5. The answer is C.

Chapter 10: Alternative and Herbal Pharmaceuticals

1. **Which of the following does NOT increase the risk of bleeding during interventional pain procedures?**
   A. Garlic
   B. Ephedra
   C. Ginseng
   D. Gingko biloba

2. **The ASA recommends that herbal medications be discontinued how early before any interventional procedure?**
   A. 1 week
   B. 2–3 weeks
   C. greater than 3 weeks
   D. They do not have to be discontinued if used in the recommended dose range

3. **White willow bark exerts its anti-inflammatory response by inhibiting which enzyme?**
   A. COX-2
   B. Lipoxygenase
   C. Both
   D. None of the above

4. **Currently what proportion of patients presenting to the pain physician for consultation are taking herbal supplements?**
   A. 1 in 3
   B. 1 in 8
   C. 1 in 20
   D. 1 in 100

Answers

1. The answer is B. Garlic, ginseng, and gingko biloba all may increase the risk of bleeding. Ephedra does not. Ephedra, however, may cause systemic and pulmonary hypertension, tachycardia, cardiomyopathy, cardiac dysrhythmias, myocardial infarction, stroke, seizures, psychosis, and death due to its inherent sympathomimetic properties.
2. The answer is B. The ASA currently recommends discontinuing all herbal medications 2–3 weeks prior to any perioperative or interventional procedure. These precautions were taken to protect patients from side effects of these herbals, since standardizations have not been formulated. There have not been many safety trials conducted to determine a safe dosage for patients to take during the perioperative period.
3. The answer is C. White willow bark, from the family of salicylates, shares the same metabolic pathway as aspirin and affects both the COX-2 and lipoxygenase enzyme. It has been suggested that prostaglandin and cytokine modulation may also contribute to its effect.

4. The answer is A. According to the recent literature, approximately one in three patients are taking herbal medications. Moreover, 70% of these patients would not disclose this information during routine preoperative questioning.

Chapter 11: Importance of Placebo Effect in Pain Management

1. **A 37-year-old man presents with a history persistent axial low back pain despite a previous lumbar spine fusion from L3–5. He has been complaining of constant, 6/10 pain even after the surgery, for which he now takes extended-release oxycodone, oxycodone immediate release, and gabapentin. He is otherwise healthy. He is in your office today to discuss enrollment in a trial testing a new type of pain medication that inhibits cytokines. The safety of this medication has been demonstrated, but efficacy has not been shown yet. Which of the following statements is correct?**
   A. His enrollment in the study will breach ethics
   B. It is safe to include him in the study even if he has expressed suicidal thoughts
   C. Participation is acceptable provided it will not produce a high level of risk to the patient or cause irreversible harm
   D. He can be enrolled provided he is in the treatment group

2. **The mechanisms whereby expectancies might produce biological effects include all of the following EXCEPT**
   A. Reduction in anxiety
   B. Changes in cognition or coping mechanisms
   C. Changes in behavior that would improve health outcomes
   D. A reduction in immunity

3. **Placebo effect can be reversed with**
   A. Flumazenil
   B. Naloxone
   C. Doxapram
   D. Neostigmine

4. **Specific therapeutic effect of an active drug is calculated by**
   A. Adding efficacies of the drug to that of the placebo
   B. Subtracting efficacy of placebo from that of the drug
   C. None of the above
   D. All of the above

5. **Perceived placebo effect could be due to:**
   A. Natural history of the disease
   B. Biologic fluctuation
   C. Increase in the skills of the physician
   D. All of the above

Answers

1. The answer is C. In designing a proposed clinical trial, it is important to consider the ethics of the study. Several criteria should be fulfilled. First, there should be important scientific

reasons to conduct the trial. Chronic pain is endemic in the community (estimates up to 50%), and the administration of placebo for chronic pain is associated with significant improvement in pain control. Studies have documented a 30–40% response rate to placebo administration alone. Moreover, several interventions for the treatment of chronic pain have been shown to be ineffective when subjected to the rigors of a randomized controlled trial. Therefore, it is important to scientifically test the investigational drug against a placebo. Second, participation in the trial should not produce a high level of risk to the patient and should not cause irreversible harm. This patient has suffered from chronic pain for several years, and there is no reason to think that he is at undue risk if his pain continues. However, patients should be screened to determine their level of risk. For example, a patient who has expressed suicidal thoughts after worsening of pain would not be appropriate for this trial. Third, the patient should be monitored closely with clinic visits or telephone interactions, as appropriate. If his clinical condition worsens beyond a predetermined threshold, he should withdraw from the trial. Finally, it is imperative that he understand the purpose and design of the trial, the consequences of his participation in the trial, and provide informed consent. In spite of fulfilling these recommendations, some would argue that the trial should compare the investigational drug to standard therapy. This philosophy is embedded in the Declaration of Helsinki, which states that, "The benefits, risks, burdens, and effectiveness of a new method should be tested against those of the best current prophylactic, diagnostic, and therapeutic methods. This does not exclude the use of the placebo, or no treatment, in studies where no proven prophylactic, diagnostic, or therapeutic method exists."

2. The answer is D. Cognitive theory of placebo effect states that patient expectations are critical in the placebo response. Anxiety and stress reduce immunity.
3. The answer is B.
4. The answer is B.
5. The answer is D.

Chapter 12: Psychological and Psychosocial Evaluation of the Chronic Pain Patient

1. **Mechanisms underlying the reciprocal relationships between pain, affective distress and stress may include**
   A. Enhancement of the response to pain by amygdala
   B. Increase in cytokine activity due to stress
   C. Up-regulation of BDNF (brain-derived neurotropic factor)
   D. Only A and B are true

2. **Regarding CBT (Cognitive-Behavioral Therapy), all are true EXCEPT**
   A. It focuses on modification of the thoughts, beliefs, and expectations
   B. It involves skills training
   C. Neuromatrix theory refutes the effectiveness of CBT
   D. CBT treatment can modify limbic activity

3. **Which of the following is true about the use of antidepressants and their analgesic effects?**
   A. Analgesic effects are only seen in patients who suffer from depression
   B. Depressed patients require higher doses for analgesic effect

C. Antidepressants do not relieve pain if the patient suffers from depression

D. Depressed patients respond faster to analgesic effects of antidepressants

4. **Fluoxetine may be contraindicated if the patient is suffering from**

A. Fibromyalgia

B. Diabetic neuropathy

C. Restless leg syndrome

D. IBS (irritable bowel syndrome)

5. **A 32-year-old man is in the emergency room with a fracture of his right forearm. He is in pain and anxious because he is worried about loosing his job. He tells you that he had undergone treatment for depression in the past. Your emergency room treatment should include**

A. Analgesics only

B. Anlagesics and anxiolytics

C. Analgesics and antidepressants

D. Analgesics, axiolytics, and antidepressants

Answers

1. The answer is D. Chronic negative affective states can increase the response of the amygdala to pain, leading to increased pain perception. Increased production of cytokines can lead to the "over shooting" of immune response. Heightened glucocorticoid activity, stress, and pain culminate in downregulation of BDNF.

2. The answer is C. With cognitive restructuring and coping skills training patients may experience less physiological arousal and less intense pain, which is consistent with the Neuromatrix Theory of pain.

3. The answer is D. Antidepressants relieve pain in patients irrespective of the fact whether they suffer from endogenous depression or not. In both these situation the dose required to produce a reduction in pain is far less than the dose needed to produce the anti depressant effect.

4. The answer is C. Exacerbation of restless legs syndrome is a possibility with fluoxetine.

5. The answer is A. This is an acute pain phase of pain, and treatment is centered on pain relief, identification and, if possible, remediation of the underlying medical condition.

Chapter 13: Interventional Pain Management

1. **Which is true of the trigeminal neurolysis procedure**

A. All three divisions of the trigeminal nerve (ophthalmic, mandibular, and maxillary can be individually blocked

B. The Gasserian ganglion block will block all the three divisions of the fifth cranial nerve

C. It can be used to treat chronic headache

D. Facial numbness is not a complication of this procedure

2. Mary is a 35-year-old female who has been suffering from a headache following whiplash injury. She says that her pain starts from the back of her head and radiates to the forehead and into both of her eyes. On examination, she has tenderness over the posterior occiput. The following statement is *not* correct:
   A. She could be suffering from occipital neuralgia
   B. Occipital nerve block is one of the treatment options
   C. Depot steroid injection can prolong the duration of occipital nerve block
   D. Peripheral nerve stimulation is not a treatment option for Mary

3. A 75-year-old man is referred to you by the orthopedic surgeon. He has been suffering from low back pain radiating to lateral side of his right calf. MRI of lumbar spine shows a herniated disc impinging right L5 nerve root. The indicated pain intervention is
   A. Right L5 nerve root block
   B. A caudal epidural
   C. Interlaminar epidural injection
   D. All of the above

4. When performing radiofrequency ablation the following does NOT occur
   A. Heating up of the tissues
   B. Nerves are stimulated first to avoid complication
   C. Temperature ranges from $42°$ to $80°$
   D. None of the above

5. Which of the following statements is *not* true regarding SCS (Spinal Cord Stimulator)?
   A. The electrodes are placed in the epidural space, stimulating the dorsal column of the spinal cord
   B. SCS is effective for pain due to ischemia
   C. Infection is a possible complication
   D. SCS uses radiofrequency waves for stimulation

Answers

1. The answer is D. Only mandibular and maxillary divisions are blocked individually. Trigeminal nerve sub serves facial sensation so the neurolysis is not useful for treating chronic headache and it can lead on to unpleasant facial numbness.
2. The answer is D. Occipital nerve stimulation can be used to treat resistant cases of occipital neuralgia.
3. The answer is D. All these interventions can produce pain relief, though a right L5 nerve root injection has the advantage of targeting directly the affected nerve root with minimal volume of the injectate.
4. The answer is D.
5. The answer is D. SCS uses lower frequencies for producing pain relief. It has been used successfully for treating angina and ischemic limb pain.

Chapter 14: Functional Restoration of Patients with Pain

1. **Which of the following is *not* one of the goals of physiotherapy in pain management?**
   A. Reduce all activities that increase pain
   B. Reduce self-perceived pain frequency, intensity, duration, disability, and depression
   C. Increase self-perceived functional status, quality of life, and health status
   D. Return to work, recreational, and home activities

2. **Moist hot packs ease pain by**
   A. Vasodilatation
   B. Relaxing muscles
   C. Decreasing muscle spasm
   D. All of the above

3. **Regarding the use of ultrasound in treating pain**
   A. Its effect on tissue blood flow is similar to application of heat
   B. It increases tissue permeability to applied medications
   C. All of the above
   D. None of the above

4. **TENS (transcutaneous electrical nerve stimulation) differs from NMES (neuromuscular electrical stimulation) in that TENS:**
   A. Uses electric current to stimulate muscles
   B. Is used in treating chronic pain
   C. Is used to identify individual muscles
   D. All of the above

Answers

1. The answer is A. The aim of physiotherapy is to minimize functional limitation due to pain.
2. The answer is D. Vasodilatation increases blood flow leading onto B and C.
3. The answer is C.
4. The answer is B. TENS and NMES both use electric current to stimulate muscle. The latter is used to identify individual muscles and enables the physical therapist to teach the patient how to contract specific muscles.

Chapter 15: Occupational Therapy in Client-Centered Pain Management

1. **All of the following indicate appropriate referrals to occupational therapy EXCEPT**
   A. Fibromyalgia
   B. Diabetic peripheral neuropathy
   C. Rotator cuff tear
   D. All of the above

2. **Occupational therapy incorporates a variety of pain management strategies to promote participation and quality of life for each client. Which strategy falls under the "environmental/contextual" category?**
   A. Personal adaptive equipment usage (such as a bathtub bench)

    B. Nerve gliding exercises done twice daily

    C. Physical agent modality usage

    D. Splinting fabrication

3. **Because there is a strong psychological component to the pain experience, which OT strategy is least likely to be effective for this component?**

    A. Stress management

    B. Home safety modification

    C. Relaxation training

    D. Cognitive-behavioral approaches

4. **Chris, a 48-year-old truck driver, has a history of ulnar neuropathy and generalized wrist pain. He is now presenting with Carpal Tunnel Syndrome symptoms. You determine the need for Occupational Therapy (OT) evaluation and intervention (see Occupational Therapy Referral form – Fig. 15.2). In addition to referring to OT for wrist cock-up splints bilaterally, iontophoresis, and therapeutic exercise, it would be appropriate to request**

    A. Home safety evaluation

    B. Relaxation education

    C. An ergonomic evaluation

    D. Myofascial release

Answers

1. The answer is D. Occupational therapists are qualified to treat a wide variety of clients including those with autoimmune, orthopedic, and neurological disorders. Appropriate client referrals include those who are experiencing acute or chronic pain, especially if there is a limitation in functional ability.

2. The answer is A. The other answers pertain to the physical management of pain; all strategies can be effective for healing of soft tissues and fall under physical interventions used by occupational therapists. Personal adaptive equipment usage (whether for dressing, bathing, grooming, or toileting) falls under the category of "environmental/contextual" adaptations for pain management. Occupational therapists are adept at analyzing people engaging in occupations within various contexts, so they can be counted on to quickly evaluate and address any such patient needs.

3. The answer is B. Stress management, relaxation training, and cognitive-behavioral approaches have all been demonstrated to promote positive psychological coping strategies for acute or chronic pain management. Thus, home safety modification, although helpful for environmental/contextual intervention, will be less likely to have an impact on a client's immediate need for positive coping strategies to address managing or lessening the impact of pain on their daily living.

4. The answer is C. Due to the symptoms of ulnar neuropathy and now carpal tunnel syndrome, it is expected that splints, iontophoresis, and therapeutic exercise will be beneficial to the client. Beyond this, the benefits of myofascial release have not been demonstrated to be effective. Relaxation may be beneficial, but the intervention most likely to bring about the needed work and lifestyle modifications would be an ergonomic evaluation. Through an ergonomic evaluation, Chris' sitting and reach in the semi-truck, along with his daily

routine and tasks can be analyzed by the occupational therapist. Together with Chris, they can develop an adaptation plan for driving, rest, self-exercise, and sleep breaks that will promote the best positions of his upper extremity joints to decrease inflammation and allow healing of the soft tissues.

Chapter 16: Acupuncture

1. **Which one of the following is not included in the traditional Chinese acupuncture theory?**
   A. The Taoism
   B. Qi
   C. Lymph systems
   D. Yin-Yang

2. **Which technique(s) is (are) used in acupuncture practice?**
   A. A medical technique using needle
   B. A medical techniques using moxa
   C. A medical technique using cupping
   D. All of the above

3. **Which one of the following has NOT been suggested as the mechanism of acupuncture analgesia?**
   A. Trigger the release of β-endorphin
   B. Trigger the release of interferon
   C. Interference with the pain pathway
   D. Reorganization of the local connective tissue

4. **Acupuncture can be used for which of the following pain disorders?**
   A. Dysmenorrhea
   B. Headache
   C. Neck and shoulder pain
   D. All of the above

Answers

1. The answer is C.
2. The answer is D. Cupping is another traditional acupuncture technique. Newer techniques include electro acupuncture, laser, and hydro injection.
3. The answer is B. All the other responses are true regarding acupuncture.
4. The answer is D.

Chapter 17: Nursing Perspective on Pain Management

1. **Unrelieved acute pain can result in**
   A. Enhanced wound healing
   B. Shorter hospital stay
   C. Serious systemic abnormalities
   D. More accurate clinical diagnosis

2. **Which of the following is true regarding the importance of having a care plan for each patient**
   A. It is the responsibility of the nurse to assess pain and provide adequate pain relief
   B. It helps to avoid frequent reassessment of pain
   C. It helps patient assess his/her own pain and take appropriate medication
   D. There is no need for discussing care plans with patients

3. **In which of the following patient assessment of pain could prove difficult?**
   A. Severely psychotic patient
   B. One-year-old child
   C. Demented octogenarian
   D. All of the above

4. **Regarding pain assessment tools:**
   A. Pain assessment tools are designed to be easy to use by the nurse, since nurses are supposed to conduct a basic assessment
   B. Tools must be appropriate for the patient's developmental, physical, emotional, and cognitive status
   C. Self-assessment of pain is most reliable
   D. B and C are true

5. **A one-year-old boy is under your care following hernia repair. He is frowning, tensing up his legs, yet lying quietly, not crying and is reassured by occasional hugging. His FLACC score is**
   A. 5
   B. 3
   C. 2
   D. 1

Answers

1. The answer is C. Unrelieved acute pain can lead to increased levels of catecholamines, which in turn can cause tachycardia, hypertension, myocardial ischemia, hypercoagulable state, abnormal breathing, and delayed gastric emptying. It can delay wound healing and suppress immunity, predisposing to infections. The end result can be delayed recovery and discharge from the hospital. Choice D is unethical.
2. The answer is A. Care plans are essential in the management of pain on the ward as it is primarily the nurse who will be providing initial assessment of pain. It involves a detailed discussion with the patient and his/her family.
3. The answer is D.
4. The answer is D. Pain assessment tools should be reliable, valid and easy for the patient, nurse, and physician to use.
5. The answer is B. Face, Legs, Activity, Cry, and Consolability (FLACC) score is 3 out of a maximum of 10.

Chapter 18: Post-surgical Pain Management

1. **Which of the following non-pharmacological modes of postoperative pain relief are NOT mediated by endorphins?**

A. Relaxation techniques
B. Application of heat or cold
C. Acupuncture
D. Application of TENS

2. **Acetaminophen is widely used to control postoperative pain because it has**
   A. Anti-inflammatory properties
   B. Opioid-sparing effect
   C. Peripheral and central actions
   D. No known renal or hepatic toxicity

3. **When administering opioids for surgical pain, enteral route is preferred whenever possible because**
   A. It is the easiest route and offers the most stable pharmacokinetics
   B. It avoids first-pass metabolism
   C. Enteral route has a higher bioavailability
   D. The dose requirement is less

4. **Which of the following properties of methadone makes it unsuitable in acute pain?**
   A. Increased bioavailability and rapid rise in plasma concentration
   B. Dose-independent action
   C. Short duration of action
   D. Patients need to be followed-up and monitored closely

5. **A morbidly obese patient is on PCA morphine following a gastric bypass procedure. Choose the most appropriate action for the situation**
   A. Supplemental oxygen should be administered
   B. Monitoring of ventilation is not mandatory if saturation is 98% on room air
   C. Give oxygen, monitor oxygen saturation, and ventilation
   D. Pulse oximetry is sufficient as it is a reliable indicator of respiratory function

Answers

1. The answer is B. The application of heat reduces muscle spasms and cold reduces inflammation, both resulting in pain relief. In the case of the other modalities, endorphins are released providing pain relief.
2. The answer is B. Acetaminophen neither has anti-inflammatory properties nor peripheral action. It can produce hepatic necrosis if an overdose occurs.
3. The answer is A. When administered enterally, opioids undergo significant first-pass metabolism in liver and hence their bioavailability by this route is less in comparison with other routes. For the same reason, when given orally, the dose requirement is substantially higher than intravenous dose.
4. The answer is D. Slow onset of action secondary to slow rise in plasma concentration and dose-dependant potency make methadone an unsuitable agent for acute surgical pain. Prolonged duration of action and the need for close follow-up are yet another reasons.
5. The answer is C. Obese patients on PCA should be monitored for both oxygenation and ventilation. Pulse oximeter does not monitor ventilation and becomes even more unreliable when oxygen is supplemented.

Chapter 19: Pain Management for Trauma

1. **A 45-year-old woman is in the emergency department following a house fire. Her pain score is 9 out of 10. Her skin is white, leathery and with mostly absent capillary refill. Chose the most appropriate statement:**
   A. She has sustained a deep second-degree burn
   B. No surgery is indicated as her wound will heal spontaneously
   C. The treatment for this type of burn is surgical excision and grafting
   D. The pain she experiences has no bearing on her age and gender

2. **Regarding the pain experienced by the above patient**
   A. She could potentially suffer four different types of pain
   B. Background pain is mild to moderate and lasts until complete healing occurs
   C. Preemptive analgesia may have a role in her pain management
   D. All of the above are true

3. **Which of the following agents are not used in the immediate acute phase of burn pain?**
   A. Anxiolytics
   B. Tricyclic antidepressants
   C. NSAIDs
   D. High potency opioids

4. **The following is *not* a causative factor in breakthrough pain in burns:**
   A. Opioid intolerance
   B. Changes in plasma protein concentration
   C. Healing process
   D. Psychosocial factors

5. **In the acute setting following trauma, which of the following is a contraindication to epidural analgesia?**
   A. Hypovolemia
   B. Coagulopathy
   C. A and B
   D. Flail chest

Answers

1. The answer is C. She has sustained a third-degree burn and the pain score can vary depending on age, gender, previous pain experience, and the degree of burn injury.
   Treatment involves resuscitation, adequate pain relief, and surgical excision along with grafting.
2. The answer is D. Burn victims can experience pain directly due to injury, breakthrough pain, procedural pain, and post-surgical pain. Preemptive analgesia should be administered sufficiently early before a planned procedure such as a dressing change.
3. The answer is B. TCA (tricyclic antidepressants) have latent onset and generally are not very useful in an acute setting.

4. The answer is A. Opioid tolerance can lead to breakthrough pain.
5. The answer is C. Thoracic epidural can be used for effective analgesia in flail chest.

Chapter 20: Regional Anesthesia Techniques

1. **For brachial plexus blockade at the axillary level, which technique yields the highest success rate?**
   A. A 2-injection transarterial technique
   B. A single-injection paresthesia technique
   C. A single-injection neurostimulation technique
   D. A 3–4-injection neurostimulation technique

2. **Which of the following sentences is true regarding local anesthetic systemic toxicity?:**
   A. Systemic toxicity is very common when used for lower extremity peripheral nerve blocks
   B. A forceful, rapid injection of local anesthetic carries a higher risk of systemic local anesthetic toxicity
   C. There are no case reports of toxicity following lumbar plexus and proximal sciatic blocks, while there are several cases reported after popliteal sciatic blockades
   D. The risk of severe toxicity can be decreased if epinephrine is not used as an intravascular marker

3. **All the following are branches of the lumbar plexus EXCEPT**
   A. Genitofemoralis nerve
   B. Femoral nerve
   C. Sural nerve
   D. Iliohypogastric nerve

4. **At the level of the popliteal fossa, the sciatic nerve is located:**
   A. Medial to the femur and anterior to the popliteal artery
   B. Between the biceps femoris and the semimembranous muscles, posterior to the popliteal artery
   C. Medial to the semimembranosus muscles and posterior to the popliteal artery
   D. Posterior to the femur and anterior to the popliteal artery

5. **Which of the following is the most common side effect following interscalene brachial plexus block?**
   A. Horner's syndrome
   B. Hemidiaphragmatic paresis
   C. Recurrent laryngeal nerve block
   D. Pneumothorax

Answers

1. The answer is D.
2. The answer is B.
3. The answer is C.
4. The answer is B.
5. The answer is B.

Chapter 21: Principles of Ultrasound Techniques

1. **The use of ultrasound during administration of a nerve block helps to visualize**
   A. Target nerve and the collateral structures
   B. Block needle
   C. Real-time spread of the local anesthetic solution
   D. All of the above

2. **An effective, precise regional anesthetic technique can make significant contribution to multimodal approach to pain management. Which of the following is FALSE regarding multimodal analgesia:**
   A. It reduces dose-dependant side effects of individual agents
   B. The combined analgesic effects are simply additive
   C. Analgesic effect is exerted through multiple pathways
   D. Improvement of overall patient satisfaction

3. **Regarding US imaging for peripheral nerve block**
   A. Long-axis view is always used
   B. Short-axis view is always used
   C. A short-axis view becomes long-axis view when the probe is rotated 90°
   D. A short-axis view becomes long-axis view when the probe is rotated 180°

4. **US-guided nerve block is specifically indicated when performing nerve blocks in:**
   A. The presence of a coagulopathy
   B. Trauma
   C. Abnormal anatomy
   D. All of the above

5. **All of the following statements regarding ultrasound waves are true EXCEPT**
   A. Waves have a frequency >20 kHz
   B. Frequencies of 7–15 mHz are used for regional anesthesia
   C. Lower frequencies attenuate more than higher frequencies
   D. Higher frequencies will provide higher resolution

Answers

1. The answer is D.
2. The answer is B. The combined effect is synergistic. The combined effect is more than the sum of the analgesic effects of individual agents.
3. The answer is C. Both short- and long-axis views are used depending on the operator preferences.
4. The answer is D.
5. The answer is C. Lower frequencies attenuate less in comparison with higher frequencies.

Chapter 22: Labor Pain Management

1. **Which is a component of labor pain?**
   A. Cervical dilatation
   B. Myometrical ischemia

   C. Vaginal distention
   D. All of the above

2. **Options for analgesia for the second stage of labor include all of the following EXCEPT**
   A. Single-dose spinal
   B. Lumbar sympathetic block
   C. Pudendal nerve
   D. Epidural block

3. **Maternal changes associated with labor include all of the following EXCEPT**
   A. Increased minute ventilation
   B. Increased cardiac output
   C. Respiratory acidosis
   D. Increased endogenous epinephrine

4. **Labor analgesia can be administered**
   A. Not before 5 cm dilatation
   B. Only when Lamaze techniques fail
   C. At maternal request
   D. Only by an anesthesiologist

Answers

1. The answer is D
2. The answer is B. Lumbar sympathetic block provides analgesia for the first stage of labor but will not provide relief for the discomfort associated with vaginal and perineal pain.
3. The answer is C.
4. The answer is C.

Chapter 23: Neuropathic Pain

1. **The approximate incidence of neuropathic pain in the general population is closest to**
   A. 1%
   B. 5%
   C. 10%
   D. 15%

2. **Signs and symptoms most suggestive of neuropathic pain include which one of the following:**
   A. Anosmia
   B. Depression
   C. Hyperalgesia
   D. Hypothermia

3. **Which of the following medications is LEAST effective in the treatment of neuropathic pain?**
   A. Gabapentin
   B. Duloxetine

C. Naproxen
D. Oxycodone

4. **Which of the following anticonvulsants has been approved by the FDA in the treatment of neuropathic pain?**
   A. Phenytoin
   B. Topirmate
   C. Valproate
   D. Gabapentin

Answers

1. The answer is B. The prevalence of neuropathic pain in the general population currently is estimated to be between 3.3 and 8.2%. The prevalence of neuropathic pain is markedly higher among patients with diseases known to cause neuropathic pain, such as diabetes (40–50%), HIV infections (38–62%), and multiple sclerosis (27.5%).
2. The answer is C. Hyperalgesia is an increased pain response to a suprathreshold noxious stimulus and is the result of abnormal processing of nociceptive input. Patients with neuropathic pain may complain, for example, that a simple pinprick and venipuncture are exquisitely painful experiences and are common clinical findings in neuropathic pain states.
3. The answer is C. Simple analgesics such as acetaminophen and non-steroidal anti-inflammatory medication are usually ineffective in pure neuropathic pain but may help with a coexisting nociceptive condition (e.g., sciatica with musculoskeletal low back pain).
4. The answer is D. There are three anticonvulsants currently approved by the FDA for the treatment of various neuropathic pain syndrome, including: 1. gabapentin approved for postherpetic neuralgia, 2. pregabalin approved for both postherpetic neuralgia and diabetic peripheral neuropathy, and 3. carbamazepine which has been approved for the treatment of trigeminal neuralgia.

Chapter 24: Ischemic and Visceral Pain

1. **Raynaud's phenomenon occurs as result of vasospasm and it has all the following features EXCEPT**
   A. Emotional stimulus is not a trigger
   B. It can affect ears and nose
   C. Signs include pain and pallor of affected part
   D. Heat can provide analgesia

2. **Which of the following is not true regarding treatment of visceral pain?**
   A. Acute visceral pain often does not require any therapeutic intervention
   B. Sympathetic blockade is an option for chronic visceral pain
   C. Ketamine has the added benefit of counteracting "wind-up phenomenon"
   D. Vagolytic agents are contra indicated

3. **In Sickle cell anemia, the following is true of a sickle cell crisis EXCEPT**
   A. Present with acute chest pain, abdominal pain, or bone pain
   B. Dehydration can worsen the effects of sickling

C. Oxygen therapy is mandatory

D. Treating pain has no effect in shortening the duration of the acute phase.

4. **The following statement is true regarding electro therapy for ischemic pain**
   A. Spinal cord stimulation is an option for relieving pain and salvaging the limb
   B. TENS has a role in rehabilitation
   C. Both A and B are true
   D. Both A and B are false

Answers

1. The answer is A. Raynaud's commonly affects fingers and toes. It is precipitated by cold and emotional stimuli and relieved by the application of heat.
2. The answer is D. Vagolytics such as atropine can be used to treat spasmodic visceral pain.
3. The answer is D. Sickling of red cells occurs when the hemoglobin becomes desaturated. Dehydration worsens the effects of sickling. Sickle cell crisis occurs secondary to vascular occlusion by the sickled red cells, leading on to ischemia. This can affect lungs, bone marrow, and the abdomen, and present as a sickle crisis. Correction of hypoxia and dehydration is vital in reversing sickling and its effects.
4. The answer is C.

Chapter 25: Fibromyalgia, Arthritic, and Myofascial Pain

1. **The following statements are true regarding fibromyalgia EXCEPT:**
   A. It more commonly affects male population
   B. It is associated with unidentifiable structural and inflammatory causes
   C. It is associated with co-morbid conditions such as anxiety and depression
   D. It affects approximately 5 million people in the United States

2. **Which of the following is (are) seen in fibromyalgia?**
   A. Decreased levels of excitatory amino acids in the CSF
   B. Hypothalamus–pituitary and adrenal axis suppression
   C. None of the above
   D. All of the above

3. **Which of the following is a feature of myofascial pain syndrome?**
   A. Presence of trigger points in the skeletal muscles
   B. Absence of referred pain from trigger points
   C. Taunt bands in the muscles are not a feature
   D. Botox injection is not an effective therapeutic option

4. **A 70-year-old woman presents with pain and morning stiffness of her right knee. She has been suffering from this for the past 6 months. She mentions that the pain and stiffness improve with activity. What would be the most likely finding if an X-ray of the right knee was ordered?**
   A. Narrowing of the joint space
   B. A hairline fracture of the patella
   C. Presence of osteophytes
   D. Both A and C

5. **In the above patient, you make a diagnosis of osteoarthritis. On routine blood testing you notice that she has elevated serum creatinine. Given this finding, the following medication can be used to control her pain:**
   A. Ketorolac
   B. Celecoxib
   C. Acetaminophen
   D. Ibuprofen

Answers

1. The answer is A. Fibromyalgia has female preponderance with a ratio of 9:1.
2. The answer is C. In fibromyalgia, there is activation of hypothalamo–pituitary–adrenal axis and elevated levels of excitatory amino acids, neurotropins, and substance P have been noted in the CSF.
3. The answer is A. Pressure on trigger points, which could be felt as taunt bands, often reproduces the typical pain experienced by the patient. Botox injection is a treatment option.
4. The answer is D. She is most likely to be suffering from osteoarthritis.
5. The answer is C. It is desirable to avoid NSAIDs in view of the elevated serum creatinine.

Chapter 26: Head, Neck, and Back Pain

1. **About 60% of patients suffer from back pain and majority of these cases have benign etiology. Which of the following symptoms/signs may indicate pathology related to a malignant/infectious disease process**
   A. Fever and night sweats
   B. Loss of bladder or bowel control
   C. Weight loss
   D. All of the above

2. **A 40-year-old male is complaining of lower back pain radiating to the buttocks and thighs. On examination, there is localized tenderness over the paravertebral muscles and the neurological examination is normal. Which of the following could be true?**
   A. He could be suffering from nerve root pain
   B. He could be suffering from facet joint pain
   C. Blocking the medial branch of the posterior rami at one level can be diagnostic
   D. B and C are true

3. **Risk factors for neck pain include**
   A. Psychological factors
   B. Presence of degenerative disc disease and facet disease
   C. Sitting for long periods at work
   D. Stress at work

4. **Which of the following statements regarding neck pain is FALSE?**
   A. Pain in the upper neck is likely to originate from C1–2
   B. Pain in the lower neck is likely from C5–6 and C6–7

C. Neck pain can be referred to the head

D. Neck pain can result from a pathological lesion in the throat

5. **Which of the following is the most effective treatment for acute neck pain?**

   A. NSAIDs combined with muscle relaxants

   B. Opioids, which are effective as potent analgesics

   C. Simple neck exercises to keep the neck mobile and increase the range of motion

   D. Immobilization of the neck using cervical collar for 3 months

Answers

1. The answer is D. History of cancer and progressive neurological deficit are other red flags.
2. The answer is B. For diagnosis, two medial branches need to be blocked at each level. Nerve root pain usually radiates below the knees.
3. The answer is D.
4. The answer is A. The upper neck pain is likely to originate from C2–3
5. The answer is C.

Chapter 27: Headache

1. **A 20-year-old woman with a BMI of 35 is complaining of a headache that she has had for the last 6 months. She feels it "all over the head" as a constant dull pain, associated with diplopia. CT scan of the head shows cerebral edema and small lateral ventricles without any midline shift. Possible diagnostic and therapeutic considerations are**

   A. She is suffering from benign intracranial hypertension and lumbar puncture is contraindicated as the intracranial pressure is elevated

   B. The diagnosis is tension headache and it is likely to respond to NSAIDS, caffeine, tricyclic antidepressants, or TENS

   C. She has a space-occupying lesion and the treatment is surgery or chemotherapy

   D. None of the above

2. **In the classic migraine**

   A. There is absence of aura

   B. There is a stronger familial inheritance

   C. One of the diagnostic criteria is at least five headaches lasting 4–72 h each

   D. scintillating lights and visual scotomas are not presenting symptoms

3. **Which of the following supports the diagnosis of a cluster headache?**

   A. Unilateral ocular pain associated with lacrimation

   B. Diplopia

   C. Headache lasting less than 15 min

   D. The headache never occurs during sleep

4. **Cluster headache is managed by**

   A. Oxygen therapy for an established headache

   B. Intranasal capsaicin to reduce the intensity of headache

   C. Ergotamine, which is useful during the acute phase

   D. Non-opioids to minimize the risk of addiction to opioids

5. **Blindness may be a presenting feature in**
   A. Retinal migraine
   B. Temporal arteritis
   C. Pseudo tumor cerebri
   D. Tension headache

Answers

1. The answer is D. The diagnosis is pseudotumor cerebri and the treatment options include acetazolamide, mannitol, digoxin, steroids, and surgical procedures like lumbar puncture. Obesity is a risk factor for this condition.
2. The answer is B. Aura is a feature of classic migraine. C is a feature of common migraine. Aura can have visual and sensory components.
3. The answer is A. Diplopia is not a feature of cluster headache. Attacks last from 15 min to hours and characterized by nightly occurrences.
4. The answer is B. Ergotamine has a preventive role while oxygen therapy is used in the early phase of the cluster headache. Opioids can be used if other agents fail to relieve pain.
5. The answer is B.

Chapter 28: Management of Cancer Pain

1. **Regarding Cancer-related pain**
   A. Radiotherapy is always curative
   B. 25% of patients with advanced cancer suffer from pain
   C. Medical treatment is effective in up to 90% of patients
   D. Interventions have a limited role in its management

2. **Which of the following statements is true regarding WHO analgesic ladder for cancer pain treatment?**
   A. Strong opioids are always indicated
   B. Severe intractable pain is treated with interventional procedures along with opioids and adjuvant agents
   C. Anticonvulsants have no role
   D. Modified analgesic ladder has five steps

3. **Combining long- and short-acting opioids to control moderate to severe cancer pain**
   A. Is indicated when the patient is on long-acting opioids and the pain is poorly controlled
   B. Is ideal when the patient experiences moderate to severe pain around the clock
   C. Can be helpful is the PRN dose of the short-acting opioid is increased gradually until it is about 20% of the total opioid intake
   D. Can be useful to treat breakthrough pain with the addition of a long-acting agent

4. **Radiotherapy for cancer pain management**
   A. Can be used for pain relief if the tumor is invading bone or soft tissue
   B. Can be used to reduce mass effect due to tumor
   C. Can be utilized as hemi-body radiation in some cases
   D. All of the above

5. **An 80-year-old man undergoes a neurolytic injection for cancer pain relief. A few hours later he complaints of voice hoarseness, weakness of all four extremities, and inability to lift his eyelid. He is most likely suffering from complications of**
   A. Celiac plexus block
   B. Subarachnoid block
   C. Stellate ganglion block
   D. Superior laryngeal nerve block

Answers

1. The answer is C. Cancer patients experience visceral, somatic, and neuropathic pain or a combination of these. Pain can result from radiotherapy. Ninety percent of patients with advanced cancer suffer from pain. Interventions have a role in controlling cancer pain which is resistant to other forms of treatment.
2. The answer is B. Opioids are not indicated if the pain is mild. Anticonvulsants can be used as adjuvants, and the modified analgesic ladder has four steps.
3. The answer is B. Short-acting opioids are introduced initially to treat moderate to severe cancer pain. Long-acting opioids are added when inadequate analgesia is suggested by the persisting pain. Small doses of long-acting opioids are added to PRN doses of short-acting opioids until the contribution from the latter is one-fifth of the total daily opioid requirement. Breakthrough pain is covered by PRN dose of a short-acting opioid.
4. The answer is D. In case of widely disseminated bone metastases, hemi-body irradiation is an option for pain relief.
5. The answer is C.

Chapter 29: Ethics in Pain Management and End of Life Care

1. **The purpose of the Guidelines for Pain Management, as defined by The American Society of Anesthesiology Task Force, is all of the following EXCEPT**
   A. Optimize pain control
   B. Minimize adverse outcomes and costs
   C. Enhance functional abilities, physical and psychological well-being
   D. Achieve a pain-free state

2. **In pain management and end-of-life care, the physician is expected to**
   A. Respect patient's autonomy
   B. Strive to preserve life
   C. Keep the patient comfortable and pain free if death is inevitable
   D. All of the above

3. **The Federal Controlled Substances Act**
   A. Addresses medical treatment issues such as the selection of prescribed drugs
   B. Regulates practice of medicine
   C. Allows properly trained medical personal to prescribe an appropriate medication in the usual course of professional practice
   D. Allows a dentist to prescribe opioids for gynecological pain in an emergency

4. **Parenteral feeding in a terminally ill cachexic patient**
   A. Improves survival
   B. Does not improve tumor response to chemotherapy or decrease chemotherapy toxicity
   C. Enhances quality of life as it satisfies hunger
   D. Improves immune response to cancer

5. **Which of the following is true regarding the "opioid contract"**
   A. It should be executed before treating chronic painful conditions with opioids
   B. It is mandatory before the start of treatment
   C. It has no role in monitoring patient's adherence to therapy
   D. Once signed, patient should not be given any other analgesics

Answers

1. The answer is D.
2. The answer is D.
3. The answer is C.
4. The answer is B.
5. The answer is A.

Chapter 30: Pediatric Pain Management

1. **Which of the following statements is FALSE regarding pediatric pain assessment tools?**
   A. FLACC scoring is validated for scoring postoperative pain in infants and children
   B. CHEOPS score can have a maximum score of 12 points
   C. PIPP is for infants of <36 weeks of gestational age
   D. COMFORT score measures distress in unconscious or ventilated infants, children, and adolescents

2. **All of the following statements are true regarding intrathecal morphine EXCEPT**
   A. Respiratory depression, if occurs, will happen in the first 2 h
   B. Its hydrophilic nature imparts prolonged analgesia
   C. Intrathecal morphine warrants monitoring for hypoxia
   D. Pruritus is a known side effect

3. **Which of the following is true regarding the use of PCA in pediatric pain management?**
   A. It is the most common form of intravenous opioid delivery
   B. It is never used below the age of 2 years
   C. Short-acting opioids are preferred
   D. Basal infusion of opioids is never used

4. **A 6-month-old infant undergoes inguinal herniotomy. The following option is not an option for postoperative pain relief:**
   A. Caudal analgesia
   B. Infiltration of wound with local anesthetic
   C. Rectal acetaminophen
   D. Intrathecal opioid

5. **The maximum recommended dose of bupivacaine in pediatric age group is**
   A. 2 mg/Kg
   B. 3 mg/Kg
   C. 4 mg/Kg
   D. 5 mg/Kg

Answers

1. The answer is B. CHEOPS can have a maximum score of 13.
2. The answer is A. Intrathecal morphine can produce biphasic respiratory depression, the delayed depression occurring after 12 h of administration.
3. The answer is A. Though controversial, it can be used in younger children. Longer-acting opioids such as morphine and hydromorphone are commonly employed in PCA.
4. The answer is D. When combining A and B, care should be taken not to exceed the total maximum dose of local anesthetic agent used.
5. The answer is B.

Chapter 31: Managing Pain in the Addicted Patient

1. **Which of the following statement is true about cocaine?**
   A. It is a directly acting sympathomimetic
   B. Cardiomyopathy is a known complication of cocaine abuse
   C. Hypertension leads to increased bleeding when used as a topical anesthetic
   D. It does not produce mydriasis

2. **Choose the matched pair from the following:**
   A. Continued use of a given dose producing diminishing effects = tolerance
   B. Drug class-specific withdrawal syndrome that can be produced by abrupt cessation = addiction
   C. Need to increase medication as a result of a progression of the disease = pseudo addiction
   D. Behaviors that may mimic those commonly associated with opioid abuse in the presence of unrelieved pain = pseudo tolerance

3. **Management of acute pain in the patient with history of opioid abuse involves**
   A. Defining the pain syndrome and treating the underlying disorder
   B. Relying only on opioid-based therapies as none of the other therapies might not work
   C. Allowing the patient to choose the drugs.
   D. Signing of opioid contract is mandatory

4. **Guidelines for prescribing drugs with a potential for addiction to a patient with a history of drug abuse include**
   A. Setting clear rules and expectations for you and the patient, and having both sign an agreement
   B. Obtaining random urine screens
   C. Monitoring for lost or stolen prescriptions
   D. All of the above

5. **Important considerations in a pregnant patient with a history of opioid abuse include**
   A. Prescribing of methadone is a standard practice
   B. The use of buprenorphine or naltrexone is not as safe as methadone
   C. Opioid detoxification is contraindicated during the second trimester
   D. Methadone metabolism decreases during pregnancy

Answers

1. The answer is B. It is an indirectly acting sympathomimetic. It produces beneficial vasoconstriction when used as a topical agent.
2. The answer is A. B is suggestive of physical dependence, C is pseudo tolerance, and D is pseudo addiction.
3. The answer is A.
4. The answer is D.
5. The answer is A.

Chapter 32: Pain Management in Elderly Patients

1. **All of the following statements regarding physiological changes in the elderly are true EXCEPT**
   A. Diastolic dysfunction is increased in the elderly.
   B. Serum creatinine level does not decrease with aging.
   C. Elderly patients have a higher volume of distribution.
   D. The lean body mass increases with age.

2. **Which of the following statements about opioid use in the elderly is true?**
   A. It is safe to use meperidine in an elderly patient with renal dysfunction.
   B. Opioid doses should not be adjusted for age.
   C. Healthy elderly patients are not more prone to respiratory depression by opioids.
   D. The opioid dose should be decreased by 10–25% in the elderly.

3. **The following statements regarding intervention techniques are true EXCEPT**
   A. Elderly patients may have a lower incidence of previously undiagnosed coagulopathy.
   B. Interventional techniques can be used in the treatment of moderate to severe acute or chronic pain.
   C. Interventional techniques are useful in the management of cancer pain.
   D. Interventional techniques may be contraindicated in patients with dementia, Alzheimer's disease, or other cognitive dysfunction.

4. **A 75-year-old man is admitted with malena and jaundice. His renal function has started to deteriorate. He is complaining of abdominal pain. Which of the following analgesics is contraindicated?**
   A. Acetaminophen
   B. Ketorolac
   C. Morphine
   D. Fentanyl citrate

5. **Normal PaO2 in an otherwise healthy 80-year-old patient would be approximately**
   A. 100 mm of Hg
   B. 90 mm of Hg
   C. 80 mm of Hg
   D. 70 mm of Hg

Answers

1. The answer is D. Lean body mass decreases with aging.
2. The answer is D.
3. The answer is A.
4. The answer is B. Ketorolac can worsen GI bleeding and renal function. Opioids need to be administered with caution.
5. The answer is C.

Chapter 33: Management of Oro-dental Pain

1. **High-intensity pain experienced in the tooth is the result of**
   A. High sensitivity of free nerve endings in the dental pulp
   B. Dense supply of free nerve endings in the dental pulp
   C. Reduced thickness of dentine
   D. Dental pulp being a vascular structure

2. **Which of the following is true regarding the nerve innervation of the tooth?**
   A. Dentine has Aδ and C fibers
   B. Pulp has Aβ and C fibers
   C. C fibers are polymodal
   D. Lingual nerve is a sensory nerve

3. **A 25-year-old woman presents with throbbing pain in her tooth which is aggravated by both hot and cold foods. Which of the following statements is FALSE?**
   A. She is suffering from acute pulpitis
   B. Pulp is undergoing degeneration and necrosis
   C. Pain is likely to BE relieved by lying down
   D. X-ray may help in diagnosis

4. **A 22-year-old woman presents with a dental abscess and she is in severe pain. Which of the following is the treatment of choice to control her pain?**
   A. NSAIDs
   B. Topical application of local anesthetic agents
   C. Nerve blocks
   D. An early surgical drainage of abscess

5. **Regarding TMJ dysfunction**
   A. Application of ultrasound is a treatment option
   B. Tricyclic antidepressants are not useful in the management of pain
   C. Occlusal splints worsen the symptoms
   D. Surgical correction is the first line of treatment

Answers

1. The answer is B. The dental pulp has a rich supply of free nerve endings.
2. The answer is C. Dentine has Aβ and Aδ fibers while dentine has Aδ and C fibers.
3. The Answer is C. She is most likely suffering from acute pulpitis and the pain is likely to worsen in supine position.
4. The answer is D. Topical anesthetic might not be effective in presence of an abscess, and NSAIDs can provide temporary relief. Nerve block in presence of infection is probably not ideal. Definitive treatment is drainage of abscess under appropriate antibiotic coverage.
5. The answer is A.

Index

Note: The letters 'f' and 't' followed by the locators refers to figures and tables cited in the text.

Bedside test
  pinprick testing, 528
  tuning fork, 528
  von Frey filament, 528
Benzocaine, 403, 412, 424, 721
Benzodiazepines, 707
  as abortive anxiolytics, 136
  disadvantages, 136
  as pure analgesics, 136
  side effects, 136
Betamethasone (Celestone®), 123, 745
Bier block, 421t, 447–448
Biofeedback, 21, 42, 216, 328, 370, 410, 534t,
        587t, 591
Biotransformation, 96–97, 120
Biplanar imaging, 247
Black box warning, 742
Black pepper
  CYP3A4 inhibition, 167
  drugs affected, 167
  excess intake, 167
  putative compounds
    acid amines, 167
    fatty acids, 167
    volatile oils, 167
  uses, 167
Blind technique, 274, 476
Blood chemistry values, 69
Blood pressure (BP), 61, 73, 112, 115,
        161–163, 192, 218t, 349, 373,
        392, 394, 448, 465, 511, 549, 598,
        643–644, 646, 653, 674, 677,
        742
"Blues," see Oxymorphone (opana)
Body mechanics training, 308
Bone scans
  benefits, 85
  conditions used as initial test, 85t
  distant metastases, identification, 82
  identifying occult fractures, 84
  images, 83f
  technetium 99-m-labeled
        diphosphonates, injection, 82
  triple-phase, 84
Boston Scientific, 285, 285f
Boswellia, 169
BP, see Blood pressure (BP)
Bradycardia, 76, 86, 244, 427, 503t, 506,
        647–648, 652–653, 679
Brain-derived neurotrophic factor (BDNF),
        205, 517
Brainstem mesencephalotomy, 292–294,
        294f

Brain-targeted surgical interventions
  cingulotomy, 294
  hypophysectomy, 294
  transsphenoidal approach, 294, 295f
Breakthrough medication, 601
Breast augmentation, 516
Bretylium, 448
Brudzinki's sign, 592
Brush test, 63
Bruxism, 578, 717, 720
Bupivacaine, 42, 51, 115, 264, 267, 287,
        289t, 390, 390t, 393, 395–396,
        420t–421t, 424, 426, 432, 434,
        437, 439, 441, 443–447, 449,
        451–453, 456, 459, 462, 471, 472t,
        506, 508–509, 508t–509t, 548,
        563, 582, 608, 612–613, 621, 622t,
        655t, 655, 657t, 661, 741
Buprenorphine therapy
  chronic pain, 686
  clinical efficacy, 687
  etiology, 686
  Finnish study, 687
  France, 687
  pregnancy, alternative, 687
  United States, 686
Bupropion, 129–130, 217, 737
  See also Wellbutrin®/Wellbutrin® SR;
        Zyban®
Burning mouth syndrome, 719, 721, 722t
Burrowing effect, 715
Buspar®, 739–740
Buspirone, see Buspar®

C
CA, see Carotid artery (CA)
CAD, see Coronary artery disease (CAD)
CADASIL, see Cerebral autosomal-
        dominant arteriopathy with
        subcortical infarcts and
        leukodystrophy (CADASIL)
Caffeine, 587t, 589, 591, 594, 657, 740
Calcitonin gene-related peptide (CGRP), 35,
        38, 47, 533
Calcium
  calcium channel blockers effects, 151
  dysrhythmias, 151
  supplementation, 151
  tetracyclines and quinolone, antibiotic
        effects, 151
  thiazide diuretics, 151
California Medical Board Statement (1993),
        632

CPSIA information can be obtained at www.ICGtesting.com
Printed in the USA
LVOW012036141011

250630LV00002B/70/P

9 780387 875781